Hematopathology of the Young

Editor

VINODH PILLAI

CLINICS IN LABORATORY MEDICINE

www.labmed.theclinics.com

September 2021 • Volume 41 • Number 3

ELSEVIER

1600 John F. Kennedy Boulevard • Suite 1800 • Philadelphia, Pennsylvania, 19103-2899

http://www.theclinics.com

CLINICS IN LABORATORY MEDICINE Volume 41, Number 3
September 2021 ISSN 0272-2712, ISBN-13: 978-0-323-79247-9

Editor: Katerina Heidhausen
Developmental Editor: Ann Gielou M. Posedio

Reprints. For copies of 100 or more, of articles in this publication, please contact the Commercial Reprints Department, Elsevier Inc., 360 Park Avenue South, New York, New York 10010-1710. Tel. 212-633-3874, Fax: 212-633-3820, E-mail: reprints@elsevier.com.

Clinics in Laboratory Medicine (ISSN 0272-2712) is published quarterly by Elsevier Inc., 360 Park Avenue South, New York, NY 10010-1710. Months of issue are March, June, September, and December. Business and Editorial offices: 1600 John F. Kennedy Blvd., Suite 1800, Philadelphia, PA 19103-2899. Periodicals postage paid at NewYork, NY and additional mailing offices. Subscription prices are $283.00 per year (US individuals), $731.00 per year (US institutions), $100.00 per year (US students), $363.00 per year (Canadian individuals), $768.00 per year (Canadian institutions), $100.00 per year (Canadian students), $404.00 per year (international individuals), $768.00 per year (international institutions), $185.00 (international students). Foreign air speed delivery is included in all Clinics subscription prices. All prices are subject to change without notice. POSTMASTER: Send address changes to *Clinics in Laboratory Medicine*, Elsevier Health Sciences Division, Subscription Customer Service, 3251 Riverport Lane, Maryland Heights, MO 63043. **Customer Service: 1-800-654-2452 (US). From outside of the US and Canada, call 1-314-447-8871. Fax: 1-314-447-8029. E-mail: journalscustomerservice-usa@elsevier.com (for print support) or journalsonlinesupport-usa@elsevier.com (for online support).**

Clinics in Laboratory Medicine is covered in *EMBASE/Exerpta Medica, MEDLINE/PubMed (Index Medicus), Cinahl, Current Contents/Clinical Medicine, BIOSIS and ISI/BIOMED.*

Contributors

EDITOR-IN-CHIEF

MILENKO JOVAN TANASIJEVIC, MD, MBA
Vice Chair for Clinical Pathology and Quality, Department of Pathology, Director of Clinical Laboratories, Brigham and Women's Hospital, Dana-Farber Cancer Institute, Associate Professor of Pathology, Harvard Medical School, Boston, Massachusetts

EDITOR

VINODH PILLAI, MD, PhD
Division of Hematopathology, The Children's Hospital of Philadelphia; Department of Pathology and Laboratory Medicine, University of Pennsylvania, Philadelphia, Pennsylvania

AUTHORS

NIDHI AGGARWAL, MD
Professor, Department of Pathology, University of Pittsburgh, School of Medicine, UPMC Presbyterian Hospital, Pittsburgh, Pennsylvania, USA

AHMED ALJUDI, MD
Department of Pathology, Children's Healthcare of Atlanta, Atlanta, Georgia, USA

XUEYAN CHEN, MD, PhD
Associate Professor, Department of Laboratory Medicine and Pathology, University of Washington, Seattle, Washington

SINDHU CHERIAN, MD
Associate Professor, Department of Laboratory Medicine and Pathology, University of Washington, Seattle, Washington

JOHN KIM CHOI, MD, PhD
Professor of Pathology, Division of Laboratory Medicine, The University of Alabama at Birmingham, Birmingham, Alabama, USA

J. GREGORY DOLAN, MD
Instructor, Division of Oncology and Cellular Therapy, The Children's Hospital of Philadelphia, Perelman School of Medicine, University of Pennsylvania, Philadelphia, Pennsylvania, USA

M. TAREK ELGHETANY, MD
Department of Pathology and Immunology, Baylor College of Medicine/Texas Children's Hospital, Houston, Texas, USA.

MOHAMED ELKHALIFA, MD, PhD
Department of Pathology, Children's Healthcare of Atlanta, Atlanta, Georgia, USA

FARAH EL-SHARKAWY, MD
Department of Pathology and Laboratory Medicine, Hospital of the University of Pennsylvania, Philadelphia, Pennsylvania, USA

MARIA FARAZ, MD
Department of Health Sciences, McMaster University

MARIAN H. HARRIS, MD, PhD
Director, Molecular Pathology, Department of Pathology, Boston Children's Hospital
Assistant Professor of Pathology, Harvard Medical School, Boston, Massachusetts, USA

ALEXANDRA E. KOVACH, MD
Division of Hematopathology, Department of Pathology and Laboratory Medicine, Children's Hospital Los Angeles (CHLA); Associate Professor, Clinical Pathology, Keck School of Medicine, University of Southern California, Los Angeles, California, USA

BRYAN KROCK, PhD
Caris Life Sciences, Phoenix, AZ, USA

DRAGOŞ C. LUCA, MD
Director of Hematopathology and Flow Cytometry, Children's National Health System, Washington, DC, USA

ANDREA N. MARCOGLIESE, MD
Department of Pathology and Immunology, Baylor College of Medicine/Texas Children's Hospital, Houston, Texas, USA

ELIZABETH MARGOLSKEE, MD, MPH
Assistant Professor, Department of Pathology and Laboratory Medicine, Hospital of the University of Pennsylvania, Department of Pathology and Laboratory Medicine, Children's Hospital of Philadelphia, Philadelphia, Pennsylvania, USA

EMILY F. MASON, MD, PhD
Assistant Professor, Department of Pathology, Microbiology & Immunology, Vanderbilt University Medical Center, Nashville, Tennessee

PAUL E. MEAD, PhD, SCYM(ASCP)
Director COVID Laboratory Operations, Technical Director of Research Operations, Technical Director of Immunopathology, Department of Pathology, St. Jude Children's Research Hospital, Memphis, Tennessee, USA

MATTHEW J. OBERLEY, MD, PhD
Caris Life Sciences, Phoenix, AZ, USA

MICHELE E. PAESSLER, DO
Associate Professor, Division of Hematopathology, The Children's Hospital of Philadelphia, Department of Pathology and Laboratory Medicine, University of Pennsylvania, Philadelphia, Pennsylvania, USA

SUNITA PARK, MD
Department of Pathology, Children's Healthcare of Atlanta, Atlanta, Georgia, USA

SANJAY S. PATEL, MD, MPH
Assistant Professor of Pathology and Laboratory Medicine, Division of Hematopathology, Department of Pathology and Laboratory Medicine, Weill Cornell Medical College, New York, New York

VINODH PILLAI, MD, PhD
Assistant Professor, Division of Hematopathology, The Children's Hospital of Philadelphia, Department of Pathology and Laboratory Medicine, University of Pennsylvania, Philadelphia, Pennsylvania, USA

JYOTINDER NAIN PUNIA, MD
Department of Pathology and Immunology, Baylor College of Medicine/Texas Children's Hospital, Houston, Texas, USA.

SUSAN R. RHEINGOLD, MD
Professor, Division of Oncology and Cellular Therapy, The Children's Hospital of Philadelphia, Perelman School of Medicine, University of Pennsylvania, Philadelphia, Pennsylvania, USA

FLAVIA G.N. ROSADO, MD
University of Texas Southwestern Medical Center, Dallas, Texas, USA

HAO-WEI WANG, MD, PhD
Flow Cytometry Unit and Hematopathology Section, Laboratory of Pathology, National Cancer Institute, National Institutes of Health, Bethesda, Maryland, USA

OLGA K. WEINBERG, MD
Associate Professor, Department of Pathology, University of Texas Southwestern, Texas, BioCenter, Dallas, Texas, USA

ELIZABETH WEINZIERL, MD, PhD
Department of Pathology, Children's Healthcare of Atlanta, Atlanta, Georgia, USA

GERALD WERTHEIM, MD, PhD
Children's Hospital of Philadelphia, Perelman School of Medicine at the University of Pennsylvania, Philadelphia, Pennsylvania, USA

TING ZHOU, MD, PhD
Flow Cytometry Unit and Hematopathology Section, Laboratory of Pathology, National Cancer Institute, National Institutes of Health, Bethesda, Maryland, USA

Contents

Preface: Hematopathology Gets Younger xiii

Vinodh Pillai

Hematopathologic Correlates of CAR T-Cell Therapy 325

J. Gregory Dolan, Michele E. Paessler, Susan R. Rheingold, and Vinodh Pillai

CD19-targeting chimeric antigen rector (CAR) T-cell products are used for the treatment of relapsed/refractory B-acute lymphoblastic leukemia, diffuse large B-cell lymphoma, and mantle cell lymphoma. The success of CD19-CAR-T cells has led to the investigation of CAR T-cell products targeting different antigens in other hematological malignancies and solid tumors. Clinical laboratories play an important role in the manufacture, distribution, and monitoring of CAR T-cell therapy. Hence, it is important for laboratory professionals to be cognizant of clinicopathologic aspects of CAR T-cell therapy.

Antigen Loss after Targeted Immunotherapy in Hematological Malignancies 341

Ting Zhou and Hao-Wei Wang

Immunotherapy marked a milestone in cancer treatment and has shown unprecedented efficacy in a variety of hematological malignancies. Downregulation or loss of target antigens is commonly seen after immunotherapy, which often causes diagnostic dilemma and represents a key mechanism that tumor escapes from immunotherapy. The awareness of phenotypic changes after targeted immunotherapy is important to avoid misdiagnosis. Further understanding of the mechanisms of antigen loss is paramount for the development of therapeutic approaches that can prevent or overcome antigen escape in future immunotherapy.

Update on Pediatric and Young Adult Mature Lymphomas 359

Emily F. Mason and Alexandra E. Kovach

After acute leukemia and brain and central nervous system tumors, mature lymphomas represent the third most common cancer in pediatric patients. Non-Hodgkin lymphoma accounts for approximately 60% of lymphoma diagnoses in children, with the remainder representing Hodgkin lymphoma. Among non-Hodgkin lymphomas in pediatric patients, aggressive lymphomas, such as Burkitt lymphoma, diffuse large B-cell lymphoma, and anaplastic large cell lymphoma, predominate. This article summarizes the epidemiologic, histopathologic, and molecular features of selected mature systemic B-cell and T-cell lymphomas encountered in this age group.

The Hematological Differential Diagnosis of Mediastinal Masses 389

Ahmed Aljudi, Elizabeth Weinzierl, Mohamed Elkhalifa, and Sunita Park

Mediastinal masses commonly present in children and may pose diagnostic challenges, particularly with limited sampling. This article aids the pathologist by reviewing the hematologic differential diagnosis of a pediatric mediastinal mass, along with ancillary testing useful for rendering the correct diagnosis. A review of the more common lymphomas is presented, including classic Hodgkin lymphoma, T-lymphoblastic leukemia/lymphoma, and primary mediastinal (thymic) large B-cell lymphoma, along with brief mentions of less common entities such as gray zone lymphoma and thymoma as well as non-neoplastic conditions such as benign cysts and infections.

Update on Lymphoblastic Leukemia/Lymphoma 405

Dragoş C. Luca

Lymphoblastic leukemias/lymphomas are predominantly diseases of childhood, where they represent almost all acute leukemias however, they are also encountered with significant frequency in the adult population. These neoplastic processes can be of B-cell or T-cell derivation and are composed of immature precursors of either lineage. The classification of B-lymphoblastic neoplasms relies predominantly on genetic and molecular findings, whereas the same is not true for those of T-lymphoid origin. Many of these recurrent cytogenetic abnormalities have important prognostic and therapeutic implications.

Inherited Bone Marrow Failure Syndromes: Biology and Diagnostic Clues 417

M. Tarek Elghetany, Jyotinder Nain Punia, and Andrea N. Marcogliese

Inherited bone marrow failure syndromes are a group of genetic disorders associated with bone marrow production defects resulting in single or multiple cytopenias. Many of these disorders predispose the patient to hematologic and nonhematologic malignancies, requiring life-long follow-up. A positive family history of hematologic disorders or malignancies is frequent, as these disorders commonly run in families, and selection of family members as potential bone marrow donors should be performed with caution to avoid transplanting potentially defective stem cells. This review highlights the most common genetic disorders associated with bone marrow failure.

Reactive Lymphadenopathies 433

Maria Faraz and Flavia G.N. Rosado

Lymphadenitis in the pediatric population frequently is benign and self-limited, often caused by infections. In children with refractory symptoms, lymph node biopsy may be indicated to rule out malignancy or obtain material for culture. Acute bacterial infections typically show a suppurative pattern of necrosis with abscess formation. Viral infections are associated with nonspecific follicular and/or paracortical hyperplasia. Granulomatous inflammation is associated with bacterial, mycobacterial, and fungal infections. Toxoplasma lymphadenitis displays follicular hyperplasia, monocytoid B-cell hyperplasia, and clusters of epithelioid histiocytes.

Autoimmune and noninfectious inflammatory disorders are included in differential diagnosis of lymphadenitis. Infectious mononucleosis and Kikuchi-Fujimoto lymphadenitis may mimic Hodgkin and non-Hodgkin lymphomas.

Update on Acute Leukemias of Ambiguous Lineage **453**

Nidhi Aggarwal and Olga K. Weinberg

Acute leukemias of ambiguous lineage are a heterogenous group of diseases that include acute undifferentiated leukemias and mixed-phenotype acute leukemias (MPALs). These leukemias pose a challenge for pathologists and clinicians alike in diagnosis, treatment, and further management. Recent genetic characterization has provided insights into their underlying biology and classification, and has offered potential for targeted therapies. This article addresses diagnosis of MPALs with examples of the most common pitfalls, recent comprehensive molecular studies, and advancement in treatment and follow-up modalities.

Role of Minimal Residual Disease Testing in Acute Myeloid Leukemia **467**

Xueyan Chen and Sindhu Cherian

Minimal or measurable residual disease (MRD) after therapy is the most important independent prognostic factor in acute myeloid leukemia. MRD measured by multiparametric flow cytometry and real-time quantitative polymerase chain reaction has been integrated into risk stratification and used to guide future treatment strategies. Recent technological advances have allowed the application of the novel molecular method, high-throughput sequencing, in MRD detection in clinical practice to improve sensitivity and specificity. Randomized studies are needed to address outstanding issues, including the optimal methods and timing of MRD testing and interlaboratory standardization to facilitate comparisons, to further improve MRD-directed interventions.

Laboratory Aspects of Minimal / Measurable Residual Disease Testing in B-Lymphoblastic Leukemia **485**

John Kim Choi and Paul E. Mead

Minimal residual disease detection provides critical prognostic predictor of treatment outcome and is the standard of care for B lymphoblastic leukemia. Flow cytometry–based minimal residual disease detection is the most common test modality and has high sensitivity (0.01%) and a rapid turnaround time (24 hours). This article details the leukemia associated immunophenotype analysis approach for flow cytometry–based minimal residual disease detection used at St. Jude Children's Research Hospital and importance of using guide gates and back-gating.

Molecular Genetics of Pediatric Acute Myeloid Leukemia **497**

Bryan Krock and Matthew J. Oberley

The genetic basis for pediatric acute myeloid leukemia (AML) is highly heterogeneous, often involving the cooperative action of characteristic chromosomal rearrangements and somatic mutations in progrowth and antidifferentiation pathways that drive oncogenesis. Although some driver mutations are shared with adult AML, many genetic lesions are unique to pediatric patients, and their appropriate identification is essential for patient care. The increased understanding of these malignancies through broad genomic studies allows for patient risk-stratification

Pediatric Myelodysplastic Syndromes **517**

Sanjay S. Patel

Pediatric myelodysplastic syndromes (MDS) comprise less than 5% of childhood malignancies. Approximately 30% to 45% of pediatric MDS cases are associated with an underlying genetic predisposition syndrome. A subset of patients present with MDS/acute myeloid leukemia (AML) following intensive chemotherapy for an unrelated malignancy. A definitive diagnosis of MDS can often only be rendered pending a comprehensive clinical and laboratory-based evaluation, which frequently includes ancillary testing in a reference laboratory. Clinical subtypes, the current diagnostic schema, and the results of more recently performed next-generation sequencing studies in pediatric MDS are discussed here.

Pediatric Myeloproliferative Neoplasms **529**

Farah El-Sharkawy and Elizabeth Margolskee

Myeloproliferative neoplasms can present early in life and may present a diagnostic challenge. Very few studies have focused on the diagnosis, prognosis, and therapy for pediatric myeloproliferative neoplasms. This article focuses on chronic myeloid leukemia, essential thrombocythemia, polycythemia vera, and primary myelofibrosis in children.

Infant Acute Leukemia **541**

Gerald Wertheim

Infant acute leukemia is a rare but aggressive disease. Although infant acute leukemia is cytologically and histologically similar to acute leukemia seen in older children and adults, it displays unique clinical and genetic characteristics. The features, as well as the extremely young age of the patients, present challenges for treatment. This review on the unique pathology of acute myeloid and lymphoid leukemia of infancy, and highlights the genetic characteristics that are frequent in these diseases.

Gene Rearrangement Detection in Pediatric Leukemia **551**

Marian H. Harris

The detection of gene rearrangements in pediatric leukemia is an essential component of the work-up, with implications for accurate diagnosis, proper risk stratification, and therapeutic decisions, including the use of targeted therapies. The traditional methods of karyotype and fluorescence in situ hybridization are still valuable, but many new assays are also available, with different strengths and weaknesses. These assays include next-generation sequencing–based assays that have the potential for highly multiplexed and/or unbiased detection of rearrangements.

CLINICS IN LABORATORY MEDICINE

FORTHCOMING ISSUES

December 2021
Updates in Blood Banking and Transfusion Medicine
Suzanne R. Thibodeaux, *Editor*

March 2022
Detection of SARS-CoV-2 Antibodies in Diagnosis and Treatment of COVID-19
Daimon P. Simmons and Peter H. Schur, *Editors*

June 2022
Covid-19 Molecular Testing and Clinical Correlates
Sanjat Kanjilal and Yi-Wei Tang, *Editors*

RECENT ISSUES

June 2021
Beyond LC MS: The Next Frontier in Clinical Mass Spectrometry
Sankha S. Basu, *Editor*

March 2021
Topics in Pediatric Transfusion Medicine
Sarah R. Vossoughi and Brie A. Stotler, *Editors*

December 2020
Current Issues in Clinical Microbiology
Nicole D. Pecora and Matthew Pettengill, *Editors*

SERIES OF RELATED INTEREST

Surgical Pathology Clinics
Available at: https://www.surgpath.theclinics.com/
Pediatric Clinics
Available at: https://www.pediatric.theclinics.com/

Preface

Hematopathology Gets Younger

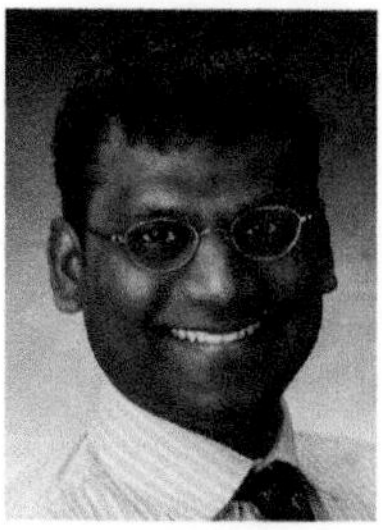

Vinodh Pillai, MD, PhD
Editor

I am honored and delighted to present the first ever series focused on "Hematopathology of the young." I chose this title instead of "pediatric hematopathology" since many of the disorders discussed in this issue straddle the pediatric, adolescent, and young adult age groups. The workup of hematologic disorders in this age group may differ from the ones in adults due to differences in presentation and differential diagnosis. Hematologic neoplasms in the young tend to have a shorter latent period, show more genetic translocations, and respond to therapy better than in adults. Many disorders, such as pediatric-type follicular lymphoma, IRF4-rearranged diffuse large B-cell lymphoma, Hodgkin lymphoma, primary mediastinal large B-cell lymphoma, Burkitt lymphoma, B- and T-lymphoblastic leukemia, acute megakaryoblastic leukemia, aplastic anemia, Rosai-Dorfman disease, Langerhan cell histiocytosis, and Kikuchi-Fujimoto lymphadenitis, are predominantly seen in the younger age group. However, they are not uncommon in older adults either. Hence, readers have the opportunity to compare and contrast the pediatric experience described here with the adult experience. The success of novel cellular immunotherapy products in B-lymphoblastic leukemia has created unique learning opportunities that can be applied to other neoplasms. Congenital bone marrow failure syndromes, such as dyskeratosis congenita and Fanconi anemia, can first present with a malignancy in the adult age group. Though acute myeloid leukemia, myelodysplastic syndromes, and myeloproliferative neoplasms are less common than in adults, they do occur in the young and have a somewhat different genetic basis. Finally, clinical trial practices of large consortia, such as the Children Oncology Group, impact laboratory assessment for minimal

Clin Lab Med 41 (2021) xiii–xiv
https://doi.org/10.1016/j.cll.2021.04.013

residual disease and genetic alterations. I hope a series that covers these aspects will be useful to the wider laboratory medicine and pathology audience.

Vinodh Pillai, MD, PhD
Division of Hematopathology
The Children's Hospital of Philadelphia
3400 Civic Center Boulevard
Philadelphia, PA 19104, USA

E-mail address:
pillaiv1@chop.edu

Hematopathologic Correlates of CAR T-Cell Therapy

J. Gregory Dolan, MD[a], Michele E. Paessler, DO[b,c], Susan R. Rheingold, MD[a], Vinodh Pillai, MD, PhD[b,c,*]

KEYWORDS

• B-ALL • CD19 • Immunotherapy • CAR T-cell therapy • Tisagenlecleucel • Hematopathology

KEY POINTS

- CD19-positive B-cell counts are an excellent surrogate marker for chimeric antigen receptor (CAR) T-cell function.
- CD19-positive relapses are generally due to loss of CAR T-cell function.
- CD19-negative relapses are due to loss of surface CD19 expression by blasts under CAR T-cell pressure.

INTRODUCTION

CD19 is a key B-cell lineage marker that is expressed almost universally on immature and mature lymphoid neoplasms.[1] CD19-targeting chimeric antigen receptor (CAR) T-cell products, tisagenlecleucel, axicabtagene ciloleucel, and brexucabtagene autoleucel, are approved by the Food and Drug Administration (FDA) for the treatment of relapsed/refractory B-acute lymphoblastic leukemia (B-ALL), diffuse large B-cell lymphoma (DLBCL), and mantle cell lymphoma (MCL),[2,3] respectively. CAR T cells are under active investigation for the treatment of other hematological malignancies (eg, acute myeloid leukemia [AML], myeloma), solid tumors, and nonmalignant diseases.[4,5]

Although 70% to 95% of patients with relapsed/refractory B-ALL go into a complete morphologic remission following CD19-targeting CAR T-cell therapy, a subset of patients relapses with CD19-negative or CD19-positive leukemia.[6–9] The cause and

[a] Division of Oncology and Cellular Therapy, The Children's Hospital of Philadelphia, Perelman School of Medicine, University of Pennsylvania, Philadelphia, PA, USA; [b] Division of Hematopathology, The Children's Hospital of Philadelphia, Philadelphia, PA, USA; [c] Department of Pathology and Laboratory Medicine, University of Pennsylvania, Philadelphia, PA, USA
* Corresponding author. The Children's Hospital of Philadelphia, 3400 Civic Center Boulevard, Philadelphia, PA 19104.
E-mail address: pillaiv1@chop.edu

Clin Lab Med 41 (2021) 325–339
https://doi.org/10.1016/j.cll.2021.03.012 **labmed.theclinics.com**

treatment of relapse varies depending on the CD19 status and immunophenotype of the relapse.

Various clinical laboratory professionals play an important role in the collection, administration, and follow-up of patients treated with CAR T-cell therapy. The blood bank is involved in the apheresis of the initial T cells, and the stem-cell laboratory is vital for administration of CAR T-cell products. Peripheral blood, bone marrow, and cerebrospinal fluid (CSF) cell counts from the hematology laboratory are important in the monitoring of patients undergoing CAR T-cell therapy. Peripheral blood B-cell and T-cell counts assessed by flow cytometry are necessary for monitoring of CAR T-cell function. Cytokine panels from the immunology laboratory aid in the evaluation of cytokine release syndrome (CRS) postinfusion. Bone marrow biopsies, tissue biopsies in conjunction with immunophenotyping, and genetic studies are necessary for characterization of responses and relapses. This review focuses on hematopathology correlates of CD19-targeted CAR T-cell therapy of B-ALL but can be extended to other targeted antigens in other hematologic malignancies.

DISCUSSION

CD19-directed CAR T-cell therapy was first approved by the FDA for relapsed/refractory B-cell leukemia and lymphoma based on the results from the global, phase 2 ELIANA trial for ALL,[7] and the JULIET trial for axicabtagene ciloleucel.[10] In the initial trials, patients with B-ALL were candidates for CAR T-cell therapy if they were refractory to chemotherapy, immunotherapy, or had experienced second or greater relapse, including post-stem cell transplant.[9,11] Newer studies are investigating the use of CD19-targeted CAR T cells earlier in therapy for specific patient populations with high-risk leukemia. The NCHOP Basket trial (CT04276870) is investigating the use of tisagenlecleucel in pediatric and young adult patients with hypodiploid or t(17;19) B-ALL, infants with very high-risk *KMT2A*-rearranged B-ALL, and patients with central nervous system (CNS) relapse. The COG AALL1721 CASSIOPEIA trial (NCT03876769) is investigating the frontline use of tisagenlecleucel in de novo high-risk pediatric and young adult B-ALL patients who are end-of-consolidation minimal residual disease positive.

PRE-CHIMERIC ANTIGEN RECEPTOR EVALUATION

The first step in evaluation for eligibility of a CD19-directed, CAR T product is confirmation of a CD19-expressing B-ALL (**Fig. 1**) or lymphoma. However, this is complicated by the fact that there are no standardized criteria for reporting antigen expression. "Dim variable" expression (see **Fig. 1**B) might be reported as "subset positive" or "subset negative" by some. Hence, review of original flow cytometric plots is important to accurately evaluate CD19, especially in patients with prior exposure to CD19-targeted therapies. History of prior exposure may be important even if CD19 is positive, as antigens are frequently reexpressed after cessation of targeted therapy but may be lost again under treatment pressure.[6] By WHO criteria,[12] at least dim CD19 expression is necessary for a diagnosis of B-ALL. Our large retrospective study of 628 cases of B-ALL indicated that CD19 is expressed in 100% of de novo B-ALL.[1] Leukemia without any CD19 (but with other B-cell markers) should raise the possibility of mixed phenotype or mixed lineage leukemia. The only true B-ALL without CD19 expression are those that have lost CD19 after treatment with a CD19-targeting agent such as blinatumomab or a CAR T-cell product.[13] Dim or variable CD19 or presence of rare (<1%) CD19-negative events show equivalent responses to CAR T-cell therapy as CD19-normal or CD19-bright B-ALL.[6] CAR

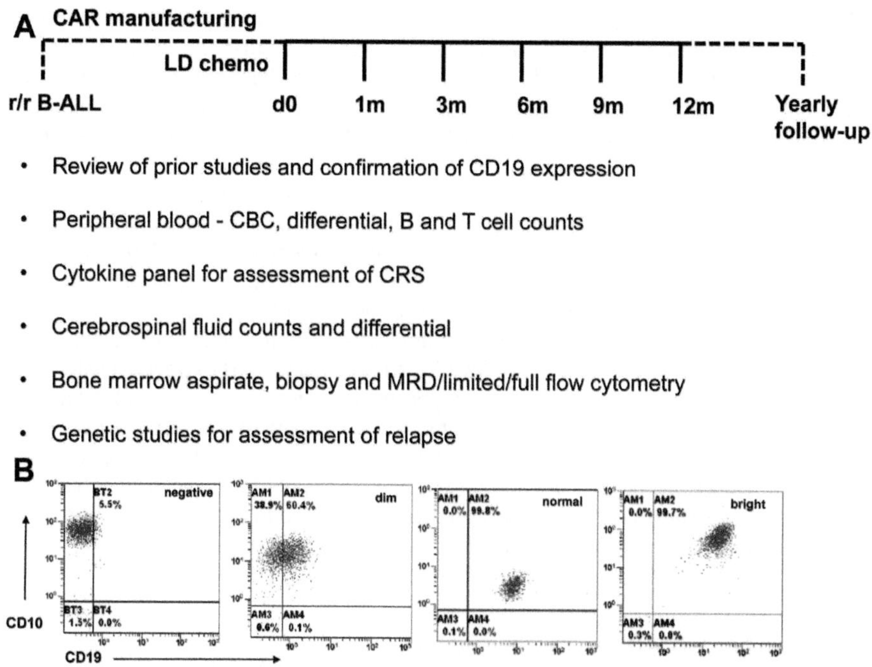

Fig. 1. (*A*) Timeline and overview of ancillary studies for CAR T-cell therapy in B-ALL. CRS, cytokine release syndrome; d, days postinfusion; LD, lymphodepleting chemotherapy; m, months postinfusion; MRD, minimal residual disease; r/r, relapsed/refractory. (*B*) Spectrum of CD19 expression in B-ALL. Examples of negative, dim, normal and bright CD19 expression in B-ALL are shown. Complete lack of CD19 (*far left*) is due to prior CD19-targeted therapy. The other examples are from de novo B-ALL.

T cells are able to recognize and lyse target cells that express very low levels of CD19.[6] Hence, pretreatment assessment of CD19 expression level is not as important for tisagenlecleucel in B-ALL if the patient has not had prior CD19-targeted therapy or their cytogenetics are not at high risk for lineage switch at relapse. It is important to note that this may not apply to other CAR T-cell products such as CD22 CAR, where the level of pretreatment antigen density by quantitative flow cytometry seems to be associated with a higher proportion of antigen-negative relapses.[14] The differences are likely due to lower CD22 expression (compared with CD19) in B-ALL.[1]

In addition to immunophenotype, documentation of diagnostic genetic abnormalities is helpful in evaluation for residual and relapsed disease should the need arise. *KMT2A*- and *ZNF384*-rearranged B-ALL have a propensity to lose B-cell makers and switch lineage to myelomonocytic leukemia after CAR T-cell therapy.[15,16] However, such genetic categories are not exclusionary criteria because many patients will achieve a complete remission, and the factors predicting lineage switch have not been elucidated. *TP53*-mutated B-ALL have a higher propensity to relapse with CD19-negative blasts after CAR T-cell therapy.[17] Additional eligibility requirements vary among CAR T-cell trials. Presence of CSF blasts are not an exclusionary criterion, but increasing CSF white-cell counts along with neurologic symptoms may be. In addition, adequate organ function and performance status are required. Active infections are also typically a contraindication to CAR T-cell infusion.

Following screening for eligibility, T cells are collected from peripheral blood by apheresis when the absolute lymphocyte count (ALC) is greater than 500/μL and the CD3 count is greater than 150 to 200 μL/mL (Kymriah [tisagenlecleucel] package insert: Novartis Pharmaceuticals Corp, East Hanover, NJ; 2018). Some patients may not have sufficient numbers of normal lymphocytes due to extensive disease or chemotherapy-induced cytopenias. For this reason, peripheral blood mononuclear cells may be collected and stored for patients at high risk of nonresponse even before they are eligible for CAR T-cell therapy. Patients without sufficient autologous T cells are also candidates for trials using allogeneic CAR T-cell products.[18] CAR T cells are typically produced at either a centralized production facility (FDA approved) or at research facilities for clinical trials. Unsorted peripheral blood mononuclear cells or sorted CD3+ T cells are activated with anti-CD3 and anti-CD28 antibodies, transduced with lentiviral vectors carrying CAR T-cell constructs and expanded with cytokines for 1 to 2 weeks.[7] They are then cryopreserved for future use. Most patients receive pre-CAR lymphodepleting chemotherapy consisting of fludarabine and cyclophosphamide the week before CAR T-cell infusion.[7] Lymphodepletion reduces disease burden and promotes CAR T-cell expansion by homeostatic mechanisms.[19] Preinfusion bone marrow and CSF analyses are performed to assess proportion of residual disease. The preinfusion marrow also helps clinicians anticipate side effects, as severe CRS is associated with higher preinfusion disease burden.[8,20,21]

POST-CHIMERIC ANTIGEN RECEPTOR EVALUATION

CAR T-cell products are released for infusion after they meet minimum criteria for viability, transduction efficiency, and lack of residual magnetic beads, endotoxins, and microbial organisms.[21] Patients are infused with 1 to 5 million transduced CAR T cells per kilogram body weight either as a single dose (day 0) or in a dose-escalation fashion depending on the trial.[7] Clearance of circulating blasts and onset of CRS are early signs of CAR T-cell activity. Although CRS is initiated by CAR T cells engaging CD19 antigen, it is propagated and sustained by monocyte/macrophage activation. Key cytokines involved in the pathogenesis of CRS include interferon-gamma (IFNγ) and granulocyte-macrophage CSF (secreted by CAR T cells) and interleukin-6 (IL-6), IL-1, and macrophage inflammatory protein (MIP) 1α (secreted by macrophages).[22] CRS has a cytokine signature based on expression of inflammatory markers such as IFNγ, MIP1α, and IL-13 that seems to differ from the cytokine signature of sepsis.[21] CRS is graded as mild, moderate, and severe using clinical criteria including the Penn and Lee grading scales or the new American Society for Transplantation and Cellular Therapy guidelines.[21,23] In a retrospective analysis, early and higher levels of the cytokines IFNγ, IL-6, soluble gp130, and soluble IL-6 receptor were associated with severe CRS.[21] Mild to moderate CRS can be managed with supportive care, but additional interventions are needed for severe CRS, which is defined by refractory hypotension, significant hypoxia, or signs of end-organ dysfunction. Cases of severe CRS typically require intensive care unit care along with IL-6 receptor inhibitor tocilizumab and steroids.[7] Broad cytokine immune assays are helpful in monitoring CRS and response to treatment but results need rapid turnaround to permit fast interventional response. We use a chemiluminescence-based assay using the MesoScale Discovery Quickplex instrument. The 10-plex proinflammatory cytokine panel measures cytokines that are important in inflammation and includes IL-1β, IL-2, IL-4, IL-6, IL-8, IL-10, IL-12p70, IL-13, tumor necrosis factor alpha, and IFNγ. The most common cytokine elevations in CRS are IL-6, IL-8, IL-10, and IFNγ. As use of cytokine panels becomes more widespread, it may become a predictive measure for development of severe CRS and allow for earlier intervention of targeted cytokine blockade. Clinically, it has been shown that early administration of the IL6-receptor inhibitor tocilizumab may mitigate severe CRS without adversely affecting the effectiveness of CD19-directed CAR T cells.[24,25]

Direct measurements of CAR using molecular and flow cytometric assessments are performed in the context of clinical trials in research laboratories and are of unclear utility for real-time assessment.[26,27] A functional assessment of B-cell aplasia (BCA) based on peripheral blood CD19 counts is an excellent surrogate for assessment of CAR T-cell function compared with direct assessment of CAR T cells by polymerase chain reaction or flow cytometry.[6] Lack of CAR T cells by peripheral blood studies does not exclude the presence of viable CAR T cells that may be sequestered in tissues. Importantly, they may be sequestered in bone marrow where they mediate aplasia of B-cell precursors at their origin. It is difficult to differentiate BCA from the effect of lymphodepleting chemotherapy in the first few weeks after CAR T-cell infusion. Normal B cells start recovering around day 28 post-CAR chemotherapy, and hence BCA cannot be used to monitor CAR T-cell function before that time point.

The flow cytometry panel for assessing BCA ("CAR T-cell panel") is a single tube assay that evaluates CD45, CD3, CD4, CD8, CD19, and CD22. Approximately 20,000 white blood cells are stained with antibodies. A red blood cell lysis step is necessary for exclusion of CD45-negative erythrocytes. A CD45 versus side scatter gate is used to identify CD45-bright lymphocytes and CD45-dim-negative blasts. The proportion of CD3+, CD3+/CD4+, and CD3+/CD8+ are reported for the lymphocyte gate. The proportion of CD19+ and CD22+ events from the lymphocyte and the blast gate is used for enumeration of B cells. Absolute B-cell and T-cell counts, which are calculated from a tandem CBC, are also reported out in addition to the percentages. The gating strategy ensures that the T-cell numbers are derived solely from the CD45-bright mature lymphocyte gate, whereas the B-cell numbers are derived from CD45-mature and CD45-dim-negative gates. Mature B lymphocytes may be absent due to chemotherapy, but CD19+ blasts or early hematogones may be present, indicating loss of CAR T-cell efficacy despite absence of mature B cells.

BCA in peripheral blood is defined at our institution as less than 3% CD19+ B cells, or an absolute B-cell count of less than 50/μL. White blood counts (WBC) may be very low in many CAR T-cell–treated patients who were heavily pretreated before CAR T infusion. The proportion of CD19+ B cells can be artifactually high due to low WBC, but absolute B-cell counts will still be low in those cases. Although BCA is easily assessed from peripheral blood, CD19-positive, B-cell precursors in the marrow precede the appearance of circulating mature B cells.[28] Loss of BCA in the marrow is defined at our institution as reappearance of more than 1% CD19+ cells among total cellularity. Many centers perform peripheral blood B-cell flow cytometry monthly for the first 1 to 2 years post-CAR T-cell infusion and then more infrequently.

In addition to its utility in following CAR T-cell functions, BCA is also a measure of immune status. In adult populations, replacement with intravenous immunoglobulin (IVIG) is not typically done because of long-lived plasma cells or memory B cells that may not express high CD19.[29] In pediatric populations, it is thought that there is less immunologic memory so replacement with IVIG for BCA is indicated.[7,9] Patients with chronic BCA (lasting longer than 6 months) should also be considered for subcutaneous immunoglobulin replacement.

Early recovery of CD19+ B cells (defined as <6 months for tisagenlecleucel) is associated with increased risk of CD19-positive ALL recurrence.[6] Patients with early recovery of B cells and no evidence of ALL recurrence on bone marrow have several therapeutic options. Patients can be reinfused with their original CAR T-cell product if doses are available[30] or may be eligible for humanized CAR T cells (NCT03792633),[30,31] with or without PD-1 inhibitors.[32] If patients are in an minimal residual disease (MRD)-negative remission, they can also be considered for stem-cell transplant.[33] Patients who exhibit B-cell recovery can have delayed reconstitution of immunoglobulin levels, so replacement is often needed following B-cell recovery.

An atypical population of CD19-negative, nonneoplastic B-cell precursors in bone marrow is sometimes prominent on MRD flow cytometry after CAR T-cell therapy.[6,34] They are characteristically CD19– CD22+ CD24– CD10var and CD34+. Lack of CD19 and CD24 distinguishes them from normal hematogones. Comparison of prior blast phenotype and genetic data can also be used to exclude a CD19-negative relapse. The appearance of CD19-negative, nonmalignant precursors is not a harbinger of early loss of BCA. They are mostly likely an early B-cell precursor that was always present but more prominent now due to lack of normal B-cell precursors and increased scrutiny for CD19-negative blasts.

Bone marrow biopsy, aspirate, and CSF analyses are often performed at day 28 and at 3, 6, 9, and 12 months (see **Fig. 1**A) following the timeline of the initial B-ALL trials.[11] MRD positivity is a sensitive harbinger of frank relapse in B-ALL. However, the widely used Children's Oncology Group (COG) MRD panels that only use common B-cell leukemia markers are not optimal for assessing CD19-negative populations, CD10-negative leukemia, switch to myeloid leukemia, or normal hematogones. Panels incorporating additional markers such as CD22 and CD24 are necessary to assess for CD19-negative relapses.[34] A full immunophenotyping of other lineages may be necessary in some cases to evaluate for a switch to myeloid or monocytic leukemia, especially in *KMT2A*- and *ZNF384*-rearranged leukemias. The utility of T-cell immunophenotyping is discussed later.

Next-generation sequencing (NGS) tracking of MRD can also be performed if the diagnostic clone was characterized.[35] Although NGS MRD has higher sensitivity, it does not determine surface CD19 expression, which is important to determine the cause of relapse and further therapy. Bone-marrow biopsy is necessary for accurate estimation of disease involvement when aspirates for flow cytometry are limited by hemodilution or fibrosis.[36] Biopsies are also useful to assess overall marrow cellularity. Prolonged cytopenias have been noted in some patients post-CAR T-cell therapy[37] and can be associated with an aplastic bone marrow. Increased T-cell aggregates or blasts are not seen in these aplastic marrows that only contain residual stromal cells.

Laboratory studies used for CAR T-cell therapy for B-ALL (see **Fig. 1**A) are also applicable for assessment of residual disease in plasma-cell disorders and mature lymphomas/leukemias that involve the marrow. However, marrow studies are of limited utility when involvement is restricted to lymph nodes or extranodal tissues as is the case in DLBCL. Radiologic PET studies are of greater utility in assessing for residual disease in such situations. Also, lymphoma studies evaluate response later at 3 months, not day 28.[10] Emerging biomarkers such as circulating tumor DNA may also be useful.[38]

CATEGORIZATION OF RESPONSES AND RELAPSES AFTER CHIMERIC ANTIGEN RECEPTOR T-CELL THERAPY

Between 70% and 93% of patients with B-ALL achieve a complete remission (CR) after CD19-directed CAR T-cell therapy.[7,8,39] CR is defined as a morphologic remission (less than 5% disease)[11] and often is further defined as an MRD-negative (<0.01%) CR[6] depending on the study. Nonresponders show persistent morphologic or MRD-level disease at day 28 post-CAR assessment. The cause of nonresponse is not clear but is likely related to the composition of the CAR T-cell product.[39] CAR T cells with memory or a stem-like phenotype or favorable integration (TET2) sites show greater efficacy.[40] Nonresponders also include partial responders who may show a transient decrease in disease burden that eventually returns. Outcome measures such as partial response or stable disease may be of greater utility in DLBCL than B-ALL. The immunophenotype of leukemia at day 28 is usually similar to pre-CAR disease but has, on occasion, shown complete loss of CD19 or lineage switch to myeloid leukemia even during the first month.[6]

Although CAR T-cell therapy induces initial complete remission rates of greater than 70%, 1-year event-free survival and overall survival are 50% to 60%.[38] Around 40% to 50% of those patients who obtained a CR will eventually relapse with CD19-negative or CD19-positive disease.[6] The cause of CD19-positive relapses is different from CD19-negative relapses. CD19-positive relapses are often preceded by early loss of BCA.[6,28] Comparison of pretherapy and posttherapy leukemic blasts showed that blasts had the same immunophenotype and immune repertoire as the pre-CAR leukemia. These findings suggest loss of CAR T-cell function and return of the pre-CAR clone as the mechanism of CD19-positive relapses. Exceptions to this pattern include isolated CNS or extramedullary relapses that showed CD19-positive relapse along with intact B-cell aplasia.[6,41] Hypotheses include a site-specific immune dysregulation instead of general CAR T-cell loss in such cases or a sanctuary site not available to the circulating CAR T cells. Most losses of BCA associated with CD19-positive relapses occur within a year of infusion and suggest a need for persistence and surveillance by CAR T cells. CAR T-cell products with a 4-1BB costimulatory molecule persist longer than those with a CD28 costimulatory molecule.[42] Other factors that affect persistence of CAR T cells include T-cell fitness and human immunogenicity to murine components of the CAR T-cell molecule. Until we understand the factors affecting CAR T-cell persistence, consolidation of CAR T-cell–induced remissions with a hematopoietic stem cell transplant could be considered in a subset of patients with short CAR T-cell persistence.[33]

In contrast to CD19-positive relapses, CD19-negative relapses occur despite ongoing B-cell aplasia. Comparison of pre-CAR and post-CAR immunophenotype showed that only CD19 expression was different—in most of the cases the immune repertoires of the malignant cells were identical (**Fig. 2**).[6] Expression of other antigens

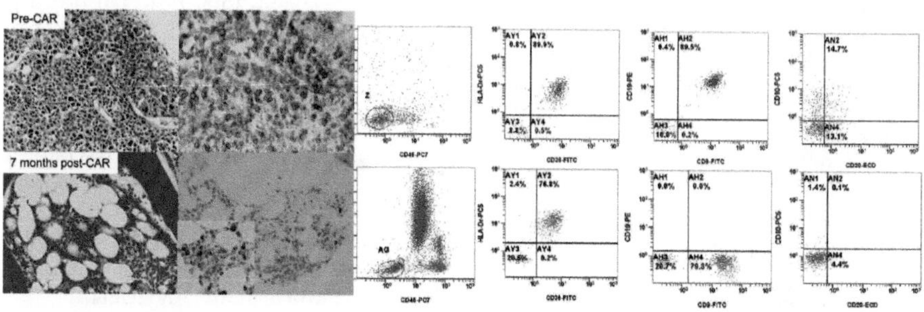

Fig. 2. CD19-negative relapse with total loss of CD19. Morphology and immunophenotype of pre-CAR (*top row*) B-ALL and relapse (bottom row). H&E and CD19 immunostains are shown at 400X. Inset shows B-cell marker CD79a in blasts. Flow cytometric plots of pre-CAR B-lymphoblastic leukemia (*top row*) and 7 months post-CAR CD19-negative B lymphoblastic leukemia (*bottom row*) showing similar immunophenotype except for CD19, which is completely negative. H&E, hematoxylin and eosin.

were mostly comparable suggesting an isolated event affecting CD19 expression. Frequently dim cytoplasmic CD19 expression may be noted by immunohistochemistry on biopsy, although it is completely absent on surface flow cytometric assessment (**Fig. 3**). Dim cytoplasmic expression likely reflects sequestration of the misfolded protein in the cytoplasm[43] or expression of alternatively spliced isoforms.[44] Although most cases show complete loss of all CD19, some patients show a subset with loss of CD19 or reduction in CD19 intensity before total loss (**Fig. 4**). Loss of surface CD19 expression after therapy is due to various mechanisms including mutations and loss of heterozygosity of *CD19* gene,[45] alternative splice isoforms,[44] sequestration of CD19 in endoplasmic reticulum,[46] evolution to plasmablastic lymphoma,[47] and switch to myeloid leukemia or sarcoma.[6,48] Trogocytosis (transfer of surface CD19 antigen from B cells to CAR T cells) has been suggested as a mechanism of CD19 loss in murine models.[49] However, the authors have not seen acquisition of CD19 on CAR T cells in their cohort, and it has never been demonstrated in humans. Also, membrane transfer of CD19 is unlikely to result in permanent loss of *CD19* gene expression. Trogocytosis is most likely a transient phenomenon of unclear real-world significance. Aberrant transduction of the CAR construct in B lymphoblasts causing in-cis masking of CD19 expression has been demonstrated in one patient.[50] However, there is no evidence that this is a widespread mechanism of relapse.

CD19-negative clones might arise from rare preexisting cells or might represent de novo loss of CD19 by blasts under CAR T-cell pressure. However, such low-level CD19-negative blasts could always be detected by MRD flow cytometry and did not correlate with the occurrence of CD19-negative relapses.[6] It is possible other factors such as CAR T-cell fitness and persistence determine which patients relapse as CD19-negative disease. Dim variable CD19 expression pre-CAR also did not predict the occurrence of CD19-negative relapses if such dim or negative CD19 was not due to prior CD19-targeted therapy. The reason for the negative impact of prior CD19-targeted therapy is unclear. It could be due to increased susceptibility to CD19-negative escape variants, or those patients might represent a subset that are refractory to T-cell–directed immunotherapies. Given the use of CD19-targeting blinatumomab upfront in B-ALL, the incidence of CD19-negative disease is likely to increase.[51]

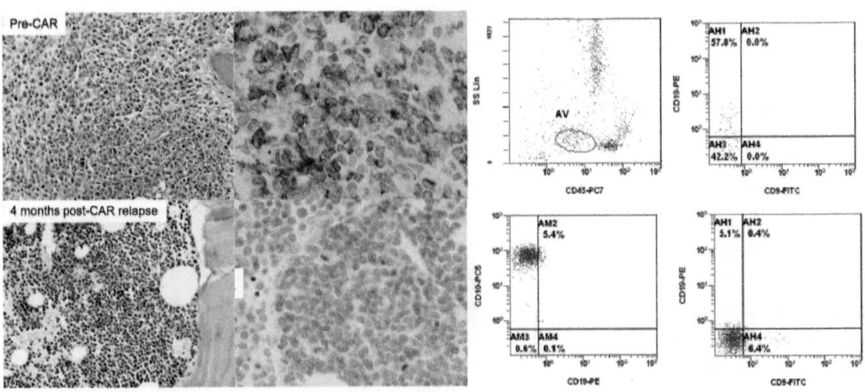

Fig. 3. CD19-negative relapse with loss of surface CD19 but retained cytoplasmic expression. Morphology and immunophenotype of pre-CAR (*top row*) B-ALL and relapse (*bottom row*). H&E (400X) and CD19 immunostains (1000X) are shown. Strong membrane expression is noted pre-CAR but only dim cytoplasmic expression noted post-CAR. Flow cytometric plots of pre-CAR B-lymphoblastic leukemia (*top row*) and 4 months post-CAR CD19-negative B lymphoblastic leukemia (*bottom row*) showing complete loss of surface CD19.

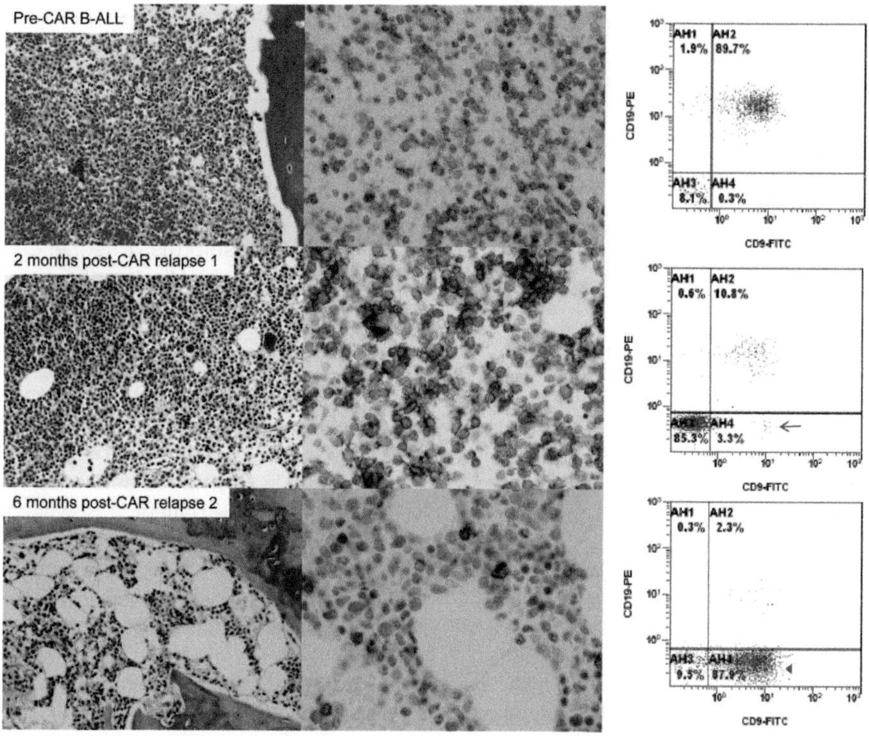

Fig. 4. Evolution of CD19-negative relapse. Morphology and immunophenotype of pre-CAR (*top row*) B-ALL, relapse 1 (*middle row*) and relapse 2 (*bottom row*). H&E (400X), CD19 immunostains (1000X), and flow cytometric CD19 expression are shown. Loss of CD19 in a minor subset (*arrow*) and major subset (*arrow head*) are shown. Patient was reinfused with CAR T cells at relapse 1.

B-ALL switch to AML after CAR T-cell therapy is noted in a subset of *KMT2A*- and *ZNF384*-rearranged B-ALL.[15,16] Typically, all B-cell markers are lost and myeloid or monocytic markers are gained during this time (**Fig. 5**). Some leukemias may not meet the criteria for B-ALL or AML during this period and are best classified as "acute leukemia" until the diagnosis is clear. Lineage switch is also a CD19 escape mechanism similar to CD19-negative relapses. Despite the dramatic difference in their immunophenotype, both pre-CAR B ALL and post-CAR AML possess identical dominant IgH gene rearrangements in addition to identical genetics.[6] Presence of identical immunoglobulin H (IgH) gene arrangements, unchanged cytogenetic alterations, and lack of dysplasia are helpful in excluding a therapy-related myeloid leukemia that is also in the differential. Lineage switch is likely due to inherent capacity for lineage plasticity in *KMT2A*- and *ZNF384*-rearranged B-ALL.

Some lymphomas and leukemias may also undergo transdifferentiation to a nonhematopoietic lineage.[52] MCL transdifferentiation into rhabdomyosarcoma under CAR T-cell pressure has been noted.[52] Characteristic t(11:14) IgH-cyclin D1 rearrangement in MCL and identical IgH gene rearrangements were noted in both sarcoma and lymphoma.

Therapeutic options for patients with CD19-negative relapse are often limited. Assessment of other antigens such as CD22, CD33, CD38, or CD123 may be helpful in identifying novel clinical trials targeting these antigens. Directed immunotherapy

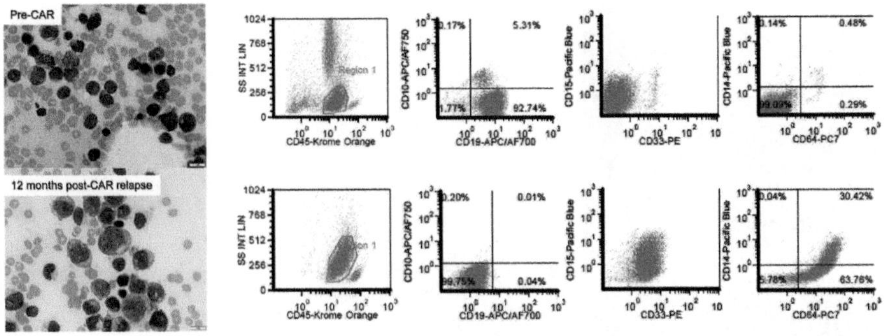

Fig. 5. Switch to myeloid leukemia post-CAR T-cell therapy. Top row: pre-CAR B-lymphoblasts are medium sized with scant cytoplasm and are positive for CD19 and negative for myelomonocytic markers. Bottom row: 12 months post-CAR acute myelomonocytic leukemia with large monocytic blasts with ample vacuolated cytoplasm show complete loss of CD19 (and all other B-cell antigens) concurrent with acquisition of myeloid and monocytic markers.

and/or conventional chemotherapy can be used depending on the immunophenotype of the leukemia. Patients with a switch to a different lineage have limited treatment options but curative attempts can be made with AML-type chemotherapy or immunotherapy, and consolidative transplant.

Routine genetic studies are not necessary for follow-up of patients treated with CAR T-cell therapy, although karyotype and fluorescence in situ hybridization (FISH) studies are useful in confirming relapsed leukemia. Single nucleotide polymorphism or copy number variation arrays for assessment of large deletions may detect deletions and loss of heterozygosity of the 16p locus where the *CD19* gene resides. NGS mutational panels may be helpful in assessing for novel targets for enrolling in clinical trials after failure of CAR T-cell therapy. Lymphoid and myeloid malignancy NGS panels do not assess for deleterious mutations in *CD19*, and the utility of such assessment is not clear. Analysis of surface CD19 expression by flow cytometry is the end result of a variety of genetic events and is more easily assessed.

IMMUNOPHENOTYPE OF CHIMERIC ANTIGEN RECEPTOR T CELLS

CAR T cells are a polyclonal population of cells at infusion, but the clonal diversity may decrease at later time points.[53] CAR T-cell products contain both CD4+ and CD8+ T cells with some institutions using unsorted CD3+ T cells and others controlling the ratio of CD4+ and CD8+ cells.[28] The transduction efficiency of CAR constructs varies widely across individual products. Low transduction efficiency does not preclude a response because even a minor population of CAR T cells may expand and engraft efficiently in vivo. CAR T-cell infusion dose is calculated based on the number of transduced cells per kilogram body weight rather than total cells in the product. Hence, the infused product contains variable numbers of nontransduced T cells in addition to transduced cells depending on the transduction efficiency. However, only the transduced cells are likely to expand, engraft, and lyse targets after infusion.

CD8 CAR T cells kill through perforin-dependent and granzyme-dependent mechanisms, whereas CD4 CAR T cells provide helper function.[54] CAR T-cell expansion is maximal 2 to 3 weeks after infusion when they comprise most of the circulating T cells. The T-cell immunophenotype at this point reflects the phenotypic of expanding

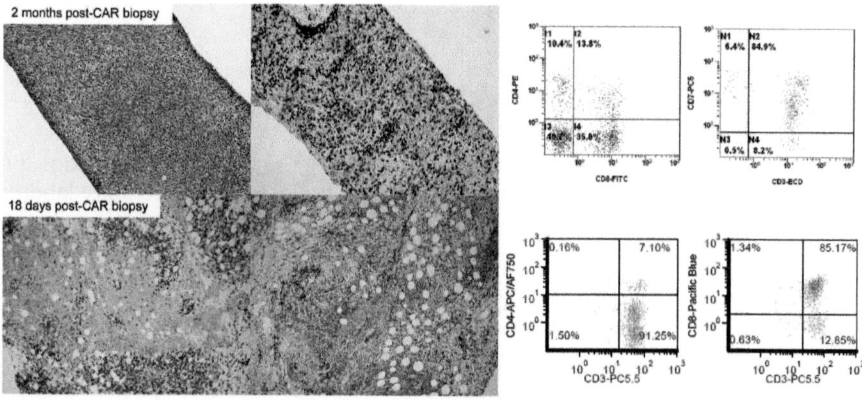

Fig. 6. Immunophenotype of CAR T cells. Top row: 2 months post-CAR renal biopsy from patient with relapsed primary mediastinal large B-cell lymphoma is shown (see Yu et al.[55] for details). H&E and CD3 stain are shown at 100X magnification. Surface CD19 expression was lost by tumor cells. Atypical CD3+ CD8-predominant T-cell infiltrate shows dim CD4 expression by flow cytometry. Bottom row: 18 days post-CAR eyelid biopsy from patient with relapsed B-ALL is shown (see Pillai et al.[56] for details). CD3 and CAR lentivirus-specific in situ hybridization is shown at 100X. Concurrent flow cytometry shows CD8 predominance with dim CD4 expression.

CAR T cells. After 1 month, CAR T cells are in a quiescent phase and only form a minor proportion of circulating T cells due to admixture with normal regenerating T cells. CAR T cells have been shown to persist in some patients for years. It is likely that long-lived CAR T cells with a memory phenotype persist in tissues rather than circulate in peripheral blood. Although we do not perform a CAR T-cell-specific flow in the clinical laboratory, we have been able to immunophenotype CAR T cells when we assess for relapsed leukemia during the first month (**Fig. 6**). CAR T cells in the expansion phase predominantly comprise of CD8 T cells that co-express dim CD4. Other immunophenotypic abnormalities noted include bright CD3 and variable CD7 expression. Clonal transformation of CAR T cells have never been seen or reported.

SUMMARY

Although CAR T products were first used in CLL and B-ALL, they have also shown efficacy in DLBCL, MCL, and multiple myeloma. They are now being investigated in upfront settings in B-ALL and in other hematopoietic malignancies. Advances in CAR T-cell technology may lead to therapeutic indications in solid tumors and even nonmalignant disorders. Laboratories that are used for assessing CAR T-cell efficacy and function in B-ALL may be adapted for use in other indications.

CLINICS CARE POINTS

- CAR T-cell function after infusion can be followed by CRS and clearance of peripheral blasts.
- CAR T-cell function after the first month is followed by B-cell aplasia.
- CAR T-cell response in B-ALL is assessed at day-28 bone marrow biopsy.
- Immunophenotype of relapsed disease after CAR T-cell therapy guides subsequent therapy.

DISCLOSURE

None.

ACKNOWLEDGMENTS

V. Pillai is a Cancer Research Institute CLIP investigator. The authors acknowledge the contributions of personnel in the hematology laboratory, the flow cytometry laboratory, and the CAR T-cell therapy team.

REFERENCES

1. Rosenthal J, Naqvi AS, Luo M, et al. Heterogeneity of surface CD19 and CD22 expression in B lymphoblastic leukemia. Am J Hematol 2018;93(11):E352–5.
2. Teachey DT, Hunger SP. Acute lymphoblastic leukaemia in 2017: immunotherapy for ALL takes the world by storm. Nat Rev Clin Oncol 2018;15(2):69–70.
3. Maus MV, Grupp SA, Porter DL, et al. Antibody-modified T cells: CARs take the front seat for hematologic malignancies. Blood 2014;123(17):2625–35.
4. June CH, O'Connor RS, Kawalekar OU, et al. CAR T cell immunotherapy for human cancer. Science 2018;359(6382):1361–5.
5. Weber EW, Maus MV, Mackall CL. The emerging landscape of immune cell therapies. Cell 2020;181(1):46–62.
6. Pillai V, Muralidharan K, Meng W, et al. CAR T-cell therapy is effective for CD19-dim B-lymphoblastic leukemia but is impacted by prior blinatumomab therapy. Blood Adv 2019;3(22):3539–49.
7. Maude SL, Laetsch TW, Buechner J, et al. Tisagenlecleucel in children and young adults with B-cell lymphoblastic leukemia. N Engl J Med 2018;378(5):439–48.
8. Lee DW, Kochenderfer JN, Stetler-Stevenson M, et al. T cells expressing CD19 chimeric antigen receptors for acute lymphoblastic leukaemia in children and young adults: a phase 1 dose-escalation trial. Lancet 2015;385(9967):517–28.
9. Gardner RA, Finney O, Annesley C, et al. Intent-to-treat leukemia remission by CD19 CAR T cells of defined formulation and dose in children and young adults. Blood 2017;129(25):3322–31.
10. Schuster SJ, Bishop MR, Tam CS, et al. Tisagenlecleucel in adult relapsed or refractory diffuse large B-cell lymphoma. N Engl J Med 2019;380(1):45–56.
11. Maude SL, Frey N, Shaw PA, et al. Chimeric antigen receptor T cells for sustained remissions in leukemia. N Engl J Med 2014;371(16):1507–17.
12. Swerdlow SHCE, Harris NL, Jaffe ES, et al. WHO classification of tumours of haematopoietic and lymphoid tissues. 4th edition. IARC; 2008.
13. Braig F, Brandt A, Goebeler M, et al. Resistance to anti-CD19/CD3 BiTE in acute lymphoblastic leukemia may be mediated by disrupted CD19 membrane trafficking. Blood 2017;129(1):100–4.
14. Fry TJ, Shah NN, Orentas RJ, et al. CD22-targeted CAR T cells induce remission in B-ALL that is naive or resistant to CD19-targeted CAR immunotherapy. Nat Med 2018;24(1):20–8.
15. Gardner R, Wu D, Cherian S, et al. Acquisition of a CD19-negative myeloid phenotype allows immune escape of MLL-rearranged B-ALL from CD19 CAR-T-cell therapy. Blood 2016;127(20):2406–10.
16. Oberley MJ, Gaynon PS, Bhojwani D, et al. Myeloid lineage switch following chimeric antigen receptor T-cell therapy in a patient with TCF3-ZNF384 fusion-positive B-lymphoblastic leukemia. Pediatr Blood Cancer 2018;65(9):e27265.

17. Pan J, Tan Y, Deng B, et al. Frequent occurrence of CD19-negative relapse after CD19 CAR T and consolidation therapy in 14 TP53-mutated r/r B-ALL children. Leukemia 2020;34(12):3382–7.
18. Margolskee E, Pillai V. Loss of surface CD3 expression in allogeneic CAR T-cells. Am J Hematol 2020;95(9):1115–6.
19. Miller JS, Weisdorf DJ, Burns LJ, et al. Lymphodepletion followed by donor lymphocyte infusion (DLI) causes significantly more acute graft-versus-host disease than DLI alone. Blood 2007;110(7):2761–3.
20. Hay KA, Hanafi LA, Li D, et al. Kinetics and biomarkers of severe cytokine release syndrome after CD19 chimeric antigen receptor-modified T-cell therapy. Blood 2017;130(21):2295–306.
21. Teachey DT, Lacey SF, Shaw PA, et al. Identification of predictive biomarkers for cytokine release syndrome after chimeric antigen receptor T-cell therapy for acute lymphoblastic leukemia. Cancer Discov 2016;6(6):664–79.
22. Giavridis T, van der Stegen SJC, Eyquem J, et al. CAR T cell-induced cytokine release syndrome is mediated by macrophages and abated by IL-1 blockade. Nat Med 2018;24(6):731–8.
23. Lee DW, Santomasso BD, Locke FL, et al. ASTCT consensus grading for cytokine release syndrome and neurologic toxicity associated with immune effector cells. Biol Blood Marrow Transplant 2019;25(4):625–38.
24. Gardner RA, Ceppi F, Rivers J, et al. Preemptive mitigation of CD19 CAR T-cell cytokine release syndrome without attenuation of antileukemic efficacy. Blood 2019;134(24):2149–58.
25. Kadauke S, Myers RM, Li Y, et al. Risk-adapted preemptive tocilizumab to prevent severe cytokine release syndrome after CTL019 for pediatric B-cell acute lymphoblastic leukemia: a prospective clinical trial. J Clin Oncol 2021;39(8):920–30.
26. Sarikonda G, Pahuja A, Kalfoglou C, et al. Monitoring CAR-T cell kinetics in clinical trials by multiparametric flow cytometry: benefits and challenges. Cytometry B Clin Cytom 2021;100(1):72–8.
27. Maryamchik E, Gallagher KME, Preffer FI, et al. New directions in chimeric antigen receptor T cell [CAR-T] therapy and related flow cytometry. Cytometry B Clin Cytom 2020;98(4):299–327.
28. Hay KA, Gauthier J, Hirayama AV, et al. Factors associated with durable EFS in adult B-cell ALL patients achieving MRD-negative CR after CD19 CAR T-cell therapy. Blood 2019;133(15):1652–63.
29. Bhoj VG, Arhontoulis D, Wertheim G, et al. Persistence of long-lived plasma cells and humoral immunity in individuals responding to CD19-directed CAR T-cell therapy. Blood 2016;128(3):360–70.
30. Maude SL, Barrett DM, Rheingold SR, et al. Efficacy of humanized CD19-targeted chimeric antigen receptor (CAR)-modified T cells in children with relapsed ALL. J Clin Oncol 2016;34(15_suppl):3007.
31. Maude SL, Hucks GE, Callahan C, et al. Durable remissions with humanized CD19-targeted chimeric antigen receptor (CAR)-modified T cells in CAR-naive and CAR-exposed children and young adults with relapsed/refractory acute lymphoblastic leukemia. Blood 2017;130(Supplement 1):1319.
32. Li AM, Hucks GE, Dinofia AM, et al. Checkpoint inhibitors augment CD19-directed chimeric antigen receptor (CAR) T cell therapy in relapsed B-cell acute lymphoblastic leukemia. Blood 2018;132(Supplement 1):556.

33. Bouziana S, Bouzianas D. Exploring the dilemma of allogeneic hematopoietic cell transplantation after chimeric antigen receptor T cell therapy: to transplant or not? Biol Blood Marrow Transplant 2020;26(8):e183–91.
34. Cherian S, Miller V, McCullouch V, et al. A novel flow cytometric assay for detection of residual disease in patients with B-lymphoblastic leukemia/lymphoma post anti-CD19 therapy. Cytometry B Clin Cytom 2018;94(1):112–20.
35. Pulsipher MA, Han X, Quigley M, et al. Molecular detection of minimal residual disease precedes morphological relapse and could be used to identify relapse in pediatric and young adult B-cell acute lymphoblastic leukemia patients treated with tisagenlecleucel. Blood 2018;132(Supplement 1):1551.
36. Shalabi H, Yuan CM, Kulshreshtha A, et al. Disease detection methodologies in relapsed B-cell acute lymphoblastic leukemia: opportunities for improvement. Pediatr Blood Cancer 2020;67(4):e28149.
37. Jain T, Knezevic A, Pennisi M, et al. Hematopoietic recovery in patients receiving chimeric antigen receptor T-cell therapy for hematologic malignancies. Blood Adv 2020;4(15):3776–87.
38. Sidaway P. ctDNA predicts outcomes in DLBCL. Nat Rev Clin Oncol 2018; 15(11):655.
39. Deng Q, Han G, Puebla-Osorio N, et al. Characteristics of anti-CD19 CAR T cell infusion products associated with efficacy and toxicity in patients with large B cell lymphomas. Nat Med 2020;26(12):1878–87.
40. Nobles CL, Sherrill-Mix S, Everett JK, et al. CD19-targeting CAR T cell immunotherapy outcomes correlate with genomic modification by vector integration. J Clin Invest 2020;130(2):673–85.
41. Willier S, Raedler J, Blaeschke F, et al. Leukemia escape in immune desert: intraocular relapse of pediatric pro-B-ALL during systemic control by CD19-CAR T cells. J Immunother Cancer 2020;8(2):e001052.
42. Philipson BI, O'Connor RS, May MJ, et al. 4-1BB costimulation promotes CAR T cell survival through noncanonical NF-kappaB signaling. Sci Signal 2020; 13(625):eaay8248.
43. Black KL, Naqvi AS, Asnani M, et al. Aberrant splicing in B-cell acute lymphoblastic leukemia. Nucleic Acids Res 2019;47(2):1043.
44. Sotillo E, Barrett DM, Black KL, et al. Convergence of acquired mutations and alternative splicing of CD19 enables resistance to CART-19 immunotherapy. Cancer Discov 2015;5(12):1282–95.
45. Orlando EJ, Han X, Tribouley C, et al. Genetic mechanisms of target antigen loss in CAR19 therapy of acute lymphoblastic leukemia. Nat Med 2018;24(10): 1504–6.
46. Bagashev A, Sotillo E, Tang CA, et al. CD19 alterations emerging after CD19-directed immunotherapy cause retention of the misfolded protein in the endoplasmic reticulum. Mol Cell Biol 2018;38(21):e00383-18.
47. Evans AG, Rothberg PG, Burack WR, et al. Evolution to plasmablastic lymphoma evades CD19-directed chimeric antigen receptor T cells. Br J Haematol 2015; 171(2):205–9.
48. Jacoby E, Nguyen SM, Fountaine TJ, et al. CD19 CAR immune pressure induces B-precursor acute lymphoblastic leukaemia lineage switch exposing inherent leukaemic plasticity. Nat Commun 2016;7:12320.
49. Hamieh M, Dobrin A, Cabriolu A, et al. CAR T cell trogocytosis and cooperative killing regulate tumour antigen escape. Nature 2019;568(7750):112–6.

50. Ruella M, Xu J, Barrett DM, et al. Induction of resistance to chimeric antigen receptor T cell therapy by transduction of a single leukemic B cell. Nat Med 2018;24(10):1499–503.
51. Zhao Y, Aldoss I, Qu C, et al. Tumor intrinsic and extrinsic determinants of response to blinatumomab in adults with B-ALL. Blood 2021;137(4):471–84.
52. Zhang Q, Orlando EJ, Wang HY, et al. Transdifferentiation of lymphoma into sarcoma associated with profound reprogramming of the epigenome. Blood 2020;136(17):1980–3.
53. Sheih A, Voillet V, Hanafi LA, et al. Clonal kinetics and single-cell transcriptional profiling of CAR-T cells in patients undergoing CD19 CAR-T immunotherapy. Nat Commun 2020;11(1):219.
54. Benmebarek MR, Karches CH, Cadilha BL, et al. Killing mechanisms of chimeric antigen receptor (CAR) T cells. Int J Mol Sci 2019;20(6):1283.
55. Yu H, Sotillo E, Harrington C, et al. Repeated loss of target surface antigen after immunotherapy in primary mediastinal large B cell lymphoma. Am J Hematol 2017;92(1):E11–3.
56. Pillai V, Maude SL. CART attack. Blood 2017;130(2):229.

Antigen Loss after Targeted Immunotherapy in Hematological Malignancies

Ting Zhou, MD, PhD[a,b], Hao-Wei Wang, MD, PhD[a,b,*]

KEYWORDS

• Antigen loss • Phenotypic change • Lineage switch • Targeted immunotherapy • CAR-T • Hematological malignancies

KEY POINTS

- Downregulation or loss of target antigens is commonly seen after targeted immunotherapy, which often causes diagnostic dilemma and represents a key mechanism that tumor escapes from immunotherapy.
- The awareness of phenotypic changes after targeted immunotherapy and the development of a multiparametric diagnostic assay is important to avoid misdiagnosis.
- Further understanding of the mechanisms of antigen loss is important to the development of future therapeutic approaches that can prevent or overcome antigen escape.

INTRODUCTION

Over the past decades, the advances in chemotherapy and hematopoietic cell transplantation have dramatically improved the outcomes of hematological malignancies, especially in the pediatric population. The 5-year survival rates have now exceeded 90% for children with acute lymphoblastic leukemia (ALL), classic Hodgkin lymphoma, and non-Hodgkin lymphomas (NHLs).[1] However, long-term survival rates for these entities have plateaued after years of steady progress, and the limitations and disadvantages of conventional therapies are becoming increasingly apparent. A significant proportion of patients are still refractory to conventional treatment, or experience relapse after an initial response. Therefore, enormous effort has been devoted to developing novel therapeutic strategies that are more effective and less toxic.

[a] Flow Cytometry Unit, Laboratory of Pathology, National Cancer Institute, National Institutes of Health, Bethesda, MD, USA; [b] Hematopathology Section, Laboratory of Pathology, National Cancer Institute, National Institutes of Health, Bethesda, MD, USA
* Corresponding author. National Institutes of Health, 10 Center Drive, Building 10, Room 3S235F, Bethesda, MD 20892.
E-mail address: hao-wei.wang@nih.gov

Clin Lab Med 41 (2021) 341–357
https://doi.org/10.1016/j.cll.2021.04.005
0272-2712/21/Published by Elsevier Inc.

Recent years have witnessed significant progress in the understanding of how the immune system interacts with tumors. This progress has led to novel immunotherapy to direct the humoral and/or cell-mediated adaptive immunity against tumor cells. The goal of immunotherapy is to enhance both the magnitude and specificity of antitumor immune responses, which can be achieved by two main approaches, namely checkpoint inhibition and targeted immunotherapies. Checkpoint inhibition aims to tip the balance from immune escape/tolerance to the antitumor immune response by blocking the T-cell inhibitory pathways through checkpoint inhibitors such as cytotoxic T lymphocyte–associated protein 4 (CTLA-4) and programmed cell death protein 1 (PD-1) blockers. Unlike checkpoint inhibition, the goal of targeted immunotherapies is to induce specific immune response against tumor antigens. Despite the remarkable breakthrough in immunotherapy, a lingering problem, as with any antineoplastic agents, is the acquired resistance developed in residual neoplastic cells, which eventually leads to disease relapse. A common mechanism is the modulation of target tumor antigens. This mechanism not only poses a tremendous challenge in the treatment because of its impact on the efficacy and durability of immunotherapy but also complicates the diagnosis of residual or relapsed diseases either by flow cytometry or immunohistochemistry, because the phenotypic changes interfere with the phenotypic characterization of neoplastic cells.

Hematological malignancies, in particular leukemia, are known to have unstable immunophenotype. Phenotypic changes at relapse, either loss of initially present aberrancies or emergence of new aberrancies, occur in 50% to 90% of patient with ALL or acute myeloid leukemia (AML) undergoing conventional chemotherapy.[2,3] The use of targeted immunotherapy adds another layer of complexity, because it frequently results in loss or downregulation of the target antigens at relapse. Importantly, the antigens targeted by immunotherapies are often the same markers used for phenotypic characterization, because of their lineage specificity; that is, cluster of differentiation (CD) 19, CD20, and CD22 in B-cell malignancies. Thus, downregulation of these antigens creates a "moving target" for disease detection and causes diagnostic dilemmas. Few studies have evaluated the dynamics of antigen expression after therapy, and some have investigated the molecular mechanisms underlying these posttherapy antigen modulations. However, many questions remain to be answered.

This article provides an overview on current targeted immunotherapies in hematological malignancies, and summarizes available data regarding how antigen loss occurs after these therapies, as well as the implications these changes have for treatment and diagnosis. It is hoped that this review will instigate more investigations in this field.

OVERVIEW OF TARGETED IMMUNOTHERAPIES

The currently available targeted immunotherapies can be divided into 4 main classes (**Table 1**): (1) conventional monoclonal antibody therapy; (2) antibody-drug conjugates, comprising monoclonal antibodies and cytotoxic agents covalently conjugated through chemical linkers; (3) engineered monoclonal antibodies, also known as bispecific T-cell engagers (BiTEs), which bind both CD3 and a surface antigen on tumor cells and direct T cells to target tumor cells; and (4) adoptive cell transfer therapy with T cells engineered to express chimeric antigen receptors (CARs) or tumor antigen-specific T-cell receptors (TCRs).

Monoclonal antibodies (mAbs) are among the earliest approved forms of anticancer immunotherapy and continue to be at the forefront of treatment regimens for hematological malignancies. These agents have shown remarkable efficacy in patients with otherwise untreatable diseases and hold great promise for the advancement of cancer

Table 1
Monoclonal antibody–based immunotherapies for hematological malignancies

Agent	Target	Type	Applications
Rituximab	CD20	Monoclonal antibody	B-NHL
Ofatumumab	CD20	Monoclonal antibody	B-NHL
Ocrelizumab	CD20	Monoclonal antibody	B-NHL
Tositumomab	CD20	Monoclonal antibody	B-NHL
Obinutuzumab	CD20	Monoclonal antibody	B-NHL
Epratuzumab	CD22	Monoclonal antibody	B-ALL, B-NHL
Daratumumab	CD38	Monoclonal antibody	PCM, B-ALL, T-ALL, AML
Isatuximab	CD38	Monoclonal antibody	B-ALL, T-ALL, AML
Inotuzumab ozogamicin	CD22	Antibody-drug conjugate	B-ALL
Moxetumomab pasudotox	CD22	Antibody-drug conjugate	B-ALL, B-NHL
Gemtuzumab ozogamicin	CD33	Antibody-drug conjugate	AML
Vadastuximab talirine	CD33	Antibody-drug conjugate	AML
Brentuximab vedotin	CD30	Antibody-drug conjugate	cHL, ALCL
Blinatumomab	CD19	BiTE	B-ALL, B-NHL
Tisagenlecleucel	CD19	CAR	B-ALL, B-NHL
Axicabtagene ciloleucel	CD19	CAR	B-ALL, B-NHL

Abbreviations: ALCL, anaplastic large cell lymphoma; BiTE, bispecific T-cell engagers; B-NHL, B-cell NHL; CAR, chimeric antigen receptor; cHL, classic Hodgkin lymphoma; NHL, non-Hodgkin lymphoma; T-ALL, T-cell ALL; PCM, plasma cell myeloma.

treatment. Monoclonal antibodies exert their tumor-killing effects through various direct and indirect mechanisms. First, the binding of mAbs to their target antigens directly activates apoptotic signaling pathways and induces apoptosis of tumor cells. The other mechanisms involve effectors from the patient's own immune system, including complement-dependent cytotoxicity, antibody-dependent cell-mediated cytotoxicity, and antibody-dependent cellular phagocytosis, either by activating the complement system or by recruiting Fc receptor–expressing effector cells, including monocytes, macrophages, and natural killer cells. In addition, the therapeutic mAbs may also elicit a vaccinal effect beyond their direct tumor-killing function. Destruction of tumor cells facilitates the release of tumor-associated antigens, improves the uptake and presentation of these antigens by dendritic cells, and triggers a cascade of antitumor immune responses.

Built on the initial success of conventional unconjugated mAbs, several mAb derivatives have been developed for clinical use over the past decades. Antibody-drug conjugates comprise tumor-specific antibodies covalently linked to cytotoxic payloads such as mitotic toxins, chemotherapeutic agents, or radiotherapeutic agents, which have the potential to increase therapeutic efficacy by selectively delivering cytotoxic agents into tumor cells. Another class of modified monoclonal antibodies, BiTEs, is designed to enhance the patient's antitumor immune response by redirecting cytotoxic T cells to tumor cells. They contain 2 linked sets of the single-chain variable fragments of antibodies; 1 binds to CD3 on T cells and the other binds to an antigen on tumor cells. This physical bridge enables optimal interaction between these 2 cell types, bypassing the requirement for major histocompatibility complex (MHC)/TCR engagement. This process results in MHC-independent activation of polyclonal T cells, while preventing undesired T-cell activation and anergy. The concept underlying the design of CAR-T therapy is similar to that of BiTEs, both directly coupling the antigen specificity of an mAb with the effector function of T cells.

Collectively, these mAb-based immunotherapeutic approaches rely on mAbs to target cancer cells, and mAbs can therefore serve as a conceptual basis for understanding the mechanisms of their action as well as resistance. A comprehensive overview of resistance to immunotherapy is beyond the scope of this article, which focuses on the role of antigen loss.

IMMUNE TARGETING AND ANTIGEN ESCAPE

Anti–CD20 Monoclonal Antibodies

CD20 is a transmembrane phosphoprotein expressed on B cells from late precursor B cell through the memory B-cell stage. Although its precise function remains obscure, CD20 has been suggested to play an important role in B-cell activation and proliferation, possibly by functioning as a calcium channel and/or interacting with the B-cell receptor (BCR) and other molecules important in B-cell signal transduction.[4,5] Despite the uncertainty in its biological role, CD20 is an attractive target for cancer immunotherapy. It is uniformly expressed at high density on almost all mature B-cell neoplasms and approximately 30% of pre–B-cell ALL (pre–B-ALL).[6] The high expression level (typically 100,000 molecules per cell) also facilitates efficient target opsonization. Importantly, it is not shed or secreted into the circulation in large amounts and is unlikely to persist as a soluble, antigenically intact molecule because of its hydrophobic nature and tetraspan structure. These features prevent the antibodies from binding primarily to freely circulating antigens without targeting the tumor cells. Another major consideration of selecting CD20 as an appropriate target is that hematopoietic stem cells, early B-cell progenitors, and plasma cells do not express CD20, and thus depleting B cells by CD20 targeting does not cause permanent B-cell aplasia and immune deficiency.

Rituximab, a chimeric mouse-human anti-CD20 antibody, was the first monoclonal antibody clinically approved for cancer therapy and a paradigm of mAbs. Since its inception in 1997, rituximab has become the cornerstone in the management of virtually all types of B-cell malignancies across different age groups. It is now routinely incorporated into almost every line of therapy, including first-line, maintenance, and salvage therapy, either as a monotherapy or in a combination with other chemotherapeutic agents. The depletion of circulating B cells occurs rapidly after administration of rituximab. Because of the long elimination half-life of rituximab of approximately 3 weeks,[7] repopulation of circulating B cells usually does not occur until 6 to 9 months after a standard dosing schedule. The absolute numbers of B cells return to baseline levels at approximately 12 months after therapy.[8] Similarly, rituximab also induces a prompt and prolonged B-cell depletion in lymphoid tissues.[9] Compared with conventional lymphoma therapies, rituximab exerts higher antitumor activity and carries reduced toxicity. Based on the success of rituximab, a second-generation of anti-CD20 mAbs, such as ofatumumab and obinutuzumab, has been developed and marketed.

Nonetheless, the ultimate effectiveness of anti-CD20 mAbs is limited by intrinsic and acquired resistance. For instance, 20% of patients with diffuse large B-cell lymphoma (DLBCL) are primarily refractory to R-CHOP (rituximab with cyclophosphamide, doxorubicin, vincristine, and prednisone), and another 30% eventually relapse after complete remission.[10,11] Decreased CD20 expression on the target cells has been reported in up to 30% of patients who received rituximab,[11,12] and is thought to be one of the major mechanisms governing resistance to such treatments. Notably, there is the potential for discordant results of CD20 expression by flow cytometry and immunohistochemistry, depending on the antibody clones used.[13,14]

Anti-CD19 Monoclonal Antibodies

CD19 belongs to the immunoglobulin superfamily and is an activating coreceptor of the BCR complex. It is expressed throughout B-cell development from the pro-B stage to plasma cells. By modulating BCR signaling, CD19 directs B-cell fate and differentiation during lymphopoiesis and promotes their survival and proliferation. CD19 is expressed on a broad variety of B-cell malignancies, including early B-cell neoplasms such as B-ALL. The broad expression pattern and biological function of CD19 makes it a promising immunotherapeutic target. Notably, CD19 is internalized more rapidly and efficiently than CD20, and thus is better suited for antibody-drug conjugate therapies.[15,16] Unconjugated CD19 mAbs showed only modest activity in preclinical trials. Hence, efforts are being made to develop novel approaches, including bispecific antibodies, antibody-drug conjugates, and Fc-engineered antibodies. The most advanced is blinatumomab, a bispecific T-cell engager, which was approved for B-ALL in 2014 and has also shown encouraging results in clinical trials of relapse/refractory DLBCL.[17]

As with rituximab, blinatumomab causes B-cell aplasia, which is reversible because the stem cells do not express CD19. Blinatumomab has a short elimination half-life and requires continuous intravenous infusion. After blinatumomab infusion, the peripheral B-cell counts rapidly decrease to less than 1 cell per microliter within an average of 2 days and remain undetectable throughout the treatment period.[18] The nonresponders tend to have incomplete or shorter duration of B-cell depletion.[19] CD19 loss is less common following blinatumomab, occurring in up to 20% of patients with B-ALL relapsing after therapy.[20,21] In a study that evaluated the dynamic changes of CD19 surface expression in pediatric patients with B-ALL after CD19-targeted therapy,[22] most (74%) of the patients with CD19-negative relapse after CD19-targeting therapies remained CD19 negative during the follow-up, but a subset regained partial or full expression of CD19. Notably, prior blinatumomab therapy has been shown to affect the effectiveness of subsequent CD19 CAR-T–cell therapy.[23]

Anti-CD22 Monoclonal Antibodies

CD22 is a transmembrane protein that physically associates with the BCR and regulates its signaling.[24] CD22 is expressed on 60% to 80% of B-cell malignancies and is detected on leukemic blasts in more than 80% of patients with ALL.[25,26] In contrast with CD20, CD22 is quickly internalized when bound by antibody and can recycle back to the cell membrane after modulation.[27] This distinct internalization property provides strong rationale for its use as a target for antibody-drug conjugates. Inotuzumab ozogamicin consists of a humanized immunoglobulin (Ig) G4 anti-CD22 mAb linked to the cytotoxic antibiotic calicheamicin. It was approved by the US Food and Drug Administration (FDA) in 2017 for the treatment of relapsed or refractory B-ALL in adults, and has also shown promising antitumor effects and a favorable safety profile in pediatric patients with B-ALL.[28]

Downregulation or loss of CD22 has been observed in more than 10% of adult patients following anti-CD22 therapy,[29] but data in the pediatric population are limited. In 1 recent study of inotuzumab ozogamicin in pediatric patients with relapsed/refractory B-ALL,[28] downregulation of surface CD22 expression was detected in 3 patients at the time of relapse, suggesting a possible escape mechanism for inotuzumab ozogamicin therapy.

Anti-CD38 Monoclonal Antibodies

CD38 is a transmembrane glycoprotein expressed in a variety of hematopoietic and other tissues. It was first recognized as a differentiation and activation marker of lymphocytes and later found to have multiple functions, including enzymatic activity and as a receptor for CD31.[30] It regulates the adhesion and migration of leukocytes through endothelial cells, as well as their activation and proliferation.[31] CD38 is robustly expressed in a variety of hematological malignancies, including multiple myeloma, B-ALL, T-cell ALL, AML, and B-cell NHL (B-NHL; Burkitt and non-Burkitt),[32,33] and has been considered as a promising target for immunotherapies. Daratumumab is a human IgG kappa mAb against CD38, which has now been widely used for the treatment of multiple myeloma. There are also newer anti-CD38 mAbs, such as isatuximab, which induces direct apoptosis independent of cross-linking.[34] There have been several ongoing clinical trials evaluating the efficacy of these anti-CD38 mAbs in pediatric hematological malignancies.

One known diagnostic problem in patients who received daratumumab is the interference of the therapeutic mAbs with the detection of residual diseases.[35] It has been shown that daratumumab may saturate the CD38 throughout the body for several months after discontinuation of mAb treatment. The daratumumab mAbs persisting on the cell surface interfere with CD38 detection, because standard diagnostic CD38 mAbs bind to epitopes overlapping with the daratumumab binding site, which results in an apparent loss of CD38 in otherwise CD38-expressing cells. This antigen-masking effect can be circumvented by the usage of multiepitope CD38 antibody or CD38 nanobody that recognizes different epitopes, or by staining other antigens.[35,36] In addition, daratumumab bound on CD38-expressing cells also causes an artifactual kappa light chain restriction pattern that may potentially lead to misdiagnosis.[37]

Chimeric Antigen Receptor T-cell Therapy

Immunotherapy with T cells genetically modified to express a CAR against CD19 represents a promising salvage approach for patients with refractory and relapsed B-cell malignancies. Several clinical trials have shown remarkable efficacy in a variety of B-cell malignancies, most notably in B-ALL, even in patients who have failed multiple lines of chemotherapy and allogenic stem cell transplant (CAR-T–cell therapy in B-ALL is reviewed separately in this issue). Similar to what is observed with anti-CD19 mAb treatment, relapse may occur because of the emergence of malignant subclones that have lost CD19 expression, which is observed in 10% to 20% of pediatric B-ALL relapsing after CAR-T–therapy.[38,39] Anti-CD22 CAR-T therapy has also shown promising efficacy for B-ALL, including the CD19-negative relapses after anti-CD19 therapy.[40,41] Most relapse after this therapy is associated with diminished surface CD22 expression, again indicating that antigen modulation is an important mechanism of immune escape. One approach to further diminish the likelihood of tumor escape through antigen loss is to target more than 1 antigen at the same time. Simultaneous targeting of CD19 and CD22 via bispecific CAR-T has been shown to be more effective in preventing antigen escape than sequential administration of anti-CD19 CAR-T and anti-CD22 CAR-T cells,[42,43] although the possibility of emergence of CD19-negative, CD22-dim blasts still exists.

IMPACT ON DIAGNOSIS

The awareness of changes in immunophenotype after targeted immunotherapy is important to avoid misdiagnosis. CD20-negative residual or relapsed disease is a well-known diagnostic pitfall in B-cell neoplasms after anti-CD20 therapies. In this scenario, the use of other B-cell antigens, including surface expression of CD19, CD79a, and CD22, as well as nuclear expression of PAX-5, OCT-2, and BOB-1, should suffice to detect the disease and confirm the B-cell origin.

Loss of CD19 in B-ALL poses significant challenges for minimal residual disease (MRD) testing by flow cytometry. Given that conventional flow cytometric gating strategies often rely on CD19 to identify B-cell lineages, residual disease or relapse of B-ALL with a CD19-negative immunophenotype may be missed. Thus, alternative strategies have been designed for residual disease detection in this setting. One example uses CD22 and CD24 in combination with CD66b (to exclude CD24-positive neutrophils) to identify the B-cell lineage,[44] from which the neoplastic blasts can be detected by their abnormal immunophenotype that deviates from the normal maturation pattern of B-cell precursors based on expression of other markers, including CD10, CD20, CD34, CD38, CD58, and CD45. Most abnormal blast populations of B lineage can be detected using this method, because they are typically positive for at least 1 of CD22 and CD24 (>95%).[6] However, it is necessary to keep in mind that several clinical scenarios and therapeutic settings can lead to downregulation of CD22 and/or CD24, which may constitute diagnostic pitfalls. Downregulation or loss of CD22 occurs following anti-CD22 therapy; transient downregulation of both CD22 and CD24 may also occasionally be seen during the course of anti-CD19 therapy. Further complicating the matter, anti-CD22 therapy is often used as salvage after failure of anti-CD19 therapy, and simultaneous CD19/CD22 targeting is also a promising future development. This dual selective pressure could potentially cause antigen loss of both targets simultaneously. Another diagnostic pitfall is the presence of CD19-negative, CD22-positive, normal precursors, which are often expanded in regenerating marrow following CD19-targeted therapy. This precursor population may mimic a residual disease and should be distinguished from B-ALL based on their distinct immunophenotypic features.[44] In addition, cases of lineage switch to AML have been reported in B-ALL following the treatment with blinatumomab and anti-CD19 CAR-T (discussed more comprehensively later). Judicious inclusion of myeloid evaluation is important to avoid misdiagnosis in this context. Overall, in the era of immunotherapy, a comprehensive flow cytometric assay to investigate multiple B-cell lineage markers is needed to increase the sensitivity of detecting neoplastic B cells. The results should not be interpreted in isolation but within the appropriate clinical context. In addition, molecular MRD testing to track clonal rearrangements of immunoglobulin genes or specific allelic variants can serve as an alternative or complementary strategy.

MECHANISMS OF ANTIGEN LOSS

The molecular mechanisms underlying antigen loss after targeted immunotherapy are multifold and not yet fully understood. Several mechanisms have been discovered, affecting different steps of surface antigen expression, including removal of antigens from the cell surface via internalization or trogocytosis, disrupted trafficking to the membrane, transcriptional downregulation, and genomic alterations (**Fig. 1**). In addition, the reduction in average expression levels of the target antigen might be in part caused by elimination of the subpopulations with the highest expression levels. In rare cases, the therapeutic pressure can also lead to lineage switch, as seen in cases of B-ALL switching to AML.

Antigen Internalization

A straightforward mechanism leading to antigen loss is antigen internalization. A prototypic example is the internalization of CD20-rituximab complexes in malignant B

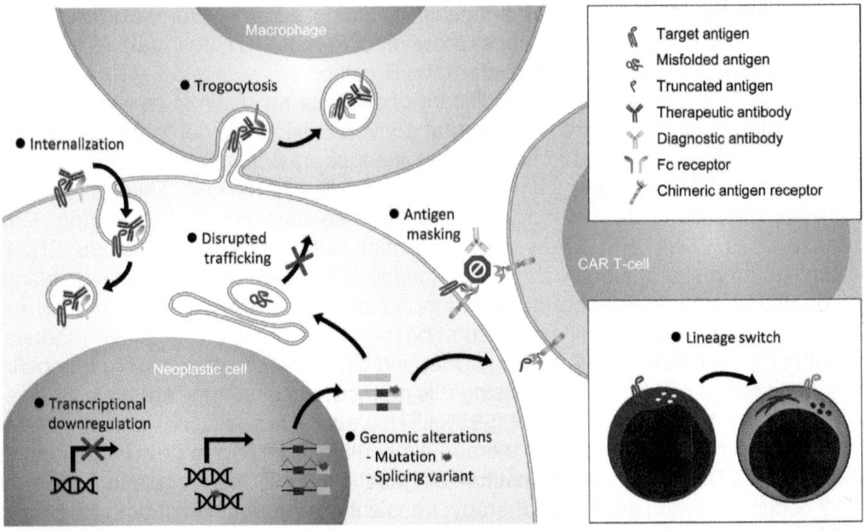

Fig. 1. Mechanisms of antigen loss after targeted immunotherapy. Loss of tumor antigens may result from removal of the antigens from cell surface by internalization or trogocytosis, or from disrupted protein trafficking. Antigens may be masked because of overlapped epitope binding, which prevents them from being recognized by the diagnostic or therapeutic antibodies. In addition, antigen loss may be a result of transcriptional downregulation. Genomic alterations, including mutations and splicing variants, may change the structure of the antigens, rendering them unrecognizable by the antibodies, or result in truncated or misfolded protein that fails to be expressed on the surface. In addition, loss of the initial tumor antigen may be caused by lineage switch, where the relapsed disease acquires a different lineage phenotype.

cells, which is known to be mediated by the Fc gamma receptor IIb (FcγRIIb or CD32B) through a cis interaction between the Fc portion of rituximab and FcγRIIb on the same cell.[45] Different types of B-cell malignancies internalize CD20-rituximab complexes at different rates, possibly because of different levels of FcγRIIb. Lymphoma subtypes with a high level of FcγRIIb, such as chronic lymphatic leukemia (CLL) and mantle cell lymphoma (MCL), show rapid CD20 internalization, whereas DLBCL cells express a lower level of FcγRIIb and are more resistant to CD20 loss.[45] Such variations may provide an explanation for the differing sensitivity of B-cell malignancies to rituximab. In concordance with their lower CD20 expression and/or rapid CD20 internalization, treatment success is more modest in CLL and MCL, compared with that in DLBCL and follicular lymphomas. Although CLL, nodal follicular lymphoma, and MCL almost never occur in children, the findings discussed earlier nonetheless provide a conceptual basis for using pretherapeutic CD20 expression, FcγRIIb expression, and extent of CD20 internalization as predictive biomarkers to identify the subset of pediatric patients who will benefit most from rituximab. Despite some controversies, several studies have shown a correlation between higher CD20 expression and longer overall survival in patients treated with rituximab. In contrast, the specific type of anti-CD20 antibodies also affects the extent of target antigen loss. Anti-CD20 mAbs are classified into 2 classes based on their ability to redistribute CD20 into lipid rafts on the plasma membrane. Type I antibodies, such as rituximab and ofatumumab, trigger clustering and recruitment of CD20 into lipid raft. The enhanced clustering of type I antibodies renders them more susceptible to internalization and subsequent proteolytic degradation. By contrast, type II antibodies do not induce efficient clustering of CD20 or antibody internalization, hence showing an increased therapeutic potency and decreased treatment resistance.[46]

Trogocytosis

Another mechanism that leads to removal of antigens from the surface of target cells is so-called shaving, otherwise termed trogocytosis, of the antigens by phagocytic cells, including monocytes, macrophages, and neutrophils.[47–49] This process is mediated through the Fcγ receptors expressed on the effector cells, which interacts in trans with the Fc portion of the antibody-antigen complex on target cells and triggers the uptake of the antibody-antigen complex. The best-studied antigen loss secondary to trogocytosis is the loss of CD20 after anti-CD20 mAbs. The relative contribution of internalization versus trogocytosis to antigen downregulation depends on the types of anti-CD20 mAbs.[46] As discussed earlier, internalization occurs mainly in type I mAbs, whereas both types are subject to trogocytosis. Notably, the loss of CD20 and bound rituximab by trogocytosis occurs faster than antigen internalization and was thought to be the key mechanism of rituximab-induced CD20 loss.[50]

Trogocytosis also contributes to antigen loss after other mAb therapies. Epratuzumab, an anti-CD22 mAb, induces reduction of B-cell antigens as a result of trogocytosis.[51] Not only is CD22 downregulated after epratuzumab but the levels of other antigens, including CD19, CD21, and CD79b, are also significantly decreased, which was thought to be caused by their close proximity to the epratuzumab-bound CD22 recruited to the lipid rafts. Trogocytosis may also play a role in resistance to CAR-T–cell therapy. In experimental cell culture and mouse models for CD19 CAR therapy, a reversible reduction of CD19 was observed on leukemia cells, as a result of trogocytic transfer of CD19 to CAR T cells, which leads to reduced T-cell activity by promoting fratricide T-cell killing and T-cell exhaustion.[52] This reversible antigen loss through trogocytosis was thought to contribute to the escape of antigen-low tumors to CAR-T cells, although its clinical significance awaits further support from clinical studies.

The trogocytic transfer deserves special consideration in the context of antibody-drug conjugates, for the concern of potential off-target effects. For instance, gemtuzumab ozogamicin, a CD33-specific mAb conjugated to calicheamicin, has been used in the treatment of adult AML. It is associated with a 9% risk of developing liver sinusoidal obstruction syndrome after therapy; the risk is even higher (14%) in patients who further received stem cell transplants.[53] This gemtuzumab ozogamicin–induced hepatotoxicity was partly attributed to direct delivery of calicheamicin to CD33-expressing cells residing in the liver sinusoids, including the sinusoidal endothelial cells.[54] In addition, it was proposed that trogocytic transfer through the FcγRIIb expressed on the liver sinusoidal endothelium may also play a role.[55]

Disrupted Membrane Trafficking

The expression of surface protein requires multiple steps of regulated trafficking from the endoplasmic reticulum through layers of Golgi apparatus. These organelles serve the places where the membrane protein is properly modified and folded before it reaches the final destinations. Thus, it is plausible that any defect in the trafficking routes may impair the surface expression of target antigens. Disrupted CD19 trafficking has been reported in a case of relapsed B-ALL, which resulted in loss of CD19 and resistance to blinatumomab.[56] In this case, the loss of CD19 was caused by the lack of CD81, which serves as a chaperone of CD19 and facilitate its transport from the Golgi to the cell surface. It is still unclear whether this is a prevalent mechanism of antigen escape and whether it also occurs in other types of targeted immunotherapy.

Antigen Masking

As discussed earlier in the example of daratumumab, the masking of antigen by therapeutic mAbs may interfere with its detection by diagnostic antibodies that bind to the same epitope, resulting in apparent loss of antigen. In rare instances, antigen masking may also result in resistance to therapy. In one case report, the CD19 CAR gene was unintentionally introduced into a leukemic B-ALL cell during the manufacture of CAR-T cells. This CAR product bound in cis to the CD19 epitope on the cell surface, masking it from recognition by CAR-T cells and resulting in resistance to the therapy.[57] This resistance mechanism caused by target antigen masking was also reproduced in an experimental model for CAR-T-cell therapy in AML.[58]

Transcriptional Downregulation

In patients with relapsed or progressive B-cell malignancies following rituximab-containing chemotherapies, the CD20 messenger RNA expression was found to be significantly lower in the rituximab-resistant cells.[11,59] Interestingly, treatment with 5-aza-2′-deoxycytidine (decitabine) was shown to restore the expression of CD20 as well as the sensitivity to rituximab in vitro, indicating that an epigenetic mechanism may be involved.[11,60] Further chromatin immunoprecipitation studies showed that the histone deacetylase (HDAC) complex is recruited to the promoter of the *CD20* gene in the CD20-negative transformed B cells, resulting in histone acetylation and repression of CD20 expression. Understanding of CD20 regulation may inform the design of novel combination regimens designed to increase the efficacy of rituximab, because the combinatory agents may affect the expression of CD20. For instance, spleen tyrosine kinase (SYK) inhibitors, Bruton's tyrosine kinase (BTK) inhibitors, phosphoinositide 3-kinase inhibitors, or C-X-C Motif Chemokine Receptor 4 (CXCR4) antagonists have been found to significantly repress CD20 expression, which largely prevents their successful combination with rituximab.[61]

Genomic Alterations

In addition to those changes described earlier that affect the level of protein expression, structural alteration at the molecular level is an important mechanism that leads to antigen escape. These alternations may result from genetic mutations, such as point mutation, insertion, and deletion, or posttranscriptional processes, including alternative splicing.

Mutations in CD20 have been shown to account partly for rituximab resistance in B-cell lymphomas. CD20 contains two extracellular loops and three cytoplasmic domains, and rituximab recognizes the large extracellular loop.[62] Mutations in the rituximab epitope disrupt the binding of rituximab to the target, although it occurs infrequently. In one study, rituximab epitope mutations were detected in only 0.4% and 6% of DLBCL biopsies taken at diagnosis and relapse following R-CHOP.[63] In addition, C-terminal mutations were shown to result in decreased presentation of the large extracellular loop and decreased rituximab binding.[64] In one study, C-terminal deletion mutations were detected in 8% of B-NHLs, which were associated with relapse/resistance after rituximab therapy.[65]

Genomic alterations have been shown to be a major mechanism of target antigen loss in CAR therapy. Next-generation sequencing, including whole-exon DNA sequencing, RNA sequencing, and copy number analyses on CD19-negative relapsed B-ALL samples after CD19 CAR-T-cell therapy, has revealed de novo genomic alterations in the *CD19* gene in most cases.[66] These mutations were found throughout exons 2 to 5. Nearly all relapsed samples contain loss-of-function mutations, including frameshift mutations, which lead to truncated protein lacking the transmembrane domain encoded by exon 5. It was proposed that these loss-of-function mutations may be the major source of CD19 loss and acquired resistance to CD19 CAR-T–cell therapy.[66] In addition, alternative splicing variants, especially exon 2 skipping and intron 2 retention, were also a common finding.[67] The Δex2 variants were shown to become trapped in the endoplasmic reticulum without trafficking to the cell surface because of protein misfolding.[68] In contrast, retention of intron 2 often introduces a premature nonsense codon, thus functionally equivalent to a nonsense mutation. The alternative splicing of CD19 was proposed as a major mechanism that contributes to the resistance to CD19 CAR therapy.[69]

Lineage Switch

Since the advent of immunotherapy, cases with lineage switch from B-ALL to AML have been described at relapses following CD19-directed therapy in both children and adults.[70–72] Almost all of these cases carry rearrangements of *KMT2A* (*MLL1*), most commonly t(4;11) translocation (*KMT2A-AFF1*). These patients often had a rapid relapse within 30 days after treatment, although lineage switch at late relapse has also been reported. The blasts at relapse showed partial or complete loss of B-lineage antigens (CD19, CD20, CD22, CD24, and cytoplasmic CD79a) and acquisition of myelomonocytic markers including CD117, CD13, CD33, MPO, CD11b, CD4, CD14, or CD64, whereas the expression of CD34 and HLA-DR is often retained. Despite immunophenotypic conversion, the relapsed disease maintained the original genetic rearrangements, confirming the clonal relationship between the original and relapsed leukemias.

Several mechanisms have been invoked to explain the lineage switch, including bipotentiality of leukemic stem cells/progenitors, cellular reprogramming, and clonal selection. The AML at relapse and original B-ALL may derive from the same leukemia-initiating cell, which has the potential to differentiate into either B-lymphoid or myeloid lineage in response to specific intrinsic and environmental signals. Exposure to anti-CD19 immunotherapy may trigger an alteration of cell fate programs and direct differentiation toward myeloid lineage. In support of this, *MLL*-rearranged B-ALL shows gene expression profiles consistent with early hematopoietic progenitors. A possible link between CD19-directed immunotherapy and modification of transcriptional factor activities is immunologic pressure and inflammatory cytokine release (notably interleukin [IL]-6). Cytokine release following CD19-directed immunotherapy is frequently observed early in the course of treatment, when T cells encounter abundant targets and become fully activated. Consistent with this time frame, the phenotypic switch mostly occurs within 30 days after therapy. In addition, IL-6 was shown to induce myeloid differentiation of a biphenotypic leukemia cell line.[73] Therefore, changes in cell fate decision in these cases are likely the results of a combination of intrinsic (genetic and epigenetic cues mediated by the leukemic translocations) and extrinsic factors (therapeutic pressure, cytokine stimulation, and so forth). Another less probable mechanism is that anti-CD19 therapy provides a growth advantage to a preexisting myeloid clone. However, flow cytometric analysis in most cases did not detect a myeloid clone at diagnosis, although this does not completely disprove the presence of myeloid clones at low frequencies. The high plasticity of the leukemic clone carrying the translocations mentioned earlier suggests that caution is warranted when treating these patients using CD19-targeted therapy. A comprehensive evaluation of the myeloid phenotype should be included during the follow-up. Additional consolidation therapy should also be considered in these patients to prevent the emergence of a myeloid clone after the initial remission.

SUMMARY

The development of immunotherapy marked a milestone in the evolution of cancer treatments and has changed the landscape of treatment of a variety of hematological malignancies. Antigen loss after therapy represents one of the most important mechanisms of therapy resistance and also causes diagnostic dilemma. Flow cytometric assays with a combination of multiple lineage-specific markers are needed to increase the sensitivity of detecting neoplastic cells that can potentially lose target antigens after immunotherapy. In contrast, attempts are being made to overcome resistance related to antigen escape, either by dual-targeting therapies or by induction of antigen expression. For instance, preclinical or phase I/II clinical trials are underway to evaluate the combination of rituximab and CD20 inducers such as histone deacetylase inhibitors, and have shown promising results.[74,75] Other preclinical studies have also shown promising results of target antigen modulation as a strategy to improve the efficacy of CAR therapy. For example, administration of bryostatin-1 has been shown to upregulate CD22 site density on leukemia and lymphoma cells and improve the functionality of CD22 CAR-T cells.[76] Nonetheless, understanding of the mechanisms, patterns, and dynamics of immunophenotypic changes following immune therapy is still at an early stage. The authors anticipate that future research will shed light on these fundamental issues. It is also expected that, with improved knowledge in this field, clinicians will be able to identify reliable predictive markers to select patients up front who are likely to benefit from immunotherapy, as well as to guide the choice of the optimal immunotherapy for each patient.

CLINICS CARE POINTS

- Antigen loss after therapy represents one of the most important mechanisms of therapy resistance and also causes diagnostic dilemma.
- A flow cytometric assay with a combination of multiple lineage-specific markers is needed to increase the sensitivity of detecting neoplastic cells.
- Developing therapeutic approaches that can prevent or overcome antigen escape remains an important goal of future research.

ACKNOWLEDGMENTS

The authors wish to thank the entire flow cytometry laboratory for the gracious support and the insightful discussions during the manuscript preparation. This work was supported by the Intramural Research Program of the National Institutes of Health (NIH).

DISCLOSURE

The authors have no relevant conflicts of interest to disclose.

REFERENCES

1. Siegel RL, Miller KD, Fuchs HE, et al. Cancer statistics, 2021. CA Cancer J Clin 2021;71(1):7–33.
2. Baer MR, Stewart CC, Dodge RK, et al. High frequency of immunophenotype changes in acute myeloid leukemia at relapse: implications for residual disease

detection (Cancer and Leukemia Group B Study 8361). Blood 2001;97(11): 3574–80.
3. Guglielmi C, Cordone I, Boecklin F, et al. Immunophenotype of adult and childhood acute lymphoblastic leukemia: changes at first relapse and clinico-prognostic implications. Leukemia 1997;11(9):1501–7.
4. Janas E, Priest R, Wilde JI, et al. Rituxan (anti-CD20 antibody)-induced translocation of CD20 into lipid rafts is crucial for calcium influx and apoptosis. Clin Exp Immunol 2005;139(3):439–46.
5. Polyak MJ, Li H, Shariat N, et al. CD20 homo-oligomers physically associate with the B cell antigen receptor. Dissociation upon receptor engagement and recruitment of phosphoproteins and calmodulin-binding proteins. J Biol Chem 2008; 283(27):18545–52.
6. Raponi S, De Propris MS, Intoppa S, et al. Flow cytometric study of potential target antigens (CD19, CD20, CD22, CD33) for antibody-based immunotherapy in acute lymphoblastic leukemia: analysis of 552 cases. Leuk Lymphoma 2011; 52(6):1098–107.
7. Regazzi MB, Iacona I, Avanzini MA, et al. Pharmacokinetic behavior of rituximab: a study of different schedules of administration for heterogeneous clinical settings. Ther Drug Monit 2005;27(6):785–92.
8. Roll P, Palanichamy A, Kneitz C, et al. Regeneration of B cell subsets after transient B cell depletion using anti-CD20 antibodies in rheumatoid arthritis. Arthritis Rheum 2006;54(8):2377–86.
9. Cioc AM, Vanderwerf SM, Peterson BA, et al. Rituximab-induced changes in hematolymphoid tissues found at autopsy. Am J Clin Pathol 2008;130(4):604–12.
10. Cunningham D, Hawkes EA, Jack A, et al. Rituximab plus cyclophosphamide, doxorubicin, vincristine, and prednisolone in patients with newly diagnosed diffuse large B-cell non-Hodgkin lymphoma: a phase 3 comparison of dose intensification with 14-day versus 21-day cycles. Lancet 2013;381(9880):1817–26.
11. Hiraga J, Tomita A, Sugimoto T, et al. Down-regulation of CD20 expression in B-cell lymphoma cells after treatment with rituximab-containing combination chemotherapies: its prevalence and clinical significance. Blood 2009;113(20): 4885–93.
12. Foran JM, Norton AJ, Micallef IN, et al. Loss of CD20 expression following treatment with rituximab (chimaeric monoclonal anti-CD20): a retrospective cohort analysis. Br J Haematol 2001;114(4):881–3.
13. Tokunaga T, Tomita A, Sugimoto K, et al. De novo diffuse large B-cell lymphoma with a CD20 immunohistochemistry-positive and flow cytometry-negative phenotype: molecular mechanisms and correlation with rituximab sensitivity. Cancer Sci 2014;105(1):35–43.
14. Walsh KJ, Al-Quran SZ, Li Y, et al. Discordant expression of CD20 by flow cytometry and immunohistochemistry in a patient responding to rituximab: an unusual mechanism. Clin Lymphoma Myeloma 2007;7(4):319–22.
15. Gerber HP, Kung-Sutherland M, Stone I, et al. Potent antitumor activity of the anti-CD19 auristatin antibody drug conjugate hBU12-vcMMAE against rituximab-sensitive and -resistant lymphomas. Blood 2009;113(18):4352–61.
16. Yan J, Wolff MJ, Unternaehrer J, et al. Targeting antigen to CD19 on B cells efficiently activates T cells. Int Immunol 2005;17(7):869–77.
17. Viardot A, Goebeler ME, Hess G, et al. Phase 2 study of the bispecific T-cell engager (BiTE) antibody blinatumomab in relapsed/refractory diffuse large B-cell lymphoma. Blood 2016;127(11):1410–6.

18. Klinger M, Brandl C, Zugmaier G, et al. Immunopharmacologic response of patients with B-lineage acute lymphoblastic leukemia to continuous infusion of T cell-engaging CD19/CD3-bispecific BiTE antibody blinatumomab. Blood 2012;119(26):6226–33.
19. Zugmaier G, Gokbuget N, Klinger M, et al. Long-term survival and T-cell kinetics in relapsed/refractory ALL patients who achieved MRD response after blinatumomab treatment. Blood 2015;126(24):2578–84.
20. Mejstrikova E, Hrusak O, Borowitz MJ, et al. CD19-negative relapse of pediatric B-cell precursor acute lymphoblastic leukemia following blinatumomab treatment. Blood Cancer J 2017;7(12):659.
21. Jabbour E, Dull J, Yilmaz M, et al. Outcome of patients with relapsed/refractory acute lymphoblastic leukemia after blinatumomab failure: no change in the level of CD19 expression. Am J Hematol 2018;93(3):371–4.
22. Libert D, Yuan CM, Masih KE, et al. Serial evaluation of CD19 surface expression in pediatric B-cell malignancies following CD19-targeted therapy. Leukemia 2020;34(11):3064–9.
23. Pillai V, Muralidharan K, Meng W, et al. CAR T-cell therapy is effective for CD19-dim B-lymphoblastic leukemia but is impacted by prior blinatumomab therapy. Blood Adv 2019;3(22):3539–49.
24. Clark EA, Giltiay NV. CD22: a regulator of innate and adaptive B cell responses and autoimmunity. Front Immunol 2018;9:2235.
25. Vitetta ES, Stone M, Amlot P, et al. Phase I immunotoxin trial in patients with B-cell lymphoma. Cancer Res 1991;51(15):4052–8.
26. Rosenthal J, Naqvi AS, Luo M, et al. Heterogeneity of surface CD19 and CD22 expression in B lymphoblastic leukemia. Am J Hematol 2018;93(11):E352–5.
27. Shan D, Press OW. Constitutive endocytosis and degradation of CD22 by human B cells. J Immunol 1995;154(9):4466–75.
28. Bhojwani D, Sposto R, Shah NN, et al. Inotuzumab ozogamicin in pediatric patients with relapsed/refractory acute lymphoblastic leukemia. Leukemia 2019;33(4):884–92.
29. Lanza F, Maffini E, Rondoni M, et al. CD22 expression in B-cell acute lymphoblastic leukemia: biological significance and implications for inotuzumab therapy in adults. Cancers (Basel) 2020;12(2). https://doi.org/10.3390/cancers12020303.
30. van de Donk NW, Janmaat ML, Mutis T, et al. Monoclonal antibodies targeting CD38 in hematological malignancies and beyond. Immunol Rev 2016;270(1):95–112.
31. Deaglio S, Morra M, Mallone R, et al. Human CD38 (ADP-ribosyl cyclase) is a counter-receptor of CD31, an Ig superfamily member. J Immunol 1998;160(1):395–402.
32. Bras AE, Beishuizen A, Langerak AW, et al. CD38 expression in paediatric leukaemia and lymphoma: implications for antibody targeted therapy. Br J Haematol 2018;180(2):292–6.
33. Tembhare PR, Sriram H, Khanka T, et al. Flow cytometric evaluation of CD38 expression levels in the newly diagnosed T-cell acute lymphoblastic leukemia and the effect of chemotherapy on its expression in measurable residual disease, refractory disease and relapsed disease: an implication for anti-CD38 immunotherapy. J Immunother Cancer 2020;8(1). https://doi.org/10.1136/jitc-2020-000630.
34. Deckert J, Wetzel MC, Bartle LM, et al. SAR650984, a novel humanized CD38-targeting antibody, demonstrates potent antitumor activity in models of multiple

myeloma and other CD38+ hematologic malignancies. Clin Cancer Res 2014; 20(17):4574–83.
35. Oberle A, Brandt A, Alawi M, et al. Long-term CD38 saturation by daratumumab interferes with diagnostic myeloma cell detection. Haematologica 2017;102(9): e368–70.
36. Wang HW, Lin P. Flow cytometric immunophenotypic analysis in the diagnosis and prognostication of plasma cell neoplasms. Cytometry B Clin Cytom 2019; 96(5):338–50.
37. Jiang XY, Luider J, Shameli A. Artifactual Kappa light chain restriction of marrow hematogones: a potential diagnostic pitfall in minimal residual disease assessment of plasma cell myeloma patients on daratumumab. Cytometry B Clin Cytom 2020;98(1):68–74.
38. Park JH, Riviere I, Gonen M, et al. Long-term follow-up of CD19 CAR therapy in acute lymphoblastic leukemia. N Engl J Med 2018;378(5):449–59.
39. Maude SL, Laetsch TW, Buechner J, et al. Tisagenlecleucel in children and young adults with B-cell lymphoblastic leukemia. N Engl J Med 2018;378(5):439–48.
40. Fry TJ, Shah NN, Orentas RJ, et al. CD22-targeted CAR T cells induce remission in B-ALL that is naive or resistant to CD19-targeted CAR immunotherapy. Nat Med 2018;24(1):20–8.
41. Shah NN, Highfill SL, Shalabi H, et al. CD4/CD8 T-cell selection affects Chimeric Antigen Receptor (CAR) T-cell potency and toxicity: updated results from a phase I anti-CD22 CAR T-cell trial. J Clin Oncol 2020;38(17):1938–50.
42. Shah NN, Johnson BD, Schneider D, et al. Bispecific anti-CD20, anti-CD19 CAR T cells for relapsed B cell malignancies: a phase 1 dose escalation and expansion trial. Nat Med 2020;26(10):1569–75.
43. Qin H, Ramakrishna S, Nguyen S, et al. Preclinical development of bivalent chimeric antigen receptors targeting both CD19 and CD22. Mol Ther Oncolytics 2018;11:127–37.
44. Cherian S, Miller V, McCullouch V, et al. A novel flow cytometric assay for detection of residual disease in patients with B-lymphoblastic leukemia/lymphoma post anti-CD19 therapy. Cytometry B Clin Cytom 2018;94(1):112–20.
45. Lim SH, Vaughan AT, Ashton-Key M, et al. Fc gamma receptor IIb on target B cells promotes rituximab internalization and reduces clinical efficacy. Blood 2011;118(9):2530–40.
46. Dahal LN, Huang CY, Stopforth RJ, et al. Shaving is an epiphenomenon of type I and II anti-CD20-mediated phagocytosis, whereas antigenic modulation limits type I monoclonal antibody efficacy. J Immunol 2018;201(4):1211–21.
47. Beum PV, Kennedy AD, Williams ME, et al. The shaving reaction: rituximab/CD20 complexes are removed from mantle cell lymphoma and chronic lymphocytic leukemia cells by THP-1 monocytes. J Immunol 2006;176(4):2600–9.
48. Pham T, Mero P, Booth JW. Dynamics of macrophage trogocytosis of rituximab-coated B cells. PLoS One 2011;6(1):e14498.
49. Valgardsdottir R, Cattaneo I, Klein C, et al. Human neutrophils mediate trogocytosis rather than phagocytosis of CLL B cells opsonized with anti-CD20 antibodies. Blood 2017;129(19):2636–44.
50. Beum PV, Peek EM, Lindorfer MA, et al. Loss of CD20 and bound CD20 antibody from opsonized B cells occurs more rapidly because of trogocytosis mediated by Fc receptor-expressing effector cells than direct internalization by the B cells. J Immunol 2011;187(6):3438–47.
51. Rossi EA, Goldenberg DM, Michel R, et al. Trogocytosis of multiple B-cell surface markers by CD22 targeting with epratuzumab. Blood 2013;122(17):3020–9.

52. Hamieh M, Dobrin A, Cabriolu A, et al. CAR T cell trogocytosis and cooperative killing regulate tumour antigen escape. Nature 2019;568(7750):112–6.
53. Tallman MS, McDonald GB, DeLeve LD, et al. Incidence of sinusoidal obstruction syndrome following Mylotarg (gemtuzumab ozogamicin): a prospective observational study of 482 patients in routine clinical practice. Int J Hematol 2013;97(4): 456–64.
54. Rajvanshi P, Shulman HM, Sievers EL, et al. Hepatic sinusoidal obstruction after gemtuzumab ozogamicin (Mylotarg) therapy. Blood 2002;99(7):2310–4.
55. Taylor RP, Lindorfer MA. Fcgamma-receptor-mediated trogocytosis impacts mAb-based therapies: historical precedence and recent developments. Blood 2015;125(5):762–6.
56. Braig F, Brandt A, Goebeler M, et al. Resistance to anti-CD19/CD3 BiTE in acute lymphoblastic leukemia may be mediated by disrupted CD19 membrane trafficking. Blood 2017;129(1):100–4.
57. Ruella M, Xu J, Barrett DM, et al. Induction of resistance to chimeric antigen receptor T cell therapy by transduction of a single leukemic B cell. Nat Med 2018; 24(10):1499–503.
58. Warda W, Da Rocha MN, Trad R, et al. Overcoming target epitope masking resistance that can occur on low-antigen-expresser AML blasts after IL-1RAP chimeric antigen receptor T cell therapy using the inducible caspase 9 suicide gene safety switch. Cancer Gene Ther 2021. https://doi.org/10.1038/s41417-020-00284-3.
59. Czuczman MS, Olejniczak S, Gowda A, et al. Acquirement of rituximab resistance in lymphoma cell lines is associated with both global CD20 gene and protein down-regulation regulated at the pretranscriptional and posttranscriptional levels. Clin Cancer Res 2008;14(5):1561–70.
60. Sugimoto T, Tomita A, Hiraga J, et al. Escape mechanisms from antibody therapy to lymphoma cells: downregulation of CD20 mRNA by recruitment of the HDAC complex and not by DNA methylation. Biochem Biophys Res Commun 2009; 390(1):48–53.
61. Pavlasova G, Mraz M. The regulation and function of CD20: an "enigma" of B-cell biology and targeted therapy. Haematologica 2020;105(6):1494–506.
62. Tomita A. Genetic and epigenetic modulation of CD20 expression in B-cell malignancies: molecular mechanisms and significance to rituximab resistance. J Clin Exp Hematop 2016;56(2):89–99.
63. Johnson NA, Leach S, Woolcock B, et al. CD20 mutations involving the rituximab epitope are rare in diffuse large B-cell lymphomas and are not a significant cause of R-CHOP failure. Haematologica 2009;94(3):423–7.
64. Mishima Y, Terui Y, Takeuchi K, et al. The identification of irreversible rituximab-resistant lymphoma caused by CD20 gene mutations. Blood Cancer J 2011; 1(4):e15.
65. Terui Y, Mishima Y, Sugimura N, et al. Identification of CD20 C-terminal deletion mutations associated with loss of CD20 expression in non-Hodgkin's lymphoma. Clin Cancer Res 2009;15(7):2523–30.
66. Orlando EJ, Han X, Tribouley C, et al. Genetic mechanisms of target antigen loss in CAR19 therapy of acute lymphoblastic leukemia. Nat Med 2018;24(10): 1504–6.
67. Sotillo E, Barrett DM, Black KL, et al. Convergence of acquired mutations and alternative splicing of CD19 enables resistance to CART-19 immunotherapy. Cancer Discov 2015;5(12):1282–95.
68. Bagashev A, Sotillo E, Tang CH, et al. CD19 alterations emerging after CD19-directed immunotherapy cause retention of the misfolded protein in the

endoplasmic reticulum. Mol Cell Biol 2018;38(21). https://doi.org/10.1128/MCB.00383-18.
69. Asnani M, Hayer KE, Naqvi AS, et al. Retention of CD19 intron 2 contributes to CART-19 resistance in leukemias with subclonal frameshift mutations in CD19. Leukemia 2020;34(4):1202–7.
70. Gardner R, Wu D, Cherian S, et al. Acquisition of a CD19-negative myeloid phenotype allows immune escape of MLL-rearranged B-ALL from CD19 CAR-T-cell therapy. Blood 2016;127(20):2406–10.
71. Jacoby E, Nguyen SM, Fountaine TJ, et al. CD19 CAR immune pressure induces B-precursor acute lymphoblastic leukaemia lineage switch exposing inherent leukaemic plasticity. Nat Commun 2016;7:12320.
72. Rayes A, McMasters RL, O'Brien MM. Lineage switch in MLL-rearranged infant leukemia following CD19-directed therapy. Pediatr Blood Cancer 2016;63(6):1113–5.
73. Cohen A, Petsche D, Grunberger T, et al. Interleukin 6 induces myeloid differentiation of a human biphenotypic leukemic cell line. Leuk Res 1992;16(8):751–60.
74. Schultz L, Gardner R. Mechanisms of and approaches to overcoming resistance to immunotherapy. Hematol Am Soc Hematol Educ Program 2019;2019(1):226–32.
75. Damm JK, Gordon S, Ehinger M, et al. Pharmacologically relevant doses of valproate upregulate CD20 expression in three diffuse large B-cell lymphoma patients in vivo. Exp Hematol Oncol 2015;4:4.
76. Ramakrishna S, Highfill SL, Walsh Z, et al. Modulation of target antigen density improves CAR T-cell functionality and persistence. Clin Cancer Res 2019;25(17):5329–41.

Update on Pediatric and Young Adult Mature Lymphomas

Emily F. Mason, MD, PhD[a,*], Alexandra E. Kovach, MD[b]

KEYWORDS

• Pediatric mature lymphoma • Hodgkin lymphoma • Aggressive B-cell lymphoma • IRF4 • Pediatric type • Anaplastic large cell lymphoma • ALK positive

KEY POINTS

- Nodular lymphocyte-predominant Hodgkin lymphoma occurs in children and must be distinguished from reactive and more aggressive neoplastic mimics.
- Mature B-cell lymphomas in children are predominantly high-grade subtypes, including Burkitt lymphoma and diffuse large B-cell lymphoma.
- Indolent B-cell lymphomas affecting children include pediatric-type follicular lymphoma and pediatric nodal marginal zone lymphoma.
- Anaplastic large cell lymphoma, anaplastic lymphoma kinase positive, represents the most common mature T-cell lymphoma in pediatrics.
- Other T-cell lymphomas are rare in children and may raise consideration for underlying immunodeficiency.

INTRODUCTION

After acute leukemia and brain and central nervous system tumors, mature lymphomas represent the third most common cancer in pediatric patients.[1] Non-Hodgkin lymphoma (NHL) accounts for approximately 60% of lymphoma diagnoses in children, with the remainder representing Hodgkin lymphomas.[1] This article summarizes the epidemiologic, histopathologic, and molecular features of selected mature systemic B-cell and T-cell lymphomas encountered in this age group (**Box 1**), including several entities introduced in the most recent update of the World Health Organization (WHO) Classification of Haematopoietic and Lymphoid Tissues.[2] Differential diagnoses are reviewed in **Table 1** (also see **Tables 3** and **5**) and are focused on the pediatric and adolescent age group.

[a] Department of Pathology, Microbiology & Immunology, Vanderbilt University Medical Center, 4603A TVC, Nashville, TN 37232-5310, USA; [b] Department of Pathology and Laboratory Medicine, Children's Hospital Los Angeles, 4650 Sunset Boulevard, Mailstop #32, Los Angeles, CA 90027, USA

* Corresponding author.
E-mail address: emily.f.mason@vumc.org

Clin Lab Med 41 (2021) 359–387
https://doi.org/10.1016/j.cll.2021.03.018
labmed.theclinics.com

Box 1
Pediatric lymphomas discussed in this article

Hodgkin lymphoma
- Nodular lymphocyte-predominant Hodgkin lymphoma[a]

B-cell NHL
- Aggressive B-cell lymphomas[a]
  - Burkitt lymphoma
  - Burkitt-like lymphoma with 11q abnormalities
  - Diffuse large B-cell lymphoma not otherwise specified
  - Epstein-Barr virus–positive diffuse large B-cell lymphoma
  - Large B-cell lymphoma with *IRF4* rearrangement
- Indolent B-cell lymphomas
  - Pediatric-type follicular lymphoma
  - Pediatric nodal marginal zone lymphoma

T-cell NHL
- Anaplastic large cell lymphoma, anaplastic lymphoma kinase positive
- Peripheral T-cell lymphoma not otherwise specified
- Hepatosplenic T-cell lymphoma

[a]For discussions on classic Hodgkin lymphoma, primary mediastinal large B-cell lymphoma, and B-cell lymphoma unclassifiable with features intermediate between diffuse large B-cell lymphoma and classic Hodgkin lymphoma, see Ahmed Aljudi and colleagues' article, "The Hematological Differential Diagnosis of Mediastinal Masses," in this issue.

HODGKIN LYMPHOMA

Hodgkin lymphoma encompasses both nodular lymphocyte-predominant Hodgkin lymphoma and classic Hodgkin lymphoma (CHL), which has 4 histologic subtypes. These distinct diseases are conceptualized together for historical and histologic reasons,[3–5] because they are both characterized by few scattered transformed tumoral lymphocytes in a predominating nonneoplastic inflammatory background (for a

Table 1
Pediatric differential diagnosis of nodular lymphocyte-predominant Hodgkin lymphoma

Diagnosis	Differential Diagnosis	Comments
Nodular lymphocyte-predominant Hodgkin lymphoma	Progressive transformation of germinal centers	No lymphocyte-predominant (popcorn) cells, may spontaneously regress
	Autoimmune lymphoproliferative syndrome	Preserved, if distorted, nodal architecture; paracortical T-cell zone hyperplasia; CD4/CD8 double-negative T cells
	Classic Hodgkin lymphoma (especially lymphocyte-rich)	Distinct morphology and immunophenotype of Reed-Sternberg cells: CD30+, CD15+/−, PAX5+ (weak)
	Peripheral T-cell lymphoma not otherwise specified	Sheetlike architectural effacement; typically immunophenotypic aberrancy among T cells; clonal T-cell receptor gene rearrangement

Abbreviation: CD, cluster of differentiation.

discussion on CHL, see the article "The Hematological Differential Diagnosis of Mediastinal Masses" in this issue).

Nodular Lymphocyte-predominant Hodgkin Lymphoma

Nodular lymphocyte-predominant Hodgkin lymphoma (NLPHL) is an uncommon, typically indolent lymphoma that represents approximately 3% to 5% of all Hodgkin lymphomas.[6,7] Unlike CHL, the neoplastic cells in NLPHL are derived from germinal center centroblasts.[8,9] Although NLPHL occurs across the age spectrum, it is more prevalent in adolescents and young adults than in older adults; in a large consensus case review, 72% of patients with NLPHL were less than 50 years of age.[10] Most NLPHLs present with limited-stage disease involving superficial lymph nodes,[10] and excision alone in select cases of stage I disease may be curative.[11] Late relapses with transformation to T cell/histiocyte–rich large B-cell lymphoma are described.[11]

NLPHL is characterized by lymph node enlargement and diffuse or near-diffuse architectural effacement by a vague follicular lymphoid proliferation, resembling progressive transformation of germinal centers (**Fig. 1**A; **Table 1**).[12,13] Variant architectural patterns of NLPHL are recognized, including classic nodular (see **Fig. 1**A), serpiginous nodular, and nodular with prominent extranodular lymphocyte-predominant (LP) cells,[14] which are seen across pediatric NLPHL.[15] The LP or popcorn cells are scattered large lymphoid cells with polylobated nuclei and vesicular chromatin (**Fig. 1**B). Variants include forms with simplified nuclei, abundant cytoplasm, and pleomorphic or Reed-Sternberg–like features, with conspicuous central nucleoli or apparent binucleation.

Immunophenotype features can readily distinguish NLPHL from CHL in most cases. Unlike the Reed-Sternberg cells of CHL, LP cells maintain expression of cluster of differentiation (CD) 45 and of B-cell markers (CD20 [**Fig. 1**C], PAX5, OCT2, BOB1) and are negative for CD15. CD30 is also typically negative on LP cells but may be weak or patchy. Epstein-Barr virus (EBV)+ NLPHL has been described in a small subset of cases, in both pediatric and adult patients, and is reported to be associated with CD30 expression.[16] The background inflammatory cells in NLPHL are typically small follicular B cells (see **Fig. 1**C) with variably intact and expanded underlying follicular dendritic cell meshworks (CD21 [**Fig. 1**D], CD23, and CD35 expressing), especially apparent in the nodular architectural variant. The LP cells stand out from the frequent background small B cells by encircling rims of T-follicular helper cells, which express CD57 and PD1 in addition to mature T-cell antigens.

NLPHLs are reported to have complex diploid karyotypes,[17] recurrent *BCL6* rearrangements,[18] and, similarly to CHL, constitutive nuclear factor kappa-B (NF-κB) activation.[19] The precise biological relationship between NLPHL and T cell/histiocyte–rich large B-cell lymphoma remains unknown.[20]

NON-HODGKIN LYMPHOMA

Mature B-cell Lymphomas

Among NHLs, mature B-cell lymphomas account for approximately 60% of cases.[21] Unlike in adults, where low-grade to intermediate-grade B-cell NHLs (B-NHLs) are most common, high-grade B-NHLs predominate among lymphomas in children.[21] In developed countries, Burkitt lymphoma (BL) accounts for approximately 80% of B-NHLs in children, and diffuse large B-cell lymphoma (DLBCL) accounts for an additional 10% to 20% of cases.[21] In the adolescent and young adult (AYA) age group (15–39 years old), the incidence of BL decreases, whereas the incidence of DLBCL

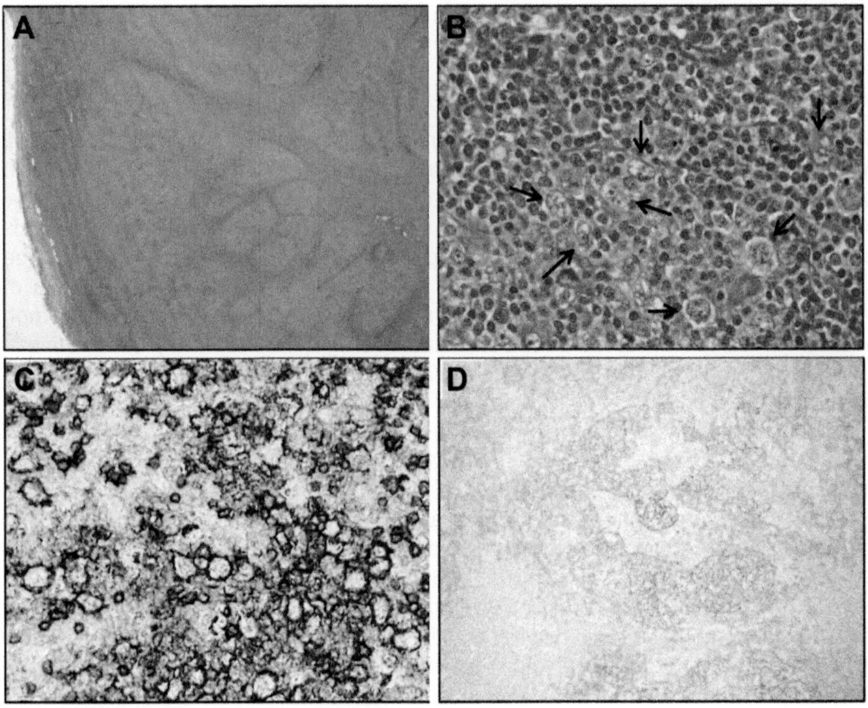

Fig. 1. Nodular lymphocyte-predominant Hodgkin lymphoma. (*A*) This enlarged submandibular lymph node from a 13-year-old boy is effaced by a nodular proliferation resembling progressive transformation of germinal centers (hematoxylin and eosin [H&E], original magnification ×20). (*B*) The nodules contain scattered large mononuclear lymphoid cells with polylobated nuclei and vesicular chromatin (lymphocyte-predominant, or popcorn, cells; *arrows*) (H&E, original magnification ×600). (*C*) The lymphocyte-predominant cells retain expression of the B-cell marker CD20. Background small B cells are also highlighted by CD20; note that the small lymphocytes immediately surrounding the lymphocyte-predominant cells are PD-1+, CD57+ T cells and therefore negative in this image (original magnification ×600). (*D*) CD21 immunostain highlights underlying expanded follicular dendritic cell networks (original magnification ×100).

increases.[21,22] The remaining cases of B-NHL in children include primary mediastinal large B-cell lymphoma (PMLBL), B-cell lymphoma unclassifiable with features intermediate between DLBCL and CHL (BCLU), EBV-positive DLBCL, large B-cell lymphoma with *IRF4* rearrangement, pediatric-type follicular lymphoma (PTFL), and pediatric-type marginal zone lymphoma (**Tables 2** and **3**) (for a discussion on PMLBL and BCLU, see the article "The Hematological Differential Diagnosis of Mediastinal Masses" in this issue).

Aggressive B-cell lymphomas

Burkitt lymphoma. BL includes 3 epidemiologic variants: endemic BL, which occurs in equatorial Africa and Papua New Guinea and is strongly linked to EBV; sporadic BL, which occurs throughout the world, predominantly in pediatric patients, and is associated with EBV in approximately 20% to 30% of cases; and immunodeficiency-associated BL, which is particularly associated with human immunodeficiency virus (HIV) infection and is associated with EBV in 25% to 40% of cases.[2] In the United States, pediatric sporadic BL has a median age at diagnosis of 7.8 years and is more common in

Table 2
Pathologic features of pediatric mature systemic B-cell non-Hodgkin lymphoma

Diagnosis	Morphology	Immunophenotype	Genetics
Aggressive B-cell Lymphomas			
BL	Medium-sized, monotonous cells with multiple nucleoli; frequent mitotic figures and apoptotic debris; starry-sky appearance	Pos: CD19, CD20, PAX5, CD10, BCL6, MYC, EBV (subset of patients); Ki67>95% Neg: CD5, TdT, BCL2 (weak BCL2 expression possible)	t(8;14) MYG-IGH rearrangement Mutations in *ID3*, *TCF3*, and *CCND3*
Burkitt-like lymphoma with 11q abnormalities	More pleomorphism than BL May show a follicular growth pattern	Pos: CD19, CD20, PAX5, CD10, BCL6, LMO2 Neg: BCL2	Proximal gain and telomeric loss of 11q Mutations in *GNA13*
DLBCL not otherwise specified	Medium-sized to large cells with centroblastic morphology	Pos: CD19, CD20, CD22, CD79a, PAX5; predominantly GCB type, positive for CD10 and BCL6; variable MUM1 staining; BCL2 (30%–40%); MYC (84%); Ki67>50% Neg: EBV	MYC rearrangement Mutations in *SOCS1*, *KMT2D*, *BTG1*, *EZH2*, *GNA13*, *MYD88*, and *PIM1*
EBV-positive diffuse large B-cell lymphoma	Various patterns resembling T-cell/histiocyte-rich large B-cell lymphoma, DLBCL-NOS, CHL, or gray-zone lymphoma. Various cytology: medium-sized to large centroblastic or immunoblastic cells, Reed-Sternberg–like cells, lymphocyte-predominant–like cells	Pos: EBV, CD19, CD20, CD22, CD79a, PAX5, MUM1, CD30, CD15 (small subset of patients), PD-L1/L2 Neg: CD10, BCL6	Chromosomal gains at 9p24.1
Large B-cell lymphoma with *IRF4* rearrangement	Variable architecture: entirely diffuse, entirely follicular, or mixed follicular and diffuse; medium-sized to large cells with relatively open chromatin and small nucleoli; mitotic figures and tingible-body macrophages are infrequent	Pos: CD20, CD79a, PAX5, IRF4/MUM1 (strong, diffuse), BCL6, CD10 (66%), BCL2 (66%), CD5 (small subset of patients), Ki67>50% Neg: EBV	Cytogenetically cryptic *IRF4* rearrangement Mutations in *IRF4*, *CARD11*, and *CCND3*

(*continued on next page*)

Table 2
(*continued*)

Diagnosis	Morphology	Immunophenotype	Genetics
Indolent B-cell Lymphomas			
Pediatric-type follicular lymphoma	Partial or total architectural effacement by large, serpiginous, coalescing follicles with a starry-sky pattern but lacking polarization; attenuated mantle zones; possible marginal zone differentiation; medium-sized to large cells with blastoid or centroblastic cytology without prominent nucleoli; patients with areas of DLBCL are excluded	Pos: CD20, CD79a, PAX5, CD10, BCL6, FOXP1, Ki67>30% Neg: IRF4/MUM1, BCL2 (may be positive in a small subset of patients)	Clonal IGH rearrangement Loss of heterozygosity/ deletion of 1p36 Mutations in *TNFRSF14* and *MAP2K1*
Pediatric nodal marginal zone lymphoma	Large follicles with infiltration of mantle zone B cells into germinal centers; expanded marginal zones; interfollicular proliferation of small to medium-sized lymphocytes, with possible diffuse areas; variable cytology: small centrocyte-like cells, monocytoid-appearing cells, admixed larger transformed cells and plasma cells	Pos: CD20, CD43, BCL2 (40%–50%) Neg: CD5, CD10, BCL6	Clonal IGH rearrangement Trisomy 18

Abbreviations: IGH, immunoglobulin heavy chain; Neg, negative; Pos, positive.

boys than in girls (male/female ratio of 3.7:1).[23] Sporadic BL presents most commonly with an abdominal mass, particularly in the ileocecal region, but involvement of other extranodal sites as well as of lymph nodes can also be seen.[2] Because of the rapid doubling time of the tumor, patients can present with high tumor burden.[2]

BL is typically composed of medium-sized cells with a monotonous appearance, with round nuclei, finely clumped chromatin, multiple nucleoli, and small to moderate amounts of cytoplasm (**Fig. 2**A, B), often with cytoplasmic vacuolization (best seen on touch preparations). Mitotic figures and apoptotic debris are frequent, and scattered tingible-body macrophages impart a classic starry-sky appearance at low power. Tumor cells are positive for B-cell markers (CD19, CD20, PAX5), germinal center markers (CD10 and BCL6), and MYC (**Fig. 2**C, D). CD38 is frequently positive. TCL1 is strongly expressed in most pediatric BL, regardless of EBV status.[24] Tumor cells are classically negative for CD5, TdT, and BCL2 (**Fig. 2**E), although cases with weak BCL2 expression have been described.[25] The Ki67 proliferative index is greater than 95% (**Fig. 2**F).

BL is characterized by rearrangement of the *MYC* locus at 8q24. The most common translocation partner is the immunoglobulin heavy-chain (*IGH*) gene at 14q32, resulting in a t(8;14)(q24q32) translocation. Less commonly, the *MYC* translocation involves the immunoglobulin kappa locus at 2p12 or lambda locus at 22q11. The *MYC* translocation is thought to be insufficient to induce lymphomagenesis, and recurrent gene mutations involving the *ID3*, *TCF3*, and *CCND3* genes, which occur in more than 80% of pediatric BLs, may be important in BL pathogenesis.[26] Signaling through the ID3-TCF3-CCND3 pathway activates B-cell receptor signaling.[26] Additional recurrently mutated genes identified in a recent large whole-exome sequencing study of pediatric BL,[27] as well as by others,[28,29] include *TP53*, *MYC*, members of the SWI/SNF complex *ARID1A* and *SMARCA4*, *FOXO1*, *GNA13*, *RHOA*, *DDX3X*, and *HIST1H1E*.

Burkitt-like lymphoma with 11q aberration. Burkitt-like lymphoma with 11q aberration (BLL) was introduced as a provisional entity in the 2017 WHO classification[2] and encompasses lymphomas that resemble BL morphologically (**Fig. 3**A, B) and immunophenotypically and show similar gene expression profiles, but that lack a MYC rearrangement[30] (**Fig. 3**C). Instead, these patients show abnormalities involving chromosome 11q, with proximal gains and telomeric losses[30,31] (**Fig. 3**D). The chromosomal abnormality is detectable by fluorescence in situ hybridization (FISH) probes specific for this region, available at commercial laboratories and distinct from the *KMT2A* (*MLL*) locus, and the diagnosis may be suggested by copy number alterations on chromosome microarray. BLL has been reported predominantly in children and young adults less than 40 years of age and seems to present frequently with nodal disease.[30–33] These lymphomas are composed of germinal center–derived B cells, with positivity for CD10, BCL6, and often LMO2, and negativity for BCL2, but may show more morphologic pleomorphism than BL and occasionally show a follicular growth pattern.[30,31] In addition to absence of a *MYC* translocation and presence of 11q aberrations, BLL shows more complex karyotypes than BL and lacks mutations in the ID3-TCF3-CCND3 or SWI/SNF pathways, but shows recurrent mutations in *GNA13*.[31,34]

Diffuse large B-cell lymphoma, not otherwise specified. Although DLBCL is rare in young children, the incidence of DLBCL increases with age, becoming more common than BL in the AYA population.[35] A large cohort of 173 cases of DLBCL in patients up to 18 years of age showed a median age at diagnosis of 11.4 years and a male/female ratio of 1.7:1.[36] Children often present with extranodal disease, although dissemination to the bone marrow or central nervous system is rare.[37]

DLBCL in children is composed of a diffuse infiltrate of intermediate-sized to large cells most commonly with centroblastic morphology, with multiple round to oval nuclei[38] (**Fig. 4**). Cells express pan–B-cell markers CD19, CD20, CD22, CD79a, and PAX5, although 1 or more of these may be negative.[2] Cells are negative for EBV; significant positivity for EBV should lead to a diagnosis of EBV-positive DLBCL, not otherwise specified (discussed later). DLBCL can be divided into 2 main cell-of-origin subtypes, germinal center B-cell (GCB) type and activated B-cell (ABC) type, based on gene expression profiling (GEP). Immunophenotypic algorithms, including the Hans algorithm,[39] have been developed to distinguish GCB from non-GCB tumors;

Table 3
Differential diagnosis of pediatric mature B-cell non-Hodgkin lymphoma

Diagnosis	Differential Diagnosis	Comments
BL	B-lymphoblastic lymphoma	Positive for TdT; typically negative for CD20 and surface light chain Can show MYC rearrangements[125]
	Diffuse large B-cell lymphoma	Often larger cells with more pleomorphism without a starry-sky pattern Can show MYC rearrangements
	Burkitt-like lymphoma with 11q aberration	More pleomorphic Absence of MYC translocation and presence of 11q aberrations
Diffuse large B-cell lymphoma	BL	Monomorphic infiltrate with starry-sky pattern
	Infectious mononucleosis	Distorted but intact nodal architecture Immunoblastic expansion in a polymorphous background of small to intermediate-sized lymphocytes and plasma cells
EBV-positive diffuse large B-cell lymphoma	Classic Hodgkin lymphoma	Typically negative for CD20, positive for CD30 and CD15
	Diffuse large B-cell lymphoma	EBV negative
	Infectious mononucleosis	Distorted but intact nodal architecture Immunoblastic expansion in a polymorphous background of small to intermediate-sized lymphocytes and plasma cells
Large B-cell lymphoma with IRF4 rearrangement	Pediatric-type follicular lymphoma	Tingible-body macrophages; Negative for MUM1 Lacks IRF4 rearrangement
	Diffuse large B-cell lymphoma	Diffuse architecture Germinal center phenotype with variable MUM1 expression Lacks IRF4 rearrangement
	Reactive follicular hyperplasia	Tingible-body macrophages and polarization of germinal centers Lacks IRF4 rearrangement

(*continued on next page*)

Table 3 (continued)

Diagnosis	Differential Diagnosis	Comments
Pediatric-type follicular lymphoma	Large B-cell lymphoma with IRF4 rearrangement	May show diffuse architecture; typically lacks tingible-body macrophages Positive for MUM1 and IRF4 rearrangement
	Reactive follicular hyperplasia	Polarization of germinal centers Negative for clonal IGH rearrangement
Pediatric nodal marginal zone lymphoma	Progressive transformation of germinal centers	Negative for CD43; lacks clonal IGH rearrangement
	Nodal marginal zone hyperplasia	Associated with *Haemophilus influenzae* infection; lacks clonal IGH rearrangement

the Hans algorithm uses immunohistochemical stains for CD10, BCL6, and MUM1. With respect to cell-of-origin classification, DLBCL represents a more homogeneous disease in pediatric patients than in adults, with 75% to 80% of pediatric cases classified as GCB type by both GEP[40] and immunohistochemistry.[38,41] As such, most pediatric patients are positive for CD10 and BCL6, with variable staining for MUM1. In contrast with adult patients, the prognostic significance of GCB versus non-GCB disease has not been established in the pediatric population, perhaps because of the small number of ABC cases in children.[22,38,41] Coexpression of BCL2 and MYC by immunohistochemistry has been associated with inferior outcomes in adults[2]; BCL2 and MYC positivity by immunohistochemistry is seen in 30% to 40% and 84% of pediatric DLBCL, respectively.[38,41] The Ki67 proliferative index is increased in most cases (>50%),[41] although the proliferation rate is often lower than that seen in BL.

Translocations involving *MYC* are more common in DLBCL in children than in adults (up to 30% vs 5%–10% of adult cases).[42–44] In contrast, rearrangements involving *BCL6* and *BCL2* are rare in pediatric patients, and tumors harboring both *MYC* and *BCL2* and/or *BCL6* rearrangements (so-called double-hit or triple-hit lymphomas) are exceedingly rare in this population.[22,38,42,43] Next-generation sequencing of 22 samples of DLBCL from patients less than 26 years old showed recurrent mutations in *SOCS1* (27%), *KMT2D* (23%), and *BTG1*, *EZH2*, *GNA13*, *MYD88*, and *PIM1* (all 14%); the frequency of *SOCS1* mutations was significantly higher than that seen in adult DLBCL.[45]

Epstein-Barr virus–positive diffuse large B-cell lymphoma, not otherwise specified. EBV-positive DLBCL represents an EBV-positive clonal B-cell proliferation occurring in patients with no documented predisposing immunodeficiency or immunosuppression.[2] Although originally introduced in the fourth edition of the WHO classification as EBV-positive DLBCL of the elderly, several studies have shown that EBV-positive DLBCL also occurs in young patients (<50 years old),[46–51] and the 2017 WHO revision adopted the term EBV-positive DLBCL, not otherwise specified.[2] A report of 46 cases of EBV-positive DLBCL in young patients less than or equal to 45 years of age showed a median age at diagnosis of 23 years (range, 4–45 years)

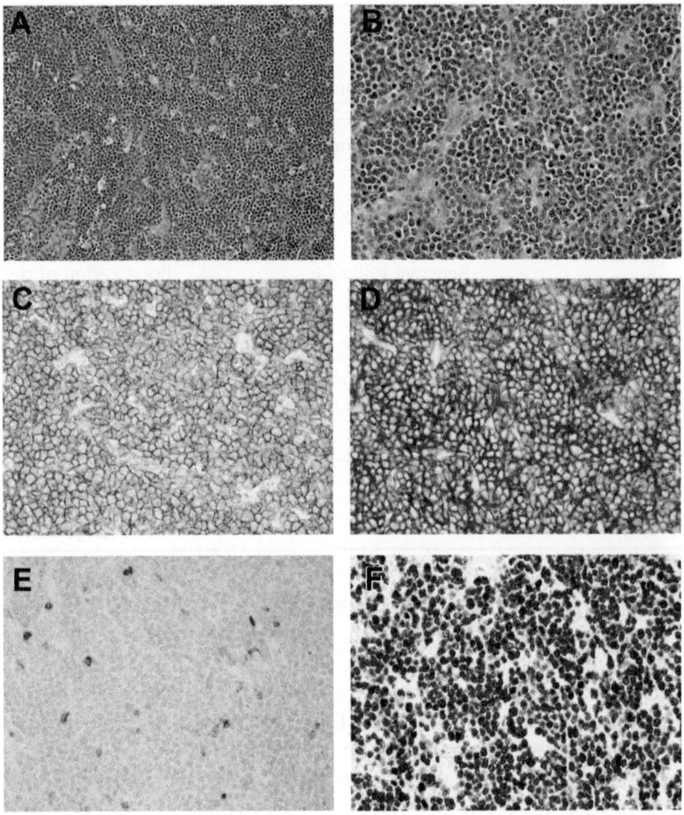

Fig. 2. Ileocecal mass in a 14-year-old patient showing BL. (*A*) A diffuse, monomorphic infiltrate with scattered tingible-body macrophages (H&E, original magnification ×200). (*B*) A high-power view shows intermediate-sized lymphocytes with round nuclei, finely clumped chromatin, multiple small nucleoli, and small amounts of cytoplasm (H&E, original magnification ×400). Neoplastic cells are positive for CD20 (*C*) and CD10 (*D*) and negative for BCL2 (*E*). (*F*) The Ki67 proliferative index is greater than 95% (all immunohistochemical stains at original magnification ×400).

and a male/female ratio of 3.6:1.[51] All patients in this cohort presented with lymphadenopathy, and 11% also had extranodal disease.

EBV-positive DLBCL shows partial or total effacement of lymph node architecture and can show various histologic patterns. In young patients, the most common pattern is the T cell/histiocyte–rich large B-cell lymphoma–like pattern (**Fig. 5**), with a minor component of large EBV-positive B cells embedded within an inflammatory background infiltrate composed predominantly of T cells and histiocytes.[51] Additional cases can morphologically resemble DLBCL not otherwise specified (NOS), CHL, or BCLU.[2,51] Admixed eosinophils and plasma cells may be present, and geographic necrosis and angioinvasion may be seen.[2] The EBV-positive B cells can range in morphology from intermediate-sized to large cells resembling centroblasts or immunoblasts to cells resembling Reed-Sternberg or lymphocyte-predominant cells.[2,51]

A diagnosis of EBV-positive DLBCL requires positivity for EBV-encoded RNA (EBER) by in situ hybridization in greater than 80% of neoplastic cells.[2] The neoplastic

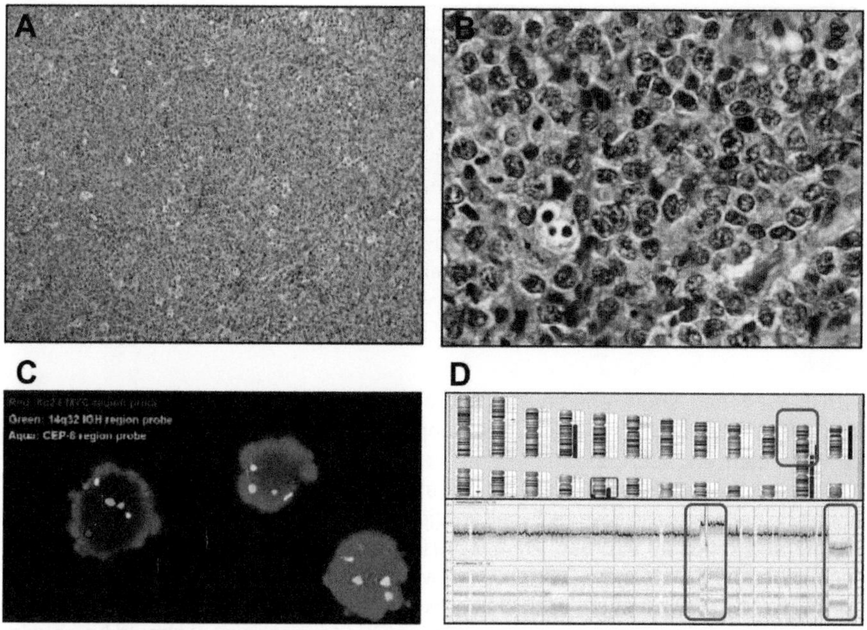

Fig. 3. Burkitt-like lymphoma with 11q aberration. Tonsillectomy specimen from a 15-year-old boy with unilateral tonsillar enlargement. (*A*) A starry-sky pattern is apparent at scanning magnification (H&E, original magnification ×20). (*B*) The lymphoma cells show more pleomorphism than typical BL (H&E, original magnification ×600). By immunohistochemistry, the cells expressed CD20, CD10, BCL6, and c-MYC and showed a Ki67 proliferation fraction approaching 100% (not shown). (*C*) No *c-MYC* rearrangement was detected by fluorescence in situ hybridization (FISH); FISH for *BCL6, IGH/BCL2,* and *IRF4/DUSP22* rearrangements was also negative (not shown). (*D*) A chromosome microarray (CMA) study detected localized copy number abnormalities diagnostic of this entity, including a terminal/telomeric deletion, several gains at chromosome 11q23, and one gain at 11q14. *FISH and CMA images courtesy of Gordana Raca MD PhD, Director, Clinical Cytogenomics Laboratory, Center for Personalized Medicine (CPM), Children's Hospital Los Angeles.*

cells are typically positive for B-cell markers CD19, CD20, CD22, CD79a, and PAX5, although 1 or more may be negative.[2,51] Lesional B cells are typically positive for MUM1 and negative for CD10, with BCL6 positivity in a small subset of cases, consistent with an ABC phenotype. CD30 is commonly positive, and CD15 is positive in a small subset of cases. Programmed death-ligand 1 (PD-L1) and PD-L2 are commonly positive on tumor cells,[51,52] which may be related to chromosomal gains at 9p24.1.[53]

Large B-cell lymphoma with *IRF4* rearrangement. Large B-cell lymphoma with *IRF4* rearrangement (LBCL-*IRF4*) was introduced in the 2017 revision of the WHO classification as a provisional entity representing an uncommon large B-cell lymphoma that occurs primarily in children and young adults.[2,54] In a large series of 20 cases, the median age at diagnosis was 12 years (range, 4–79 years).[54] This entity is characterized by a cytogenetically cryptic rearrangement of *IRF4* in most cases, most commonly involving translocation with the *IGH* locus, although rare cases involving the immunoglobulin light-chain loci have been described.[2,54] Patients frequently present with lymphadenopathy in the head and neck or with involvement of Waldeyer ring.[33,54–56]

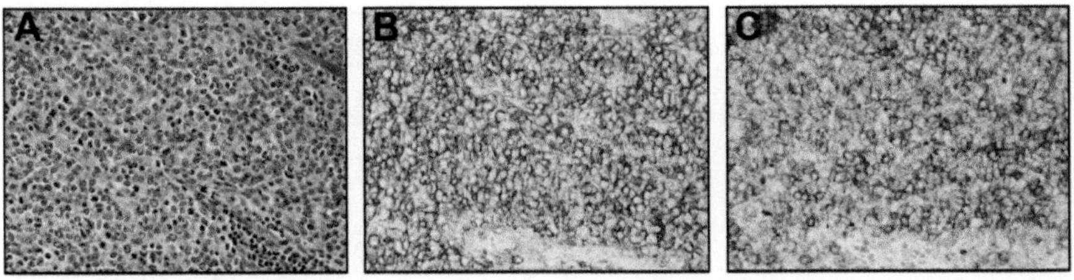

Fig. 4. DLBCL. (*A*) High-power view showing sheets of intermediate-sized to large cells with round to oval nuclei, distinct nuclei, and small to moderate amounts of cytoplasm (H&E, original magnification ×400). Neoplastic cells are positive for CD20 (*B*) and CD10 (*C*) (Both immunohistochemical stains, original magnification ×400).

LBCL-*IRF4* can show entirely diffuse, entirely follicular, or mixed follicular and diffuse architecture[2] (**Fig. 6**A, B). The neoplastic cells are intermediate to large in size with relatively open chromatin and small nucleoli. Mitotic figures and tingible-body macrophages are infrequent, and a starry-sky pattern is typically not present. Neoplastic cells express mature B-cell antigens CD20, CD79a, and PAX5 and typically strongly and diffusely express IRF4/MUM1 (**Fig. 6**C, D). BCL6 is positive in most cases, whereas CD10 and BCL2 are positive in approximately two-thirds of cases[54] (**Fig. 6**E, F). In the appropriate clinical context, screening of patients with coexpression of IRF4/MUM1, BCL6, and CD10 with FISH for *IRF4* rearrangement should be considered.[2] CD5 expression has been reported in a subset of patients,[54] whereas EBV in situ hybridization (EBER) is negative.[45] The Ki67 proliferative index is generally increased (>50%).[33,54]

Recent large-scale molecular analysis of LBCL-*IRF4* showed recurrent mutations in *IRF4* (76%), *CARD11* (35%), and *CCND3* (24%) as well as somatic intronic *BCL6* mutations (50%) predicted to affect IRF4 binding sites.[45] In addition, 6 of 17 analyzed

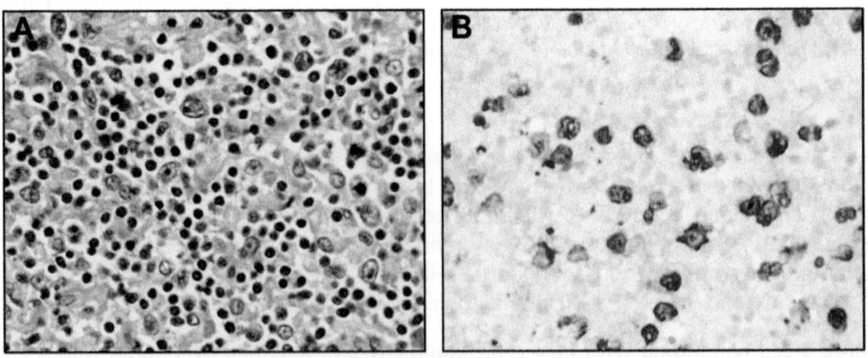

Fig. 5. EBV-positive DLBCL, not otherwise specified. Neck mass from an otherwise healthy 18-year-old man with lymphadenopathy, B symptoms, and no known immunodeficiency. (*A*) The lymph node is enlarged and effaced by a polymorphous lymphoid proliferation including frequent large lymphoid cells, some resembling Reed-Sternberg-cell variants, amid a delicate vascular proliferation without sclerosis (H&E, original magnification ×400). (*B*) EBER (EBV-encoded RNA, in situ hybridization, (original magnification ×400 is positive in the large cells. In addition, the abnormal lymphoid cells express CD20, CD79a, and MUM1; show weak CD30 expression in a subset of cells (most cells negative); and are negative for CD15 (not shown).

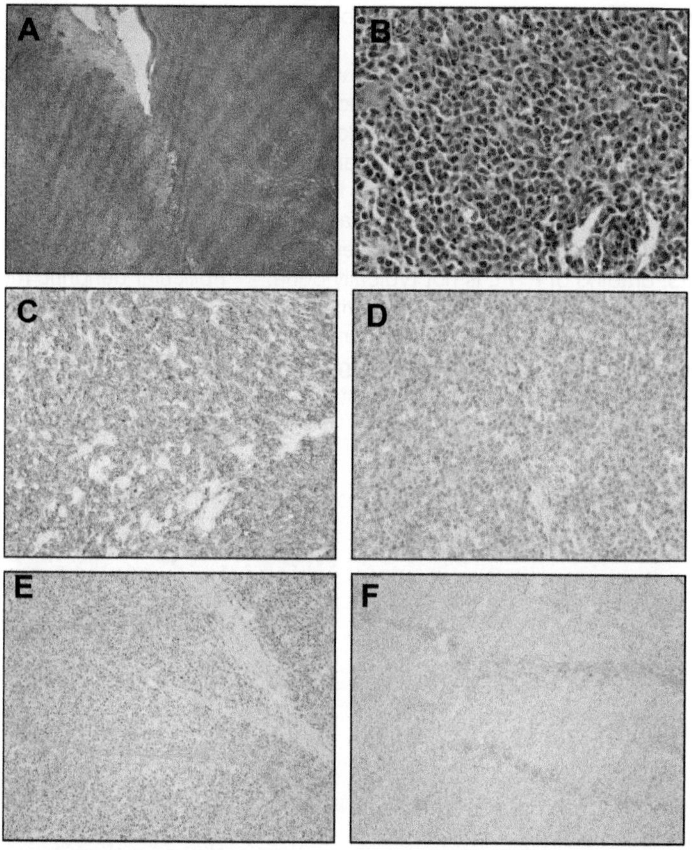

Fig. 6. Large B-cell lymphoma with *IRF4* rearrangement in a tonsillectomy specimen from a 23 year-old woman. (*A*) A low-power view shows follicular and diffuse architecture (H&E, original magnification ×40). (*B*) A high-power view shows medium-sized cells with relatively open chromatin and small nucleoli (H&E, original magnification ×400). Neoplastic cells are diffusely positive for CD20 (*C*), MUM1 (*D*), and BCL6 (*E*) and are negative for CD10 (F) (*C* and *D*, original magnification ×200; *E* and *F*, original magnification ×100).

cases showed mutations thought to result in NF-κB activation (*CARD11*, *CD79B*, and *MYD88*). *MAP2K1* mutations, frequently seen in PTFL (discussed later) were present in 2 cases with a predominantly follicular growth pattern and confirmed *IRF4* rearrangement.

Indolent B-cell lymphomas

Pediatric-type follicular lymphoma. PTFL is a rare nodal B-cell lymphoma, accounting for less than 2% of pediatric NHL,[57] with follicular architecture that occurs predominantly in young patients and is distinct from usual follicular lymphoma (FL) in adults. In cohorts of patients less than or equal to 18 years of age, the median age at diagnosis of PTFL ranges from 11 to 15 years.[58–62] PTFL is more common in boys and typically presents with isolated, asymptomatic peripheral lymphadenopathy, with most reported cases involving lymph nodes of the head and neck.[63] The presence of disseminated disease precludes a diagnosis of PTFL.[2,57] The prognosis for PTFL is excellent, with overall survival of 100% in children and adolescents reported in the literature,[63] and, for patients with completely resected disease, a watch-and-wait approach may be appropriate.[2,57,63]

Lymph nodes involved by PTFL show partial or total effacement of architecture by large, expansile, often serpiginous, and sometimes coalescing follicles[55,59,64] (**Fig. 7**A). Follicles contain frequent tingible-body macrophages (starry-sky pattern), lack polarization, and have attenuated or absent mantle zones. Marginal zone differentiation may be seen at the periphery of follicles. Neoplastic cells are intermediate to large in size with blastoid or centroblastic cytology without prominent nucleoli (**Fig. 7**B). In some cases, smaller centrocytes may predominate. However, unlike usual FL in adults, grading of PTFL is not typically done.[2,57] Follicular dendritic meshworks may be expanded or fragmented; cases with areas of DLBCL are excluded from this category.[2,57] Lesional cells are positive for B-cell markers CD20, CD79a, and PAX5 and are positive for CD10 and BCL6[2,61] (**Fig. 7**C, D). IRF4/MUM1 is typically negative; strong expression by immunohistochemistry should raise suspicion for LBCL-*IRF4*.

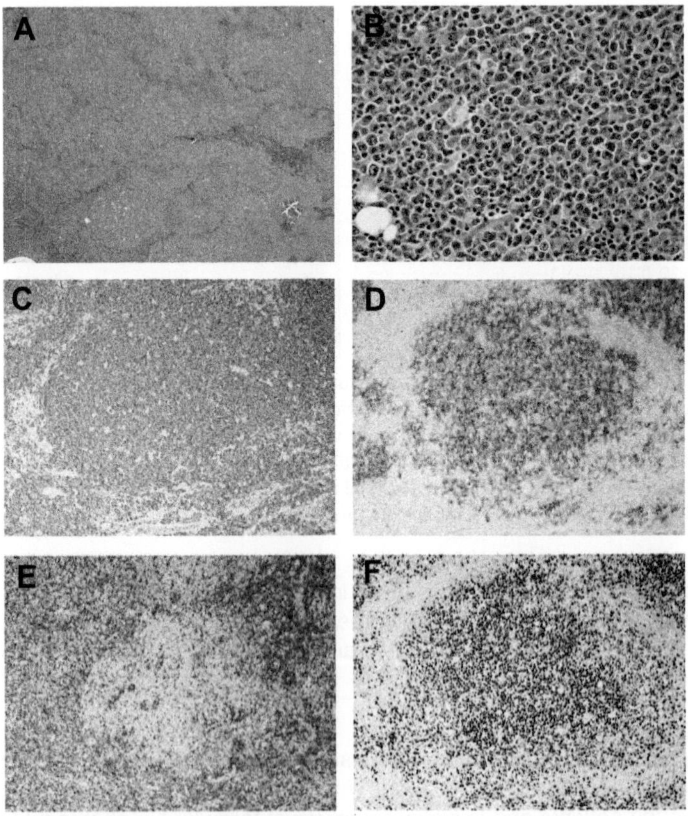

Fig. 7. PTFL. (*A*) A low-power view of this cervical lymph node from a 9-year-old boy shows effacement of nodal architecture by large coalescing follicles (H&E, original magnification ×20). (*B*) A high-power view shows intermediate-sized to large cells with round to irregular nuclei and distinct nucleoli (H&E, original magnification ×400). The neoplastic cells are positive for CD20 (*C*) and CD10 (*D*). (*E*) BCL2 is predominantly negative within the follicles. (*F*) The Ki67 proliferative index is increased within follicles (all immunohistochemical stains original magnification ×100).

BCL2 may be positive in a minority of cases (**Fig. 7**E). The Ki67 proliferative index is typically moderate to high within follicles (>30%) (**Fig. 7**F). Recent work has suggested that FOXP-1 expression may be useful to differentiate PTFL from reactive follicular hyperplasia (FH).[65]

Molecular testing is positive for clonal *IGH* rearrangements in PTFL, which may help distinguish PTFL from cases of florid FH. Rearrangements involving *BCL2*, *BCL6*, and *IRF4/MUM1* are not present in PTFL. Instead, studies have shown recurrent loss of heterozygosity or deletion of 1p36 (approximately 15%–25% of cases), often in association with mutations in *TNFRSF14* (approximately 30%–40% of cases overall).[60,61] Recurrent mutations in exons 2 and 3 of *MAP2K1* are also present in approximately 40% of cases.[61]

Pediatric nodal marginal zone lymphoma. Pediatric nodal marginal zone lymphoma (NMZL) is a provisional entity in the WHO classification that presents with limited-stage disease predominantly in adolescent boys, with a median age at diagnosis of 15 to 16 years.[2,57,63,66,67] Patients typically present with asymptomatic, localized lymphadenopathy, most commonly involving head and neck lymph nodes. Similar to PTFL, pediatric NMZL is associated with an excellent prognosis, with low relapse rates following complete resection.[2,57,63]

Involved lymph nodes show residual large follicles with infiltration of mantle zone B cells into germinal centers, resembling progressive transformation of germinal centers, as well as expanded marginal zones and an interfollicular proliferation of small to medium-sized lymphocytes, with possible diffuse areas[2,57,63,68] (**Fig. 8**A). The cytology of the lesional cells may be variable, including small centrocytelike cells as well as monocytoid-appearing cells with more abundant cytoplasm; admixed larger transformed cells and plasma cells may also be present.[69,70] Lesional cells are positive for CD20 (**Fig. 8**B), with frequent coexpression of CD43, and are negative for CD5, CD10, and BCL6. BCL2 is positive in approximately 40% to 50% of cases.[63,69]

Molecular testing is positive for a clonal *IGH* gene rearrangement in most cases.[67] Limited genetic analysis has shown overall low levels of genomic complexity; approximately 20% of cases show trisomy 18,[67] whereas recurrent point mutations have not been identified in pediatric NMZL.[71] Cases of nodal marginal zone hyperplasia, some with skewed light-chain expression by immunohistochemistry or flow cytometry, have

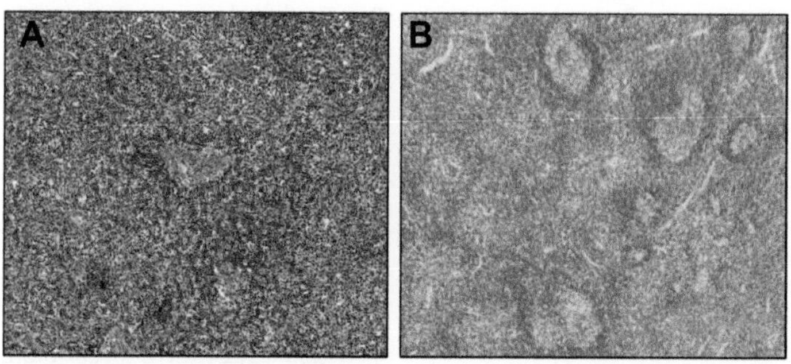

Fig. 8. Pediatric NMZL. Excisional biopsy of an isolated submandibular mass from a 13-year-old asymptomatic boy. (*A*) Sections show a lymph node enlarged by an interfollicular expansion of atypical intermediate-sized lymphocytes with moderately abundant cytoplasm (H&E, original magnification ×100). (*B*) The atypical cells are B cells that expand but do not obliterate B-cell follicles (CD20, original magnification ×20). The Ki67 proliferation fraction was low (not shown).

been described in association with *Haemophilus influenzae* infection; however, in contrast with NMZL, these cases showed polyclonal patterns by *IGH* molecular testing.[72]

Mature T-cell Lymphomas

With the exception of anaplastic large cell lymphoma, which is common in children, mature T-cell (and natural killer [NK]--cell) lymphomas in the pediatric age group are generally rare and diverse and therefore often pose diagnostic dilemmas.[73] In children, certain clinicopathologic entities occur almost exclusively (hydroa vacciniforme–like lymphoproliferative disorder), others raise consideration for underlying immunodeficiency (eg, peripheral T-cell lymphoma, not otherwise specified), and some are typically adult diseases but do occur and must be approached with a high index of suspicion in children (eg, mycosis fungoides)[74–76] (**Tables 4** and **5**). Most other entities described in children occur on the order of case reports and series. Because of their association with primary EBV infection, systemic pathologic manifestations of EBV infection involving T cells disproportionately affect children and adolescents compared with adults; discussion of this spectrum of diseases, the EBV-positive

Table 4
Pathologic features of pediatric mature systemic T-cell non-Hodgkin lymphoma

Diagnosis	Morphology	Immunophenotype	Genetics
Anaplastic large cell lymphoma, ALK positive	Variably numerous large hallmark cells in sheets or amid variably dense inflammatory, histiocytic, or fibroblastic background; subtle sinusoid involvement in early nodal disease and bone marrow	Pos: CD30, ALK1, granzyme and/or TIA1 and/or perforin, +/− CD4 Neg: variable loss of T-cell markers (sCD3, CD2, CD5, CD7) Rare: CD8	*ALK1* rearrangement; most common partner gene: *NPM1*
Peripheral T-cell lymphoma not otherwise specified	Patternless sheets of variably sized lymphoid cells, with or without a granulomatous or lymphoepithelioid background	Pos: T-cell markers (sCD3, CD2, CD5, CD7) with variable loss; variable CD4 and/or CD8 expression or neither Rare: few EBV+ cells	Complex; 2 putative subgroups defined by GEP in adults
Hepatosplenic T-cell lymphoma	Hepatic and bone marrow sinusoidal involvement, and splenic sinus and cord involvement, by intermediate-sized monomorphous lymphoid cells	Pos: CD3, CD56 +/−, TCR gamma-delta (rarely TCR alpha-beta) Neg: CD5, EBER, CD4/CD8 (typical)	Isochromosome 7q *STAT5B* alterations

Abbreviation: EBER, EBV-encoded RNA.

Table 5
Differential diagnosis of pediatric mature systemic T-cell non-Hodgkin lymphoma

Diagnosis	Differential Diagnosis	Comments
Anaplastic large cell lymphoma, ALK positive	Classic Hodgkin lymphoma	Limited-stage and/or isolated mediastinal presentation; nodules and sclerosis (nodular sclerosis subtype); Reed-Sternberg cells and variants without hallmark cells (may show overlap); CD15 expression, PAX5 and variable B-cell marker expression, EBV expression (subset)
	Infectious or autoimmune lymphadenitis	Preserved, if obscured, nodal architecture; CD30 expression variable in intensity and size of reactive cells (immunoblasts); +/− identifiable organism
	Spindle cell sarcoma	Not lymph node based, even at metastasis; associated translocation or other defining feature
	Metastatic nonhematopoietic tumor	Evidence of morphologic differentiation; positive immunophenotypic expression of differentiation (eg, melanocytic, germ cell)
	ALK-positive large B-cell lymphoma	Immunoblast-like neoplastic cells; plasmacytic immunophenotype
	ALK-positive histiocytosis	Rare; systemic (nonnodal) presentations; foamy and/or phagocytic-type histiocyte morphology
Peripheral T-cell lymphoma, not otherwise specified	Anaplastic large cell lymphoma	Hallmark cells; sinusoidal pattern in bone marrow and lymph node capsule; uniform strong CD30 expression; ALK positive in most pediatric patients
	Nodular lymphocyte-predominant Hodgkin lymphoma	Serpiginous or other variant growth patterns, including progressive transformation of germinal center–type features (nondiffuse); lymphocyte-predominant (popcorn) cells. Caution: may have frequent CD4/CD8 double-positive T cells
	Paracortical T-cell zone hyperplasia	Preserved nodal architecture, nonfollicular nodules, polymorphous lymphocytes, scattered Langerhans cells; preserved T-cell immunophenotype; polyclonal gene rearrangements

(*continued on next page*)

Table 5
(continued)

Diagnosis	Differential Diagnosis	Comments
Hepatosplenic T-cell lymphoma	EBV hepatitis[126]	EBV+, CD8+, smaller cells than those in hepatosplenic T-cell lymphoma (intermediate size)

T-cell and NK-cell lymphoproliferative diseases of childhood,[77,78] is beyond the scope of this article.

Anaplastic large cell lymphoma, anaplastic lymphoma kinase positive

Anaplastic large cell lymphoma (ALCL) is the most common mature T-cell lymphoma of childhood, representing 10% to 30% of all pediatric lymphomas,[1,79] and has a generally favorable prognosis, even at relapse.[80] It most commonly presents with high-stage lymphadenopathy and B symptoms but may have extranodal involvement, including skin, liver, lung, and bone. Rare presentations of ALCL described in children include leukemic phase, brain involvement, associated hemophagocytosis, and isolated skin involvement.[73,81] Most pediatric ALCLs express the anaplastic lymphoma kinase 1 (ALK1) protein through *ALK1* rearrangements (ALK1+ ALCL). ALK1-negative ALCLs,[82] including those with *DUSP22*[83,84] or *TP63* abnormalities,[85,86] primary cutaneous ALCL, and breast implant/seroma–associated ALCL, are primarily adult diseases, and as such there are limited data on their prognostic significance in the pediatric age group.

A wide histologic spectrum of ALCL is recognized throughout the life span, including in ALK-positive ALCL in children.[87] A uniform feature is the horseshoe-shaped nuclear morphology in at least a subset of the lymphoma cells (hallmark cells) (**Fig. 9**A).[88] Cases with sheets of tumor cells (see **Fig. 9**A) raise a differential diagnosis of DLBCL or peripheral T-cell lymphoma not otherwise specified, whereas cases with few scattered tumor cells obscured by a lymphohistiocytic or fibroblastic background may resemble CHL, infectious or autoimmune lymphadenitis such as Kikuchi-Fujimoto lymphadenopathy (see the article, "Pediatric Lymphadenitis," in this issue), or even a sarcoma.[89] The small cell pattern of ALCL,[90] together with the lymphohistiocytic pattern, has been associated with adverse prognosis in children.[91] Early or limited nodal involvement and bone marrow involvement show a sinusoidal pattern, mimicking metastatic carcinoma or melanoma, and may be small and focal. These subtle morphologic variants and settings require a high index of suspicion.

ALK-positive ALCL is defined by expression of CD30 and ALK1 (**Fig. 9**B, C); as such, anti-CD30 (eg, brentuximab vedotin) and ALK inhibitor (eg, crizotinib) therapy may supplement or follow multiagent chemotherapy in relapsed/refractory disease.[92–94] The ALK1 protein is expressed in both the cytoplasm and nucleus of cells with the t(2;5);*NPM1-ALK1* rearrangement (see **Fig. 9**C); alternative (non-*NPM1*) *ALK1* fusions and the small cell histologic variant show other patterns of protein expression.[79,87] Cytogenetic studies and documentation of an *ALK1* fusion is generally not required for diagnosis. Few other lesions express ALK1 (eg, ALK-positive large B-cell lymphoma, ALK-positive histiocytosis, inflammatory myofibroblastic tumor, a subset of rhabdomyosarcoma), and their morphologic and other immunophenotypic features are generally distinct from those of ALCL. CD30 is typically uniformly strong but may show a spectrum of intensity, with the largest tumor cells showing the strongest staining.[87] Inclusion of CD30 in an initial immunostain panel for cell lineage assessment in subtle lesions, such as the lymphohistiocytic variant, is recommended to uncover

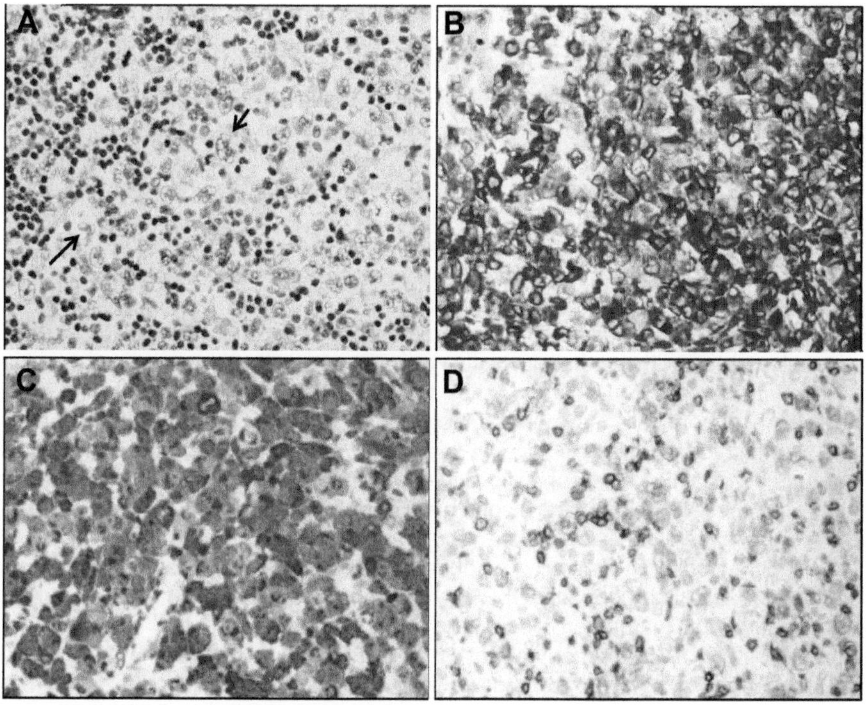

Fig. 9. Anaplastic large cell lymphoma, ALK positive. Excisional cervical lymph node biopsy from a 7-year-old girl with diffuse lymphadenopathy and B symptoms. (*A*) The lymph node architecture is effaced by sheets of large pleomorphic cells with abundant cytoplasm and vesicular chromatin; a subset show curved or horseshoe-shaped nuclei, hallmark cells (*arrows*) (H&E). (*B*) The neoplastic cells are uniformly positive for CD30 by immunohistochemistry. (*C*) ALK1 expression is strong and uniform, and both nuclear and cytoplasmic, suggestive of an *ALK1-NPM1* fusion. (*D*) CD3 expression is weak to negative in the neoplastic cells, a common feature of ALCL that may cause diagnostic confusion; the small cells with strong CD3 expression are infiltrating nonneoplastic T cells. (All images, original magnification ×200)

ALCL. In addition, ALCL shows variable loss of leukocyte common antigen (CD45) and of pan–T-cell antigens (so-called null phenotype), including CD3 (>75% of cases; see **Fig. 9**D)[88]; this may especially raise the differential diagnosis of a nonhematopoietic neoplasm. ALCL typically expresses CD4 (weakly); rare patients express CD8, which has been associated with variant histologies and prognostic significance in a pediatric series.[95] Variable expression of cytotoxic T-cell antigens (granzyme B, perforin, TIA-1) is evident in most ALCLs.

ALK-positive ALCL is molecularly distinct from ALK-negative ALCL,[96,97] with a gene expression profile enriched in STAT3 pathway–related signaling.[98] Variant (non-*NPM1*) *ALK1* fusion partners have no known prognostic implications among ALK-positive ALCL.[99,100] Molecular detection of clonal T-cell receptor (TCR) gene rearrangements and *ALK1* fusion transcripts has an emerging role in minimal residual disease monitoring.[101]

Peripheral T-cell lymphoma not otherwise specified

A minority of cases of T-cell lymphoma in pediatric patients do not meet WHO criteria for ALCL and typically require classification as peripheral T-cell lymphoma, not otherwise specified (PTCL-NOS).[57,102] PTCL-NOS, a diverse group of neoplasms related by their lack of other clinicopathologic features of currently recognized lymphomas, is most prevalent in older adults.[2] When encountered in a pediatric patient, like any lymphoma rarely encountered in a child, PTCL-NOS may raise consideration for an underlying immunodeficiency.[103,104] The prognosis of PTCL-NOS in children is reported to be less favorable than that of ALCL using ALCL-type treatment regimens,[105] although limited-stage disease is often cured.[106] Angioimmunoblastic T-cell lymphoma and related T-follicular helper cell neoplasms generally do not occur in children.

PTCL-NOS is most commonly a nodal disease, with patternless sheets of neoplastic cells with a moderate to high proliferation fraction.[107] The histologic features of PTCL-NOS are heterogeneous, ranging from monomorphous large cells resembling DLBCL, to granulomatous with epithelioid histiocytes (lymphoepithelioid pattern, so-called Lennert lymphoma) (**Fig. 10**), to cases with small cells. PTCL-NOS with small neoplastic lymphoid cells may raise a differential diagnosis of reactive lymphadenopathy, with paracortical T-cell zone hyperplasia,[108] and NLPHL, which may have numerous atypical but nonneoplastic CD4/CD8 double-positive T cells.[109] Rigorous exclusion of these more common diagnoses, use of TCR gene rearrangement clonality studies, and expert consultation are recommended before making a diagnosis of PTCL-NOS in a child. In particular, a subset of T-lymphoblastic leukemia/lymphoma (T-ALL/LBL) lacks immunophenotypic markers of immaturity,[110,111] and, moreover, immunophenotypic maturation of T-ALL/LBL may occur after therapy[112,113]; both scenarios may raise a differential diagnoses of PTCL-NOS and, in some clinical and immunophenotypic settings, hepatosplenic T-cell lymphoma. Nevertheless, T-cell immunophenotypic aberrancies are common but not universal in PTCL-NOS, and rare cases are CD30 positive but lack other defining features of ALCL.

PTCL-NOS is heterogeneous and genetically complex, and efforts toward prognosis-driven subclassification of PTCL-NOS are ongoing. GEP studies have identified 2 subgroups,[114,115] for which immunophenotypic surrogate markers have been developed.[116] The significance of this classifier in pediatric PTCL-NOS is unknown.

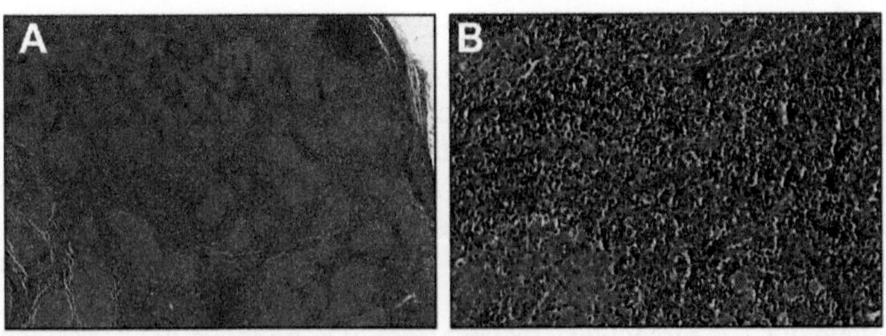

Fig. 10. Peripheral T-cell lymphoma, not otherwise specified. Cervical lymph node excision from a 6-year-old boy with diffuse lymphadenopathy, subsequently found to harbor biallelic germline variants in the *ATM* gene, consistent with a diagnosis of ataxia telangiectasia. (*A*) A low-power view shows effacement of nodal architecture by numerous nonnecrotizing granulomata with an associated abnormal lymphoid infiltrate (H&E, original magnification ×50). (*B*) At higher power, the lymphoid infiltrate is composed of small to intermediate-sized cells with round to irregular nuclei, indistinct nucleoli, and moderate amounts of cytoplasm (H&E, original magnification ×200). The neoplastic cells were positive for CD2, CD3, CD4, and TCR alpha-beta and negative for CD30, PD1, and TCR gamma-delta (not shown). Molecular studies were positive for a clonal TCR gene rearrangement.

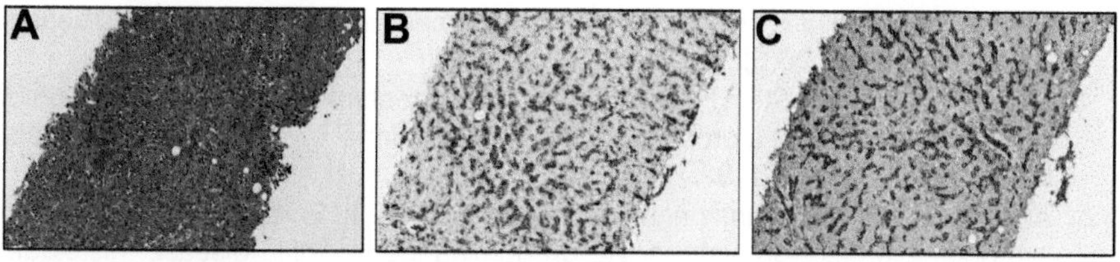

Fig. 11. Liver core biopsy with involvement by hepatosplenic T-cell lymphoma. (*A*) H&E stain showing a sinusoidal infiltrate composed of small to intermediate-sized T cells that are positive for CD3 (*B*) and CD56 (*C*) (All images, original magnification ×20).

Hepatosplenic T-cell lymphoma

Hepatosplenic T-cell lymphoma (HSTCL) is an uncommon, aggressive clinicopathologic entity characterized by systemic symptoms, frequent cytopenias, hepatosplenomegaly, bone marrow involvement, and poor overall survival. The median age of HSTCL presentation is 35 years, and pediatric and adolescent cases are well described.[117,118]

Histopathologically, HSTCL shows a characteristic sinusoidal pattern in liver (similar to that seen in EBV hepatitis) (**Fig. 11**), spleen (sinuses and cords), and bone marrow. The neoplastic cells are monomorphous intermediate-sized lymphoid cells; bone marrow biopsy with flow cytometry has replaced splenectomy for first-line diagnostic specimens, and bone marrow involvement may be focal and subtle and require multiple tissue levels together with immunostains for identification. Phenotypically, the neoplastic T cells of HSTCL show a gamma-delta T-cell phenotype, with expression of CD3, CD56 (+/−), and TCR gamma-delta, no expression of CD5, and typically no expression of CD4 or CD8. A minority of cases show an alpha-beta T-cell phenotype.[119] EBV is negative at presentation.

The pathogenesis of HSTCL is unknown. Isochromosome 7q[120,121] and *STAT5B* mutations[122] are recurrent genetic abnormalities. Immunodeficiency, including from chronic immunosuppression such as tumor necrosis factor alpha inhibitor therapy, is a known risk factor.[123,124]

CLINICS CARE POINTS

- Lymphomas affecting children, adolescents, and young adults represent a subset of all recognized lymphomas, and are optimally managed by pediatric hematology-oncology.
- Nodular lymphocyte predominant Hodgkin lymphoma is a unique clinicopathologic entity distinct from classic Hodgkin lymphoma, with its own stage-specific treatment guidelines.
- Rare lymphoma subtypes presenting in children should prompt evaluation for underlying immunodeficiency as applicable.

DISCLOSURE

The authors have nothing to disclose.

REFERENCES

1. Sandlund JT, Downing JR, Crist WM. Non-Hodgkin's lymphoma in childhood. N Engl J Med 1996;334(19):1238–48.
2. Swerdlow SH, Campo E, harris NL, et al. WHO classification of tumours of haematopoietic and lymphoid tissues. Revised 4th edition. Lyon: IARC; 2017.

3. Lukes RJ, Butler JJ. The pathology and nomenclature of Hodgkin's disease. Cancer Res 1966;26(6):1063–83.
4. Harris NL, Jaffe ES, Stein H, et al. A revised European-American classification of lymphoid neoplasms: a proposal from the International Lymphoma Study Group. Blood 1994;84(5):1361–92.
5. Anagnostopoulos I, Hansmann ML, Franssila K, et al. European Task Force on Lymphoma project on lymphocyte predominance Hodgkin disease: histologic and immunohistologic analysis of submitted cases reveals 2 types of Hodgkin disease with a nodular growth pattern and abundant lymphocytes. Blood 2000;96(5):1889–99.
6. Bazzeh F, Rihani R, Howard S, et al. Comparing adult and pediatric hodgkin lymphoma in the Surveillance, Epidemiology and End results Program, 1988-2005: an analysis of 21 734 cases. Leuk Lymphoma 2010;51(12):2198–207.
7. Xing KH, Savage KJ. Modern management of lymphocyte-predominant Hodgkin lymphoma. Br J Haematol 2013;161(3):316–29.
8. Ashton-Key M, Thorpe PA, Allen JP, et al. Follicular Hodgkin's disease. Am J Surg Pathol 1995;19(11):1294–9.
9. Chan WC. Cellular origin of nodular lymphocyte-predominant Hodgkin's lymphoma: immunophenotypic and molecular studies. Semin Hematol 1999;36(3):242–52.
10. Diehl V, Sextro M, Franklin J, et al. Clinical presentation, course, and prognostic factors in lymphocyte-predominant Hodgkin's disease and lymphocyte-rich classical Hodgkin's disease: report from the European Task Force on Lymphoma Project on Lymphocyte-Predominant Hodgkin's Disease. J Clin Oncol 1999;17(3):776–83.
11. Spinner MA, Varma G, Advani RH. Modern principles in the management of nodular lymphocyte-predominant Hodgkin lymphoma. Br J Haematol 2019;184(1):17–29.
12. Osborne BM, Butler JJ, Gresik MV. Progressive transformation of germinal centers: comparison of 23 pediatric patients to the adult population. Mod Pathol 1992;5(2):135–40.
13. Miles RR, Cairo MS. A pediatric translational perspective on the entity "progressive transformation of germinal centers (PTGC)". Pediatr Blood Cancer 2013;60(1):3–4.
14. Fan Z, Natkunam Y, Bair E, et al. Characterization of variant patterns of nodular lymphocyte predominant hodgkin lymphoma with immunohistologic and clinical correlation. Am J Surg Pathol 2003;27(10):1346–56.
15. Untanu RV, Back J, Appel B, et al. Variant histology, IgD and CD30 expression in low-risk pediatric nodular lymphocyte predominant Hodgkin lymphoma: a report from the Children's Oncology Group. Pediatr Blood Cancer 2018;65(1). https://doi.org/10.1002/pbc.26753.
16. Huppmann AR, Nicolae A, Slack GW, et al. EBV may be expressed in the LP cells of nodular lymphocyte-predominant Hodgkin lymphoma (NLPHL) in both children and adults. Am J Surg Pathol 2014;38(3):316–24.
17. Stamatoullas A, Picquenot JM, Dumesnil C, et al. Conventional cytogenetics of nodular lymphocyte-predominant Hodgkin's lymphoma. Leukemia 2007;21(9):2064–7.
18. Wlodarska I, Nooyen P, Maes B, et al. Frequent occurrence of BCL6 rearrangements in nodular lymphocyte predominance Hodgkin lymphoma but not in classical Hodgkin lymphoma. Blood 2003;101(2):706–10.

19. Schumacher MA, Schmitz R, Brune V, et al. Mutations in the genes coding for the NF-kappaB regulating factors IkappaBalpha and A20 are uncommon in nodular lymphocyte-predominant Hodgkin's lymphoma. Haematologica 2010; 95(1):153–7.
20. Hartmann S, Doring C, Jakobus C, et al. Nodular lymphocyte predominant hodgkin lymphoma and T cell/histiocyte rich large B cell lymphoma–endpoints of a spectrum of one disease? PLoS One 2013;8(11):e78812.
21. Egan G, Goldman S, Alexander S. Mature B-NHL in children, adolescents and young adults: current therapeutic approach and emerging treatment strategies. Br J Haematol 2019;185(6):1071–85.
22. Sandlund JT, Martin MG. Non-Hodgkin lymphoma across the pediatric and adolescent and young adult age spectrum. Hematol Am Soc Hematol Educ Program 2016;2016(1):589–97.
23. Mbulaiteye SM, Biggar RJ, Bhatia K, et al. Sporadic childhood Burkitt lymphoma incidence in the United States during 1992-2005. Pediatr Blood Cancer 2009; 53(3):366–70.
24. Teitell MA, Lones MA, Perkins SL, et al. TCL1 expression and Epstein-Barr virus status in pediatric Burkitt lymphoma. Am J Clin Pathol 2005;124(4):569–75.
25. Masque-Soler N, Szczepanowski M, Kohler CW, et al. Clinical and pathological features of Burkitt lymphoma showing expression of BCL2–an analysis including gene expression in formalin-fixed paraffin-embedded tissue. Br J Haematol 2015;171(4):501–8.
26. Rohde M, Bonn BR, Zimmermann M, et al. Relevance of ID3-TCF3-CCND3 pathway mutations in pediatric aggressive B-cell lymphoma treated according to the non-Hodgkin Lymphoma Berlin-Frankfurt-Munster protocols. Haematologica 2017;102(6):1091–8.
27. Grande BM, Gerhard DS, Jiang A, et al. Genome-wide discovery of somatic coding and noncoding mutations in pediatric endemic and sporadic Burkitt lymphoma. Blood 2019;133(12):1313–24.
28. Panea RI, Love CL, Shingleton JR, et al. The whole-genome landscape of Burkitt lymphoma subtypes. Blood 2019;134(19):1598–607.
29. Giulino-Roth L, Goldman S. Recent molecular and therapeutic advances in B-cell non-Hodgkin lymphoma in children. Br J Haematol 2016;173(4):531–44.
30. Salaverria I, Martin-Guerrero I, Wagener R, et al. A recurrent 11q aberration pattern characterizes a subset of MYC-negative high-grade B-cell lymphomas resembling Burkitt lymphoma. Blood 2014;123(8):1187–98.
31. Gonzalez-Farre B, Ramis-Zaldivar JE, Salmeron-Villalobos J, et al. Burkitt-like lymphoma with 11q aberration: a germinal center-derived lymphoma genetically unrelated to Burkitt lymphoma. Haematologica 2019;104(9):1822–9.
32. Rymkiewicz G, Grygalewicz B, Chechlinska M, et al. A comprehensive flow-cytometry-based immunophenotypic characterization of Burkitt-like lymphoma with 11q aberration. Mod Pathol 2018;31(5):732–43.
33. Au-Yeung RKH, Arias Padilla L, Zimmermann M, et al. Experience with provisional WHO-entities large B-cell lymphoma with IRF4-rearrangement and Burkitt-like lymphoma with 11q aberration in paediatric patients of the NHL-BFM group. Br J Haematol 2020;190(5):753–63.
34. Wagener R, Seufert J, Raimondi F, et al. The mutational landscape of Burkitt-like lymphoma with 11q aberration is distinct from that of Burkitt lymphoma. Blood 2019;133(9):962–6.
35. Hochberg J, El-Mallawany NK, Abla O. Adolescent and young adult non-Hodgkin lymphoma. Br J Haematol 2016;173(4):637–50.

36. Burkhardt B, Zimmermann M, Oschlies I, et al. The impact of age and gender on biology, clinical features and treatment outcome of non-Hodgkin lymphoma in childhood and adolescence. Br J Haematol 2005;131(1):39–49.
37. Jaglowski SM, Linden E, Termuhlen AM, et al. Lymphoma in adolescents and young adults. Semin Oncol 2009;36(5):381–418.
38. Oschlies I, Klapper W, Zimmermann M, et al. Diffuse large B-cell lymphoma in pediatric patients belongs predominantly to the germinal-center type B-cell lymphomas: a clinicopathologic analysis of cases included in the German BFM (Berlin-Frankfurt-Munster) Multicenter Trial. Blood 2006;107(10):4047–52.
39. Hans CP, Weisenburger DD, Greiner TC, et al. Confirmation of the molecular classification of diffuse large B-cell lymphoma by immunohistochemistry using a tissue microarray. Blood 2004;103(1):275–82.
40. Szczepanowski M, Lange J, Kohler CW, et al. Cell-of-origin classification by gene expression and MYC-rearrangements in diffuse large B-cell lymphoma of children and adolescents. Br J Haematol 2017;179(1):116–9.
41. Miles RR, Raphael M, McCarthy K, et al. Pediatric diffuse large B-cell lymphoma demonstrates a high proliferation index, frequent c-Myc protein expression, and a high incidence of germinal center subtype: report of the French-American-British (FAB) international study group. Pediatr Blood Cancer 2008;51(3): 369–74.
42. Minard-Colin V, Brugieres L, Reiter A, et al. Non-Hodgkin lymphoma in children and adolescents: progress through effective collaboration, current knowledge, and challenges ahead. J Clin Oncol 2015;33(27):2963–74.
43. Poirel HA, Cairo MS, Heerema NA, et al. Specific cytogenetic abnormalities are associated with a significantly inferior outcome in children and adolescents with mature B-cell non-Hodgkin's lymphoma: results of the FAB/LMB 96 international study. Leukemia 2009;23(2):323–31.
44. Deffenbacher KE, Iqbal J, Sanger W, et al. Molecular distinctions between pediatric and adult mature B-cell non-Hodgkin lymphomas identified through genomic profiling. Blood 2012;119(16):3757–66.
45. Ramis-Zaldivar JE, Gonzalez-Farre B, Balague O, et al. Distinct molecular profile of IRF4-rearranged large B-cell lymphoma. Blood 2020;135(4):274–86.
46. Beltran BE, Morales D, Quinones P, et al. EBV-positive diffuse large b-cell lymphoma in young immunocompetent individuals. Clin Lymphoma Myeloma Leuk 2011;11(6):512–6.
47. Cohen M, De Matteo E, Narbaitz M, et al. Epstein-Barr virus presence in pediatric diffuse large B-cell lymphoma reveals a particular association and latency patterns: analysis of viral role in tumor microenvironment. Int J Cancer 2013; 132(7):1572–80.
48. Cohen M, Narbaitz M, Metrebian F, et al. Epstein-Barr virus-positive diffuse large B-cell lymphoma association is not only restricted to elderly patients. Int J Cancer 2014;135(12):2816–24.
49. Hong JY, Yoon DH, Suh C, et al. EBV-positive diffuse large B-cell lymphoma in young adults: is this a distinct disease entity? Ann Oncol 2015;26(3):548–55.
50. Uccini S, Al-Jadiry MF, Scarpino S, et al. Epstein-Barr virus-positive diffuse large B-cell lymphoma in children: a disease reminiscent of Epstein-Barr virus-positive diffuse large B-cell lymphoma of the elderly. Hum Pathol 2015;46(5):716–24.
51. Nicolae A, Pittaluga S, Abdullah S, et al. EBV-positive large B-cell lymphomas in young patients: a nodal lymphoma with evidence for a tolerogenic immune environment. Blood 2015;126(7):863–72.

52. Chen BJ, Chapuy B, Ouyang J, et al. PD-L1 expression is characteristic of a subset of aggressive B-cell lymphomas and virus-associated malignancies. Clin Cancer Res 2013;19(13):3462–73.
53. Yoon H, Park S, Ju H, et al. Integrated copy number and gene expression profiling analysis of Epstein-Barr virus-positive diffuse large B-cell lymphoma. Genes Chromosomes Cancer 2015;54(6):383–96.
54. Salaverria I, Philipp C, Oschlies I, et al. Translocations activating IRF4 identify a subtype of germinal center-derived B-cell lymphoma affecting predominantly children and young adults. Blood 2011;118(1):139–47.
55. Liu Q, Salaverria I, Pittaluga S, et al. Follicular lymphomas in children and young adults: a comparison of the pediatric variant with usual follicular lymphoma. Am J Surg Pathol 2013;37(3):333–43.
56. Chisholm KM, Mohlman J, Liew M, et al. IRF4 translocation status in pediatric follicular and diffuse large B-cell lymphoma patients enrolled in Children's Oncology Group trials. Pediatr Blood Cancer 2019;66(8):e27770.
57. Attarbaschi A, Abla O, Arias Padilla L, et al. Rare non-Hodgkin lymphoma of childhood and adolescence: a consensus diagnostic and therapeutic approach to pediatric-type follicular lymphoma, marginal zone lymphoma, and nonanaplastic peripheral T-cell lymphoma. Pediatr Blood Cancer 2020;67(8):e28416.
58. Lorsbach RB, Shay-Seymore D, Moore J, et al. Clinicopathologic analysis of follicular lymphoma occurring in children. Blood 2002;99(6):1959–64.
59. Oschlies I, Salaverria I, Mahn F, et al. Pediatric follicular lymphoma–a clinicopathological study of a population-based series of patients treated within the Non-Hodgkin's Lymphoma–Berlin-Frankfurt-Munster (NHL-BFM) multicenter trials. Haematologica 2010;95(2):253–9.
60. Martin-Guerrero I, Salaverria I, Burkhardt B, et al. Recurrent loss of heterozygosity in 1p36 associated with TNFRSF14 mutations in IRF4 translocation negative pediatric follicular lymphomas. Haematologica 2013;98(8):1237–41.
61. Louissaint A Jr, Schafernak KT, Geyer JT, et al. Pediatric-type nodal follicular lymphoma: a biologically distinct lymphoma with frequent MAPK pathway mutations. Blood 2016;128(8):1093–100.
62. Attarbaschi A, Beishuizen A, Mann G, et al. Children and adolescents with follicular lymphoma have an excellent prognosis with either limited chemotherapy or with a "Watch and wait" strategy after complete resection. Ann Hematol 2013; 92(11):1537–41.
63. Woessmann W, Quintanilla-Martinez L. Rare mature B-cell lymphomas in children and adolescents. Hematol Oncol 2019;37(Suppl 1):53–61.
64. Louissaint A Jr, Ackerman AM, Dias-Santagata D, et al. Pediatric-type nodal follicular lymphoma: an indolent clonal proliferation in children and adults with high proliferation index and no BCL2 rearrangement. Blood 2012;120(12): 2395–404.
65. Agostinelli C, Akarca AU, Ramsay A, et al. Novel markers in pediatric-type follicular lymphoma. Virchows Arch 2019;475(6):771–9.
66. Makarova O, Oschlies I, Muller S, et al. Excellent outcome with limited treatment in paediatric patients with marginal zone lymphoma. Br J Haematol 2018;182(5): 735–9.
67. Rizzo KA, Streubel B, Pittaluga S, et al. Marginal zone lymphomas in children and the young adult population; characterization of genetic aberrations by FISH and RT-PCR. Mod Pathol 2010;23(6):866–73.
68. Quintanilla-Martinez L, Sander B, Chan JK, et al. Indolent lymphomas in the pediatric population: follicular lymphoma, IRF4/MUM1+ lymphoma, nodal

marginal zone lymphoma and chronic lymphocytic leukemia. Virchows Arch 2016;468(2):141–57.
69. Taddesse-Heath L, Pittaluga S, Sorbara L, et al. Marginal zone B-cell lymphoma in children and young adults. Am J Surg Pathol 2003;27(4):522–31.
70. Swerdlow SH. Pediatric follicular lymphomas, marginal zone lymphomas, and marginal zone hyperplasia. Am J Clin Pathol 2004;122(Suppl):S98–109.
71. Ozawa MG, Bhaduri A, Chisholm KM, et al. A study of the mutational landscape of pediatric-type follicular lymphoma and pediatric nodal marginal zone lymphoma. Mod Pathol 2016;29(10):1212–20.
72. Kluin PM, Langerak AW, Beverdam-Vincent J, et al. Paediatric nodal marginal zone B-cell lymphadenopathy of the neck: a Haemophilus influenzae-driven immune disorder? J Pathol 2015;236(3):302–14.
73. Jaffe ES. Mature T-cell and NK-cell lymphomas in the pediatric age group. Am J Clin Pathol 2004;122(Suppl):S110–21.
74. Pillai V, Tallarico M, Bishop MR, et al. Mature T- and NK-cell non-Hodgkin lymphoma in children and young adolescents. Br J Haematol 2016;173(4):573–81.
75. Windsor R, Stiller C, Webb D. Peripheral T-cell lymphoma in childhood: population-based experience in the United Kingdom over 20 years. Pediatr Blood Cancer 2008;50(4):784–7.
76. Al Mahmoud R, Weitzman S, Schechter T, et al. Peripheral T-cell lymphoma in children and adolescents: a single-institution experience. J Pediatr Hematol Oncol 2012;34(8):611–6.
77. Coffey AM, Lewis A, Marcogliese AN, et al. A clinicopathologic study of the spectrum of systemic forms of EBV-associated T-cell lymphoproliferative disorders of childhood: a single tertiary care pediatric institution experience in North America. Pediatr Blood Cancer 2019;66(8):e27798.
78. Huang W, Lv N, Ying J, et al. Clinicopathological characteristics of four cases of EBV positive T-cell lymphoproliferative disorders of childhood in China. Int J Clin Exp Pathol 2014;7(8):4991–9.
79. Stein H, Foss HD, Durkop H, et al. CD30(+) anaplastic large cell lymphoma: a review of its histopathologic, genetic, and clinical features. Blood 2000;96(12):3681–95.
80. Prokoph N, Larose H, Lim MS, et al. Treatment options for paediatric anaplastic large cell lymphoma (ALCL): current standard and beyond. Cancers (Basel) 2018;10(4):99.
81. Oschlies I, Lisfeld J, Lamant L, et al. ALK-positive anaplastic large cell lymphoma limited to the skin: clinical, histopathological and molecular analysis of 6 pediatric cases. A report from the ALCL99 study. Haematologica 2013;98(1):50–6.
82. Lamant L, de Reynies A, Duplantier MM, et al. Gene-expression profiling of systemic anaplastic large-cell lymphoma reveals differences based on ALK status and two distinct morphologic ALK+ subtypes. Blood 2007;109(5):2156–64.
83. Parrilla Castellar ER, Jaffe ES, Said JW, et al. ALK-negative anaplastic large cell lymphoma is a genetically heterogeneous disease with widely disparate clinical outcomes. Blood 2014;124(9):1473–80.
84. Hapgood G, Ben-Neriah S, Mottok A, et al. Identification of high-risk DUSP22-rearranged ALK-negative anaplastic large cell lymphoma. Br J Haematol 2019;186(3):e28–31.
85. Vasmatzis G, Johnson SH, Knudson RA, et al. Genome-wide analysis reveals recurrent structural abnormalities of TP63 and other p53-related genes in peripheral T-cell lymphomas. Blood 2012;120(11):2280–9.

86. Zeng Y, Feldman AL. Genetics of anaplastic large cell lymphoma. Leuk Lymphoma 2016;57(1):21–7.
87. Falini B, Bigerna B, Fizzotti M, et al. ALK expression defines a distinct group of T/null lymphomas ("ALK lymphomas") with a wide morphological spectrum. Am J Pathol 1998;153(3):875–86.
88. Benharroch D, Meguerian-Bedoyan Z, Lamant L, et al. ALK-positive lymphoma: a single disease with a broad spectrum of morphology. Blood 1998;91(6): 2076–84.
89. Chan JK, Buchanan R, Fletcher CD. Sarcomatoid variant of anaplastic large-cell Ki-1 lymphoma. Am J Surg Pathol 1990;14(10):983–8.
90. Kinney MC, Collins RD, Greer JP, et al. A small-cell-predominant variant of primary Ki-1 (CD30)+ T-cell lymphoma. Am J Surg Pathol 1993;17(9):859–68.
91. Lamant L, McCarthy K, d'Amore E, et al. Prognostic impact of morphologic and phenotypic features of childhood ALK-positive anaplastic large-cell lymphoma: results of the ALCL99 study. J Clin Oncol 2011;29(35):4669–76.
92. National comprehensive cancer network. T cell lymphoma (Version 1.2021). Available at: https://www.nccn.org/professionals/physician_gls/pdf/t-cell.pdf. Accessed October 30, 2020.
93. Turner SD, Lamant L, Kenner L, et al. Anaplastic large cell lymphoma in paediatric and young adult patients. Br J Haematol 2016;173(4):560–72.
94. Sekimizu M, Iguchi A, Mori T, et al. Phase I clinical study of brentuximab vedotin (SGN-35) involving children with recurrent or refractory CD30-positive Hodgkin's lymphoma or systemic anaplastic large cell lymphoma: rationale, design and methods of BV-HLALCL study: study protocol. BMC Cancer 2018;18(1):122.
95. Abramov D, Oschlies I, Zimmermann M, et al. Expression of CD8 is associated with non-common type morphology and outcome in pediatric anaplastic lymphoma kinase-positive anaplastic large cell lymphoma. Haematologica 2013; 98(10):1547–53.
96. Salaverria I, Bea S, Lopez-Guillermo A, et al. Genomic profiling reveals different genetic aberrations in systemic ALK-positive and ALK-negative anaplastic large cell lymphomas. Br J Haematol 2008;140(5):516–26.
97. Thompson MA, Stumph J, Henrickson SE, et al. Differential gene expression in anaplastic lymphoma kinase-positive and anaplastic lymphoma kinase-negative anaplastic large cell lymphomas. Hum Pathol 2005;36(5):494–504.
98. Nasr MR, Laver JH, Chang M, et al. Expression of anaplastic lymphoma kinase, tyrosine-phosphorylated STAT3, and associated factors in pediatric anaplastic large cell lymphoma: a report from the children's oncology group. Am J Clin Pathol 2007;127(5):770–8.
99. Brugieres L, Quartier P, Le Deley MC, et al. Relapses of childhood anaplastic large-cell lymphoma: treatment results in a series of 41 children–a report from the French Society of Pediatric Oncology. Ann Oncol 2000;11(1):53–8.
100. Falini B, Pileri S, Zinzani PL, et al. ALK+ lymphoma: clinico-pathological findings and outcome. Blood 1999;93(8):2697–706.
101. Krumbholz M, Woessmann W, Zierk J, et al. Characterization and diagnostic application of genomic NPM-ALK fusion sequences in anaplastic large-cell lymphoma. Oncotarget 2018;9(41):26543–55.
102. Mellgren K, Attarbaschi A, Abla O, et al. Non-anaplastic peripheral T cell lymphoma in children and adolescents-an international review of 143 cases. Ann Hematol 2016;95(8):1295–305.
103. Shapiro RS. Malignancies in the setting of primary immunodeficiency: implications for hematologists/oncologists. Am J Hematol 2011;86(1):48–55.

104. Haas OA. Primary immunodeficiency and cancer Predisposition Revisited: Embedding two Closely related Concepts into an Integrative conceptual Framework. Front Immunol 2018;9:3136.
105. Kontny U, Oschlies I, Woessmann W, et al. Non-anaplastic peripheral T-cell lymphoma in children and adolescents–a retrospective analysis of the NHL-BFM study group. Br J Haematol 2015;168(6):835–44.
106. Hutchison RE, Laver JH, Chang M, et al. Non-anaplastic peripheral t-cell lymphoma in childhood and adolescence: a Children's Oncology Group study. Pediatr Blood Cancer 2008;51(1):29–33.
107. Went P, Agostinelli C, Gallamini A, et al. Marker expression in peripheral T-cell lymphoma: a proposed clinical-pathologic prognostic score. J Clin Oncol 2006;24(16):2472–9.
108. Attygalle AD, Cabecadas J, Gaulard P, et al. Peripheral T-cell and NK-cell lymphomas and their mimics; taking a step forward - report on the lymphoma workshop of the XVIth meeting of the European Association for Haematopathology and the Society for Hematopathology. Histopathology 2014;64(2):171–99.
109. Sohani AR, Jaffe ES, Harris NL, et al. Nodular lymphocyte-predominant hodgkin lymphoma with atypical T cells: a morphologic variant mimicking peripheral T-cell lymphoma. Am J Surg Pathol 2011;35(11):1666–78.
110. Borowitz MJ, Pullen DJ, Winick N, et al. Comparison of diagnostic and relapse flow cytometry phenotypes in childhood acute lymphoblastic leukemia: implications for residual disease detection: a report from the children's oncology group. Cytometry B Clin Cytom 2005;68(1):18–24.
111. Weiss LM, Bindl JM, Picozzi VJ, et al. Lymphoblastic lymphoma: an immunophenotype study of 26 cases with comparison to T cell acute lymphoblastic leukemia. Blood 1986;67(2):474–8.
112. Gaipa G, Basso G, Maglia O, et al. Drug-induced immunophenotypic modulation in childhood ALL: implications for minimal residual disease detection. Leukemia 2005;19(1):49–56.
113. Roshal M, Fromm JR, Winter S, et al. Immaturity associated antigens are lost during induction for T cell lymphoblastic leukemia: implications for minimal residual disease detection. Cytometry B Clin Cytom 2010;78(3):139–46.
114. Iqbal J, Wright G, Wang C, et al. Gene expression signatures delineate biological and prognostic subgroups in peripheral T-cell lymphoma. Blood 2014;123(19):2915–23.
115. Heavican TB, Bouska A, Yu J, et al. Genetic drivers of oncogenic pathways in molecular subgroups of peripheral T-cell lymphoma. Blood 2019;133(15):1664–76.
116. Amador C, Greiner TC, Heavican TB, et al. Reproducing the molecular subclassification of peripheral T-cell lymphoma-NOS by immunohistochemistry. Blood 2019;134(24):2159–70.
117. Cooke CB, Krenacs L, Stetler-Stevenson M, et al. Hepatosplenic T-cell lymphoma: a distinct clinicopathologic entity of cytotoxic gamma delta T-cell origin. Blood 1996;88(11):4265–74.
118. Belhadj K, Reyes F, Farcet JP, et al. Hepatosplenic gammadelta T-cell lymphoma is a rare clinicopathologic entity with poor outcome: report on a series of 21 patients. Blood 2003;102(13):4261–9.
119. Macon WR, Levy NB, Kurtin PJ, et al. Hepatosplenic alphabeta T-cell lymphomas: a report of 14 cases and comparison with hepatosplenic gammadelta T-cell lymphomas. Am J Surg Pathol 2001;25(3):285–96.

120. Alonsozana EL, Stamberg J, Kumar D, et al. Isochromosome 7q: the primary cytogenetic abnormality in hepatosplenic gammadelta T cell lymphoma. Leukemia 1997;11(8):1367–72.
121. Wlodarska I, Martin-Garcia N, Achten R, et al. Fluorescence in situ hybridization study of chromosome 7 aberrations in hepatosplenic T-cell lymphoma: isochromosome 7q as a common abnormality accumulating in forms with features of cytologic progression. Genes Chromosomes Cancer 2002;33(3):243–51.
122. Nicolae A, Xi L, Pittaluga S, et al. Frequent STAT5B mutations in gammadelta hepatosplenic T-cell lymphomas. Leukemia 2014;28(11):2244–8.
123. Vega F, Medeiros LJ, Gaulard P. Hepatosplenic and other gammadelta T-cell lymphomas. Am J Clin Pathol 2007;127(6):869–80.
124. Parakkal D, Sifuentes H, Semer R, et al. Hepatosplenic T-cell lymphoma in patients receiving TNF-alpha inhibitor therapy: expanding the groups at risk. Eur J Gastroenterol Hepatol 2011;23(12):1150–6.
125. Wagener R, Lopez C, Kleinheinz K, et al. IG-MYC (+) neoplasms with precursor B-cell phenotype are molecularly distinct from Burkitt lymphomas. Blood 2018;132(21):2280–5.
126. Schechter S, Lamps L. Epstein-barr virus hepatitis: a review of clinicopathologic features and differential diagnosis. Arch Pathol Lab Med 2018;142(10):1191–5.

[illegible]

The Hematological Differential Diagnosis of Mediastinal Masses

Ahmed Aljudi, MD*, Elizabeth Weinzierl, MD, PhD, Mohamed Elkhalifa, MD, PhD, Sunita Park, MD

KEYWORDS

- Pediatric mediastinal mass • Hematopathologic differential diagnosis
- Classic Hodgkin lymphoma • T-lymphoblastic leukemia/lymphoma
- Primary mediastinal lymphoma • Thymoma • Non-hematopoietic • Non-neoplastic

KEY POINTS

- Pediatric mediastinal masses are often due to hematologic malignancy.
- Most common pediatric hematologic malignancies in the mediastinum include T-lymphoblastic leukemia/lymphoma, classic Hodgkin lymphoma, and primary mediastinal large B-cell lymphoma.
- Although biopsy of the mediastinal mass is sometimes required, alternate sources such as pleural fluid, peripheral blood, and/or extramediastinal tissue biopsy can help establish the diagnosis.

INTRODUCTION

The timely diagnosis of mediastinal masses in children is of critical importance. Although the mass may produce no symptoms, more commonly at least some respiratory symptoms are present, including dyspnea, cough, or orthopnea, although fatigue, fever, and pain may also be presenting symptoms.[1] Mediastinal masses can present at any age in children, although neural tumors are much more common in very young children (<5 years) and lymphomas and germ cell tumors are more commonly seen in older children.[2]

The differential diagnosis of pediatric mediastinal masses is diverse, and 70% to 75% are malignant.[3] The precise anatomic location of the mass can be very helpful. The anterior mediastinum is often the site of lymphomas, germ cell tumors, and thymic lesions, whereas the posterior mediastinum gives rise more exclusively to neurogenic tumors, which are outside the scope of this review. The middle mediastinum can

A. Aljudi and E. Weinzierl Contributed equally to this work.
Department of Pathology, Children's Healthcare of Atlanta, 1405 Clifton Road Northeast, Tower One, First Floor, Atlanta, GA 30322, USA
* Corresponding author.
E-mail address: ahmed.aljudi@choa.org

Clin Lab Med 41 (2021) 389–404
https://doi.org/10.1016/j.cll.2021.03.011
labmed.theclinics.com

demonstrate general lymphadenopathy from a variety of tumors, or be the site of benign etiologies such as bronchogenic cysts.

The distribution of findings in pediatric mediastinal tumors differs somewhat from that in adults, with most studies demonstrating a predominance of non-Hodgkin lymphoma, classic Hodgkin lymphoma (CHL), and neuroblastoma/ganglioneuromas.[1,4,5] **Table 1** summarizes the distribution of mediastinal biopsy diagnoses at our institution; however, a limitation of this review is that we included direct mediastinal biopsies only, and did not account for diagnoses obtained through other means, such as peripheral lymph nodes, pleural effusions (PE), or extramediastinal tissue biopsies.

PEs can be seen in the setting of mediastinal masses. Among neoplastic causes of PE in children, lymphoma is the most common pediatric malignancy, although other malignancies, including germ cell tumors, neurogenic tumors, and pulmonary neoplasms can also give rise to PEs. T-lymphoblastic leukemia/lymphoma (T-ALL/LBL) is by far the most common malignancy diagnosed by PE alone in the pediatric population.[6,7] In our experience, we have outright made this diagnosis numerous times based solely on pleural fluid. In contrast, although CHL can give rise to a PE, it rarely produces malignant cells in the pleural fluid for diagnosis.[8]

Peripheral blood (PB) flow cytometry can also be helpful if blasts are noted on the smear,[9] but may still be diagnostic even in the absence of morphologic involvement if a small (<1%) suspicious abnormal T-cell population (generally CD7 bright and CD45 dim) is identified (**Fig. 1**); however, we recognize that, for most pathologists, this finding may not suffice to comfortably make an outright diagnosis. Outside of T-ALL/LBL, PB studies in the workup of mediastinal masses are not informative.

Because mediastinal tumors can compress vital structures, sedation can be risky owing to the possibility of cardiopulmonary compromise and, therefore, alternate sources for diagnostic tissue should first be considered, where possible,[10] because these may present with an extramediastinal tumor that is more amenable to biopsy.

In many cases, however, actual tissue biopsy of the mediastinal mass is required for confirmatory diagnosis. There are several approaches to a mediastinal mass biopsy, including video-assisted thoracoscopic surgery, computed tomography (CT)-guided transthoracic needle biopsy, mediastinotomy, and open surgical biopsy. If airway compromise precludes such a biopsy, preoperative treatment with steroids or low-dose localized radiation can be considered; however, a biopsy should be performed as soon as the associated risks are alleviated to decrease the possibility of distorted histomorphologic findings.

Although core biopsies are being performed increasingly, we caution their diagnostic yield, because many mediastinal tumors are associated with fibrosis. For all tissue biopsies of mediastinal masses, we suggest preparing at least 1 air-dried Diff-Quik stained smear/touch imprint and, based on the findings, potentially submitting a small portion for flow cytometry, and the remainder in formalin.

We discuss here the hematopathological differential diagnosis of mediastinal masses in children. For lymphomas covered by other reviews in this journal issue, we mention them briefly and refer the reader to the other reviews for more details.

DISCUSSION

CLASSIC HODGKIN LYMPHOMA

Characterized by the pathognomonic Reed-Sternberg (RS) cells, a clonal neoplastic population reminiscent of late or postgerminal center B cells, CHL is one of the leading causes of a malignant mediastinal mass in the pediatric age group. According to the latest available National Cancer Institute's Surveillance, Epidemiology, and End

Table 1
Mediastinal biopsies performed at Children Healthcare of Atlanta from October 2000 to October 2020 broken down by diagnosis

Pathologic Diagnosis	Number of Cases	Percentage of Total
CHL	33	12.5%
B-cell neoplasms	21	7.9%
Primary mediastinal and diffuse large B-cell lymphomas	17	
Post-transplant lymphoproliferative disorder	2	
Burkitt lymphoma	1	
Gray zone lymphoma	1	
T-cell neoplasms	18	6.8%
T-lymphoblastic lymphoma	16	
Peripheral T-cell lymphoma, NOS	1	
Anaplastic large cell lymphoma, ALK+	1	
Thymic pathology	18	6.8%
Thymoma	5	
Thymic hyperplasia	3	
Lipoma/thymolipoma	3	
Thymic cyst	2	
Nonspecific findings	5	
Neurogenic tumors	37	14.0%
Neuroblastoma	17	
Ganglioneuroma	14	
Ganglioneuroblastoma	3	
Paraganglioma	3	
Myeloid neoplasms	4	1.5%
Teratomas	26	9.8%
Other malignant neoplasms	28	10.5%
Foregut duplication cysts	34	12.8%
Bronchogenic cyst	25	
Esophageal duplication cyst	9	
Granulomatous and fibroblastic lesions	19	7.2%
Granulomas	10	
Inflammatory myofibroblastic tumor	2	
Sclerosing mediastinitis	1	
Other fibroinflammatory lesions	6	
Vascular malformation	5	1.9%
Benign nonspecific pathology	22	8.3%
Total	265	100%

Patient ages ranged from 6 weeks to 20 years of age (average, 11.15 years). Sixty percent were males and 40% were females. Hematologic malignancies accounted for 28.7% of total.

Results Cancer Statistics Review (2013–2017), the incidence is greatest among adolescents aged 15 to 19 years. Children aged 10 to 14, 5 to 9, and 1 to 4 have approximately 3-fold, 8-fold, and 32-fold lower rates, respectively.

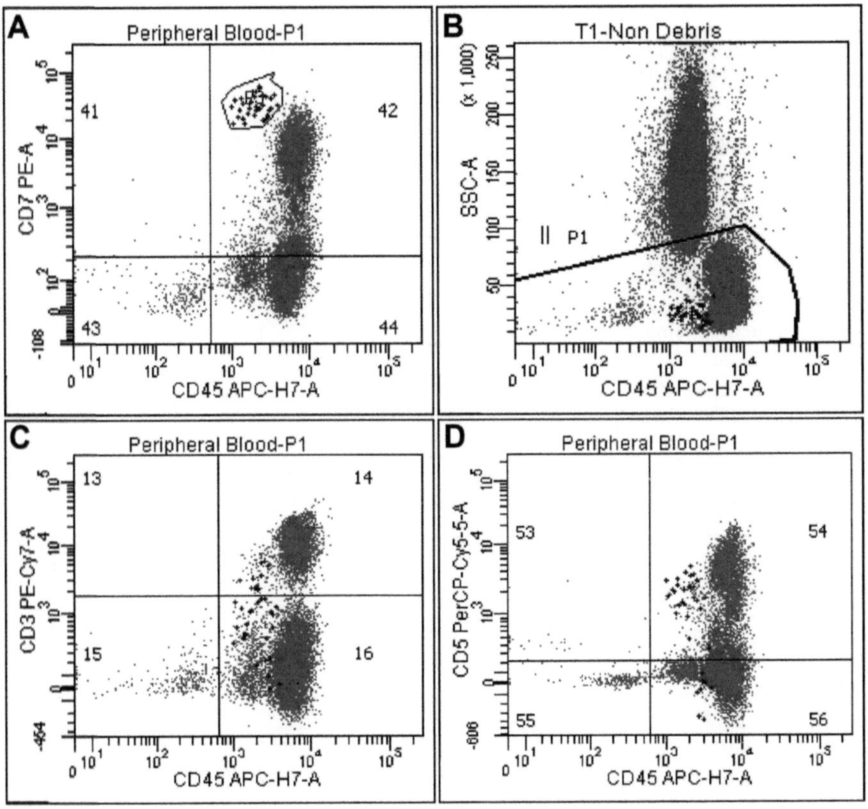

Fig. 1. Minimal PB involvement by T-lymphoblastic leukemia/lymphoma presenting as a large mediastinal mass in a 10-year-old boy. (*A, B*) Flow cytometry of the PB demonstrates a very small (0.08% of total events) CD45 dim population expressing bright CD7. (*C*) This population is negative to dimly positive for surface CD3. (*D*) CD5 is expressed, excluding natural killer cells. Tissue biopsy confirmed the diagnosis.

Although overall childhood cancer mortality decreased by more than 50% between 1975 and 2010; for CHL, the 5-year survival rate has increased from 81% to more than 95% over the same preriod.[11] Nevertheless, the prognosis of relapsed/refractory disease remains dismal.

Most patients present with painless adenopathy, most commonly involving the supraclavicular or cervical area. Mediastinal disease is present in about 75% of adolescents and young adults and may be asymptomatic, although only 35% of young children have mediastinal involvement. B symptoms, which include fatigue, anorexia, weight loss, pruritus, fever, and night sweats, occur in approximately 25% of cases. Fifteen percent to 20% of patients have concomitant extranodal involvement, most commonly in the lung, liver, and/or bone marrow (BM).

The diagnosis of CHL requires a tissue biopsy. Fine needle aspiration cytology alone is not recommended, and flow cytometry is unrevealing. The diagnostic finding is the hallmark uninucleated, binucleated, and multinucleated RS cells (**Fig. 2**) interspersed in a background of inflammatory cells (small lymphocytes, histiocytes, eosinophils, neutrophils, and plasma cells), stromal cells, and vessels. These components are present in different proportions depending on the histologic subtype. RS cells can

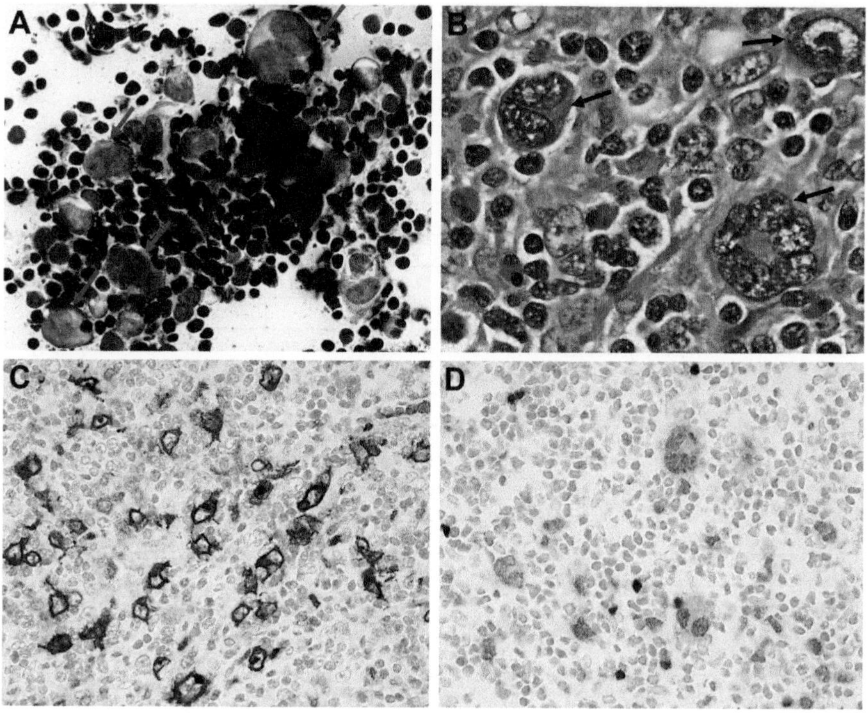

Fig. 2. CHL. (*A*) Touch preparation of a mediastinal mass demonstrating few RS cells (*arrows*) in a background of small lymphocytes and rare eosinophils (variant of Romanowsky stain; original magnification ×600). (*B*) Similar to A in hematoxylin and eosin stain. (*C*) CD30 showing strong membranous and Golgi pattern (original magnification ×400). (*D*) PAX5 showing dim reactivity in RS cells compared to small lymphocytes (original magnification ×400).

occasionally form cohesive aggregates, for which the term syncytial variant has been used. Reactive granuloma formation can also be seen.

By immunohistochemistry, RS cells almost always express CD30 with dim PAX5 and absent CD45. Approximately 75% of cases express at least partial CD15, and up to 40% express heterogeneous CD20. Any deviation from this aggregate immunoprofile should prompt extensive workup to exclude other entities that can have RS-like cells (**Table 2**). Generally, unlike mimics, RS cells do not express typical B-cell markers such as CD19 and CD79a (the latter can be rarely expressed). B-cell transcription factors OCT2 and BOB-1 are typically negative (or positive for one but not both). MUM1 is typically positive, but is nonspecific. Aberrant expression of common T-cell markers by RS cells is uncommon but well-documented. In such instances, PAX5 reactivity is telling. ALK1 is performed judiciously at our institution in CHL workups to completely exclude ALK-positive anaplastic large cell lymphoma, which can very rarely show PAX5 expression.

The 4 subtypes of CHL (from most to least common in children and adolescents) are nodular sclerosis, mixed cellularity, lymphocyte rich, and lymphocyte depleted.

Nodular sclerosis

Nodular sclerosis account for approximately 80% of CHL in older children and adolescents, but only 55% in younger children in the United States.[12] Nodular sclerosis is the

Table 2
Distinguishing features between RS cells of CHL versus other conditions that may harbor RS-like cells[a]

	CHL	NLPHL	PMBCL	THRLBCL[b]	ALK + Anaplastic large cell lymphoma[c]	Reactive Immuno-blasts
CD45	–	+	+	+	+/–	+
CD30	+	–/rarely +	+/–	–/rarely +	+	+
PAX5	+ (dim)	+	+	+	–	+ (– if T)
CD15	+/–	–	–	–	–	–
CD20	–/heterogeneous +	+	+	+	–	+ (– if T)
CD79a	–/rarely +	+	+	+	–	+ (– if T)
OCT2	–/dim focal	+	+	+	–	+ (– if T)
BOB1	–/dim focal	+	+	+	–	+ (– if T)
EMA	–	+/–	–	–/+	+/–	–
MUM1	+	–	+/–	–/+	+	Variable
EBER	–/+	–	–	–	–	– (+in IM)
ALK1	–	–	–	–	+	–
Eosinophils	+/–	–	–	–	–/+	–
T-cell markers	Occasionally +	–	–	–	Most + for at least 1	– (+if T)
PD1+ rosettes	–/+ (lymphocyte-rich)	+	–	–	–	–
Background lymphocytes	Mostly T	Mostly B	Mostly T (if any)	Nearly all T	Variable	Mostly T

Abbreviations: ALCL, anaplastic large cell lymphoma; DLBCL, Diffuse large B-cell lymphoma; IM, infectious mononucleosis; NLPHL, nodular lymphocyte predominant Hodgkin lymphoma; PMBCL, primary mediastinal (thymic) large B-cell lymphoma; THRLBCL, T-cell/histiocyte-rich large B-cell lymphoma.

[a] Gray zone lymphoma (B-cell lymphoma, unclassifiable, with features intermediate between DLBCL and CHL) as well as post-transplant lymphoproliferative disorders (PTLD) are other entities with potential RS-like cells (not presented here).

[b] If EBV-positive then then a diagnosis of EBV-positive DLBCL is warranted.

[c] ALK-negative ALCL is an uncommon occurrence in children. PAX5 reactivity should sway you away from ALCL in most instances, but it can be expressed very rarely. Note that other peripheral T-cell lymphoma subtypes may show RS-like cells but are rare in children.

most common subtype in mediastinal CHL and is characterized by broad fibrocollagenous bands traversing through the tumor forming nodules. The RS cells may exhibit a variant called lacunar cells, an artifact resulting from retraction of the cytoplasmic membrane in formalin-fixed tissue.

Mixed cellularity

Mixed cellularity is more common in young children than in adolescents and young adults, accounting for approximately 20% of patients younger than 10, but approximately 9% of patients aged 10 to 19 years in the United States.[12] Mediastinal involvement is uncommon. It is characterized by frequent more classic appearing RS cells in a background of abundant reactive inflammatory cells. Epstein–Barr virus (EBV) positivity is most common in this subtype.

Lymphocyte rich

Lymphocyte-rich CHL may have a nodular appearance and may be difficult to distinguish from nodular lymphocyte predominant Hodgkin lymphoma and T-cell/histiocyte-rich large B-cell lymphoma, but immunohistochemistry can readily resolve this differential (see **Table 2**). Notably, this subtype can also show PD1–positive T cells forming rosettes around RS cells, similar to those seen in nodular lymphocyte predominant Hodgkin lymphoma.[13] Moreover, a parafollicular or interfollicular pattern may be seen with mostly preserved nodal architecture, making it difficult to differentiate from immunoblasts in reactive LNs, especially in limited biopsies. The absent eosinophils and neutrophils complicate matters further.

Lymphocyte depleted

Lymphocyte-depleted CHL is rare in children (common in HIV+ adults), characterized by numerous large, bizarre malignant cells and few lymphocytes, and can be difficult to initially distinguish from diffuse large B-cell lymphoma (DLBCL), anaplastic large cell lymphoma, and even sarcoma.

BM involvement is relatively rare in pediatric CHL; hence, bilateral BM biopsy has extremely low yield and may be unnecessary. Moreover, PET-CT scanning has been shown to have a high sensitivity (96.9%) and specificity (99.7%) in detecting BM involvement.[14] Adverse prognostic factors include advanced stage, bulky disease (especially mediastinal), male sex, B symptoms, effusions (pericardial/pleural), and hypoalbuminemia. With contemporary treatment protocols, EBV status, and histologic subtype mostly have no significant prognostic value.

The initial response to chemotherapy by PET-CT scan also seems to be important prognostically. However, using risk stratification methods at the time of diagnosis, such as the Childhood Hodgkin International Prognostic Score, for choosing limited versus augmented treatment regimens (instead of early response assessment by imaging) may allow earlier intervention and decrease costs.[15]

Targeted therapies are being investigated in several clinical trials, mostly for high-risk as well as relapsed or refractory disease. Examples of these targeted therapies include brentuximab vedotin (anti-CD30 antibody–drug conjugate), bortezomib (indirect nuclear factor-κB pathway activation inhibitor), nivolumab (monoclonal antibody, PD1 receptor blocker), and T-cell therapies including CD30-directed chimeric antigen receptor T cells as well as (CAR) T cells directed against EBV antigens, specifically for EBV-positive CHL.[16,17]

PRIMARY MEDIASTINAL (THYMIC) LARGE B-CELL LYMPHOMA AND GRAY ZONE LYMPHOMA (B-CELL LYMPHOMA, UNCLASSIFIABLE, WITH FEATURES INTERMEDIATE BETWEEN DIFFUSE LARGE B-CELL LYMPHOMA AND CLASSIC HODGKIN LYMPHOMA)

Primary mediastinal (thymic) large B-cell lymphoma (PMBCL) was previously considered a subtype of DLBCL, then acknowledged as a separate entity in the 2008 World Health Organization classification, because it was shown to have a distinct gene expression profile that is closer to CHL. As the name implies, it arises in the mediastinum from thymic B cells and shows a diffuse large-cell proliferation (**Fig. 3**). The tumor can be invasive locally and can be associated with superior vena cava syndrome. It can also rarely disseminate outside the thoracic cavity with nodal and extranodal involvement, with a predilection to the kidneys, liver, and brain. BM involvement is exceedingly rare.[13] PMBCL is typically encountered in young adults with a female predominance.

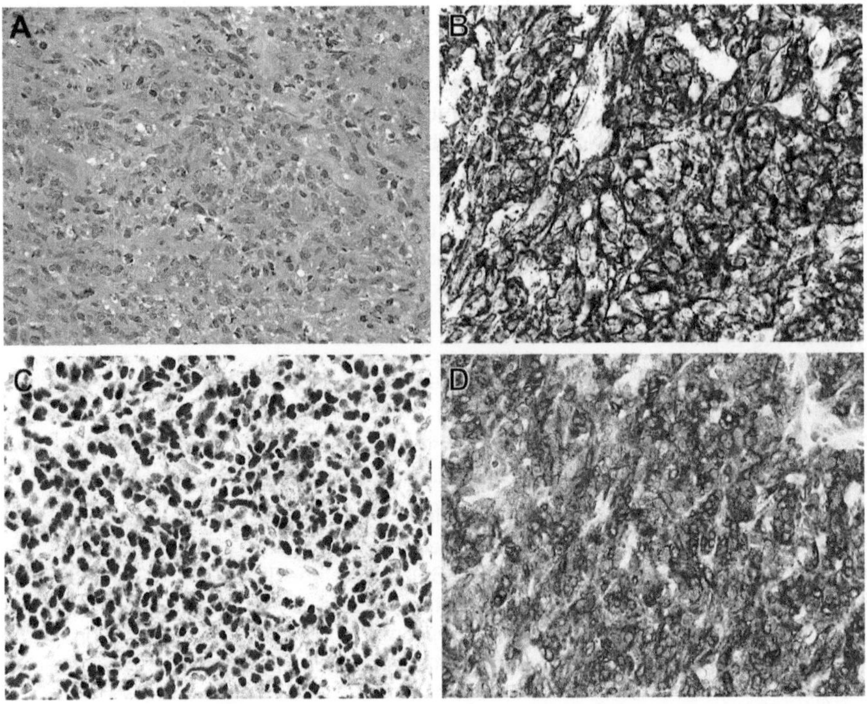

Fig. 3. Primary mediastinal (thymic) large B-cell lymphoma. (*A*) Sheets of large cells shaped by delicate collagenous fibrosis (stain: hematoxylin and eosin; original magnification ×400). (*B*) CD20 (original magnification ×400). (*C*) PAX5 (original magnification ×400). (*D*) CD30 (original magnification ×400).

It occasionally occurs in adolescents but is rare in young children. Analysis of the National Cancer Institute's Surveillance, Epidemiology, and End Results cancer statistics review (2008–2017) shows a total of 73 cases in the 0 to 19 age group.

This entity can be difficult to distinguish from systemic DLBCL with secondary mediastinal involvement. The malignant cells typically display nonspecific findings such as clear cytoplasm, background compartmentalizing sclerosis, frequent expression of CD23 and CD30 by immunohistochemistry, and mostly absent surface immunoglobulin light chain expression by flow cytometry. Because these features can also be seen in DLBCL, the bulk of resolving this differential relies on clinical and imaging findings.

There is no single standard of care for frontline PMBCL treatment owing to paucity of data. Because it is lumped in the category of aggressive mature B-cell lymphomas, it has been historically treated similar to DLBCL and Burkitt; however, clinical trial outcomes have been inferior in PMBCL. Thus, a DA-EPOCH-R regimen is preferred by many centers in the United States.

RS-like cells can be seen in PMBCL; however, the differential with CHL can be resolved by immunohistochemistry in most cases, because PMBCL shows a preserved B-cell program (see **Table 2**). Instances where an extensive workup is equivocal or overlapping may warrant a diagnosis of gray zone lymphoma (**Fig. 4**), which is very rare in children, has a male predilection, and portends a worse prognosis than either PMBCL or CHL alone. A diagnosis of gray zone lymphoma is usually not warranted if suggested by only 1 marker, or if the bulk of the disease is outside the mediastinum, especially in children. Cases of composite (concurrent) CHL and PMBCL, as well as cases of

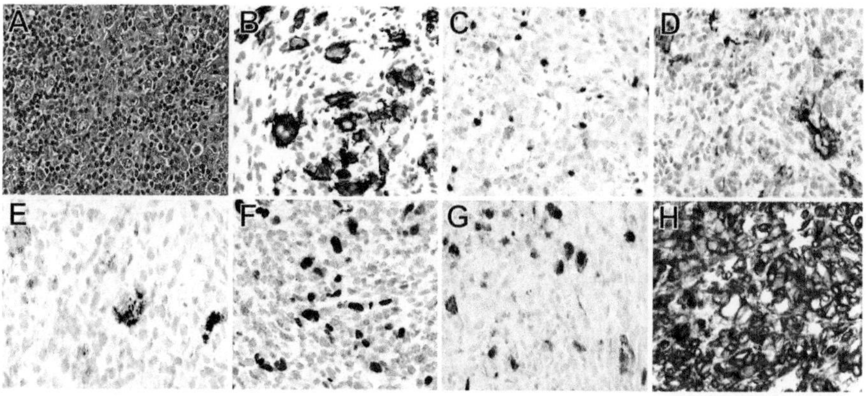

Fig. 4. Mediastinal mass in a 19-year-old man consistent with gray zone lymphoma. (*A*) Frequent large RS–like cells (stain: hematoxylin and eosin; 400) showing strong CD20 (*B*; original magnification ×400), very dim PAX5 (*C*; original magnification ×400), positive CD30 (*D*; original magnification ×400), positive CD15 in at least a subset (*E*; original magnification ×600), strong OCT2 (*F*; original magnification ×400), and strong BOB1 (*G*; original magnification ×400). CD45 is difficult to interpret but appears positive in the large cells (*H*; original magnification ×600). CD79a is also positive (not shown).

sequential (consecutive) CHL and PMBCL are not strictly accepted as examples of gray zone lymphoma, but are thought to be biologically related phenomena.[13] EBV positivity essentially excludes PMBCL and (for the most part) gray zone lymphoma, and points toward CHL or EBV-positive DLBCL. Notably, the latter usually shows a T-cell/histiocyte-rich large B-cell lymphoma-like (rather than a sheet-like) pattern in children.[18]

T-LYMPHOBLASTIC LEUKEMIA/LYMPHOMA

T-ALL/LBL is a neoplasm of immature T lineage cells, and represents approximately 15% of all pediatric ALLs.[13] Presentation as a mediastinal mass is common, as the normal counterpart to T-lymphoblasts, normal thymocytes, reside, and mature in the thymus. The classic presentation of T-LBL is an anterior mediastinal mass in an adolescent boy and is often accompanied by PE. The optimal specimen for diagnosis is either PB or pleural fluid, because sampling the mediastinal mass is not only invasive, but maturing thymocytes of a thymoma may mimic T-ALL/LBL.[19] If PB flow cytometry is unrevealing, cytology with flow cytometry of the pleural fluid can often yield a diagnostic result.

Although T lymphoblasts can rarely morphologically resemble mature lymphocytes, they typically range from small to large in size with scant agranular basophilic cytoplasm, a high nuclear to cytoplasmic ratio, irregular nuclear contours, condensed or dispersed chromatin, and occasionally small nucleoli. These blasts diffusely infiltrate the tissue in monomorphic sheets, and show frequent mitotic figures (**Fig. 5**). By flow cytometry the blasts express cytoplasmic CD3, and may express CD1a, CD2, surface CD3 (often dim), CD4, CD5, CD7, CD8, CD10, CD38, TDT, and dim to moderate CD45. The expression of CD7 is often the same as or brighter than normal T cells. The expression of myeloperoxidase is always absent.

Pitfalls in the sampling of a mediastinal mass to diagnose T-ALL/LBL include normal thymus and thymoma. Differentiating flow cytometry and immunohistochemical features are described in more detail in the following "Thymic lesions" section.

T-ALL/LBL is discussed in greater detail in the article "Update on lymphoblastic lymphoma/leukemia" in this issue.

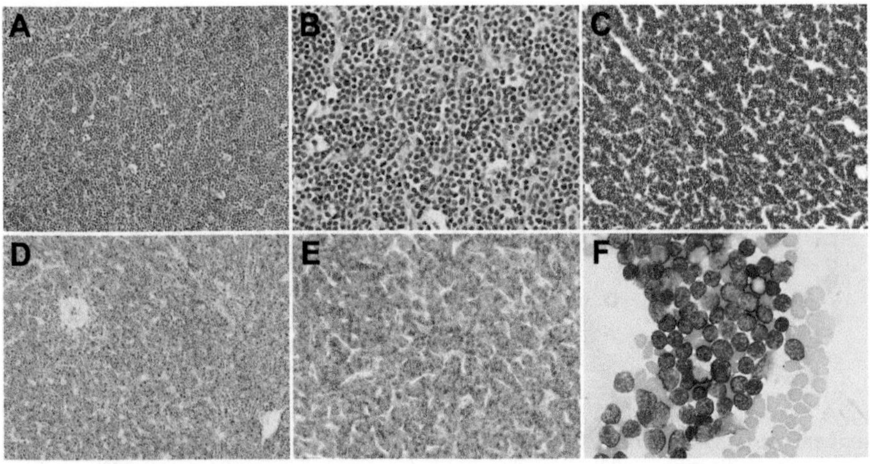

Fig. 5. T-lymphoblastic leukemia/lymphoma. (*A*) Low-power image (original magnification ×200) demonstrating diffuse effacement by monomorphic lymphoid cells (stain: hematoxylin and eosin). (*B*) High power (original magnification ×500) showing frequent mitotic figures (*arrows*) (stain: hematoxylin and eosin). (*C–E*) Immunohistochemistry positive for CD3 (*C*), TDT (*D*), and CD1a (*E*), confirming an immature T lymphoid immunophenotype. (*F*) Wright-Giemsa stain of the pleural fluid (original magnification ×1000).

THYMIC LESIONS

Thymic lesions are rare in children, but can present as anterior mediastinal masses. Such lesions include thymic cysts, thymic hyperplasia, thymolipomas, and thymomas (see **Table 1**). Thymic cysts are relatively easy to identify histologically, because they are epithelial lined cysts involving the thymus and may be unilocular or multilocular. Thymolipomas are mass forming lesions composed of well-circumscribed mature adipose tissue in the setting of histologically unremarkable thymus. Thymic hyperplasia results in an increase in thymic size, but otherwise the thymic histology is normal.

Thymomas account for less than 1% of pediatric mediastinal masses, and our experience reinforces this rarity; we have only seen a few cases in the past 20 years. In addition to symptoms associated with an enlarging mediastinal mass, thymomas can also cause paraneoplastic syndromes, although this association is rarer in children than it is with adults.[20] In some cases, a chest CT scan can indicate the diagnosis without a biopsy.

Thymomas in children can be either benign or malignant, with estimates in the literature essentially equal between the 2 entities. The World Health Organization histologic classification is the most commonly used system, which classifies thymomas into the A-B3 nomenclature based on the proportions of polygonal shaped epithelial cells and immature T cells. Thymomas are generally staged through the modified Masaoka–Koga system, based on invasion and metastatic status.

Thymoma can be morphologically difficult to distinguish from T-ALL/LBL, especially in core biopsies in which only a small fraction of the mass is sampled. Helpful distinguishing features include the presence of the cytokeratin network in thymomas, which can be demonstrated with numerous stains, such as pancytokeratin, CK5/6, p40, and p63, among others, as well as flow cytometry of the lesion. The immature T cells of thymoma generally coexpress CD4 and CD8 with a tapering smear into smaller populations of CD4 and CD8-only thymocytes (**Fig. 6**). Additionally, immature thymocytes can be divided into 3 stages, similar to the 3 hematogone stages of B-cell development, with the earliest expressing dim CD45, CD10, and CD34, but negative for CD1a and surface

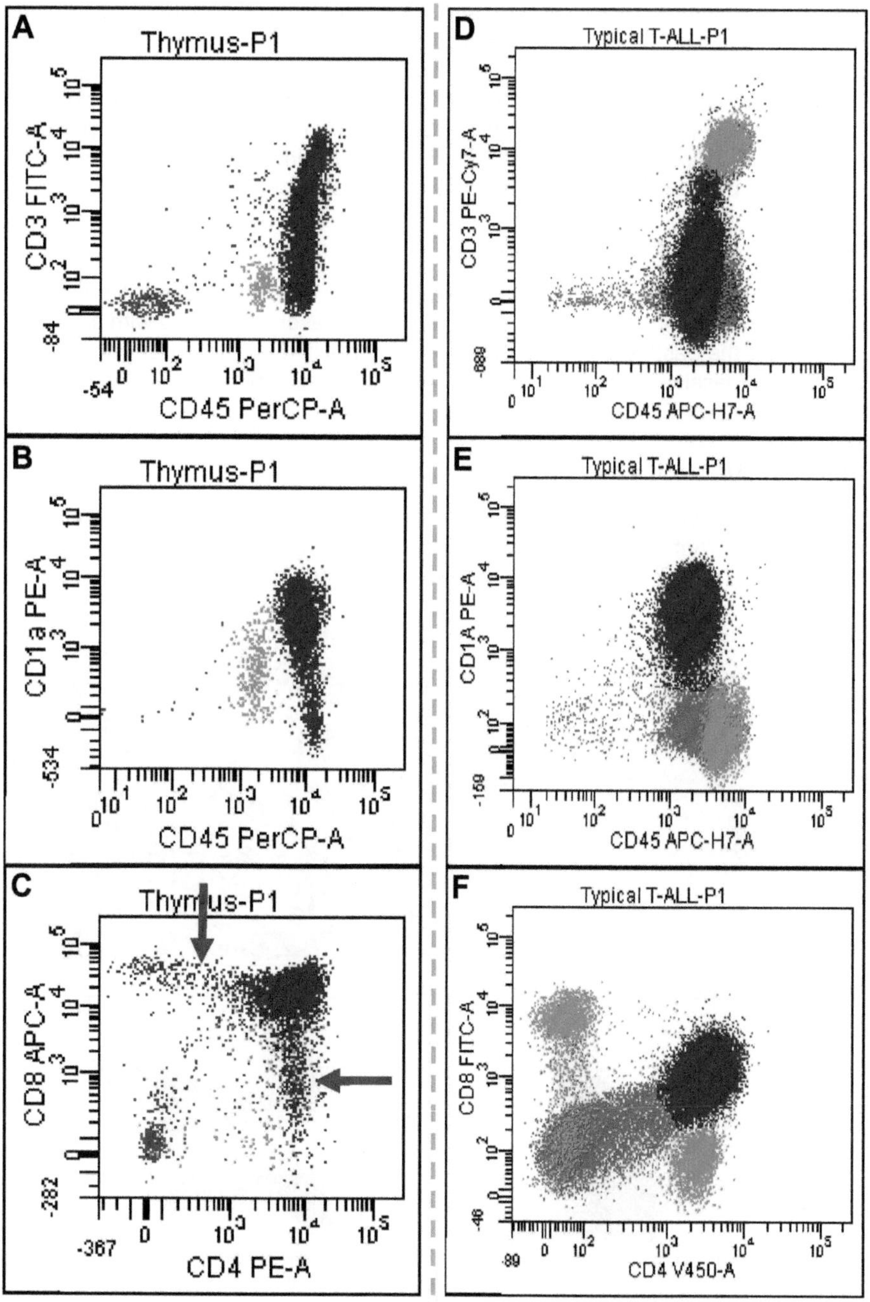

Fig. 6. Normal thymus (left) versus T-lymphoblastic leukemia/lymphoma (right) flow cytometry. (*A–C*) Normal thymus demonstrates a characteristic 3-stage maturation pattern with early thymocytes in green, cortical thymocytes in blue, and more mature lymphocytes in purple. Note the "smear" pattern on *C* as the cortical thymocytes mature into either CD4 or CD8 positive T cells (*arrows*). (*D–F*) T-ALL/LBL shows T-lymphoblasts (blue) lacking the smear pattern (*F*). Background normal T-cells are in green.

CD3. The next stage is most populous and demonstrates intermediate CD45 with heterogeneous surface CD3 and CD1a expression, without CD10 or CD34. The third stage expresses brightest CD45 and surface CD3, with normal density of other T-cell markers.[19] In contrast, malignant T lymphoblasts generally display a tight cluster of immunoreactivity without the CD4/CD8 smearing pattern seen in immature thymocytes (see **Fig. 6**), and also can demonstrate aberrant T-cell marker intensity.[19] A typical type B1 thymoma biopsied from a pediatric patient is presented in **Fig. 7**.

ANAPLASTIC LARGE CELL LYMPHOMA

Anaplastic large cell lymphoma can rarely present with mediastinal lymph node enlargement. In our institution, we have seen only 2 cases presenting with a mediastinal mass in the past 20 years (**Fig. 8**). Both patients had significant effusions; 1 patient had a massive pericardial effusion without observable tumor cells, and the other had a large PE containing numerous tumor cells.

OTHER HEMATOLOGIC MALIGNANCIES

Peripheral T-cell lymphomas, EBV-positive large B-cell lymphoma, Burkitt lymphoma, and post-transplant lymphoproliferative disorders can rarely present with mediastinal masses in children. Those entities are covered by other reviews in this journal issue.

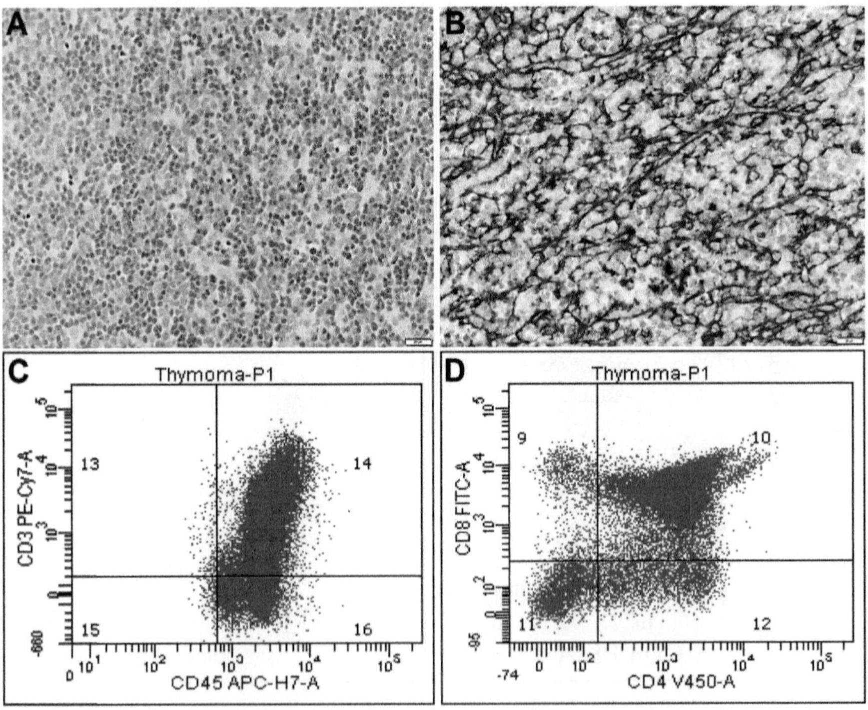

Fig. 7. Core biopsy of an anterior mediastinal mass demonstrating a proliferation of immature appearing lymphoid cells (*A*) (stain: hematoxylin and eosin; original magnification ×400). Pancytokeratin immunostain highlighting occasional epithelial cells as well as a rich cytokeratin network (*B*; original magnification ×400). Flow cytometry demonstrates varying levels of surface CD3 and CD45 expression (*C*) as well as tapering of the CD4/CD8 double-positive population into smaller populations of CD4 and CD8-only thymocytes (*D*).

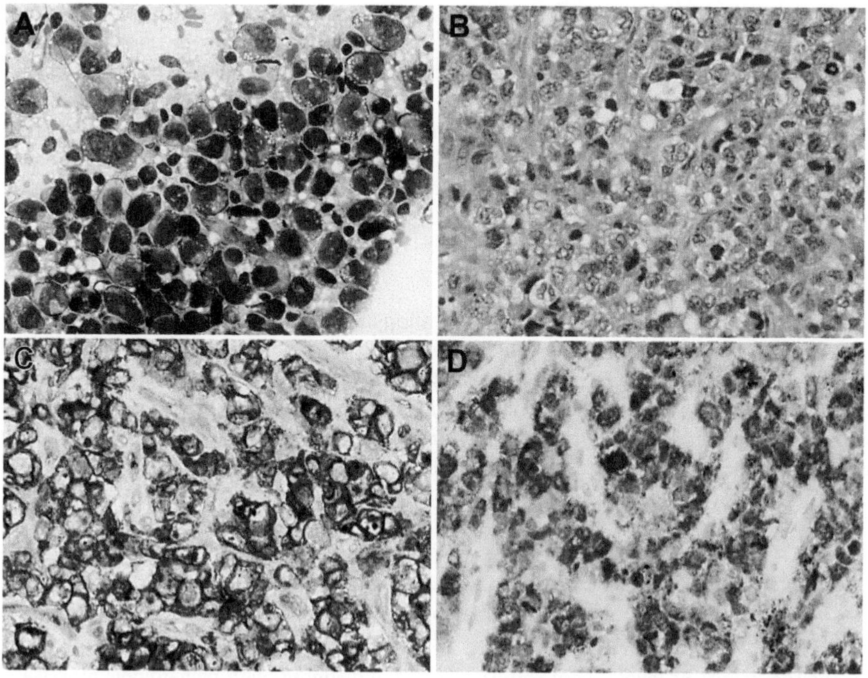

Fig. 8. Anaplastic large cell lymphoma, ALK positive. (*A*) Touch preparation of a mediastinal mass demonstrating sheets of large cells, some with hallmark morphology (variant of Romanowsky stain; original magnification ×400). (*B*) Histologic section demonstrating diffuse large anaplastic cells with vesicular nuclei and ample cytoplasm (stain: hematoxylin and eosin; original magnification ×400). (*C*) CD30 demonstrating strong membranous and Golgi immunoreactivity (original magnification ×400). (*D*) ALK immunostain demonstrating strong nuclear and cytoplasmic immunoreactivity original magnification ×400).

BENIGN MEDIASTINAL LESIONS

Overall, non-neoplastic mediastinal lesions represented 35% of all mediastinal biopsies performed at our institution during the past 20 years, with foregut duplication cysts representing the majority (see **Table 1**). Chronic mediastinitis accounted for approximately 7%, with one-half of the cases representing necrotizing granulomatous inflammation. Although an infectious etiology was suspected, special stains for

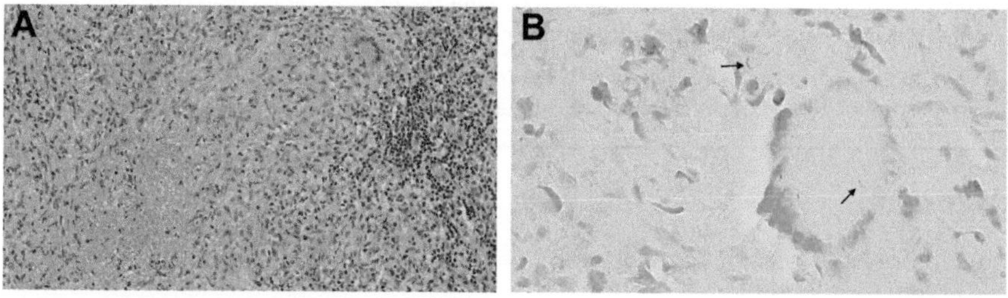

Fig. 9. Mediastinal lymph node biopsy from a 3-month-old girl. (*A*) Caseating granuloma with a multinucleated giant cell (stain: hematoxylin and eosin; original magnification ×200). (*B*) AFB stain demonstrating rare acid-fast bacilli (*arrows*) (original magnification ×1000).

microorganisms failed to pinpoint any except for 2 cases, where rare acid-fast bacilli were identified (**Fig. 9**). Tuberculous mediastinal lymphadenitis is usually seen in immunocompromised children[21] and in patients from developing countries. The differential diagnosis of mediastinal granulomata should also include Histoplasmosis, especially in endemic regions.[22] Regardless of the etiology, these granulomas may become fibrotic and calcified. Variable degrees of mediastinal fibrosis, including sclerosing mediastinitis, may occur as a secondary host response to the granulomatous inflammation.[23]

SUMMARY

Mediastinal masses are a common presentation in children, and may arise owing to a variety of neoplastic and non-neoplastic causes, with hematologic causes being more common in the anterior and middle mediastinum. The most common lymphomas are classic Hodgkin lymphoma, T-lymphoblastic leukemia/lymphoma, and primary mediastinal (thymic) large B-cell lymphoma. Correlation of morphology with flow cytometry and/or immunohistochemistry is essential in establishing the correct diagnosis.

CLINICS CARE POINTS

- Mediastinal masses are common presentations in children, and may present with respiratory symptoms owing to airway compression.
- The specific site of involvement correlates with the diagnosis, with hematologic processes occurring in the anterior and middle mediastinum, and neurogenic tumors occurring in the posterior mediastinum.
- For all fresh tissue biopsies of mediastinal masses, we suggest triaging the sample with a Diff-Quik stained smear/touch imprint.
- The most common type of lymphomas to involve the mediastinum are CHL, T-LBL, and PMBCL.
- CHL shows Hodgkin and RS cells, with an immunophenotype that is, positive for CD30, PAX-5 (weak), and CD15 (majority), but negative for CD3, CD45, and ALK-1. CD20, if expressed, is heterogenous. The common subtypes are nodular sclerosis and mixed cellularity.
- PMBCL must be differentiated from systemic DLBCL with mediastinal involvement, which is best done by clinical and imaging data.
- PB or PE flow cytometry may be diagnostic in T-ALL/LBL and may prevent invasive sampling of the mediastinal mass.
- A pitfall when a mediastinal mass is sampled is to overcall normal thymocytes or benign thymocytes in a thymoma as T-LBL. Understanding the differences by flow cytometry is essential, and demonstration of cytokeratin networks may be helpful in thymomas.
- Benign and infectious conditions, such as granulomatous mediastinitis, also occur in the mediastinum, with foregut duplication cysts as the most common in our experience.

DISCLOSURE

The authors have nothing to disclose.

REFERENCES

1. Gun F, Erginel B, Unuvar A, et al. Mediastinal masses in children: experience with 120 cases. Pediatr Hematol Oncol 2012;29(2):141–7.

2. Liu T, Al-Kzayer LFY, Xie X, et al. Mediastinal lesions across the age spectrum: a clinicopathological comparison between pediatric and adult patients. Oncotarget 2017;8(35):59845–53.
3. Verma SK, Kaushal, Rastogi S, et al. Clinical approach to childhood mediastinal tumors and management. Mediastinum 2020;4(21).
4. Freud E, Ben-Ari J, Schonfeld T, et al. Mediastinal tumors in children: a single institution experience. Clin Pediatr (Phila) 2002;41(4):219–23.
5. Simpson I, Campbell PE. Mediastinal masses in childhood: a review from a paediatric pathologist's point of view. Prog Pediatr Surg 1991;27:92–126.
6. Patel T, Patel P, Mehta S, et al. The value of cytology in diagnosis of serous effusions in malignant lymphomas: an experience of a tertiary care center. Diagn Cytopathol 2019;47(8):776–82.
7. Das DK. Serous effusions in malignant lymphomas: a review. Diagn Cytopathol 2006;34(5):335–47.
8. McCarten KM, Nadel HR, Shulkin BL, et al. Imaging for diagnosis, staging and response assessment of Hodgkin lymphoma and non-Hodgkin lymphoma. Pediatr Radiol 2019;49(11):1545–64.
9. Malik R, Mullassery D, Kleine-Brueggeney M, et al. Anterior mediastinal masses - a multidisciplinary pathway for safe diagnostic procedures. J Pediatr Surg 2019; 54(2):251–4.
10. Anghelescu DL, Burgoyne LL, Liu T, et al. Clinical and diagnostic imaging findings predict anesthetic complications in children presenting with malignant mediastinal masses. Paediatr Anaesth 2007;17(11):1090–8.
11. Smith MA, Altekruse SF, Adamson PC, et al. Declining childhood and adolescent cancer mortality. Cancer 2014;120(16):2497–506.
12. Bazzeh F, Rihani R, Howard S, et al. Comparing adult and pediatric Hodgkin lymphoma in the surveillance, epidemiology and end results program, 1988-2005: an analysis of 21 734 cases. Leuk Lymphoma 2010;51(12):2198–207.
13. Swerdlow SH, Campo E, Harris NL, et al. WHO classification of tumours of haematopoietic and lymphoid tissues. Lyon (France): IARC; 2017.
14. Adams HJ, Kwee TC, de Keizer B, et al. Systematic review and meta-analysis on the diagnostic performance of FDG-PET/CT in detecting bone marrow involvement in newly diagnosed Hodgkin lymphoma: is bone marrow biopsy still necessary? Ann Oncol 2014;25(5):921–7.
15. Schwartz CL, Chen L, McCarten K, et al. Childhood Hodgkin international prognostic Score (CHIPS) predicts event-free survival in Hodgkin lymphoma: a report from the Children's Oncology Group. Pediatr Blood Cancer 2017;64(4). https://doi.org/10.1002/pbc.26278.
16. Nagpal P, Akl MR, Ayoub NM, et al. Pediatric Hodgkin lymphoma: biomarkers, drugs, and clinical trials for translational science and medicine. Oncotarget 2016;7(41):67551–73.
17. Munz C. Redirecting T cells against Epstein-Barr virus infection and associated oncogenesis. Cells 2020;9(6):1400.
18. Nicolae A, Pittaluga S, Abdullah S, et al. EBV-positive large B-cell lymphomas in young patients: a nodal lymphoma with evidence for a tolerogenic immune environment. Blood 2015;126(7):863–72.
19. Li S, Juco J, Mann KP, et al. Flow cytometry in the differential diagnosis of lymphocyte-rich thymoma from precursor T-cell acute lymphoblastic leukemia/lymphoblastic lymphoma. Am J Clin Pathol 2004;121(2):268–74.
20. Saha S, Suhani S, Basak A, et al. Pediatric thymoma with a difference: report of a case and review of literature. J Surg Tech Case Rep 2014;6(2):64–6.

21. De Wet DR, Wright CA, Schubert PT, et al. Mediastinal granulomatous lymphadenitis in a population at risk for HIV and tuberculosis. Diagn Cytopathol 2015;43(9):696–700.
22. Demkowicz R, Procop GW. Clinical significance and histologic characterization of histoplasma granulomas. Am J Clin Pathol 2020;155(4):581–7.
23. Mole TM, Glover J, Sheppard MN. Sclerosing mediastinitis: a report on 18 cases. Thorax 1995;50(3):280–3.

Update on Lymphoblastic Leukemia/Lymphoma

Dragoş C. Luca, MD

KEYWORDS

• Lymphoblastic leukemia • Lymphoblastic lymphoma • Pediatric leukemia

KEY POINTS

- Most lymphoblastic leukemias show a B-cell phenotype, whereas most lymphoblastic lymphomas are of T-lymphoid origin.
- Morphologically, distinguishing between B and T lymphoblasts is virtually impossible; therefore, immunophenotypic analysis is required for diagnosis.
- The classification of B-lymphoblastic processes relies heavily on genetic and/or molecular findings, unlike T-lymphoblastic processes, which are not subclassified based on such criteria.
- Cytogenetic abnormalities in B-lymphoblastic leukemia have major prognostic implications; however, early response to therapy remains the most important outcome indicator.

INTRODUCTION

Lymphoblastic neoplastic processes include lymphoblastic leukemias as well as lymphoblastic lymphomas (LBLs) and represent clonal proliferations of lymphoid precursors of generally B-cell or T-cell derivation even though, rarely, natural killer (NK) phenotype might be observed. In general, if a lymphoblastic neoplasm presents in the form of acute leukemia, the likelihood of B-lymphoid origin is significantly higher (80%–85%) compared with T-cell derivation (10%–15%), whereas the opposite is true in cases with lymphomatous presentation. The distinction between leukemia and lymphoma is generally based on the degree of peripheral blood and/or bone marrow involvement. If the initial diagnosis is based on peripheral blood and/or bone marrow, a threshold of 20% is recommended by the World Health Organization (WHO) and the term acute lymphoblastic leukemia (ALL) is used; however, if the malignant process shows exclusively or predominantly tissue involvement, then the term LBL is preferred.[1] The situation becomes slightly more complicated if both tissue and bone marrow/blood involvement are present. As a rule of thumb, if the initial diagnosis is that of LBL and subsequent bone marrow analysis performed usually for staging purposes shows no or limited involvement, the diagnosis remains LBL; however, if significant involvement is present, the diagnosis becomes lymphoblastic leukemia. The

Children's National Health System, 111 Michigan Avenue Northwest, Washington, DC 20010, USA
E-mail address: d-luca@msn.com

Clin Lab Med 41 (2021) 405–416
https://doi.org/10.1016/j.cll.2021.04.003

threshold between limited and significant is arbitrary and is generally set at a value of 25% given that patients with LBL accompanied by bone marrow involvement that is greater than 25% do better with leukemia rather than lymphoma therapy protocols.[2]

TERMINOLOGY

Historically, the terms precursor B-cell lymphoblastic leukemia/lymphoma and precursor T-cell lymphoblastic leukemia/lymphoma have been used. Beginning with the fourth edition of its *Classification of Tumours of Haematopoietic and Lymphoid Tissues*, the WHO recommended a simplified nomenclature, B-lymphoblastic leukemia/lymphoma (B-ALL/LBL) and T-lymphoblastic leukemia/lymphoma (T-ALL/LBL), respectively.[1] Given the inherently precursor character of lymphoblasts as immature lymphoid elements, the word precursor was considered redundant.[2] Also, even though Burkitt lymphoma previously designated as L3 by the now-obsolete French American British (FAB) classification was excluded from this category, there are still rare cases of bona fide B-ALL with light-chain production and lack of blast markers that are sometimes referred to as mature B-ALL where the neoplastic cells have moved past the purely precursor stage. In addition, this particular word, besides being superfluous, introduced a certain degree of confusion because most health care professionals used the term pre–B-ALL as if pre were an abbreviation for precursor, whereas this prefix actually had a more specific meaning, indicating a certain degree of maturity along the immature spectrum of early precursor, common precursor, and pre–B-ALL. Moreover, the word acute can also be considered redundant because a lymphoblastic process implies rapid progression and therefore it is virtually impossible for it to behave in a chronic manner. In contrast, even though the word acute does not appear in the official name anymore, it is still present, in a manner of speaking, in the abbreviation (ALL).

CLASSIFICATION

The modern classification of lymphoblastic leukemia relies heavily on genetic and molecular abnormalities associated with variable immunophenotypes and sometimes, even though rarely, with distinct morphologic features. These recurrent abnormalities are frequently strong predictors of clinical behavior, including response to therapy as well as long-term prognosis.[1] However, these statements are mostly applicable to B-ALL and to a much lesser extent in the case of T-ALL, which is not currently subclassified function of various genetic and/or molecular abnormalities. **Box 1** summarizes these categories based on the WHO classification, including prognostic notes.

Lymphoblastic leukemias are predominantly diseases of the pediatric population. The most common cancer of childhood is leukemia, and the most frequent leukemia in terms of timeline is acute leukemia, and the most common acute leukemia function of phenotype is ALL; furthermore, the most common type of ALL is B-ALL. Approximately 80% of childhood acute leukemias are lymphoblastic but only 20% of adult acute leukemias show immature lymphoid lineage. The majority of cases (~75%) occur before the age of 6 years.[1–3]

B-LYMPHOBLASTIC LEUKEMIA/LYMPHOMA

B-ALL/LBL is a neoplasm of precursor B cells, also known as B lymphoblasts. Most ALL cases are of B-cell lineage (80%–85%). Clinically, B-ALL shows frequent extramedullary tissue involvement, including the central nervous system (CNS), lymph nodes, spleen, liver, and testes.[3] In contrast, its LBL counterpart tends to show predilection for skin, soft tissue, bone, and sometimes lymph nodes.[4] The patients

Box 1
Classification of lymphoblastic leukemia/lymphoma

B-lymphoblastic leukemia/lymphoma
- B-lymphoblastic leukemia/lymphoma, not otherwise specified (NOS)
- B-lymphoblastic leukemia/lymphoma with recurrent genetic abnormalities:
  - * B-lymphoblastic leukemia/lymphoma with t(12;21) (p13.2;q22.1); *ETV6-RUNX1*
  - * B-lymphoblastic leukemia/lymphoma with hyperdiploidy
  - † B-lymphoblastic leukemia/lymphoma with t(9;22) (q34.1;q11.2); *BCR-ABL1*
  - † B-lymphoblastic leukemia/lymphoma with t(v;11q23.3); *KMT2A*-rearranged
  - † B-lymphoblastic leukemia/lymphoma with hypodiploidy
  - † B-lymphoblastic leukemia/lymphoma, *BCR-ABL1*–like
  - † B-lymphoblastic leukemia/lymphoma with iAMP21
  - ‡ B-lymphoblastic leukemia/lymphoma with t(1;19) (q23;p13.3); *TCF3-PBX1*
  - ○ B-lymphoblastic leukemia/lymphoma with t(5;14) (q31.1;q32.1); *IGH/IL3*
- B-lymphoblastic leukemia/lymphoma with newly described oncogenic fusions (unofficial)
- B-lymphoblastic leukemia/lymphoma with other significant mutations (unofficial)

T-lymphoblastic leukemia/lymphoma
- T-lymphoblastic leukemia/lymphoma, NOS
  §Early T-cell precursor lymphoblastic leukemia

NK-lymphoblastic leukemia/lymphoma

*, favorable; †, unfavorable; ‡, intermediate; ○, probably indifferent; §, debatable.

frequently present with nonspecific findings, including fever, fatigue, lack of appetite, and weight loss; however, other findings may be more worrisome and those are usually represented by localized or generalized lymphadenopathy, hepatosplenomegaly, and bone pain. The peripheral blood shows 1 or more cytopenias (frequently thrombocytopenia) but the white blood cell (WBC) count may be variable and range from leukopenia with few or no circulating blasts to marked leukocytosis with numerous circulating blasts. Morphologically, the classic appearance of lymphoblasts, irrespective of lineage, is described as small to medium-sized cells with very high nucleocytoplasmic ratio, slightly irregular and frequently notched or cleaved nuclear contour, finely dispersed chromatin, visible but generally inconspicuous nucleoli, and a minimal amount of basophilic cytoplasm with variable vacuolization and no significant granularity. Auer rods are never present. The lymphoblast morphology is generally similar in peripheral blood and bone marrow; however, the presence of blasts with unipolar cytoplasmic pseudopod (uropod) formation (so-called hand-mirror cells) is usually easier to appreciate in aspirate smears (**Fig. 1**A, B). The morphologic and even immunophenotypic distinction between leukemic B lymphoblasts and hematogones (normal B-cell precursors) may be particularly difficult. Hematogones usually show very homogeneous purple chromatin without visible nucleoli. By flow cytometry, unlike B lymphoblasts, they show a spectrum of maturation without marker aberrancy.[2] The morphologic distinction is frequently unreliable even with the use of immunohistochemistry and therefore is not recommended. In core biopsy sections, the presence of increased numbers of cluster of differentiation (CD) 19–positive and terminal deoxynucleotidyl transferase (TdT)–positive cells may be a cause of concern for residual disease. Hematogones, even when increased, tend to be uniformly distributed within the marrow space, whereas leukemic blasts are usually clustered or in sheets; however, this distinction is unreliable and should not be used in lieu of flow cytometry. Lymphoblastic leukemia tends to show extensive involvement of the bone marrow space and consequently marked reduction of the residual normal trilineage hematopoiesis. The core biopsy is virtually 100% cellular most of the time and

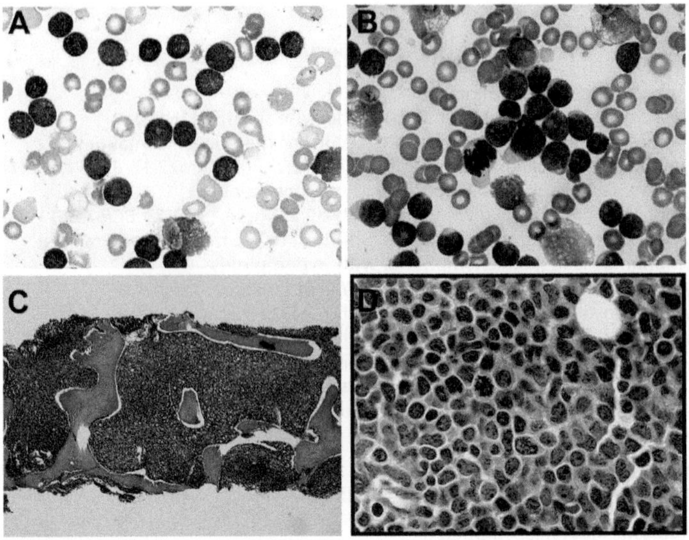

Fig. 1. Lymphoblasts in peripheral blood (*A*; Giemsa, original magnification ×1000, oil immersion) and bone marrow aspirate (*B*; Giemsa, original magnification ×1000, oil immersion); hypercellular bone marrow biopsy (*C*; hematoxylin-eosin [H&E], original magnification ×20); increased mitotic activity with abnormal mitoses (*D*; H&E, original magnification ×400).

may show areas of necrosis (**Fig. 1**C). Acute leukemia is the most common cause of bone marrow necrosis in the pediatric population.[1] At high magnification, a very monotonous blast population can be appreciated along with increased mitotic activity and frequent abnormal mitotic figures (**Fig. 1**D).

Irrespective of how carefully the morphologic assessment is performed, the diagnosis relies heavily on immunophenotyping, which is optimally performed via multiparameter flow cytometry. Lymphoblasts of any lineage tend to show low side scatter with variable but generally dimmer than normal mature lymphocyte expression of CD45. In the particular case of B lymphoblasts, the immunophenotypic findings are generally constant among patients and consist of expression of B-cell markers as well as markers of immaturity. Commonly seen B-cell markers include CD19, CD22 (surface and cytoplasmic), CD24, and CD79a. CD20 is variable and frequently negative given that immature B-lymphoid precursors may not have had the chance to acquire full intensity or any degree of expression of this mature B-cell marker. In tissue sections, PAX5 shows nuclear expression in B lymphoblasts (**Fig. 2**A). Blast (immature) markers are usually represented by CD34, TdT, and Human Leukocyte Antigen - DR isotype. In cases where 1 or more of these are missing, useful surrogate markers of immaturity include CD9, CD38, and CD58. CD99 can be successfully used in tissue sections to show immaturity irrespective of lineage (**Fig. 2**B). CD10, formerly known as the common acute lymphoid leukemia antigen (CALLA), is characteristically expressed but may be absent, especially in certain subtypes of B-ALL. Because B lymphoblasts are immature precursors incapable of performing their cytoplasmic function of immunoglobulin production, light-chain expression is absent; however, clonal light-chain expression may be encountered very rarely and does not exclude the diagnosis.[2] Because of the advent of targeted therapies, it has become increasingly important to report specifically and even quantify the presence or absence of certain markers such as CD19, CD20, or surface CD22. As in any other neoplastic

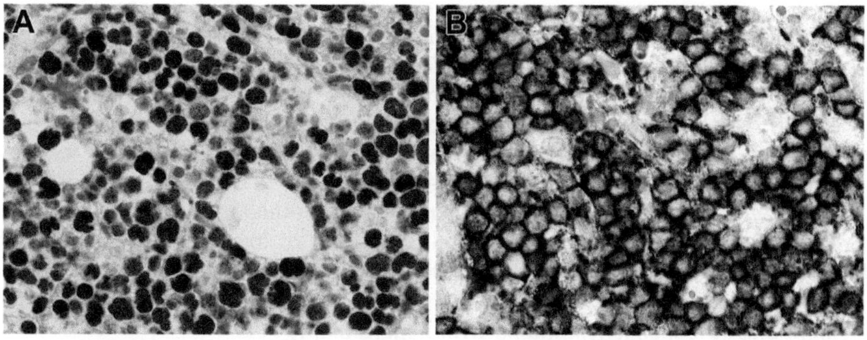

Fig. 2. PAX5 in marrow biopsy (*A*; immunohistochemistry [IHC], original magnification ×400); CD99 in marrow biopsy (*B*; IHC, original magnification ×400).

process, phenotypic aberrancies are commonly encountered in cases of B-ALL, and those usually include myeloid markers, most commonly CD13 and/or CD33, as well as occasional T-cell markers. As a rule, myeloperoxidase (MPO) should be absent; however, MPO is detected in rare cases and should not completely exclude the diagnosis even though this finding usually indicates acute myeloid leukemia (AML) with aberrant expression of B-lymphoid antigens or mixed-phenotype acute leukemia (B/myeloid).[1] This finding represents a significant change compared with the criteria in place before the 2016 WHO classification, when the unquestionable presence of MPO completely excluded a diagnosis of B-ALL and necessarily implied the presence of myeloid lineage.

Lumbar puncture to obtain and examine cerebrospinal fluid (CSF) for the presence of blasts is virtually always performed in addition to bone marrow aspiration with or without biopsy at the time of the initial diagnosis as well as subsequent follow-up studies. The identification of CSF blasts ranges from very easy, in cases with abundant involvement, to difficult, in situations where their presence is subtle and frequently represented by only 1 to 2 malignant cells. Flow cytometry may be helpful; however, it tends to be diagnostic mostly in cases with significant involvement where the cytology is obvious and is not reliable in cases with low cellularity and minimal blast presence, where it would actually be needed.

In terms of prognosis, B-ALL has a very favorable outcome in the pediatric population, with an overall complete remission rate of more than 95% and an apparent cure rate of approximately 80%.[2] The situation is not as good in adult patients, in whom the complete remission rate varies between 60% and 85%, with a cure rate of less than 50%.[2] Better outcomes are associated with more intensive therapy regimens and there is evidence that younger adults may do better with pediatric-type protocols.[2] Adverse prognosis is associated with infancy, older age, high WBC count at presentation, diminished response to initial therapy, CNS involvement, and certain genetic abnormalities. Although the outcome depends heavily on genetics, the most important prognostic factor remains an early response to therapy.[1]

Genetics

B-lymphoblastic leukemia/lymphoma with t(12;21) (p13;q22);ETV6-RUNX1

This subtype of B-ALL is one of 2 prognostically favorable groups of B-ALLs with recurrent cytogenetic abnormalities. It occurs commonly in the pediatric population, where it represents approximately 25% of cases; however, it is rarely seen in adults (~3%).[1] Morphologically, this subtype does not show any particularities compared with the common appearance of lymphoblasts. Immunophenotypically, there may be mild differences from the classic makeup, including frequent aberrant expression of myeloid markers as well as lack of CD9 and partial positivity for CD20. The (12;21) translocation resulting in the abnormal *ETV6-RUNX1* fusion is cryptic in most cases and therefore cannot be identified by karyotyping because of the insufficient resolution of regular G banding. Consequently, molecular studies (usually fluorescence in situ hybridization [FISH]) are necessary in order to detect this abnormality. The Children's Oncology Group (COG) requires FISH testing for this abnormality on the initial diagnosis of B-ALL. The overall prognosis of this particular subtype of B-ALL is very favorable, with more than 90% cure or longtime remission.[1]

B-lymphoblastic leukemia/lymphoma with hyperdiploidy

This condition is the other subtype of B-ALL with favorable prognosis and, similar to the previous one, is commonly encountered in pediatric patients (25%) but rarely in adults (7%–8%).[2] Again, there are no morphologic particularities specific to this group, and the immunophenotype shows virtually no differences compared with the common one, with the possible exception of more frequent absence of CD45. By definition, karyotyping must show at least 51 chromosomes in order to qualify as hyperdiploid. Minimal increases in the number of chromosomes (47–50) are not included in this subtype. This situation, even though possible, does not represent a practical problem because most cases show more than 66 chromosomes.[1] Typically, numerical increases are the sole abnormality and no associated translocations, deletions, or other structural alterations are present. The most common nonrandom extra copies are those of chromosomes 21, X, 14, and 4.[2] Similar to the other good prognostic group, the outcome is favorable, with more than 90% cure or longtime remission. Moreover, simultaneous trisomies of chromosomes 4, 10, and 17 have been associated with an even better prognosis. Recently, only extra copies of chromosomes 4 and 10, rather than 17, seem to be more consistently associated with a favorable effect.[3] These numerical abnormalities can be easily appreciated via karyotyping; however, the COG also requires FISH studies for these 3 particular chromosomes, which are usually performed using chromosome enumeration probes.

B-lymphoblastic leukemia/lymphoma with t(9;22) (q34;q11.2);BCR-ABL1

B-ALL with the Philadelphia chromosome represented historically the worst prognostic subgroup among various types of B-ALL with recurrent cytogenetic abnormalities. Fortunately, it is rare in children and represents only 2% to 4% of pediatric cases. In contrast, approximately 25% of adult cases of B-ALL show this abnormality.[1] Morphologically, increased blast size, more prominent granularity, conspicuous nucleoli, and more abundant cytoplasm are frequently seen. In these cases, the morphologic appearance is more myeloid than lymphoid; however, flow cytometry shows an immature B-cell phenotype confirming the diagnosis. Aberrant myeloid antigen expression is frequent in this subtype and CD25 may be seen, especially in adult patients.[2] Infrequently, this translocation may be associated with T-ALL.[1] Traditionally, on molecular studies, if the major breakpoint is involved, the resulting protein product is p210, which is classically associated with chronic myelogenous leukemia, whereas the minor breakpoint is classically associated with a smaller protein product, p190, and B-ALL. In practice, p190 is detected in almost all pediatric cases; however, approximately half of the adult cases of B-ALL show the presence of the p210 product.[2,3] In very rare cases, the 2 proteins coexist in variable proportions. The Philadelphia chromosome may be associated with other cytogenetic abnormalities. *BCR-ABL1* FISH analysis is another requirement of the COG for the initial diagnosis of B-ALL. Despite the generally unfavorable outcome, therapy with tyrosine kinase inhibitors may have a dramatic effect in a significant proportion of cases.

B-lymphoblastic leukemia/lymphoma with t(v;11q23); MLL (KMT2A) rearranged
This unfavorable prognostic group shows several particularities. In terms of epidemiology and clinical features, this subtype represents the most common leukemia before 1 year of age and may even occur in utero. It is usually accompanied by very high WBC count at presentation (>100,000/μL) and shows frequent CNS involvement.[5] There are no morphologic particularities but immunophenotypically these cases typically show lack of CD10 and various degrees of aberrant CD15 expression (**Fig. 3**). Also noted commonly are lack of CD24 and presence of CD65.[1] Of note, the *MLL* gene can have a multitude of possible fusion partners and therefore a specific dual-fusion FISH probe fails to identify numerous cases. Consequently, the use of a break-apart FISH probe (also a COG requirement) is necessary to identify the rearrangement irrespective of partner. The most common translocation is the t(4;11)(q21;q23); *AFF(AF4)-KMT2A(MLL)* along with those partnering *MLL* with *MLLT3(AF9)*, and *MLLT1(ENL)*.[5] Importantly, this cytogenetic subgroup does not include cases with 11q23 (*MLL*) deletion, which have an intermediate prognosis. As stated earlier, the prognosis is generally poor, especially in infants less than 6 months of age. This subtype is characterized by relative resistance to corticosteroids and L-asparaginase therapy, but is sensitive to cytarabine.[5]

B-lymphoblastic leukemia/lymphoma with hypodiploidy
This condition is a rare type of B-ALL with a reported frequency of about 5%, and likely as low as 1% if a strict criterion of fewer than 45 chromosomes is applied.[2] Furthermore, the group is subdivided as a function of the number of chromosomes in near haploid (23–29 chromosomes, limited to children), low hypodiploid (33–39 chromosomes), high hypodiploid (40–43 chromosomes), and near diploid (44–45 chromosomes). There are no particular features morphologically or immunophenotypically. Unlike cases with hyperdiploidy, the numerical abnormalities encountered in hypodiploid B-ALL may also be accompanied by various structural alterations. Importantly, the phenomenon of endoreduplication must be kept in mind in the context of this type of leukemia. This process results in an intranuclear duplication of the hypodiploid neoplastic clone in a variable proportion of malignant cells. Consequently, if only FISH is used for diagnosis without karyotype correlation, the otherwise lower-than-normal number of chromosomes, which is now doubled, may be easily misinterpreted as hyperdiploidy. This confusion needs to be avoided at all costs given the dramatically different prognostic implications. In most cases, both true hypodiploid and pseudohyperdiploid clones are present in variable proportions and therefore could be confirmed by karyotyping; however, a small subset of patients may only show the pseudohyperdiploid clone, a

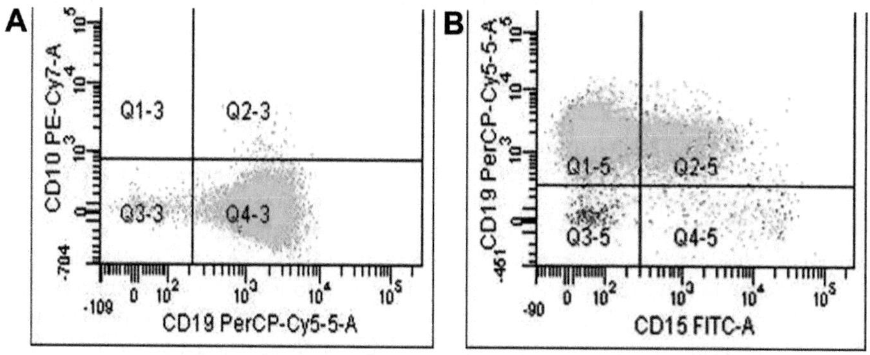

Fig. 3. Flow cytometric dot plots showing lack of CD10 (*A*) and partial aberrant CD15 (*B*).

situation in which molecular methods such as next-generation sequencing are necessary for definitive confirmation. Prognosis is generally poor, but a spectrum is noted as a function of the degree of hypodiploidy, with near-diploid cases showing the best outcome versus near-haploid cases, which are associated with the worst prognosis in this group.[1]

B-lymphoblastic leukemia/lymphoma, BCR-ABL1–like (provisional entity)

By definition, this is a subtype of B-ALL that lacks the *BCR-ABL1* translocation but shows a pattern of gene expression similar to that seen in Philadelphia chromosome-positive B-ALL (WHO).[1] This condition is a common subtype found in 10% to 25% of all patients with B-ALL but shows a spectrum of frequencies with very low percentages among children with standard-risk B-ALL that progressively increase in children with high-risk B-ALL, followed by adolescents, and then adults.[2] Certain inherited *GATA3* variants are associated with an increased risk and are encountered with increased frequency in Hispanic patients as well as patients of Native American ancestry.[1–3,6,7] These leukemias usually show a high WBC count at presentation. There is nothing particular characteristic morphologically or immunophenotypically. The genetic and molecular makeup is highly variable, including frequent translocations involving genes controlling other tyrosine kinases than those seen in *BCR-ABL1* cases (*ABL1*, *ABL2*, *PDGFRB*, *NTRK3*, *PTK2B*, *TSLP*, *TYK2*, *CSF1R*, and *JAK2*). In approximately 50% of cases, rearrangements involving *CRLF2*, including *CRLF2-P2RY8* and *CRLF2-IGH*, are present. Also noted are rearrangements of *EPOR* (*EPOR-IGH*). There is a very high frequency of *CRLF2* rearrangements in patients with Down syndrome. The abnormalities mentioned earlier are frequently associated with *IKZF1* and *CDKN2A/B* mutations or deletions.[1] Besides rearrangements, sequence mutations involving *FLT3*, *IL7R*, or *SH2B3* have also been described. Cytokine-independent proliferation and activation of phosphorylated STAT5 were present in cases with *ABL1*, *ABL2*, *CSF1R*, *JAK2*, and *PDGFRB* fusions. These types (except *JAK2*) were sensitive in vitro to dasatinib, whereas *EPOR* and *JAK2* rearrangements were sensitive to ruxolitinib, and *ETV6-NTRK3* fusions were sensitive to crizotinib.[8,9] The initial diagnosis of this subtype is particularly challenging given that these variable abnormalities are difficult to identify without complex analysis and, even more importantly, it is difficult to screen and determine which cases need such analysis. At present, 2 methods are used to identify these patients: RNA sequencing to identify a signature associated with *BCR-ABL1*, and low-density microarray containing small groups of 8 or 15 genes that can be analyzed rapidly.[10] The COG recommends that patients categorized as high risk at presentation (WBC count >50,000/μL or aged 10–16 years) be screened for these abnormalities.[8] Besides molecular methods, overexpression of the CRLF2 protein in patients with *CRLF2* rearrangements may be identified by flow cytometry and therefore provide a useful method of screening.[8] The overall prognosis is generally poor, but patients with tyrosine kinase activation may show dramatic response to therapy with tyrosine kinase inhibitors.

B-lymphoblastic leukemia/lymphoma with iAMP21

This condition is a rare (~2%) type of B-ALL that tends to present in older children and shows a low WBC count. Its frequency in the adult population seems to be significantly lower. Individuals with the rare constitutional robertsonian translocation rob(15;21)(q10;q10) have a tremendous risk increase (almost 3000-fold) for developing this type of leukemia. The underlying mechanism seems to involve chromothripsis and is likely to represent the driving factor in sporadic cases as well.[1] There is nothing special morphologically or immunophenotypically. FISH analysis using a probe for *RUNX1* shows at least 5 copies of the gene or at least 3 extra copies on the same chromosome

21.[2] The prognosis is poor, but more intensive therapy seems to overcome the adverse risk.[1]

B-lymphoblastic leukemia/lymphoma with t(1;19)q23;p13.3); TCF3-PBX1
This subtype is uncommon (6%) in the pediatric population, with an even lower frequency in adults.[1] Morphologically there are no particularities; however, immunophenotypically, several features are frequently identified, including the production of a truncated immunoglobulin chain (cytoplasmic μ) that can be identified by flow cytometry. Also noted is strong expression of CD9 as well as lack of CD34. As part of the more mature status of these neoplasms (often described as pre–B-ALL rather than precursor-B-ALL), CD20 is more commonly expressed and lymphomatous presentations are common. An alternative translocation may be present in a subset of cases, t(17;19); *TCF3-HLF*, associated with a dismal prognosis. Initially, this subtype was associated with an unfavorable prognosis; however, current intensive therapy protocols consistently overcome the previously described poor outcome. Of note, the alternative translocation mentioned earlier is still associated with a poor prognosis.[1,2]

B-lymphoblastic leukemia/lymphoma with t(5;14) (q31;q32); IL3-IGH
This condition is a rare subtype of B-ALL with recurrent cytogenetic abnormalities accounting for less than 1% of the cases.[1] Morphologically, the most striking feature is prominent reactive eosinophilia (not clonal) that may obscure the presence of lymphoblasts and hinder the diagnosis by generating confusion with other entities, including hypereosinophilic syndrome or chronic eosinophilic leukemia. The juxtaposition of *IL3* next to *IGH* amplifies the activity of the former, resulting in marked cytokine-driven eosinophilic proliferation. The prognostic implication of this particular abnormality is probably indifferent, but a definitive statement regarding its prognostic value is difficult to make given the rarity of this subtype.

B-lymphoblastic leukemia/lymphoma with newly described oncogenic fusions
A significant proportion (20%–30%) of pediatric B-ALL cannot be classified into any of the established cytogenetic and/or molecular subcategories. Several oncogenic fusions, including *DUX4* rearrangements (4%–5% of pediatric B-ALL, not otherwise specified [NOS]; favorable), *ETV6-RUNX1*–like gene expression (1%–3%; uncertain, possibly favorable), *MEF2D* rearrangements (1%–4%; unfavorable), and *ZNF384* rearrangements (1%–6%; intermediate to favorable) have been identified recently and seem to be present in approximately half of the NOS pediatric B-ALL cases.[11]

B-lymphoblastic leukemia/lymphoma with other significant mutations described recently
PAX5 (major B-lymphoid transcription-factor gene) alterations constitute an important subgroup and are estimated to represent approximately 10% of B-ALL, NOS. They define 2 main subtypes of B-ALL; namely, those with *PAX5* p.Pro80Arg and those with diverse *PAX5* alterations (rearrangements, intragenic amplifications, or mutations), collectively named *PAX5*alt. These subtypes show a variable outcome with different treatment protocols but are considered generally as having an intermediate to poor prognosis in children and adults. *IKZF1* p.Asn159Tyr alteration defines another B-ALL subtype with a distinctly inferior outcome. Several studies have linked *IKZF1* deletions to an unfavorable clinical outcome for B-ALL in various treatment protocols.[12,13] The prognostic value of *IKZF1* seems to show a strong association with the minimal residual disease (MRD) status. In postinduction MRD-negative patients,

IKZF1 did not show a distinctly negative prognostic implication, whereas MRD-positive patients showed a 10-fold higher relapse rate, according to 1 study.[13]

T-lymphoblastic Leukemia/Lymphoma

T-ALL/LBL is a neoplasm of precursor T cells, also known as T lymphoblasts. Unlike B-lymphoblastic processes, only a minority (10%–15%) of ALLs are of T-cell lineage, whereas most LBLs are of T-cell derivation (85%–90%). A slightly higher percentage (25%) of T-ALL is observed in the adult population.[1,2,4] The lymphomatous presentation is seen more frequently in adolescents than in children and shows a male predilection. The classic presentation of T-ALL/LBL is that of a rapidly growing anterior mediastinal mass with frequent respiratory and/or circulatory impairment in a teenage boy. Given the usually high WBC count at presentation, T-ALL is generally considered a higher-risk disease compared with B-ALL. The morphology of T lymphoblasts is virtually indistinguishable from their B-lineage counterparts. Occasionally, lymphoblasts of T-cell origin may show a more irregular nuclear contour and prominent nucleoli as well as more vigorously increased mitotic activity in tissue sections. Similar to B-ALL, T-lymphoblastic processes show an immunophenotype consistently composed of several T-cell markers as well as markers of immaturity; however, the exact combination of T-cell antigens is highly variable from case to case, unlike B-ALL, which tends to be significantly more uniform phenotypically. Pan–T-cell markers (CD2, CD3, CD5, and CD7) are generally expressed, but frequent aberrant loss of 1 or more of these antigens is commonly encountered. Importantly, aberrant loss of CD3 only affects the surface domain of the antigen but not the intracellular component. Cytoplasmic CD3 expression is considered the most specific indicator of T-cell lineage. Unlike normal mature T cells, which are either CD4 or CD8 positive, T lymphoblasts almost always show aberrant patterns regarding these two markers. The classic situation is that of significant coexpression of both CD4 and CD8 on the population in question (**Fig. 4**A); however, other abnormal variants are often seen, including double negativity (**Fig. 4**B) as well as virtually exclusive expression of one or the other. Intuitively, a parallel may be drawn between the immunoglobulin light chains in B-cell populations and the pattern of expression for CD4 and CD8 in T-cell populations. Similar to normal mature B lymphocytes, which are always represented by a mixture of either kappa-positive or lambda-positive cells in certain proportions, normal mature T lymphocytes can only show expression of CD4 or CD8 in certain proportions, never both (with the exception of normal thymic T-cell precursors or cortical thymocytes), and never neither. Besides T-cell markers, blast markers are also seen in variable proportions and combinations and include CD1a, CD34, TdT, and HLA-DR. It is worth mentioning that CD1a, unlike most other antigens that provide either lineage or degree of maturity information but usually never both, indicates

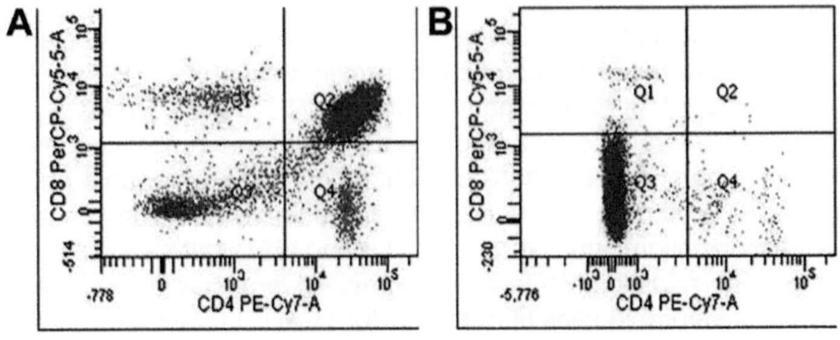

Fig. 4. Flow cytometric dot plots showing the more classic double CD4/CD8 expression (*A*), along with the less traditional possibility of double negativity (*B*).

both lineage (T cell) and degree of maturity (immature or blast), and therefore is a valuable T-lymphoblastic identifier. CD10 (CALLA) is expressed in many instances but not as frequently as in the case of B-ALL. The most commonly expressed aberrant antigens are myeloid, usually CD13 and/or CD33. When expression of CD117 is detected, the possibility of a particular subtype of T-ALL, namely early T-cell precursor ALL, should be considered and is discussed later. B-cell antigens are less frequently identified, but virtually any of them may be seen in the context of T-ALL, including cytoplasmic CD79a, which was considered for a long time a highly specific B-cell marker.[1] On occasion, these leukemias show a mature phenotype by flow cytometry with no identifiable blast markers. Such cases may be difficult to diagnose and require additional work-up, including repeating blast markers via immunohistochemistry. The clinical presentation, the microscopic blast morphology, as well as the characteristic weak expression of CD45 by flow are helpful in establishing the diagnosis. The genetic and molecular abnormalities identified in T-lymphoblastic processes span a wide spectrum but several are detected with a degree of consistency, including rearrangements of the *TCR* gene loci, the *HOX* group of genes, *TAL1 (SCL)*, *CDKN2A*, and *NOTCH1*. Abnormal karyotypes are present in 50% to 70% of cases. Surprisingly, also noted with significant frequency (~20%) are immunoglobulin gene rearrangements.[1–3] Unlike B-ALL, T-ALL is not subcategorized as a function of certain recurrent cytogenetic and molecular abnormalities.

Early T-cell–precursor lymphoblastic leukemia

This entity represents a particular subtype of T-ALL with unique immunophenotypic features supporting only limited early T-cell differentiation. It is uncommon both in pediatric (10%–13%) and adult (5%–10%) patients.[1,2] There is nothing particular from a morphologic standpoint; however, the immunophenotype tends to be characteristic. Among the pan–T-cell markers, CD7 is consistently expressed as well as cytoplasmic CD3, but surface CD3 is frequently lost. CD2 may be expressed but CD5 is frequently negative. Although expression of CD4 is noted in a subset of cases, CD8 and CD1a are virtually always negative. Another characteristic finding is represented by aberrant expression of 1 or more myeloid markers, including CD13, CD33, CD11b, and CD65. Also present are 1 or more blast markers (CD34, CD117, and HLA-DR).[1,2] Notably, CD117 is also a myeloid marker; therefore, similar to CD1a in T lymphoblasts, it represents another double indicator of both lineage (myeloid) and degree of maturity (immature, blast). The genetic makeup of these leukemias also shows certain particularities because many of the abnormally expressed genes are those usually associated with either myeloid or stem cell neoplasms rather than T-lymphoid malignancies.[1] Importantly, this group of genes includes *FLT3*, similar to AML. For practical purposes, it is recommended that *FLT3* analysis should be performed in this subgroup of T-ALL even though its prognostic significance is not yet clearly defined, unlike AML. Once this subtype was described, initial studies suggested a much worse outcome compared with other types of T-ALL; however, more recent data suggest that the difference is minimal, if any.[1]

Natural killer lymphoblastic leukemia/lymphoma

This type of lymphoblastic process represents a provisional subcategory that is not only rare but also difficult to define precisely. Many of the NK-cell markers are also common T-cell markers, including CD2, cytoplasmic CD3-epsilon, CD5, and CD7. CD56 is frequently expressed but other, more mature, and specific antigens such as CD16 are rarely seen in these immature processes. Because of the coexpression of CD4 and CD56, NK-lymphoblastic processes may be confused with blastic plasmacytoid dendritic cell neoplasms.[1]

CLINICS CARE POINTS

- B-lymphoblastic processes present most commonly as leukemias, whereas their T-cell counterparts are usually diagnosed as lymphomas, most frequently mediastinal.
- Immunophenotyping via flow cytometry is of paramount importance in lineage identification and distinction from normal immature counterparts.
- B-lymphoblastic neoplasms with hyperdiploidy or *ETV6-RUNX1* fusion are associated with favorable prognosis, whereas those with *BCR-ABL1* fusion, *KMT2A(MLL)* rearrangement, and hypodiploidy, as well as the more recently described *BCR-ABL1*–like and iAMP21 subtypes, confer an unfavorable prognosis.

DISCLOSURE

The author has nothing to disclose.

REFERENCES

1. Borowitz MJ, Chan JKC, Downing JR, et al. Precursor lymphoid neoplasms. In: Swerdlow SH, Campo E, Harris NL, et al, editors. WHO classification of Tumours of haematopoietic and lymphoid tissues (revised 4th edition). Lyon (France): IARC; 2017. p. 199–213.
2. Duffield AS, Racke FK, Borowitz MJ, et al. Precursor B- and T-cell neoplasms. In: Jaffe ES, Arber DA, Campos E, et al, editors. Hematopathology. 2nd edition. Philadelphia: Elsevier; 2017. p. 761–82.
3. Malard F, Mohty M. Acute lymphoblastic leukemia. Lancet 2020;395:1146–62.
4. Cortelazzo S, Ferreri A, Hoelzer D, et al. Lymphoblastic lymphoma. Crit Rev Oncol Hematol 2017;113:304–17.
5. El Chaer F, Keng M, Ballen KK. MLL-rearranged acute lymphoblastic leukemia. Curr Hematol Malig Rep 2020;15(2):83–9.
6. Walsh KM, de Smith AJ, Chokkalingam AP, et al. GATA3 risk alleles are associated with ancestral components in Hispanic children with ALL. Blood 2013; 122(19):3385–7.
7. Tran TH, Loh ML. Ph-like acute lymphoblastic leukemia. Hematol Am Soc Hematol Educ Program 2016;2016(1):561–6.
8. Jain S, Abraham A. *BCR-ABL1*-like B-acute lymphoblastic leukemia/lymphoma: a comprehensive review. Arch Pathol Lab Med 2020;144:150–5.
9. Roberts KG, Li Y, Payne-Turner D, et al. Targetable kinase-activating lesions in Ph-like acute lymphoblastic leukemia. N Engl J Med 2014;371(11):1005–15.
10. Reshmi SC, Harvey RC, Roberts KG, et al. Targetable kinase gene fusions in high-risk B-ALL: a study from the Children's Oncology Group. Blood 2017; 129(25):3352–61.
11. Lilljebjörn H, Fioretos T. New oncogenic subtypes in pediatric B-cell precursor acute lymphoblastic leukemia. Blood 2017;130(12):1395–401.
12. Gu Z, Churchman ML, Roberts KG, et al. PAX5-driven subtypes of B-progenitor acute lymphoblastic leukemia. Nat Genet 2019;51(2):296–307.
13. Stanulla M, Dagdan E, Zaliova M, et al. IKZF1^{plus} defines a new minimal residual disease-dependent very-poor prognostic profile in pediatric B-cell precursor acute lymphoblastic leukemia. J Clin Oncol 2018;36(12):1240–9.

Inherited Bone Marrow Failure Syndromes

Biology and Diagnostic Clues

M. Tarek Elghetany, MD*, Jyotinder Nain Punia, MD,
Andrea N. Marcogliese, MD

KEYWORDS

- Bone marrow failure • Inherited • Fanconi • Diamond-Blackfan
- Shwachman-Diamond • Dyskeratosis • Cytopenias • Laboratory studies

KEY POINTS

- Inherited bone marrow failure disorders (IBMFSs) are genetic in nature, mostly familial.
- IBMFSs are usually but not always present in infancy or childhood.
- IBMFSs may predispose to hematologic and nonhematologic malignancies.
- IBMFSs require life-long follow-up, usually annually, or as needed.
- Bone marrow transplantation may cure the marrow defect, after trial of prednisone, anabolic steroids, or growth factors in some of these entities.

OVERVIEW

The inherited bone marrow failure syndromes (IBMFSs) are a group of genetic disorders associated with inadequate bone marrow (BM) production of 1 or more blood cell lineages (**Table 1**). Although mostly inherited, a de novo gene mutation may occur during early embryogenesis. These disorders are rare, but are clinically important due to life-threatening cytopenias and propensity to progress to severe aplastic anemia (AA), myelodysplastic syndromes (MDS), acute leukemia (AL), and other nonhematologic malignancies. Traditionally, IBMFSs have been divided into multilineage cytopenias, such as Fanconi anemia (FA), dyskeratosis congenita, Shwachman-Diamond syndrome, congenital amegakaryocytic thrombocytopenia, and unilineage cytopenia, such as Diamond-Blackfan anemia, severe congenital neutropenia, thrombocytopenia with absent radii, and congenital dyserythropoietic anemia. However, with advances in molecular and genetic studies, these disorders may be classified according to their impact on cellular function, such as DNA repair, telomere

Conflict of Interest: No conflict of interest is reported by any of the authors.

Department of Pathology and Immunology, Baylor College of Medicine/Texas Children's Hospital, 6621 Fannin Street, Suite WB1100, Houston, TX 77030, USA
* Corresponding author.
E-mail address: txelghet@texaschildrens.org

Clin Lab Med 41 (2021) 417–431
https://doi.org/10.1016/j.cll.2021.04.014

Table 1
Inherited bone marrow failure syndromes

Disorder	Inheritance	Genetics	Affected Cellular Pathway	Associated Clinical Features	Associated Malignancies
Fanconi anemia	AR (except *FANCB* X-linked, *FANCR/RAD51*, AD)	At least 22 genes in FA/BRCA DNA repair pathway *FANCA* 60%–65% *FANCC* 15%	DNA repair	Thumb abnormalities, short stature, pigmentation abnormalities, café au lait spots	MDS, AML, SCC, Wilms tumor, brain tumors
Dyskeratosis congenita	XL, AD, AR, sporadic	*DKC1* (25%), *TERT, TERC*	Telomere maintenance	Reticular skin pigmentation, mucosal leukoplakia, nail dystrophy	MDS, AML, SCC, other solid tumors
Shwachman-Diamond syndrome	AR	*SBDS* (90%), *DNAJC21*, *SRP54*	Ribosomal assembly	Exocrine pancreatic insufficiency, skeletal abnormalities	MDS, AML, possibly ALL, ovarian tumors
Diamond-Blackfan anemia	AD (except *GATA1* related, X-linked)	Ribosomal proteins, small and large; *RPS19* (25%)	Ribosomal biogenesis	Short stature, thumb abnormalities	MDS, AML, osteosarcoma, colon, possibly others
Congenital dyserythropoietic anemia (CDA)	AR (types I and II), AD (types III and IV)	*CDAN1* (CDA I), *SEC23B* (CDA II), *KIF23* (CDA III) *KLF1* (CDA IV)	Unfolded protein response, cytokinesis, erythroid transcription factor	Possible splenomegaly, jaundice, iron overload	Possible myeloma with type III
Severe congenital neutropenia *ELANE* mutation	AD	*ELANE* (neurophil elastase) (50%–75% of all cases)	Unfolded protein response	Pneumonia, skin infection, omphalitis	MDS/AML
Congenital amegakaryocytic thrombocytopenia	AR	*MPL* (thrombopoietin receptor)	Megakaryopoiesis	No specific findings	Aplastic anemia, MDS, AML
Thrombocytopenia with absent radii	AR	*RBM8A*	Possible mRNA processing/binding	Skeletal abnormalities, cow milk intolerance	AML, possibly ALL

Abbreviations: AD, autosomal dominant; ALL, acute lymphoblastic leukemia; AML, acute myeloid leukemia; AR, autosomal recessive; DNA, deoxyribose nucleic acid; MDS, myelodysplastic syndrome; mRNA, messenger ribose nucleic acid; SCC, squamous cell carcinoma; XL-X, linked.

maintenance, and ribosomal biogenesis. The estimated annual incidence of IBMFS is approximately 65 per million live births.[1]

IBMFSs are commonly associated with physical abnormalities due to the impact of gene alterations on more global cell function. These abnormalities may be observed before the diagnosis of BM failure. Cytopenias may be present at birth (congenital) or may manifest at a later stage of life and may be the presenting feature that brings a patient to attention and initiates the diagnostic workup. If bone marrow transplantation (BMT) is to be considered, family members need to be screened for their disease status before they are considered as potential donors. BMT may cure the marrow defect but will not impact other tissues affected by the same genetic defect.

Several of these disorders are now recognized in the 2017 updated World Health Organization Classification of Hematopoietic Neoplasms under the category "myeloid neoplasms with germline predisposition."[2]

FANCONI ANEMIA: A DNA REPAIR DISORDER

FA is a chromosomal instability disorder with an incidence of 1:200,000 in most populations but is higher in Ashkenazi Jewish (1:30,000) and African (1:22,000) individuals. The carrier frequency is approximately 1 in 180 in North America.[3–5] The diagnosis of FA should be considered in patients with congenital anomalies, aplastic anemia, or a family history of BM failure or cancer susceptibility. The median age of diagnosis is 6.5 years. Approximately 15% to 40% of patients have no physical findings. The male-to-female ratio is 1.2:1.0. Aplastic anemia or malignancy may be the presenting features. The manifestations of FA can vary among affected members of the same family, suggesting that additional genetic, epigenetic, or environmental factors likely influence the disease characteristics and clinical course.[6] Short stature and cutaneous manifestations, such as generalized hyperpigmentation, café au lait spots, and hypopigmentation are seen in approximately 40% of patients.[7] Thumb abnormalities are also common and are seen in approximately 35% of patients. Classical congenital abnormalities include those described in the VACTERL-H association (Vertebral, Anal, Cardiac, Tracheo-esophageal fistula, Esophageal atresia, Renal, upper Limb, and Hydrocephalus). From 5% to 30% of patients with FA meet 3 of the 8 features. A recent study has correlated the presence of the entire VACTERL-H findings with *FANCB* gene mutation.[3]

Progressive BM failure is one of the hallmarks of FA. Thrombocytopenia and macrocytosis of red blood cells often precede anemia and neutropenia. Most patients with FA (53%) already have pancytopenia at the time of diagnosis.[7] The cumulative incidence of pancytopenia has been reported as 90% by age 40 years.[8] Elevated hemoglobin F levels and elevated expression of "i" antigen on red cells usually coincide with the macrocytosis and are likely manifestations of stress hematopoiesis. Serum alpha-fetoprotein levels are consistently elevated in patients with FA irrespective of the presence of liver abnormalities. Because these patients are at a higher risk for developing MDS and acute myeloid leukemia (AML), surveillance BM examinations are performed regularly, often annually to evaluate for morphologic progression and dysplasia as well as cytogenetics and molecular diagnostics (usually mutation panel testing by next generation sequencing methods) to detect development of an abnormal clone or significant somatic mutations.

The risk of cancer is approximately 500 to 700 times higher than in the healthy population. By the age of 40 years, the cumulative incidence of solid tumors is estimated to be 26% to 30%.[9] The median age at development of cancer is 16 years, contrasting with 68 years for the same types of cancer in the general population. The crude risk of

MDS in patients with FA is approximately 5% to 10% and that of AL is about 3% to 10% with cumulative incidence of leukemia and nonhematologic cancers of 33% and 28% by the age of 40 to 50 years.[1,9] The leukemias occur at a relatively young age with a median age of 17 years and are usually AML. BMT is the only curative therapy for the hematologic manifestations of FA. Androgens, transfusions, and growth factors have also been tried with variable results.[1] Follow-up surveillance for solid malignant tumors is important. The most common solid tumors in patients with FA are head and neck carcinoma, hepatocellular carcinoma, and gynecologic malignancies.

Morphologic and Other Findings

Evaluation of BM at earlier stage, such as in infancy or early childhood is usually normocellular with megaloblastic changes. The BM becomes aplastic by mid to late childhood and shows reduced or completely depleted trilineage hematopoiesis, findings that are indistinguishable from those of idiopathic/acquired AA (**Fig. 1**). Rare patients present first with MDS or AML. Paroxysmal nocturnal hemoglobinuria clones are usually not detected in IBMFS, including FA.[10,11]

Diagnostics and Molecular Mechanisms

The diagnosis of FA is based on the demonstration of increased chromosomal breakage of peripheral blood lymphocytes in the presence of DNA cross-linking agents, such as mitomycin C or diepoxybutane. Patients with mosaic FA may require testing skin fibroblasts.

Pathogenetic variants in at least 22 different DNA repair genes of the FA/BRCA pathway have been reported.[3,12] FA is usually inherited in an autosomal recessive manner. There is only one gene to date (*FANCB*) that is inherited in an X-linked manner; *FANCR/RAD51* is autosomal dominant.[3] Occasionally, hematopoietic reversion, in which a point mutation or intragenic recombination in a hematopoietic stem cell leads to correction of one FA allele and a consequent recovery of a normal or

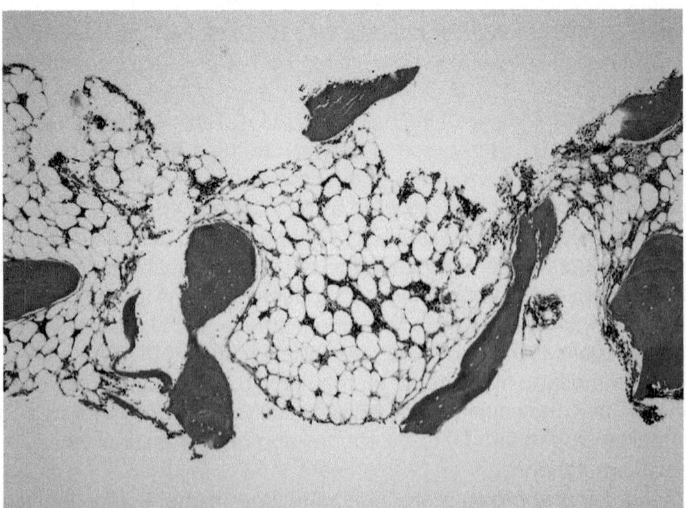

Fig. 1. BM biopsy from a patient with FA in severe aplastic anemia phase showing markedly hypocellular marrow (hematoxylin-eosin, original magnification ×40).

subnormal protein activity may occur.[13] *FANCA* is the most common mutation (approximately 60%–65%) followed by *FANCC* (approximately 15%). The FA/BRCA pathway repairs DNA interstrand crosslinks, which are covalent links between strands of DNA that interfere with DNA replication and transcription during cell mitosis. The interstrand crosslinks are produced by endogenous chemicals, such as reactive aldehydes, and environmental exposures.[14] The *FANCD1/BRCA2* subtype constitutes 1% to 2% of all patients with FA and manifests an especially high rate of early-onset AML and specific solid tumors (brain tumors and Wilms tumor) compared with other FA subtypes.

Clonal cytogenetic abnormalities are found in 34% to 48% of patients with FA. The most frequent chromosomal abnormalities in MDS occurring in patients with FA are 1q+, 3q+, −7/7q, 11q− 20q−, 6, 13, and 21q−. Aberrations of chromosomes 3 and 7 are associated with increased risk for MDS/AML.[15] Somatic mutations affecting several genes, such as *RUNX1* and *SF3B1*, have been reported in patients with FA and other IBMFS and may precede the development of cytogenetic abnormalities.[16]

DYSKERATOSIS CONGENITA: A TELOMEROPATHY

Dyskeratosis congenita (DC) is a disorder of telomere maintenance system. Telomeres are the nucleoprotein complex at the chromosomal ends with essential roles in maintaining chromosomal integrity.[17] DC is a multi-organ disorder of the mucocutaneous and hematopoietic systems associated with a wide variety of other somatic abnormalities. The traditional diagnostic ectodermal triad of reticular skin pigmentation of the upper body, mucosal leukoplakia, and nail dystrophy is usually not present at birth but may appear during the first 10 years of life. The incidence of DC in childhood is approximately 4 cases per million per year. The male:female ratio is 3.2:1.0, reflecting the X-linked recessive mode of inheritance in some patients.[7]

Clinical Features

The skin pigmentation is typically reticular and mottled, affecting approximately 70% of patients; it may be localized or widespread. Nail dystrophy is also frequent (approximately 70% of patients). Mucosal leukoplakia occurs less frequently (approximately 50% of patients) and typically involves the tongue, buccal mucosa, and oropharynx. The next most common physical abnormality is eye manifestations (30%), including lacrima duct stenosis, epiphora, exudative retinopathy, and cataracts. Approximately 20% of patients develop pulmonary disease with pulmonary fibrosis and vascular abnormalities, and pulmonary disease accounts for nearly 10% of deaths; pulmonary complications may also occur after hematopoietic stem cell transplantation (HSCT).

Cytopenias of 1 or more lineages are seen in approximately 85% of patients at presentation. Thrombocytopenia and anemia are often the first signs. Cytopenias in early childhood may be also immune mediated. Overall, the median age of onset of pancytopenia is 8 years, with 50% developing pancytopenia before age 10 and 95% by age 40. Severe aplastic anemia affects approximately 50% by age 50.[7] Among patients in the DC registry, malignancies were noted in 27 (14%) of 197 patients. These malignancies developed in older patients, generally after the second decade of life. Cancer risks have cumulative incidences of 20% to 30% for solid tumors by age 65 years and less than 10% for AML by age 70 years. Most tumors in DC are head and neck squamous cell carcinoma.[9]

The only curative treatment for BM failure, MDS, and AML in DC remains HSCT. Androgens improve BM function in approximately 50% to 70% of patients. A small number of patients may respond to G-CSF administration, with significant increase in neutrophil counts.

Morphology

BM cellularity may be normal or increased early in the disease. At advanced stages, the BM is typically hypocellular with depletion of all 3 lineages. Rarely, hypoplastic MDS or AML may be the presenting feature.

Diagnostics and Molecular Mechanisms

Telomere length analysis using multicolor flow cytometric fluorescence in situ hybridization (Flow-FISH) is a common tool, and it shows very short telomeres (less than first percentile of age-matched controls) in multiple lymphocyte subsets.[1,7] Because telomer length tends to decrease by age, telomere length studies are plotted against the patient age (**Fig. 2**). Lymphocytes have been studied as the standard lineage to assess telomere length. Rapidly proliferating cells, such as granulocytes, may give false results of having short telomeres. DC is caused by abnormalities in the telomere maintenance system or its protective cap, also known as sheltrin. Telomerase is an enzyme that adds DNA sequences to the ends of chromosomes (the telomeres) to prevent loss of terminal repeats (TTAGG) during DNA replication. Telomerase enzyme contains 2 core components, a reverse transcriptase, also known as TERT (telomere reverse transcriptase) and a ribose nucleic acid (RNA) molecule, also known as TERC (telomerase RNA component), which acts as a template for the synthesis of telomere repeats.

There are 4 distinct genetic forms of DC: X-linked, autosomal dominant, autosomal recessive, and sporadic. The X-linked mutation in the *DKC1* (Xq28) gene encoding the protein dyskerin, is the most common (25%–30%).[1] Autosomal dominant forms may be caused by mutations in the *TERT*, *TERC*, or *TINF2* genes. The latter encodes a sheltrin component known as TIN2 and may be associated with a severe form of DC and also with Revesz syndrome, which manifests as exudative retinopathy in association with DC. Biallelic *TERT* mutations can result in a severe form of DC called Hoyeraal Hreidarsson syndrome, which is characterized by hematologic and dermatologic manifestations of DC in addition to cerebellar hypoplasia. DC may also arise sporadically, without a family history.

Management of DC-associated aplastic anemia is similar to FA with androgens, growth factors, and consideration for BMT.

SHWACHMAN-DIAMOND SYNDROME: A RIBOSOMAL BIOGENESIS DISORDER

Shwachman-Diamond syndrome (SDS) is a rare autosomal recessive multisystem disorder characterized by exocrine pancreatic insufficiency, BM dysfunction, and

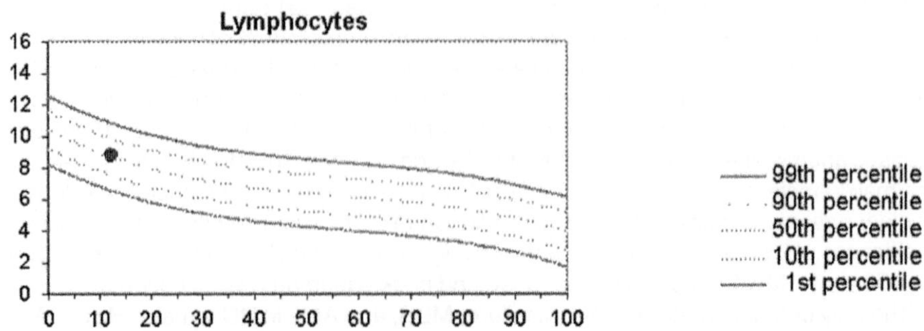

Fig. 2. A telomere length study of peripheral blood lymphocytes showing normal telomere length. The lower limit of the graph indicates the first percentile, which is the standard threshold for short telomere.

frequent skeletal abnormalities. SDS has an incidence of 8.5 cases per million live births with male:female ratio of approximately 1.5:1.0.[1]

Clinical Features

SDS is characterized by the combination of exocrine pancreatic insufficiency and BM failure. Exocrine pancreatic insufficiency typically presents in infancy with failure to thrive and steatorrhea. The latter may improve in a subset of patients with age. Imaging studies show fatty replacement of the exocrine pancreatic acini, with preservation of the ducts and islets. Exocrine pancreatic insufficiency can be tested by serum trypsinogen, which is generally depressed in patients with SDS at any age, although it may improve with time. Isoamylase levels remain low after the age of 3 and are useful in this older age group.

Neutropenia (absolute neutrophil count $<1.5 \times 10^9/L$) is most common and has been reported in 80% to 100% of patients, with approximately 50% of patients manifesting severe neutropenia (absolute neutrophil count $<0.5 \times 10^9/L$).[1] Neutropenia may be either intermittent or persistent. In some patients with SDS, neutrophils demonstrate abnormalities in chemotaxis and migration.[18] Patients are predisposed to infections, particularly bacterial and fungal. Macrocytic anemia and/or thrombocytopenia also may be seen, and a subset of patients with SDS develop aplastic anemia. SDS is characterized by a high propensity to develop MDS and leukemia, particularly AML,[18] with a risk for MDS/AML development of 18.8% by age 20 years and 36.1% by age 30.[19] Nonhematologic malignancies, such as ovarian tumors, may occur. Skeletal imaging studies may reveal a wide variety of abnormalities, such as metaphyseal dysostosis.[6] Many patients with SDS suffer from neurocognitive deficits and psychosocial dysfunction.

At present, the only curative option for severe BM failure in SDS is HSCT, which may be indicated in patients with severe or symptomatic cytopenia, MDS with excess blasts, or AL.[2]

Morphology

The BM is usually hypocellular, but cases showing normal or even increased cellularity have also been observed, particularly early in the course of disease. The BM usually shows granulocytic hypoplasia with left-shifted granulopoiesis. Mild dysplastic changes, particularly in the granulocytic lineage, are commonly observed.[20]

Diagnostics and Molecular Mechanisms

Two international consensus reports have provided guidelines for the diagnosis of SDS, using clinical and laboratory data. One report was published before the identification of the *SBDS* gene,[20] whereas a more recent report has included the use of genetic confirmation in the diagnostic criteria.[18] SDS is inherited as autosomal recessive. It is caused by mutation in the *SBDS* gene on chromosome 7q11. SBDS protein plays a major role in ribosomal assembly by preparing the nascent large (60S) ribosomal subunit to join the small subunit (40S) and form an active translating ribosomal unit (80S).[21] Other genes, such as *DNAJC21* and *SRP54*, also involved in ribosomal subunit biogenesis and stabilization, may produce an SDS-like picture when mutated.[22]

Differential Diagnosis

The differential diagnosis includes other inherited and acquired causes of marrow failure, as well as other causes of exocrine pancreatic insufficiency, such as cystic fibrosis, Pearson syndrome, and cartilage hair hypoplasia. Pearson syndrome is caused by mitochondrial DNA abnormalities, either due to large deletions or rearrangements. Patients with Pearson syndrome present with pancytopenia, pancreatic insufficiency, lactic acidosis, and failure to thrive. Unlike SDS, the BM Pearson syndrome often shows normal cellularity, numerous ring sideroblasts, and cytoplasmic vacuoles in myeloid precursors; the pancreas shows fibrosis rather than lipomatosis.

DIAMOND-BLACKFAN ANEMIA: A RIBOSOMAL BIOGENESIS DISORDER

Diamond-Blackfan Anemia (DBA) is a rare inherited BM failure syndrome of early infancy, affecting 7 per million live births.[1] The disorder manifests as severe and isolated anemia due to pure red cell aplasia in a normocellular marrow. Recent studies have identified the genes involved in this entity as mostly related to ribosome biogenesis and function.[23]

Clinical Features

Patients develop severe isolated anemia at a median age of 3 months, with ≥ 95% identified within the first year of life[7]; a very small subset of patients may present later in life (up to 64 years), making the diagnosis very challenging.[24] Asymptomatic carriers have been reported, reflecting incomplete penetrance.[25] There is no gender predilection.

Patients with DBA have reticulocytopenia, increased hemoglobin F, and elevated erythrocyte adenosine deaminase (eADA). White blood cells and platelets are within normal limits. One-quarter of patients have a physical birth defect, the most common being short stature followed by thumb abnormalities.[7] Additional defects include asymmetric scapula, fusion of cervical vertebrae, webbed neck, and genitourinary and heart defects.[1]

Anemia responds to corticosteroid therapy in up to 80% of patients. The median survival is 67 years.[9] Approximately 20% of patients experience spontaneous remission.[1] HSCT is the only cure for DBA. Patients with DBA are at a fivefold increased risk of developing cancer compared with the general population, with the highest risk observed for MDS, followed by colon carcinoma, osteosarcoma, AML, and genitourinary cancers.[9]

Morphology

BM examination shows a normocellular marrow with isolated erythroid hypoplasia/aplasia and no significant dysplastic features; occasional very early erythroid precursors may be seen. Myeloid and megakaryocytic lineages are usually normal (**Fig. 3**).

Diagnostics and Molecular Mechanisms

A combination of clinical and laboratory criteria has been prosed for the diagnosis of DBA.[26] DBA is inherited as autosomal dominant with more than 50% of cases being sporadic.[1] Most cases are caused by heterozygous mutations in 1 of at least 20 genes of ribosomal proteins (for both the small 40S and large 60S).[23] Rarely, patients presenting clinically as DBA have had mutations reported in the erythropoietin receptor, adenosine deaminase, *GATA1,* or *TSR2* genes with the latter 2 having X-linked inheritance.[23] *RPS19* mutations are the most common (25%) followed by *RPL5, RPL11,* and *RPS26*.[23]

The mutations may lead to accumulation of free unassembled ribosomal proteins, which in turn lead to release and stabilization of p53, causing cell cycle arrest or apoptosis.[1] Some severe phenotypes may be associated with reduced expression of heat shock protein 70 (HSP70). The latter protects GATA1 from degradation by

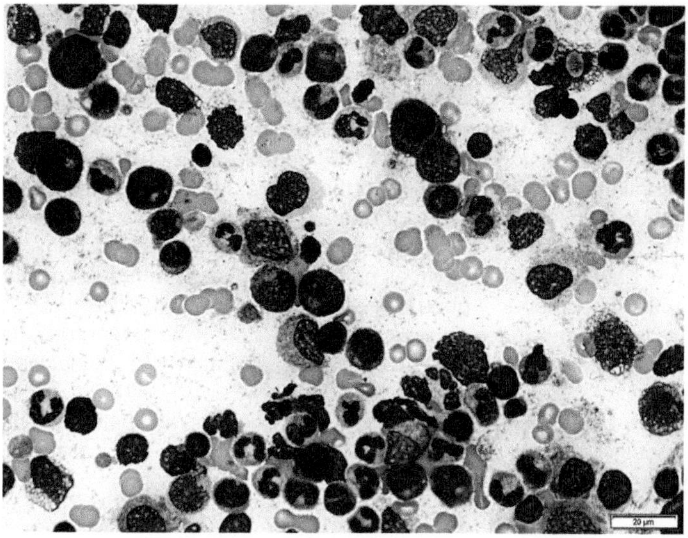

Fig. 3. BM aspirate showing absence of erythroid precursors in a patient newly diagnosed with DBA (Giemsa, original magnification ×600).

caspase 3 and when GATA1 levels are decreased, erythroid precursors will undergo apoptosis.[27] Recent studies also suggest that cytosolic and mitochondrial accumulation of heme in DBA cells is toxic and may activate the apoptotic process.[28]

Differential Diagnosis

The major differential diagnosis of DBA is transient erythroblastopenia of childhood (TEC), which shows no obvious morphologic differences; however, TEC usually manifests in early childhood (typically at approximately 2 years of age) and is transient with spontaneous recovery after 1 or 2 transfusions.[7]

CONGENITAL DYSERYTHROPOIETIC ANEMIAS

Congenital dyserythropoietic anemias (CDAs) are a group of rare hereditary disorders characterized by congenital anemia and ineffective erythropoiesis with distinct morphologic features of late erythroblasts, plus a hemolytic component and secondary hemosiderosis.

Classification and Features

CDA has 4 major subtypes (CDA I-IV). Patients with CDA I have macrocytic anemia. The BM shows incompletely divided erythroid cells with internuclear chromatin bridges. Binucleate erythroblasts are seen in 3% to 7% of nucleated red cells. Electron microscopic studies demonstrate a "Swiss cheese" appearance in which the cytoplasm may penetrate through widened pores of the nuclear envelope. CDA I is autosomal recessive with most cases being associated with mutations in *CDAN1* (CDA Ia), which is located on chromosome 15 and encodes a 134-kDa ubiquitous protein (codanin-1). Homozygous mutations in *CDIN1* (formerly known as *C15ORF41*) (CDA Ib) have been reported in some pedigrees.[1,29]

CDA II is the most common form of CDA and has autosomal recessive inheritance. It may present as normocytic anemia, combined with jaundice (90%), splenomegaly

(70%), and hepatomegaly (45%), features that may overlap with hereditary spherocytosis. Binucleated erythroid precursors are common, affecting 10% to 30% with only rare multinucleation. Electron microscopy shows erythroblasts with double plasma membranes. *SEC23 B*, located on chromosome 20, is mutated in CDA II.

CDA III is rare, with autosomal dominant inheritance. It is caused by mutations in *KIF23,* located on chromosome 15q21. *KIF23* encodes a kinesin-superfamily protein, which is essential for proper formation of the central spindle and midbody in cytokinesis. Defective cytokinesis leads to formation of large multinucleated erythroblasts (**Fig. 4**).

CDA IV has been reported in a small number of patients with autosomal dominant mutations (E325 K) in the *KLF1* gene located at chromosome 19p13.2. *KLF1* (erythroid Kruppel-like factor) produces a severe form of CDA with basophilic stippling of erythroid precursors and erythrocytes in addition to trinucleation and multinucleation.[1,29]

CDA variants other than I-IV have been described in rare patients, such as the X-linked recessive variant of *GATA1,* which may be associated with thrombocytopenia.[1,29]

Morphology

Patients usually have normocytic anemia, except CDA I, which has macrocytic anemia. BM iron stain shows increased iron as a feature of ongoing low-grade hemolysis and morphologically shows erythroid hyperplasia with abnormal-appearing normoblasts. Each subtype has some key unique morphologic features that are listed as follows:

- CDA I: internuclear bridges
- CDA II: increased binucleated erythroblasts and rare multinucleated forms
- CDA III: increased multinucleated erythroblasts
- CDA IV: internuclear bridges

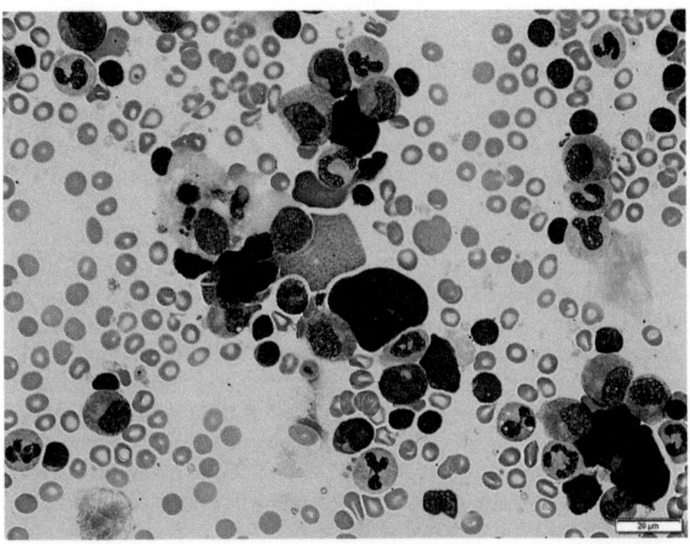

Fig. 4. BM aspirate from a patient with CDA III showing several multinucleated erythroid precursors (Giemsa, original magnification ×600).

SEVERE CONGENITAL NEUTROPENIA

Severe congenital neutropenia (SCN) is a heterogeneous group of disorders characterized by severe neutropenia presenting in the neonatal period or early infancy. Hemoglobin and platelet counts are usually normal. There are no distinctive physical features associated with most cases.[30] The incidence of SCN is approximately 1 to 2 cases per million and both sexes are affected equally.[1]

Features and Molecular Basis

Patients present with recurrent bacterial infections, such as skin infections, abscesses, omphalitis, and pneumonia. Affected patients usually have isolated severe neutropenia (absolute neutrophil count $<0.5 \times 10^9/L$), sometimes with relative monocytosis and increased monocyte percentage in the marrow. In most cases, BM examination shows normal or slightly decreased cellularity with maturation arrest of the myeloid cells at the promyelocyte/myelocyte stage (**Fig. 5**). Myelocytes and promyelocytes may show atypical nuclei and cytoplasmic vacuolization with sometimes marrow eosinophilia.

Heterozygous mutations in *ELANE* are found in 50% to 75% of patients and produce defective neutrophil elastase, triggering unfolded protein stress response resulting in apoptosis. The autosomal recessive form, Kostmann syndrome, is caused by biallelic mutations in the *HAX1* gene causing mitochondrial-induced apoptosis. An X-linked form of SCN is caused by activating mutations *WAS* gene resulting in increased actin polymerization. Mutations in *G6PC3*, a gene involved in the glucose-6-phosphate pathway has also been associated with congenital neutropenia; these patients manifest developmental anomalies of the cardiac and genitourinary systems. SCN is managed through administration of granulocyte colony-stimulating factor (G-CSF) to induce increased neutrophil counts and prevent infections. HSCT is the only curative treatment. Patients with SCN are at increased risk of developing MDS and AML, with a cumulative incidence of MDS/AML of 21% by age 10 years.

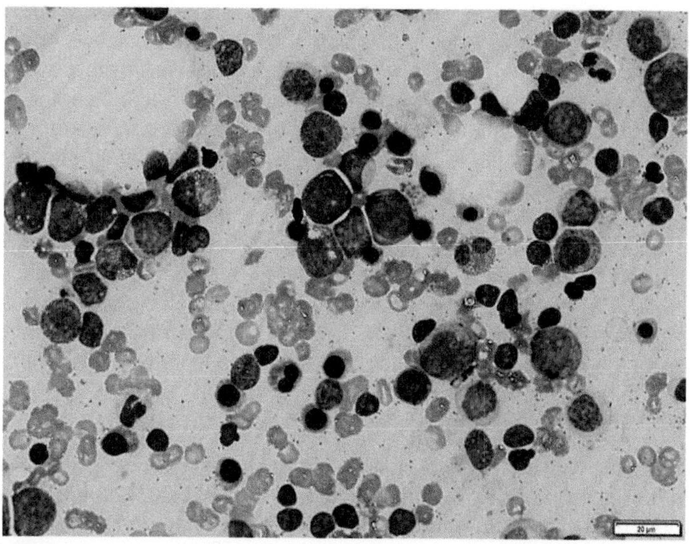

Fig. 5. BM aspirate from a patient with SCN showing granulocytic maturation arrest at the stage of promyelocyte/myelocyte with some degree of eosinophilia (Giemsa, original magnification ×600).

During the course of disease progression to MDS or AML, approximately 80% of patients acquire somatic mutations in the gene encoding the G-CSF receptor (G-CSFR), *CSF3R,* specifically in marrow myeloid cells, leading to truncation of G-CSFR C-terminus. These findings suggest that *CSF3R* mutations contribute to leukemogenesis in SCN patients.[31]

Differential Diagnosis

The most common causes of neutropenia, even in infants, are due to infections, medications/drugs, nutritional deficiency, and autoimmune neutropenia.

Cyclic neutropenia is a rare, autosomal dominantly inherited disorder characterized by neutropenia that recurs in a median of 21-day cycle (range 14–35 days). Most of the patients present with neutropenia in the first year of life. The neutrophil count waxes and wanes contrasting with the persistent neutropenia seen in SCN. Therefore, it is recommended to check white blood cell count and differentials 2 to 3 times a week for 6 weeks to understand the pattern of neutropenia. Subsequent genetic testing helps in the identification of the specific causative gene mutation. Compared with SCN, an even higher frequency of *ELANE* mutations (90%–100%) is found in cyclic neutropenia with significant overlap between both entities. Rarely, cyclic neutropenia leads to clonal evolution.[31]

The presentation in early life, the maturation arrest of granulocytic precursors at the promyelocyte/myelocyte stage, and the absence of antineutrophil antibodies are helpful in considering SCN diagnosis.

CONGENITAL AMEGAKARYOCYTIC THROMBOCYTOPENIA

Congenital amegakaryocytic thrombocytopenia (CAMT) is a rare disorder characterized by thrombocytopenia present at birth or in the neonatal period, associated with megakaryocytic hypoplasia/aplasia in the BM, without any other significant morphologic abnormalities. When present, megakaryocytes are rare with normal morphology. Thus far, there are more than 100 cases reported.

There are no characteristic congenital physical abnormalities associated with CAMT, except rare cases with neurologic or skeletal abnormalities. Approximately 70% of patients with CAMT have severe thrombocytopenia in the neonatal period causing petechiae and intracranial or intestinal mucus membrane bleeding. The major treatment for bleeding is platelet transfusion. The disease progresses to BM aplasia within the first few years of life (median age 3.7 years). Occasional patients may present with aplastic anemia, MDS, or AML without a preceding documented history of thrombocytopenia. HSCT remains the only curative therapy for CAMT.[1,7] CAMT is autosomal recessive and caused by homozygous or compound heterozygous mutations in *MPL,* which encodes the thrombopoietin (TPO) receptor. Patients with complete loss of *MPL* function have permanently low platelet counts (patients with CAMT I), whereas those with residual *MPL* activity demonstrate a transient amelioration of thrombocytopenia within the first year of life (patients with CAMT II).[1]

THROMBOCYTOPENIA WITH ABSENT RADII

Thrombocytopenia with absent radii (TAR) is a rare genetic disorder presenting in newborns as thrombocytopenia with characteristically absent bilateral radii but preserved thumbs. There are no consistent data about frequency, although an estimate of 0.42 cases per 100,000 live births was reported from Spain.[32] Patients may have other birth defects, such as hypoplastic ulnae, hypoplastic humeri, and renal malformations. Gastroenteritis and cow's milk intolerance are frequent.[7] There is typically no anemia

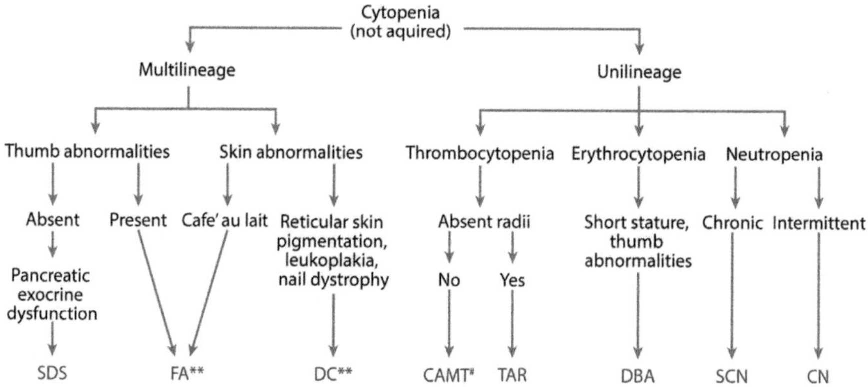

Fig. 6. Algorithmic approach to diagnosis of IBMFSs. CN, cyclic neutropenia. **May present with unilineage cytopenia; # may present with multilineage cytopenia).

or leukopenia. BM megakaryocytes may be decreased, absent, or immature-appearing, small sized, and with basophilic, vacuolated cytoplasm. It is to be noted that small and immature-appearing megakaryocytes are a normal finding in young children younger than 2 years.[33]

Approximately 60% of affected infants develop severe thrombocytopenia in the first few weeks of life, which may cause fatal hemorrhages. Platelet counts tend to increase over time, reaching normal values by adult life, although there may be fluctuation of platelet counts both in childhood and adult life. Platelet transfusions are given as needed and usually are no longer required beyond the first year of life, when the platelet count improves. Early deaths are from bleeding, with a plateau of survival of 80% by age 1 to 2 years. HSCT is rarely required.[7] Leukemoid reactions have been reported in as high as 50% of cases and are usually transient.[34] The development of aplastic anemia has not been observed, but rare cases of AML and acute lymphoblastic leukemia (ALL) have been reported.[1]

TAR is inherited in an autosomal recessive fashion. Recently, a combination of comparative genomic hybridization and next generation sequencing revealed a 200 kb microdeletion of chromosome 1q21.1 in 1 allele and 2 single nucleotide polymorphisms in *RBM8A* in the nondeleted allele.[1]

SUMMARY

IBMFS diagnosis and classification require a combination of clinical and family history, physical examination, laboratory and BM findings, and specialized testing, including molecular diagnostics. **Fig. 6** demonstrates a general approach for patients with possible IBMFS.

CLINICS CARE POINTS

- Detailed physical examination of children and young individuals with cytopenia, particularly skeletal abnormalities or skin changes, are excellent clues to an IBMFS.
- Detailed family history of transfusions, malignancies, or even premature greying of hair may also provide additional clues.
- The presence of macrocytic anemia may point to a chronic bone marrow failure process, if nutritional deficiencies and absorption defects are excluded.

REFERENCES

1. Dror Y. Inherited bone marrow failure syndromes. In: Hoffman RB, Silberstain LE, et al, editors. Hematology: basic principles and practice. 7th Ed. Philadelphia: Elsevier Health Sciences; 2018. p. 350–93.
2. Swerdlow SH, Campo E, Harris NL, et al. WHO classification of tumours of haematopoietic and lymphoid tissues (revised 4th edition). Lyon: IARC; 2017. p. 121–8.
3. Fiesco-Roa MO, Giri N, McReynolds LJ, et al. Genotype-phenotype associations in Fanconi anemia: a literature review. Blood Rev 2019;37:100589.
4. Dufour C. How I manage patients with Fanconi anemia. Br J Haematol 2017;178: 32–47.
5. Fares F, Badarneh K, Abosaleh M, et al. Carrier frequency of autosomal-recessive disorders in the Ashkenazi Jewish population: should the rationale for mutation choice for screening be reevaluated? Prenat Diagn 2008;28:236–41.
6. Furutani E, Shimamura A. Inherited aplastic anemia syndromes germline. In: Greer JP, Rodgers GM, Glader B, et al, editors. Wintrobes's clinical hematology. 14th Ed. Philadelphia: Wolters Kluwer; 2019. p. 1–46.
7. Shimamura A, Alter BP. Pathophysiology and management of inherited bone marrow failure syndromes. Blood Rev 2010;24:101–22.
8. Kutler DI, Singh B, Satagopan J, et al. A 20-year perspective on the international fanconi anemia registry (IFAR). Blood 2003;101:1249–56.
9. Alter BP, Giri N, Savage SA, et al. Cancer in the National Cancer Institute inherited bone marrow failure syndrome cohort after fifteen years of follow-up. Haematologica 2018;103:30–9.
10. DeZern AE, Symons HJ, Resar LS, et al. Detection of paroxysmal nocturnal hemoglobinuria clones to exclude inherited bone marrow failure syndromes. Eur J Haematol 2014;92:467–70.
11. Keller P, Debaun MR, Rothbaum RJ, et al. Bone marrow failure in Shwachman-Diamond syndrome does not select for clonal haematopoiesis of the paroxysmal nocturnal haemoglobinuria phenotype. Br J Haematol 2002;119:830–2.
12. Wegman-Ostrosky T, Savage SA. The genomics of inherited bone marrow failure: from mechanism to the clinic. Br J Haematol 2017;177:526–42.
13. Waisfisz Q, Morgan NV, Savino M, et al. Spontaneous functional correction of homozygous fanconi anaemia alleles reveals novel mechanistic basis for reverse mosaicism. Nat Genet 1999;22:379–83.
14. Clauson C, Scharer OD, Niedernhofer L. Advances in understanding the complex mechanisms of DNA interstrand cross-link repair. Cold Spring Harb Perspect Biol 2013;5:a012732.
15. Mehta PA, Harris RE, Davies SM, et al. Numerical chromosomal changes and risk of devlopment of myelodysplastic syndrome-acute myeloid leukemia in patients with Fanconi anemia. Cancer Gernet Cytogenet 2010;203:180–6.
16. Noy-Lotan S, Krasnov T, Dgany O, et al. Incorporation of somatic panels for the detection of haematopoietic transformation in childrens and young adults with leukemia predisposition syndromes and with acquired cytopenias. Br J Haematol 2021;193(3):570–80.
17. Savage SA. Beginning at the ends: telomeres and human disease. F1000Research 2018;7:524.
18. Dror Y, Donadieu J, Koglmeier J, et al. Draft consensus guidelines for diagnosis and treatment of Shwachman-Diamond syndrome. Ann N Y Acad Sci 2011;1242: 40–55.

19. Donadieu J, Fenneteau O, Beaupain B, et al. Classification of and risk factors for hematologic complications in a French national cohort of 102 patient with Shwachman-Diamond syndrome. Haematologica 2012;97:1312–9.
20. Rothbaum R, Perrault J, Vlachos A, et al. Shwachman-Diamond syndrome: report from an international conference. J Pediatr 2002;141:266–70.
21. Warren AJ. Molecular basis of the human ribosomopathy Shwachman-Diamond syndrome. Adv Biol Regul 2018;67:109–27.
22. Oyarbide U, Corey S. SRP54 and a need for a new neutropenia nosology. Blood 2018;132:1220–2.
23. Da Costa L, Leblanc T, Mohandas N. Diamond-Blackfan anemia. Blood 2020;136: 1262–73.
24. Flores Ballester E, Gil-Fernandez JJ, Vazquez Blanco M, et al. Adult-onset Diamond-Blackfan anemia with a novel mutation in the exon 5 of RPL11: too late and too rare. Clin Case Rep 2015;3:392–5.
25. Dietz AC, Mehta PA, Vlachos A, et al. Current knowledge and priorities for future research in late effects after hematopoietic cell transplantation for inherited bone marrow failure syndromes: consensus statement from the second pediatric blood and marrow transplant consortium international conference on late effects after pediatric hematopoietic cell transplantation. Biol Blood Marrow Transpl 2017; 23:726–35.
26. Vlachos A, Ball S, Dahl N, et al. Diagnosing and treating Diamond Blackfan anaemia: results of an international clinical consensus conference. Br J Haematol 2008;142:859–76.
27. Gastou M, Rio S, Dussiot M, et al. The severe phenotype of Diamond-Blackfan anemia is modulated by heat shock protein 70. Blood Adv 2017;1:1959–76.
28. Elghetany MT. Diamond-Blackfan anemia: death by heme toxicity? Eur J Haematol 2016;96:333–4.
29. Gambale A, Iolascon A, Andolfo I, et al. Diagnosis and management of congenital dyserythropoietic anemias. Expert Rev Hematol 2016;9:283–96.
30. Khincha PP, Savage SA. Neonatal manifestations of inherited bone marrow failure syndromes. Semin Fetal Neonatal Med 2016;21:57–65.
31. Qiu Y, Zhang Y, Hu N, et al. A truncated granulocyte colony-stimulating factor receptor (G-CSFR) inhibits apoptosis induced by neutrophil elastase G185R mutant: implication for understanding *CSF3R* gene mutations in severe congenital neutropenia. J Biol Chem 2017;292:3496–505.
32. Dufour C, Miano M, Fioredda F. Old and new faces of neutropenia in children. Haematologica 2016;101:789–91.
33. Fuchs DA, McGinn SG, Cantu CL, et al. Developmental differences in megakaryocyte size in infants and children. Am J Clin Pathol 2012;138:140–5.
34. Bonsi L, Marchionni C, Alviano F, et al. Thrombocytopenia with absent radii syndrome: from hemopoietic progenitor to mesenchymal stromal cell disease? Exp Hematol 2009;37:1–7.

Reactive Lymphadenopathies

Maria Faraz, MD[a,1], Flavia G.N. Rosado, MD[b,*]

KEYWORDS

• Reactive • Lymphadenopathy • Lymphadenitis • Infections • Lymph node
• Pediatric

KEY POINTS

- Infections are the leading cause of lymphadenitis in children.
- The histopathologic patterns may suggest a specific etiology in some cases of pediatric lymphadenitis; however, confirmation requires correlation with clinical findings and results of other laboratory testing.
- A pattern of immunoblastic paracortical hyperplasia is associated with viral infections, such as infectious mononucleosis and immunodeficiency-associated lymphoproliferative disorders.
- Granulomatous inflammation in cervical lymph nodes of young children frequently is caused by atypical mycobacterial infections.
- Some features seen in infectious or reactive disorders may mimic those seen in Hodgkin and non-Hodgkin lymphomas.

INTRODUCTION

Peripheral lymphadenopathy leading to palpable lymph nodes is a frequent finding in the pediatric population.[1,2] In infants, occipital and postauricular lymph nodes are more commonly palpable, whereas in children over 2 years of age, cervical and sometimes inguinal lymph nodes are affected more frequently.[3] In at least 75% of cases, peripheral lymphadenopathy is benign, self-limited, and managed conservatively.[4,5] A more comprehensive diagnostic investigation, including blood testing, serology, and imaging studies, may be required in refractory or symptomatic cases.[5] Clinical studies of pediatric cervical lymphadenopathy reveal no identifiable etiology in as many as 67% of cases.[2] Infections represent the most common identifiable cause, in particular viral upper respiratory infections and Epstein-Barr virus (EBV).[2,5]

The authors have no conflicts of interest to disclose.

[a] Department of Health Sciences, McMaster University; [b] University of Texas Southwestern Medical Center, 2330 Inwood Road, Biocenter EB3.234, Dallas, TX 75390-9317, USA
[1] Present address: 325 Dalgleish Garden, Milton, Ontario L9T 6Z6, Canada.
* Corresponding author.
E-mail addresses: Flavia.rosado@utsouthwestern.edu; flaviarosado7@gmail.com

Clin Lab Med 41 (2021) 433–451
https://doi.org/10.1016/j.cll.2021.04.001 labmed.theclinics.com

Autoimmune or inflammatory diseases, such as systemic lupus erythematous (SLE), Kikuchi-Fujimoto lymphadenitis, Castleman disease, and sarcoidosis, are uncommon, representing fewer than 1% of cases of pediatric lymphadenopathy worldwide.[2]

A tissue biopsy typically is recommended when there is clinical or parental concern for malignancy.[5] In samples negative for malignancy, histopathologic examination seldom reveals the specific etiology of the lymphadenitis. In cases of positive identification using microbiologic studies, bacteria and nontuberculous mycobacteria are reported most frequently.[6]

In this article, the histopathologic patterns associated with pediatric lymphadenitis are reviewed. Patterns that mimic malignancies are discussed. Recognizing the etiology associated most frequently with each of these patterns may be helpful in narrowing down a clinical differential diagnosis and guide additional testing.

DISCUSSION

Histopathologic patterns described in association with pediatric lymphadenitis can be divided into 4 categories based on the most predominant morphologic pattern: follicular hyperplasia, paracortical hyperplasia, suppurative and granulomatous, and histiocytic. Patterns of follicular and paracortical hyperplasia overlap with what is considered "normal" in a lymph node, representing a patient's normal immunologic response to nonspecific antigenic insults.[7] Although sinus histiocytosis also is considered a variation of normal lymph node reaction, the presence of granulomas and necrosis usually is indicative of an underlying pathologic process.

Follicular Hyperplasia Pattern

The follicular hyperplasia pattern is characterized by hyperplasia of lymphoid follicles with formation of prominent germinal centers. Recognizing the normal follicular architecture is important in the distinction from follicular lymphoma. Normal lymphoid follicles show a distinct rim of mantle zone small lymphocytes delineating germinal center cells in a polarized arrangement (**Fig. 1**). Normal germinal center cells comprise

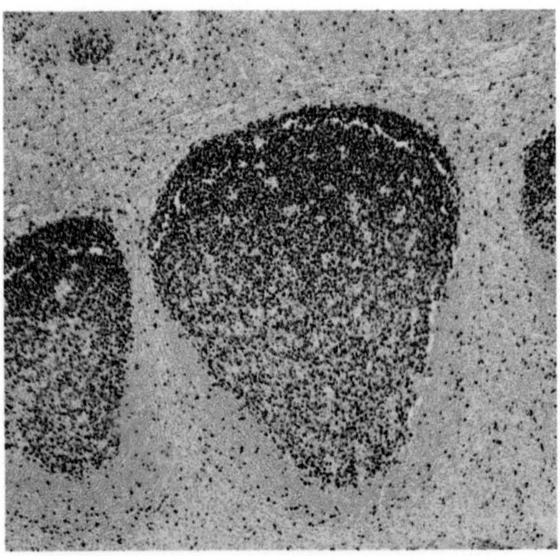

Fig. 1. A Ki-67 immunohistochemical stain highlights the normal polarization of germinal center cells in a reactive lymph node with follicular hyperplasia. Normal polarization is helpful to distinguish reactive and neoplastic follicles. Ki-67 immunostain, original magnification ×10.

a mixture of centroblasts, centrocytes, follicular dendritic cells, and tingible body macrophages.[7]

Utilizing immunohistochemical stains, the expression of CD10 and Bcl-6 is confined to the germinal center cells, and there is no coexpression of Bcl-2. Ki-67 proliferation rate is high within germinal centers (>95%) but is extremely low (<10%) otherwise. Uniform expression of CD5, CD23, CD43, or diminished CD20 on PAX5-positive B cells is considered aberrant. A low Ki-67 proliferation rate within a germinal center should be considered atypical. CD21 or CD23 may demonstrate expanded follicular dendritic cell meshworks, yet sharply delineated within the germinal centers. Flow cytometric studies are helpful to demonstrate B-cell surface kappa/lambda light chain expression in a polytypic pattern. Immunoglobulin gene rearrangement studies are polyclonal. These morphologic and phenotypic features of normal follicular hyperplasia are important in the distinction with follicular lymphoma.[7,8]

When approaching the differential diagnosis of follicular hyperplasia and follicular lymphoma, it is important to recognize that pediatric-type follicular lymphoma shows unique features that may make this distinction more challenging. Unlike systemic non-pediatric follicular lymphoma, most cases of pediatric-type follicular lymphoma are negative for Bcl2 by immunohistochemistry and fluorescence in situ hybridization, similar to follicular hyperplasia. Follicular lymphoma should be suspected even if Bcl2 staining is negative if there are expansile follicles that display other atypical features, such as attenuation or loss of mantle zones, a starry sky appearance of germinal center cells with loss of polarity, and a uniform proliferation of medium sized cells. The immunostain Foxp1 has emerged as a potential tool to differentiate between follicular hyperplasia and pediatric-type follicular lymphoma.[9] A positive polymerase chain reaction (PCR) study for immunoglobulin gene rearrangements helps establish a diagnosis, when in correlation with abnormal clinical and histologic findings.[10]

Although flow cytometry typically is a useful tool to demonstrate B-cell clonality through light chain restriction, prominent light chain–restricted B-cell populations occasionally may be identified by flow cytometry in the setting of follicular lymphoid hyperplasia. Such populations otherwise are similar to normal polyclonal germinal center cells in that they are negative for Bcl2 and express CD10 at a low to moderate level. The occurrence of these populations represents a diagnostic pitfall and illustrates the importance of correlating flow cytometric findings with clinical and morphologic findings for diagnosis of lymphoma.[11]

Follicular hyperplasia commonly is a nonspecific pattern but also is seen in association with viral infections as well as autoimmune and inflammatory diseases.[12] Isolated florid follicular hyperplasia is the hallmark of acute human immunodeficiency virus (HIV) lymphadenitis, with irregularly shaped germinal centers resembling the outlines of continents or animal crackers. Measles lymphadenitis may cause florid follicular hyperplasia in the gastrointestinal tract and an increased risk of acute appendicitis. Warthin-Finkeldey giant cells, large multinucleated cells with numerous nuclei distributed in grape-like clusters, can be seen in acute HIV and in measles lymphadenitis[13] (**Fig. 2**). Lymphadenopathy associated with untreated autoimmune diseases, such as systemic juvenile idiopathic arthritis and early-onset rheumatoid arthritis, display a pattern of marked follicular hyperplasia, with or without immunoblastic paracortical hyperplasia, accompanied by an interfollicular increase in polytypic plasma cells and occasional neutrophils. Associated hepatosplenomegaly and systemic symptoms, such as fever and fatigue, are typical of systemic juvenile idiopathic arthritis.[14] In patients who undergo immunomodulant therapy, there is regression of the lymphoid follicles with paracortical hyperplasia. The differential diagnosis in sexually active adolescents may include syphilitic lymphadenitis. In these patients, the

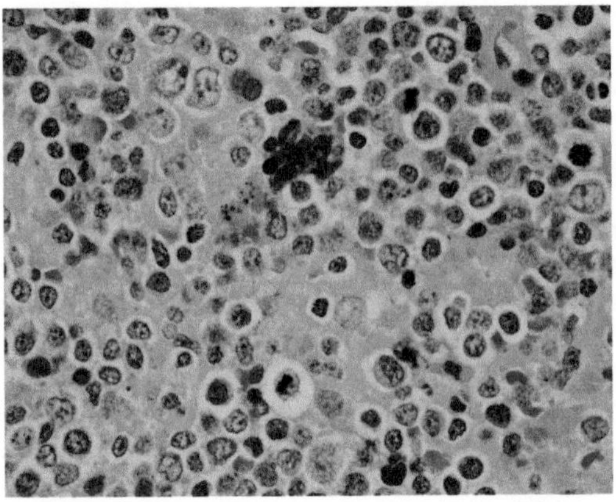

Fig. 2. Warthin-Finkeldey cells are multinucleated cells with nuclei arranged in grape-like clusters. These cells typically are seen in acute viral lymphadenitis caused by the HIV, measles, or herpesvirus. Hematoxylin-eosin, original magnification ×100 oil.

differential diagnosis also includes drug-induced lymphadenitis and EBV-related lymphoid proliferations.[14]

Castleman disease

Castleman disease is a type of lymphoproliferative disorder rarely diagnosed in children, presenting most typically as mediastinal or intra-abdominal masses or localized cervical, axillary, or inguinal lymphadenopathy.[15] Multicentric Castleman disease is a life-threatening form of Castleman disease with the occurrence of systemic inflammatory symptoms, lymphadenopathy, cytopenias, and multiorgan system dysfunction.[16] The clinical presentation significantly overlaps with those of autoimmune and infectious disorders. Multicentric Castleman disease in children usually is idiopathic (human herpesvirus 8–negative). The more recently described variant of idiopathic multicentric Castleman disease, named TAFRO syndrome (Castleman-Kojima disease), is defined by associated thrombocytopenia, anasarca, myelofibrosis/fever, renal dysfunction/reticulin fibrosis, and organomegaly and has been reported in adolescents.[17,18] Cases of Castleman disease reported in children display features of hyaline-vascular type of Castleman disease, with follicular hyperplasia, including expanded concentric mantle zones and regressed germinal centers penetrated by hyalinized vessels, interfollicular vascular proliferation, and variable degrees of interfollicular polytypic plasmacytosis.[15–19]

IgG4-related lymphadenopathy

IgG4-related disease is systemic inflammatory disorder that may be associated with lymphadenopathy (IgG4-related lymphadenopathy). Lymphadenopathy also may be the initial presentation of systemic disease in some patients.[20] There are several reports of this disease in the pediatric population, particularly in adolescents. Most cases in this age group were of orbital and pancreatic involvement, with lymphadenopathy reported less frequently.[21] In lymph node biopsies, IgG4-related lymphadenopathy is defined by plasmacytosis with a predominance of IgG4-positive polytypic plasma cells, sometimes with increase in eosinophils.[22] Additional morphologic findings are used to characterize 5 morphologic subtypes: pattern I, multicentric Castleman-like; pattern II, the most common form overall, with reactive follicular hyperplasia and intragerminal center plasma cells; pattern III, interfollicular expansion with normal to regressed follicles; pattern IV, mimics progressive transformation of germinal center (PTGC), is the most common form in pediatric patients, and may be accompanied by immunoblasts and characteristic rimming by epithelioid histiocytes; and pattern V, inflammatory pseudotumor-like, characterized by fibrosis, occasionally storiform, accompanied by small lymphocytes, plasma cells, eosinophils, and histiocytes.[20–22] Clinical correlation is necessary for a diagnosis of IgG4-related disease, because none of these patterns is specific. An increase in IgG4-positive plasma cells has been described nonspecifically as an incidental finding. The histopathologic differential diagnosis includes Castleman disease, especially in cases presenting as mediastinal and intraabdominal masses, and rheumatoid arthritis. IgG4-related lymphadenopathy typically lacks the severe systemic symptoms of multicentric Castleman disease and autoimmune diseases. In cases of increased number of histiocytes, a diagnosis of Rosai-Dorfman disease may be considered in the differential.[22]

Progressive transformation of germinal center

PTGC, a reactive pattern sometimes identified in the setting of nonspecific follicular hyperplasia, occurs frequently in children.[23] It is characterized by nodules of small lymphocytes due to the dissolution of germinal centers by the infiltration of mantle zone lymphocytes. Although PTGC is a nonspecific pattern, it may mimic or coexist with lesions of nodular lymphocyte predominant Hodgkin lymphoma[24] (**Fig. 3**).

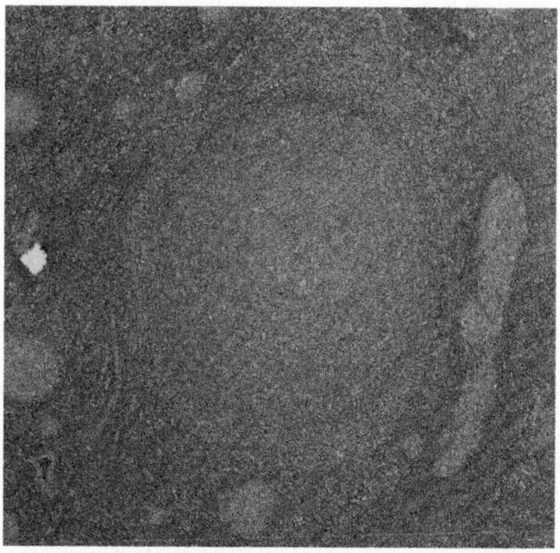

Fig. 3. Progressive transformation of germinal center is a nonspecific reactive alteration of follicles and is characterized by dissolution of the germinal center due to infiltration of mantle zone lymphocytes. This finding must be distinguished from the neoplastic nodules seen in nodular lymphocyte predominant Hodgkin lymphoma. Hematoxylin-eosin, original magnification ×4.

Paracortical Hyperplasia Pattern

The pattern of paracortical hyperplasia is characterized by prominent expansion of the lymph node paracortex (interfollicular space), leading to attenuation of lymphoid follicles. This pattern commonly is seen in association with variable degrees of follicular hyperplasia or histiocytosis. In many patients, an etiology cannot be identified[25]; viral infections may be seen in association with this pattern in children with cervical lymphadenitis.[2] Noninfectious etiologies associated with this pattern include iatrogenic lymphoproliferative disorders and immunodeficiency-associated lymphoid proliferations. Florid immunoblastic paracortical hyperplasia is seen in infectious mononucleosis and following treatment with antiepileptics and some antibiotics in susceptible individuals, often accompanied by other systemic symptoms.[26] Lymphadenopathy with paracortical hyperplasia, in the past associated with smallpox vaccination, also is seen following immunization against other viral infections, such as measles and varicella.[27]

Immunodeficiency-associated lymphoproliferative disorders

Immunodeficiency-associated lymphoproliferative disorders are uncommon causes of lymphadenopathy in children but may be seen more frequently in specialized centers. This group encompasses all lymphoid lesions that arise in the setting of a primary immune disorder (PID). These lymphoproliferative lesions are common and often indolent in autoimmune lymphoproliferative syndrome (ALPS) and common variable immune deficiency (CVID) but may be clinically aggressive in other types of PID.[28] In patients with X-linked lymphoproliferative disease and severe combined immunodeficiency, EBV-driven infectious mononucleosis and hemophagocytic lymphohistiocytosis (HLH) are important causes of mortality.[28]

Although many patients with lymphadenopathy in this setting are managed conservatively, the increased risk of lymphomas in these patients prompts a biopsy to rule out malignancy in selected individuals.[28] Given this increased risk, pathologists may choose to obtain a more comprehensive panel of ancillary studies when evaluating lymph node biopsies in this setting. Clonality testing may be useful to confirm malignancy in selected cases but is not diagnostic in isolation.[28] An EBV in situ hybridization study to demonstrate the association of EBV often is helpful.

As in other immunodeficiency-associated disorders, a lymph node biopsy in patients with PIDs is likely to show EBV-associated lesions that fall within a spectrum of benign reactive hyperplasia, ranging from florid polymorphous infiltrates with various degree of atypia, to a proliferation of clonal cells that fulfill diagnostic of malignant lymphomas.[29] The non-neoplastic lesions typically are characterized by florid immunoblastic paracortical hyperplasia similar to infectious mononucleosis, with or without follicular hyperplasia.

The various degrees of atypia may represent a diagnostic pitfall when the diagnosis of PID is unknown.[30] In ALPS, there typically is paracortical expansion with atypical T cells mimicking T-cell lymphoma. Prominent follicular hyperplasia may be present, raising concern for follicular lymphoma. In some cases, PTGCs may coexist with nodular lymphocyte-predominant Hodgkin lymphoma or T-cell/histiocyte-rich large B-cell lymphoma.[30] In CVID, there is a typical EBV-related immunoblastic paracortical hyperplasia with Reed-Sternberg (RS)-like cells mimicking classic Hodgkin lymphoma. Patients with CVID also may show prominent gastrointestinal tract nodular lymphoid hyperplasia mimicking lymphomatous polyposis.[28]

Infectious mononucleosis lymphadenitis

Infectious mononucleosis (EBV) lymphadenitis is caused by acute EBV infection. It is characterized morphologically by an expansion of the interfollicular space by inflammatory cells, which vary according to specific underlying disorders. For example, in viral infections, namely EBV and herpesvirus infections, the proliferation is described as polymorphic, because it often includes a mixture of variably sized lymphocytes, some with distinct nucleoli (immunoblasts), and occasional histiocytes and plasma cells. Necrosis may be present[31–33] (**Fig. 4**A).

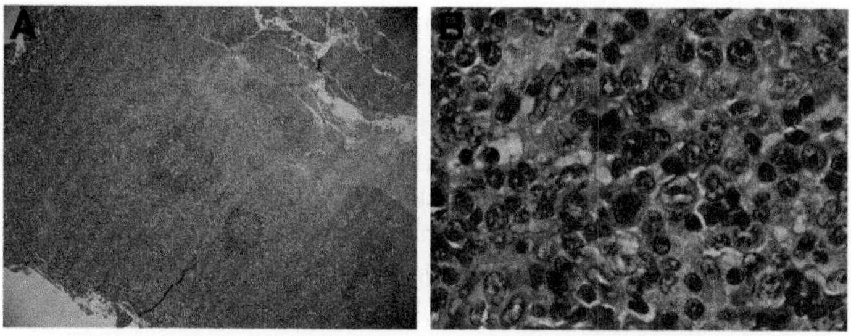

Fig. 4. Immunoblastic paracortical hyperplasia characterized by widening of the interfollicular space due to a polymorphic inflammatory infiltrate comprising predominantly variably sized lymphocytes and histiocytes (*A*). A few of the immunoblasts may be binucleate mimicking RS cells seen in classic Hodgkin lymphoma (*B*). (*A*) Hematoxylin-eosin, original magnification ×2. (*B*) Hematoxylin-eosin, original magnification ×100 oil.

In some cases, the florid immunoblastic proliferation includes few large binucleated cells with prominent nucleoli mimicking RS cells[32] (**Fig. 4**B). In such cases, the presence of features, such as intact nodal architecture and a spectrum of variably sized immunoblasts and mixture of B-immunoblasts and T-immunoblasts, are indicative of a reactive process.[33] In addition, careful correlation with immunohistochemical stains and clinical history often is helpful, because, unlike classic Hodgkin lymphoma, immunoblasts tend to retain CD20 and CD45 expression, more variably express CD30, and are negative for CD15.[33] The association with EBV easily is demonstrated with EBV-encoded RNA in situ hybridization studies (EBER) performed on tissue sections. Rare, small EBV-positive cells may be seen in healthy individuals and typically is not considered evidence of an EBV-driven process. In some cases, the predominance of large B-immunoblasts or a marked decrease in the CD4:CD8 ratio raises concern for large B-cell lymphoma or T-cell lymphoma, respectively. As such, caution in making a diagnosis of B and T-cell non-Hodgkin lymphoma in children with known EBV coinfection is advised. Utilization of molecular clonality studies is helpful to demonstrate the polyclonal nature of the process.[31,33] In children presenting with lymphadenopathy, a diagnosis of polymorphous EBV-related lymphoid proliferations outside of the clinical context of infectious mononucleosis may suggest an underlying immunodeficiency.[28]

Herpesvirus lymphadenitis

Herpesvirus lymphadenitis is an uncommon complication of herpes simplex virus (HSV)-1 or HSV-2 infections, which can occur from either primary exposure or, more commonly, reactivation.[34,35] HSV-1 infections are more common in children, whereas HSV-2 is more frequent in sexually active adolescents.[34–36] Lymph node biopsies are more likely to be performed in patients with prior diagnosis of malignancies who are undergoing surveillance for recurrence or in immunocompromised patients with disseminated infections.[35] Lymph node biopsies reveal prominent immunoblastic paracortical hyperplasia similar to that seen in infectious mononucleosis, sometimes with RS-like cells or Warthin-Finkeldey cells.[35,37] Additional features of HSV lymphadenitis include sharply circumscribed areas of necrosis and sinus histiocytosis. Adjacent to areas of necrosis, multinucleated cells with ground-glass chromatin and intranuclear inclusions with a halo (Cowdry type A inclusions) may be seen and are considered diagnostic of HSV.[34,35,37] A positive HSV immunohistochemical stain or in situ hybridization can be used to confirm the diagnosis histologically. The positive cells may be described to be more frequently lymphocytes or endothelial cells.[34]

The differential diagnosis includes other viral infections discussed in this article, including EBV, cytomegalovirus (CMV), and HIV infections. If there is necrosis, the differential diagnosis includes suppurative and necrotic types of infectious lymphadenitis, such as those caused by bacterial infections. HSV lymphadenitis typically does not elicit granulomatous type of inflammation, thus distinguishing HSV from bacterial infections, cat-scratch disease (CSD), mycobacteria, and fungal infections. The necrosis in HSV typically is neutrophilic, allowing for the distinction with Kikuchi-Fujimoto lymphadenitis.[34,38,39]

Varicella lymphadenitis

Varicella infections, both chickenpox and varicella-zoster, may lead to cervical, supraclavicular, or axillary lymphadenopathy in children, but it is rarely biopsied due to the characteristic clinical findings that do not require tissue diagnosis. Histologically, the findings are similar to all herpesvirus infections, with prominent polymorphic paracortical hyperplasia, although in the recovery phase, there may be only follicular hyperplasia. Intranuclear inclusions with halo also may be seen.[40]

Cytomegalovirus lymphadenitis

Primary infections with CMV occur often in childhood and are asymptomatic, albeit in some children they may present with an infectious mononucleosis-like picture.[1,41] Immunosuppressed children may experience CMV lymphadenitis due to reactivation.[1–3,41] The histopathology of affected lymph nodes overlaps with that described in other viral infections, such as infectious mononucleosis and HIV, although monocytoid B-cell hyperplasia is a frequent finding.[42,43] The characteristic owl's eye central intranuclear inclusions with a halo (owl's eye) seen in some cases.[43] Cells infected with CMV often are T cells and may be positive for CD15.[44] The histopathology diagnosis can be established utilizing CMV immunohistochemical stain, which is positive in the inclusions.

Measles

Measles commonly affects unvaccinated children aged 5 years to 7 years and tends to be more severe in older children and adolescents, sometimes with lymphadenopathy.[45] Histologically, affected lymph nodes may display follicular hyperplasia with multinucleated Warthin-Finkeldey cells similar to those seen in HIV lymphadenitis. More characteristic, however, is the pattern of immunoblastic paracortical hyperplasia with features that overlap with those of infectious mononucleosis and other viral lymphadenitides.[45]

Kimura disease is an uncommon chronic inflammatory disease prevalent in male individuals of Asian descent. It is seen more frequently in young adults and rarely affects children.[31–46] The disease presents as subcutaneous masses of head and neck along with regional lymphadenopathy. Histologically, lymph node shows follicular hyperplasia with abundant eosinophils in the paracortex, sinusoids, and germinal centers.[46,47]

Drug-induced lymphadenopathy

Drug-induced lymphadenopathy generally is accompanied by systemic symptoms, such as fever and fatigue, and, in some patients, skin rash; signs of hepatitis, nephritis, or arthritis; and laboratory abnormalities, including leukocytosis or leukopenia and eosinophilia. The overall findings overlap with those of HLH with increase in ferritin and LDH.[48] In the presence of eosinophilia, the above-described clinical picture may be due to drug reaction with eosinophilia and systemic symptoms (DRESS) syndrome, a rare life-threatening condition that has been reported in the pediatric population, although less frequently than in adults.[49,50]

Antiepileptic drugs are implicated most commonly in the pediatric groups.[50] The symptoms start approximately 1 week to 8 weeks after the administration of the medication or as soon as 24 hours in patients with prior exposure to the medication.[48] Lymphadenopathy may be generalized or localized, with more frequent involvement of cervical and axillary lymph nodes. A lymph node biopsy is characterized by T-cell immunoblastic paracortical hyperplasia, sometimes accompanied by some modest follicular hyperplasia, vascular proliferation, foci of neutrophilic necrosis, and eosinophils.[48] In late-onset cases, the number of immunoblasts increases, there are few eosinophils, no necrosis, and regression of follicles. The T cells may display phenotypic alterations and cytologic atypia, including occasionally RS-like cells, raising concern for T-cell lymphoma.[48] Features that may be helpful in the distinction from lymphoma is the intact nodal architecture, a mixture of scattered B-cell and T-cell immunoblasts with weak and variable CD30-expression, and negative T-cell clonality help in establishing the diagnosis, although oligoclonal and clonal T cells have been reported.[48] Correlation with clinical findings is key, because in most cases, there are other symptoms of drug-induced reaction, discussed previously. The B-cell immunoblasts cells and RS-like cells show variable CD30-expression and do not lack the CD20 and CD45 expression, unlike the RS cells in classic Hodgkin lymphoma. In addition, EBV typically is negative in drug-induced lymphadenopathies.

Methotrexate commonly is used in the pediatric population to treat systemic juvenile idiopathic arthritics, psoriasis, lupus, and other autoimmune disorders. Therapy with methotrexate and other immunosuppressant and cytotoxic agents is associated with a spectrum of changes ranging from polyclonal hyperplastic proliferations to overt lymphoma, akin to what is seen in post-transplant lymphoproliferative disorders. These abnormal lymphoproliferative reactions are classified under the umbrella term, "other iatrogenic immunodeficiency-associated lymphoproliferative disorders" in the World Health Organization classification of hematolymphoid malignancies.[51] The clinical and histopathologic findings tend to regress with discontinuation of immunosuppressant therapy, except in patients using tumor necrosis factor blockers.[51]

Granulomatous and Suppurative Patterns

Suppurative patterns frequently are caused by bacteria streptococci and staphylococci, whereas necrotizing granulomatous types of lymphadenitis are associated with mycobacterial infections, CSD, and, less frequently, fungal infections.[1–4,26] Other less frequent bacterial infections leading to abscess formation and/or poorly formed granulomas include *Haemophilus influenzae*, *Pasteurella multocida*, *Francisella tularensis* (tularemia), *Yersinia* sp, and *Brucella* sp.[6,14] Inflammatory/autoimmune disorders, such as Kikuchi-Fujimoto lymphadenitis and SLE, occasionally are diagnosed in older children.[1–4,26]

Non-necrotizing granulomas may be seen as a nonspecific finding in benign lymph nodes and may be seen in early forms of the necrotizing infections. Sarcoidosis rarely is diagnosed in children and is characterized by numerous non-necrotizing granulomas depleted of surrounding lymphocytes (naked granulomas). Clusters of epithelioid histiocytes without discrete granuloma formation are part of a diagnostic triad of toxoplasmosis.[6,52]

Bacterial lymphadenitis

Acute unilateral lymphadenitis, in particular cervical, commonly is caused by bacteria *Staphylococcus aureus* and *Streptococcus* sp.[53] Early stages of infection typically are treated and diagnosed clinically without histopathologic examination. Incision and drainage or excision may be indicated in refractory and severe cases to alleviate symptoms and determine the etiology. Histologically, severe advanced cases show extensive coalescent areas of suppurative necrosis with abscess formation, with viable non-necrotic areas showing reactive follicular hyperplasia. In clinically refractory patients with negative aerobic and anaerobic and fungal cultures, less common infectious agents and noninfectious etiologies may be considered, such as Kawasaki lymphadenopathy.[54]

Cat-scratch disease

CSD is an infectious lymphadenitis caused by *Bartonella henselae*, commonly manifesting in children as localized self-limited lymphadenitis.[1–4] *B henselae* is a slow-growing fastidious bacterium that is difficult to isolate by culture.[6] A diagnosis is made based on clinical findings and serologic testing in most cases.[55] Serologic testing, however, lacks ideal sensitivity and specificity; therefore, molecular testing with PCR may be appropriate for confirmation.[56]

Histologically, CSD shows the characteristic irregularly shaped stellate microabscesses, which are sharply delineated granulomas with small central neutrophilic necrosis. The granulomas are composed of palisading histiocytes without multinucleated giant cells.[6,57] Some cases of CSD may lack this characteristic finding and show nonspecific types of necrotizing or non-necrotizing granulomatous inflammation.[6,55–57] A special stain, Warthin-Starry, may be used in an attempt to demonstrate the organisms, but, due to poor sensitivity and specificity, PCR testing of paraffin embedded tissue is a superior option to establish the diagnosis of CSD.[57]

Mycobacterial and fungal infections

In areas of low prevalence of tuberculosis, nontuberculous mycobacterial infections, specifically, *Mycobacterium avium intracellulare* and *Mycobacterium scrofulaceum*, are the leading cause of cervical lymphadenitis in immunocompetent children younger than 6 years of age.[5,6]

Microscopic examination of affected lymph nodes typically shows well-formed granulomas with central acellular necrosis (grossly, caseating) and numerous multinucleated giant cells[6] (**Fig. 5**). Visualization of the acid-fast bacilli with Ziehl-Neelsen special stain may be difficult due to the paucity of organisms[6] and Gomori methenamine silver stain (GMS) special stain is negative. In the appropriate clinical and epidemiologic context, a diagnosis of nontuberculous mycobacteria may be suggested and confirmed with appropriate tissue culture. In immunocompromised individuals, the mycobacteria tend to be more numerous and identified more easily with special stains on tissue sections.[58]

Fungal infection is a less frequent cause of lymphadenitis in children.[1–5] Affected lymph nodes show a necrotizing granulomatous pattern similar to mycobacterial infections.[58] A diagnosis can be made on visualization of the fungal forms in tissue sections with a GMS special stain, with more specific identification obtained with fungal culture and serologic testing.[5]

Toxoplasmosis

Toxoplasma lymphadenitis is caused by the protozoan *Toxoplasma gondii* and is the most common parasitic infection in the United States.[59] Serologic studies indicate that most infections are asymptomatic and occur in childhood.[1,2,59,60] The definitive host of the parasite is the cat, and humans are intermediate hosts infected through the ingestion of oocysts from contaminated soil or undercooked meat. Transmission also occurs transplacentally from mother to fetus or through solid organ transplant.[59,60]

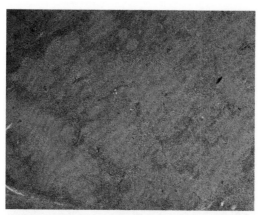

Fig. 5. Necrotizing granulomatous inflammation with acellular (grossly caseating) necrosis and numerous giant cells are seen in tuberculous and nontuberculous mycobacterial and fungal infections. Hematoxylin-eosin, original magnification ×2.

The histologic features of toxoplasma lymphadenitis include 3 key findings: (1) clusters of epithelioid histiocytes encroaching onto reactive lymphoid follicles, (2) follicular hyperplasia, and (3) aggregates of monocytoid B cells.[59] Upon identification of these findings, a diagnosis of toxoplasmosis is highly likely, and serologic testing then may be suggested for confirmation.[52,59]

Kawasaki disease

Kawasaki disease is an acute febrile exanthematous pediatric disease characterized by disseminated vasculitis of small and medium-sized vessels.[54] Unilateral acute cervical lymphadenitis is a frequent manifestation, particularly in older children. A biopsy of affected lymph nodes shows characteristic necrotic foci located immediately beneath the lymph node capsule, frequently with associated infiltration of the capsule with chronic inflammatory cells and sometimes extension into adjacent soft tissue.[54] The nodal parenchyma may show hyperplastic or atrophic lymphoid follicles and fibrin thrombi in the small vessels and perivascular nuclear debris. Acute inflammation and granulomas typically are absent.

Kikuchi-Fujimoto lymphadenitis and systemic lupus erythematosus (SLE)

Kikuchi-Fujimoto lymphadenitis (also known as necrotizing histiocytic lymphadenitis) and SLE lymphadenitis are histologically similar and occur more frequently in young female patients, although older children may be affected.[2] Unlike SLE, Kikuchi-Fujimoto lymphadenitis is a self-limited localized cause of lymphadenopathy and is of unknown etiology.[38,39] Histologically, Kikuchi-Fujimoto lymphadenitis is characterized by ill-defined histiocyte aggregates with prominent necrosis containing apoptotic nuclear debris and no neutrophils (**Fig. 6**). Clusters of immunoblasts or plasmacytoid dendritic cells may be seen, and an increase of $CD8^+$ T cells, mimicking non-Hodgkin lymphoma. Morphologic variants lacking necrosis have been described.[38,39]

Histiocytic Pattern

An increase in histiocytes seen along the sinuses is known as sinus histiocytosis and is a normal finding, especially in mediastinal lymph nodes. A diffuse proliferation of histiocytes that involves the paracortex, however, may be a sign of disorders, such as Rosai-Dorfman disease and HLH. Langerhans cell histiocytosis is a clonal neoplastic

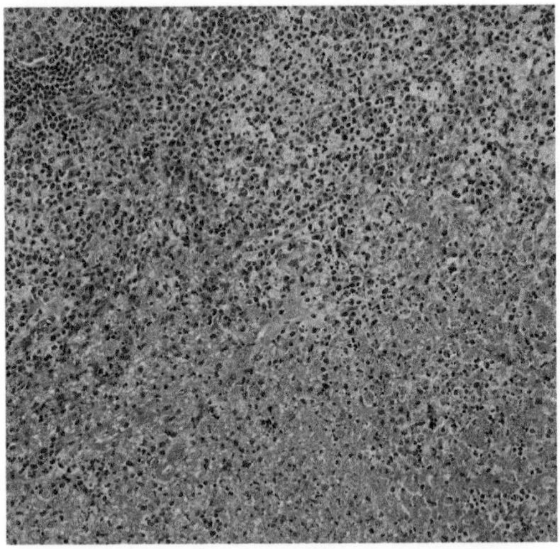

Fig. 6. Kikuchi-Fujimoto lymphadenitis is characterized by ill-defined clusters of histiocytes with acellular necrosis containing abundant nuclear debris but, unlike the granulomas of CSD. There are no neutrophils. Hematoxylin-eosin, original magnification ×20.

proliferation of Langerhans cells that is on the differential for histiocytic lesions in lymph nodes, although nodal involvement is uncommon.[61] Although malignant histiocytosis are exceedingly rare, a reactive proliferation of histiocytes often is seen accompanying a variety of Hodgkin and non-Hodgkin lymphomas, sometimes to a degree that masks the lymphoma cells.

Rosai-Dorfman disease

Rosai-Dorfman disease originally was described as "sinus Histiocytosis with massive lymphadenopathy" presenting as cervical lymphadenopathy in children, but later it was recognized as the etiology of pseudotumor in extranodal sites in patients with a wide age range.[62] Involved lymph nodes are characterized histologically by marked sinus distention that alters the nodal architecture. Distended sinus contains a mixture of histiocytes, small lymphocytes, and plasma cells. The histiocytes characteristically display abundant granular eosinophilic cytoplasm, some of which with numerous intact inflammatory cells within the cytoplasm (emperipolesis).

Immunohistochemical stains help confirm the diagnosis and highlight the emperipolesis. The histiocytes of Rosai-Dorfman disease are S100-positive but, unlike the LCH cells of Langerhans cell histiocytosis, are CD1a-negative and langerin-negative. Focal CD30 expression reflects cell activation and may be seen.[63] In Rosai-Dorfman disease, there is normal expression of histiocyte markers, such as weak CD4, CD68, and CD163, although lysozyme may be weak or absent.[62] Recurrent mutations in the *MAPK/ERK* pathway detected in Langerhans cell histiocytosis and Erdheim-Chester disease also have been described in one-third of cases of Rosai-Dorfman disease.[64]

Hemophagocytic lymphohistiocytosis

HLH is a clinical syndrome characterized by sudden development of sepsis-like symptoms. Five of the following 8 clinical-pathologic criteria are needed for the diagnosis: fever, splenomegaly, bicytopenia or pancytopenia, hyperferritinemia, hypofibrinogenemia, elevated soluble CD25, reduced or absent natural killer (NK) cell activity, and

Table 1
Differential diagnosis for the histologic patterns seen in pediatric lymphadenopathies

Histologic Pattern	Differential Diagnosis	Key Features
Isolated follicular hyperplasia	Nonspecific reactive pattern Viral infections HIV lymphadenitis Measles Follicular lymphoma Primary immunodeficiencies	Multinucleated Warthin-Finkeldey cells seen in both HIV and measles Expansile irregular follicles in acute HIV Normal polarization of germinal center cells and phenotyping helpful to rule out follicular lymphoma
Follicular hyperplasia with PTGC	Nonspecific reactive pattern Nodular lymphocyte predominant Hodgkin lymphoma	Cytologically atypical cells seen in nodular lymphocyte predominant Hodgkin lymphoma are absent in PTGC
Paracortical hyperplasia	EBV infectious mononucleosis HSV1/2 CMV Varicella Measles Classic Hodgkin lymphoma Drug-induced lymphadenopathy Primary immunodeficiencies Non-Hodgkin B-cell and T-cell lymphoma	Polymorphic with numerous immunoblasts RS-like cells express CD20, unlike RS cells of classic Hodgkin lymphoma Warthin-Finkeldey cells may be seen in measles and HSV lymphadenitis Well delineated necrosis in HSV Intranuclear inclusions may be seen in CMV, HSV, and varicella Associated monocytoid B-cell hyperplasia seen in CMV lymphadenitis
Suppurative	Bacterial lymphadenitis, Staphylococcus, Streptococcus, Haemophilus, Yersinia, *Francisella tularensis*, Brucella HSV lymphadenitis Kawasaki	Poorly formed granulomas also may be seen in bacterial infections Necrotic foci beneath the capsule seen in Kawasaki
Necrotizing granulomas	Mycobacteria, tuberculous, and nontuberculous Fungal infections CSD Kikuchi-Fujimoto lymphadenitis/SLE	Acellular (caseating) necrosis with numerous giant cells seen in mycobacterial and fungal infections CSD palisading histiocytes with neutrophilic microabscesses Kikuchi-Fujimoto lymphadenitis/SLE necrosis with nuclear debris and absence of neutrophils; C-shaped histiocytes; clusters of immunoblasts and plasmacytoid dendritic cells

(*continued on next page*)

Table 1
(continued)

Histologic Pattern	Differential Diagnosis	Key Features
Non-necrotizing granulomas	Sarcoidosis; infections; nonspecific	
Histiocytoses	HLH, Rosai-Dorfman disease	
Miscellaneous	Toxoplasmosis • Triad: follicular hyperplasia, monocytoid B-cell hyperplasia, epithelioid histiocytes extend into lymphoid follicles Kimura • Follicular hyperplasia and interfollicular eosinophils	

hemophagocytosis in the bone marrow or other tissues.[65] HLH is a fatal complication seen in children with genetic disorders affecting NK/T-cell granules exocytosis (familial HLH) and in children with primary immunodeficiencies.[66] In patients without a known HLH-predisposing condition, it may be important to rule out an associated triggering malignant lymphoma that could be masked by the lymphohistiocytic infiltrate of HLH.[66–68]

Bone marrow biopsies are the procedure of choice to demonstrate hemophagocytosis in cases of suspected HLH; however, abnormal hemophagocytosis may be seen in other tissues, such as spleen and liver. Fine-needle lymph node aspiration may show numerous hemophagocytic histiocytes.[67] Histologic examination of a lymph node biopsy may demonstrate distended sinuses due to an infiltrate of small lymphocytes and histiocytes, many of which exhibit hemophagocytosis.[69]

Although clinically distinct, HLH may be on the histopathologic differential diagnosis of Rosai-Dorfman disease and Langerhans cell histiocytosis. A single histiocyte exhibiting hemophagocytosis in isolation is a nonspecific finding, but the presence of numerous such histiocytes in a clinical and laboratorial context of suspected HLH can be diagnostic.

Table 1 summarizes the differential diagnosis for the histologic patterns of pediatric lymphadenitis discussed in this review.

CLINICS CARE POINTS

- Follicular hyperplasia must be distinguished from follicular lymphoma and other B cell neoplasms.
- In immunoblastic paracortical hyperplasia, the presence of Reed-Sternberg like cells mimic classic Hodgkin lymphoma.
- Mutations in the MAPK/ERK pathway may help to distinguish Rosai-Dorfman disease and other clonal histiocytoses from reactive non-specific proliferations.

REFERENCES

1. Peters TR, Edwards KM. Cervical lymphadenopathy and adenitis. Pediatr Rev 2000;21(12):399–405.
2. Deosthali A, Donches K, DelVecchio M, et al. Etiologies of pediatric cervical lymphadenopathy: a systematic review of 2687 subjects. Glob Pediatr Health 2019;6. 2333794X19865440.
3. Herzog LW. Prevalence of lymphadenopathy of the head and neck in infants and children. Clin Pediatr (Phila) 1983;22(7):485.
4. Yaris N, Cakir M, Sözen E, et al. Analysis of children with peripheral lymphadenopathy. Clin Pediatr (Phila) 2006;45(6):544–9.
5. McClain KL. Peripheral lymphadenopathy in children: evaluation and diagnostic approach. Uptodate Website; 2020. Available at: https://www.uptodate.com/contents/peripheral-lymphadenopathy-in-children-evaluation-and-diagnostic-approach?topicRef=6061&source=see_link. Accessed December 18, 2020.
6. Rosado FG, Stratton CW, Mosse CA. Clinicopathologic correlation of epidemiologic and histopathologic features of pediatric bacterial lymphadenitis. Arch Pathol Lab Med 2011;135(11):1490–3.

7. Ioachin HL, Medeiros LJ. Chapter 1: the normal lymph node. In: Ioachin HL, Medeiros LJ, editors. Ioachin's lymph node pathology. 4th edition. Lippincott Williams & Wilkins; 2009. p. 2–13.
8. Jaffe ES, Harris NL, Swerdlow SH, et al. Follicular lymphoma. In: Swerdlow SH, Campo E, Harris NL, et al, editors. WHO classification of tumors of haematopoietic and lymphoid tissues. Revised 4th edition. Lyon (France): IARC; 2017. p. 432.
9. Agostinelli C, Akarca AU, Ramsay A, et al. Novel markers in pediatric-type follicular lymphoma. Virchows Arch 2019;475(6):771–9.
10. Jaffe ES, Harris NL, Siebert R. Pediatric-type follicular lymphoma. In: Swerdlow SH, Campo E, Harris NL, et al, editors. WHO classification of tumors of haematopoietic and lymphoid tissues. Revised 4th edition. Lyon (France): IARC; 2017. p. 278–9.
11. Kussick SJ, Kalnoski M, Braziel RM, et al. Prominent clonal B-cell populations identified by flow cytometry in histologically reactive lymphoid proliferations. Am J Clin Pathol 2004;121(4):464–72.
12. Miranda RN, Khoury JD, Medeiros LJ. Reactive follicular hyperplasia. In: Miranda RN, Khoury JD, Medeiros LJ, editors. Atlas of lymph node pathology. Atlas of anatomic pathology. Springer; 2013. p. 11–3.
13. Ioachin HL, Medeiros LJ. Chapter 15: human immunodeficiency virus lymphadenitis. In: Ioachin HL, Medeiros LJ, editors. Ioachin's lymph node pathology. 4th edition. Lippincott Williams & Wilkins; 2009. p. 99–105.
14. Munro R, Porter DR, Sturrock RD. Lymphadenopathy in a patient with systemic onset juvenile chronic arthritis. Ann Rheum Dis 1998;57(9):513–7.
15. Zawawi F, Varshney R, Haegert DG, et al. Castleman's disease: a rare finding in a pediatric neck. Int J Pediatr Otorhinolaryngol 2014;78(2):370–2.
16. Fajgenbaum DC, Uldrick TS, Bagg A, et al. International, evidence-based consensus diagnostic criteria for HHV-8–negative/idiopathic multicentric Castleman disease. Blood 2017;129(12):1646–57.
17. Hawkins JM, Pillai V. TAFRO syndrome or Castleman-Kojima syndrome: a variant of multicentric Castleman disease. Blood 2015;126(18):2163.
18. Igawa T, Sato Y. TAFRO syndrome. Hematol Oncol Clin North Am 2018;32(1): 107–18.
19. Farruggia P, Trizzino A, Scibetta N, et al. Castleman's disease in childhood: report of three cases and review of the literature. Ital J Pediatr 2011;37:50.
20. Sato Y, Yoshino T. IgG4-related lymphadenopathy. Int J Rheumatol 2012;2012: 572539.
21. Karim F, Loeffen J, Bramer W, et al. IgG4-related disease: a systematic review of this unrecognized disease in pediatrics. Pediatr Rheumatol Online J 2016; 14(1):18.
22. Wick MR, O'Malley DP. Lymphadenopathy associated with IgG4-related disease: diagnosis & differential diagnosis. Semin Diagn Pathol 2018;35(1):61–6.
23. Shaikh F, Ngan BY, Alexander S, et al. Progressive transformation of germinal centers in children and adolescents: an intriguing cause of lymphadenopathy. Pediatr Blood Cancer 2013;60(1):26–30.
24. Stein H, Swerdlow SH, Gascoyne RD, et al. Nodular lymphocyte predominant Hodgkin lymphoma. In: Swerdlow SH, Campo E, Harris NL, et al, editors. WHO classification of tumors of haematopoietic and lymphoid tissues. Revised 4th edition. Lyon (France): IARC; 2017. p. 432.

25. Miranda RN, Khoury JD, Medeiros LJ. Reactive paracortical hyperplasia. In: Miranda RN, Khoury JD, Medeiros LJ, editors. Atlas of lymph node pathology. Atlas of anatomic pathology. Springer; 2013. p. 15–7.
26. Lang S, Kansy B. Cervical lymph node diseases in children. GMS Curr Top Otorhinolaryngol Head Neck Surg 2014;13:Doc08.
27. Ioachim HL, Medeiros LJ. Vaccinia lymphadenitis. In: Ioachim's lymph node pathology. 4th edition. Lippincott Williams & Wilkins; 2009. p. 95–6.
28. van Krieken JH, Onciu M, Elenitoba-Johnson KSJ, et al. Lymphoproliferative diseases associated with primary immune disorders. In: Swerdlow SH, Campo E, Harris NL, et al, editors. WHO classification of tumors of haematopoietic and lymphoid tissues. Revised 4th edition. Lyon (France): IARC; 2017. p. 444–8.
29. Tinguely M, Vonlanthen R, Müller E, et al. Hodgkin's disease-like lymphoproliferative disorders in patients with different underlying immunodeficiency states. Mod Pathol 1998;11(4):307–12.
30. Lim MS, Straus SE, Dale JK, et al. Pathological findings in human autoimmune lymphoproliferative syndrome. Am J Pathol 1998;153(5):1541–50.
31. Niedobitek G, Herbst H, Young LS, et al. Patterns of Epstein-Barr virus infection in non-neoplastic lymphoid tissue. Blood 1992;79(10):2520–6.
32. Dorfman RF, Warnke R. Lymphadenopathy simulating the malignant lymphomas. Hum Pathol 1974;5(5):519–50.
33. Ioachim HL, Medeiros LJ. Infectious mononucleosis lymphadenitis. In: Ioachim's lymph node pathology. 4th edition. Lippincott Williams & Wilkins; 2009. p. 76–82.
34. Gaffey MJ, Ben-Ezra JM, Weiss LM. Herpes simplex lymphadenitis. Am J Clin Pathol 1991;95(5):709–14.
35. Ioachim HL, Medeiros LJ. Herpes simplex virus lymphadenitis. In: Ioachim's lymph node pathology. 4th edition. Lippincott Williams & Wilkins; 2009. p. 87–91.
36. Xu F, Lee FK, Morrow RA, et al. Seroprevalence of herpes simplex virus type 1 in children in the United States. J Pediatr 2007;151(4):374–7.
37. Tamaru J, Mikata A, Horie H, et al. Herpes simplex lymphadenitis. Report of two cases with review of the literature. Am J Surg Pathol 1990;14(6):571–7.
38. Rosado FG, Tang YW, Hasserjian RP, et al. Kikuchi-Fujimoto lymphadenitis: role of parvovirus B-19, Epstein-Barr virus, human herpesvirus 6, and human herpesvirus 8. Hum Pathol 2013;44(2):255–9.
39. Ioachim HL, Medeiros LJ. Kikuchi lymphadenopathy. In: Ioachim's lymph node pathology. 4th edition. Lippincott Williams & Wilkins; 2009. p. 199–202.
40. Miranda RN, Khoury JD, Medeiros LJ. Herpes simplex virus lymphadenitis and varicella-herpes zoster lymphadenitis. In: Miranda RN, Khoury JD, Medeiros LJ, editors. Atlas of lymph node pathology. Atlas of anatomic pathology. Springer; 2013. p. 65–9.
41. Cannon MJ, Schmid DS, Hyde TB. Review of cytomegalovirus seroprevalence and demographic characteristics associated with infection. Rev Med Virol 2010;20(4):202–13.
42. Joubert M, Morin C, Moreau A, et al. Aspects histopathologiques de la lymphadénite à cytomégalovirus chez le sujet "immunocompétent". A propos de 7 observations. [[Histopathologic features of cytomegalovirus lymphadenitis in the "immunocompetent" patient. Report of 7 cases]]. Ann Pathol 1996;16(4):254–60.
43. Ioachim HL, Medeiros LJ. Cytolomegalovirus lymphadenitis. In: Ioachim's lymph node pathology. 4th edition. Lippincott Williams & Wilkins; 2009. p. 83–6.
44. Rushin JM, Riordan GP, Heaton RB, et al. Cytomegalovirus-infected cells express Leu-M1 antigen. A potential source of diagnostic error. Am J Pathol 1990;136(5): 989–95.

45. Ioachim HL, Medeiros LJ. Measles lymphadenitis. In: Ioachim's lymph node pathology. 4th edition. Lippincott Williams & Wilkins; 2009. p. 97–8.
46. Viswanatha B. Kimura's disease in children: a 9 years prospective study. Int J Pediatr Otorhinolaryngol 2007;71(10):1521–5.
47. Miranda RN, Khoury JD, Medeiros LJ. Kimura lymphadenopathy. In: Miranda RN, Khoury JD, Medeiros LJ, editors. Atlas of lymph node pathology. Atlas of anatomic pathology. Springer; 2013. p. 101–3.
48. Weiss LM, O'Malley D. Benign lymphadenopathies. Mod Pathol 2013;26(Suppl 1):S88–96.
49. Silva-Feistner M, Ortiz E, Rojas-Lechuga MJ, et al. Síndrome de sensibilidad a fármacos con eosinofilia y síntomas sistémicos en pediatría: Caso clínico [DRESS syndrome in paediatrics: clinical case]. Rev Chil Pediatr 2017;88(1):158–63.
50. Mori F, Caffarelli C, Caimmi S, et al. Drug reaction with eosinophilia and systemic symptoms (DRESS) in children. Acta Biomed 2019;90(3-S):66–79.
51. Gaulard P, Swerdlow SH, Harris NL, et al. Other iatrogenic immunodeficiency-associated lymphoproliferative disorders. In: Swerdlow SH, Campo E, Harris NL, et al, editors. WHO classification of tumors of haematopoietic and lymphoid tissues. Revised 4th edition. Lyon (France): IARC; 2017. p. 462–4.
52. Eapen M, Mathew CF, Aravindan KP. Evidence based criteria for the histopathological diagnosis of toxoplasmic lymphadenopathy. J Clin Pathol 2005;58(11):1143–6.
53. Fraser IP. Suppurative lymphadenitis. Curr Infect Dis Rep 2009;11(5):383–8.
54. Yokouchi Y, Oharaseki T, Harada M, et al. Histopathological study of lymph node lesions in the acute phase of Kawasaki disease. Histopathology 2013;62(3):387–96.
55. Margileth AM. Recent advances in diagnosis and treatment of cat scratch disease. Curr Infect Dis Rep 2000;2(2):141–6.
56. Hansmann Y, DeMartino S, Piémont Y, et al. Diagnosis of cat scratch disease with detection of Bartonella henselae by PCR: a study of patients with lymph node enlargement. J Clin Microbiol 2005;43(8):3800–6.
57. Jabcuga CE, Jin L, Macon WR, et al. Broadening the morphologic spectrum of bartonella henselae lymphadenitis: analysis of 100 molecularly characterized cases. Am J Surg Pathol 2016;40(3):342–7.
58. Ferry JA. Infectious lymphadenitis. In: Diagnostic pathology of infectious disease. 2nd edition. Elsevier; 2018. p. 323–51.
59. Ioachim HL, Medeiros LJ. Toxoplasmas lymphadenitis. In: Ioachim's lymph node pathology. 4th edition. Lippincott Williams & Wilkins; 2009. p. 159–64.
60. Jones JL, Kruszon-Moran D, Wilson M, et al. Toxoplasma gondii infection in the United States: seroprevalence and risk factors. Am J Epidemiol 2001;154(4):357–65.
61. Weiss LM, Jaffe R, Facchetti F. Tumours derived from Langerhans cells. In: Swerdlow SH, Campo E, Harris NL, et al, editors. WHO classification of tumors of haematopoietic and lymphoid tissues. Revised 4th edition. Lyon (France): IARC; 2017. p. 470.
62. Ioachin HL, Medeiros LJ. Chapter 36: sinus histiocytosis with massive lymphadenopathy. In: Ioachin HL, Medeiros LJ, editors. Ioachin's lymph node pathology. 4th edition. Lippincott Williams & Wilkins; 2009. p. 193–8.
63. Eisen RN, Buckley PJ, Rosai J. Immunophenotypic characterization of sinus histiocytosis with massive lymphadenopathy (Rosai-Dorfman disease). Semin Diagn Pathol 1990;7(1):74–82.

64. Garces S, Medeiros LJ, Patel KP, et al. Mutually exclusive recurrent KRAS and MAP2K1 mutations in Rosai-Dorfman disease. Mod Pathol 2017;30(10):1367–77.
65. Lehmberg K, Nichols KE, Henter JI, et al. Consensus recommendations for the diagnosis and management of hemophagocytic lymphohistiocytosis associated with malignancies. Haematologica 2015;100(8):997–1004.
66. Rosado FG, Kim AS. Hemophagocytic lymphohistiocytosis: an update on diagnosis and pathogenesis. Am J Clin Pathol 2013;139(6):713–27.
67. Rekha TS, Kiran HS, Nandini NM, et al. Cytology of secondary hemophagocytic lymphohistiocytosis masquerading as lymphoma in a nonimmunocompromised adult. J Cytol 2014;31(4):239–41.
68. Suresh N, Uppuluri R, Geetha J, et al. Hemophagocytic lymphohistiocytosis masking the diagnosis of lymphoma in an adolescent male. Indian J Hematol Blood Transfus 2014;30(Suppl 1):135–7.
69. Gupta AP, Parate SN, Bobhate SK, et al. Hemophagocytic syndrome: a cause for fatal outcome in tuberculosis. Indian J Pathol Microbiol 2009;52:260–2.

Update on Acute Leukemias of Ambiguous Lineage

Nidhi Aggarwal, MD[a,*], Olga K. Weinberg, MD[b]

KEYWORDS

• Ambiguous lineage • MPAL • Acute leukemia • Molecular typing

KEY POINTS

- Mixed-phenotype acute leukemias is a heterogenous group of leukemias that are difficult to diagnose, treat, and follow minimal residual disease.
- It is a diagnosis of exclusion after leukemias with specific diagnostic categories are excluded.
- The genetic abnormalities to look for include rearrangements involving *KMT2A*, *BCR-ABL1*, *ZNF384*, *FGFR1*, *PICALM*, *BCR-ABL1*–like, and *WT1* mutations.
- Although the line of treatment is controversial, most clinicians prefer to start treatment with a lymphoblastic regimen rather than an acute myeloblastic leukemia regimen.

INTRODUCTION

Acute leukemia of ambiguous lineage (ALAL) either shows no commitment to either the myeloid B-lymphoid or T-lymphoid lineages (acute undifferentiated leukemia [AUL]) or simultaneously shows commitment to more than 1 lineage (mixed-phenotype acute leukemia [MPAL]).[1–3] These conditions have been difficult to diagnose and treat and have historically been referred to by different terminologies, including bilineage acute leukemia (presence of 2 morphologically and immunophenotypically separate blasts) and biphenotypic acute leukemias (single blast population expressing mixed phenotypic markers).[4] To create a standardize approach, different classification systems have been proposed over the years. The European Group for the Immunological Characterization of Leukemias (EGIL) algorithm was developed in 1995 to 1998 and was based on a point system with a requirement of more than 2 points in 2 separate lineages for a diagnosis of MPAL.[5] In 2008, the World Health Organization (WHO) classification system grouped bilineal and biphenotypic acute leukemias into a unified heading of MPAL and further provided more stringent criteria using fewer but more

[a] Department of Pathology, University of Pittsburgh, School of Medicine, Hill Building, 3477 Euler Way, Pittsburgh, PA 15213, USA; [b] Department of Pathology, University of Texas Southwestern, Texas, BioCenter, 2230 Inwood Road, EB03.220G, Dallas, TX 75235, USA
* Corresponding author.
E-mail address: aggarwaln2@upmc.edu

Clin Lab Med 41 (2021) 453–466
https://doi.org/10.1016/j.cll.2021.03.016

lineage-specific antibodies. The most recently updated 2017 WHO classification recommends the use of a total of 10 antibodies for such a diagnosis.[6,7] Two genetically defined subgroups are recognized within the MPAL group: t(9;22)/BRC-ABL MPAL and KMT2A (MLL) rearranged MPAL. These 2 subgroups make up a total of 19% to 28% of all MPAL cases, leaving most MPALs defined as B-myeloid, T-myeloid, and not otherwise specified subsets, which includes exceedingly rare T/B MPAL.[8] This article discusses the various antigens suggested and the issues surrounding their use. Because of the rarity of pediatric MPAL, studies limited to children and adolescent cohorts are sparse. B-lymphoblastic leukemia (B-ALL) is the most common pediatric malignancy and expression of myeloperoxidase (MPO) by otherwise typical patients with B-ALL has been well documented, and caution is now advised in avoiding a diagnosis of MPAL in these patients.

INCIDENCE

ALAL represents a heterogeneous group of orphan diseases and accounts for about 2% to 3% of all leukemias and 0.35 cases per 1 million person-years.[9,10] Among MPAL, B lymphoid/myeloid is the most frequent and accounts for 59%; T/myeloid, B/T, and trilineage phenotype account for 35%, 4%, and 2% respectively.[1,9,11]

MORPHOLOGY

Blasts in MPAL are morphologically diverse and range from small to intermediate in size with variable cytoplasm, and they occasionally show hand-mirror morphology (**Fig. 1**A, **Fig. 2**A). Sometimes, 2 types of blasts with distinctive size, morphology, and phenotype can be identified.[12]

IMMUNOPHENOTYPING

Extensive immunophenotyping (including flow cytometry, immunohistochemistry, and cytochemistry) is essential for an accurate diagnosis of MPAL. Unlike EGIL, WHO does not provide a threshold for percentage of cells for lineage-specific antigens. In the WHO classification, the intensity of antigen expression is considered to be more lineage specific. The general principles in evaluating the flow cytometry data when coexpression of markers is being evaluated include exclusion of doublets and addressing compensation (process of correcting for fluorescence spillover) and autofluorescence issues so that dim populations can be differentiated from negative populations. One way of confirming antigen expression is doing a fluorescence minus 1 tube, which involves repeating the analysis but without the antibody in question[13,14] (see **Fig. 1** for an example).

B-cell markers

The current WHO classification requires the strong expression of cluster of differentiation (CD) 19 along with 1 other marker or weak CD19 expression with expression of 2 other markers (CD79a, CD10, cytoplasmic CD22),[6] making CD19 expression a required but not a sufficient criterion for assigning of B-cell lineage. CD19 expression (and other B-cell markers, including PAX5, CD10, CD22, and CD79a) in acute myeloid leukemias (AMLs) with t(8;21) is well documented in the literature and acknowledged in WHO classification.[6,15,16] The authors studied AMLs for expression of CD19 and found it expressed in about 7% of all non-acute promyelocytic leukemia AMLs. This expression was not restricted to t(8;21) but was also seen in AMLs with *RUNX1* mutations and AMLs with mutated *NPM1*, among other AMLs.[17] In addition, although most

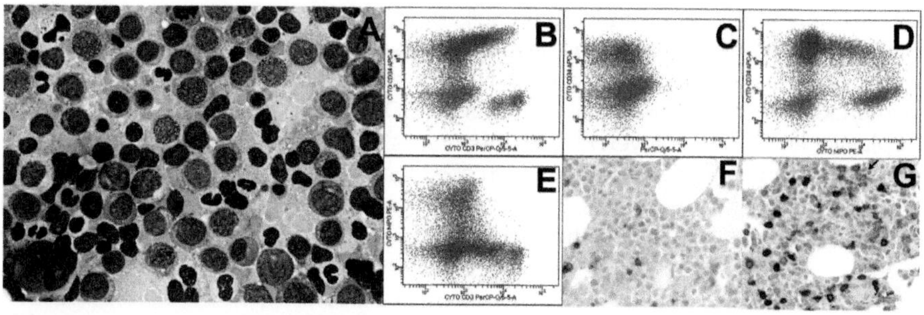

Fig. 1. A 70-year-old woman with a history of breast carcinoma and therapy-related myeloid neoplasm transformed to acute leukemia. Final diagnosis: therapy-related acute myeloid leukemia (secondary notation added: blasts show mixed phenotype). (*A*) Morphology (Wright Giemas, original magnification ×100): many blasts with a background of dysplasia (hypogranular and hypolobated neutrophils and small hypolobated megakaryocytes). (*B*) Flow cytometric studies show partial expression of cytoplasmic cluster of differentiation (CD) 3 on a subset of CD34+ blasts. (*C*) Fluorescence minus 1 tube with no cytoplasmic CD3 added (no blasts show nonspecific/autofluorescence) staining with the PerCP-Cy5.5 dye. (*D*) Subset of blasts shows MPO staining. (*E*) No blast population that coexpresses MPO and cytoplasmic CD3. (*F*) CD2 (original magnification ×50) shows scattered T cells. (*G*) CD3 (original magnification ×50) shows more staining than CD2 with few weakly positive cells, likely the blasts (*arrow*).

B-ALLs express CD19, expression levels can be variable in both de novo and relapsed settings.[18] CD19-negative recurrences are also frequently seen after chimeric antigen receptor (CAR) T-cell therapy[19] and, thus, these WHO criteria for lineage assignment do not apply. The CD22 marker is listed by the WHO as being specific for MPAL;

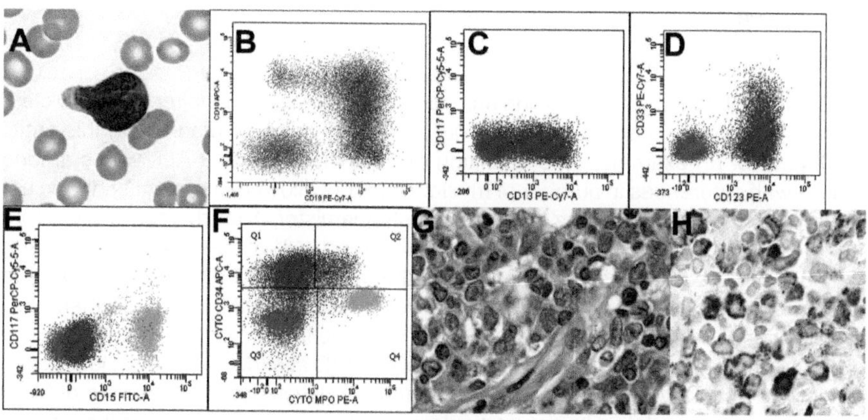

Fig. 2. A 26-year-old man with a history of sarcoma at age 17 years, after resection, no chemotherapy. MPAL versus B-lymphoblastic leukemia with isolated MPO. (*A*) Peripheral blood smear showing the typical blast (Wright Giemas, original magnification ×100). (*B–E*) Flow cytometric analysis shows blasts are CD19+, CD10 partial+, CD11−, CD13−, CD33 partial+, and CD15−. (*F*) A subset of blasts appears to be MPO positive (8%–10% of blasts on PB and 13%–15% on the BM). (*G*) HE (original magnification ×100) shows BM with sheets of blasts. (*H*) MPO immunohistochemistry (IHC) (original magnification ×100) (cytoplasmic polyclonal rabbit; Ventana antibody) showing many positive blasts BM, bone marrow; PB, peripheral blood; He, hematoxylin and eosin.

however, it is also expressed in some cells other than B-cell lineage; namely, basophils. CD79a expression in B-cell development spans from being one of the earliest to the plasma cell stage. However, CD79a expression has been described in T-lymphoblastic leukemias[20] and AMLs.[21] CD79a expression is also seen in neoplastic and normal myeloid cell precursors and megakaryocytes in a clone-dependent manner[22] and in patients with solid tumor malignancies.[23] Terminal deoxynucleotidyl transferase (TdT) is a nonspecific marker and can be seen in any of the acute leukemias, and is frequently seen in AUL.[24]

T-cell markers

CD3 cytoplasmic expression is considered essential for assigning T-cell lineage,[6,25] although it can also be seen in natural killer (NK) lymphoblastic leukemias.[26] The fluorochrome used for the determination of cytoplasmic CD3 should yield strong fluorescence (for instance, phycoerythrin or allophycocyanin) and the brightest expression should be comparable with the normal T cells.[12] Other T-cell markers, including CD2, CD7, and CD56, are not specific and have been found in many AMLs.[25]

Myeloid lineage

MPO expression by immunohistochemistry, cytochemistry, or flow cytometry, or monocytic differentiation, is considered a requirement for assigning the myeloid lineage when considering a diagnosis of MPAL.[6] Although older studies suggest a cutoff of 3% for cytochemistry based on expert opinion, no formally established cutoff guidelines exist for immunohistochemistry and flow cytometry. The issue is further compounded by the availability of many MPO clones, known nonspecific staining patterns, and lack of criteria for evaluating the stains if a significant number of nonblast myeloid cells are present. **Table 1** shows the variability of the antibody used and cutoffs taken in the literature for defining MPO positivity among cases included in the study. As shown, the cutoff for flow cytometry varies from 5.4% to 20%[27] of the blasts and has been investigated in several studies.[28,29]

B-Lymphoblastic Leukemia

B-ALL with isolated MPO expression has been acknowledged in the recent WHO classification[6]; however, there are no clear guidelines provided for diagnosing this entity (see **Fig. 2** for an example). The definition of otherwise typical B-ALL varies among studies, with differences in number of myeloid markers allowed in this entity. When using polyclonal MPO antibodies by immunohistochemistry, 1 study found that about 23% of the adult B-ALLs showed immunoreactivity and 84% of these cases had greater than 10% MPO-positive cells.[30] The B-ALLs that expressed MPO were more likely to express CD13 or CD15 and about 42% had evidence of t(9;22), although there was no difference in the immunoreactivity by type of tissue fixation or survival. It has been shown that 56% of the infant pre–B-ALLs showed MPO at either the protein level using monoclonal antibody or the messenger RNA (mRNA) level, but this presence of MPO was not found to correlate with any particular clinical, cytogenetic, or laboratory pattern and did not influence the outcome.[31] Presence of MPO mRNA in adult acute lymphoblastic leukemia (ALL) has been found to be associated with t(9;22), and likely represented CML in blast crisis rather than de novo ALL.[32] On mRNA analysis, the incidence of MPO expression ranged from 0% to 25% in the myeloid marker–negative cases to as much as 83% in ALLs that coexpress myeloid markers.[33–36] Strong MPO staining by flow cytometry and cytochemistry in otherwise typical B-ALLs that lacked CD13, CD33, and/or CD117 expression seemed to be present in a Burkitt-like entity.[37] Other studies suggested that survival of pediatric B/myeloid

Table 1
Myeloperoxidase antibodies used and the cutoff recommended in various studies

Study	Antibody/Clone Used	Cutoff Recommended
Manivannan et al,[27] 2015	Flow cytometry BD Biosciences, clone 5B8, Ms IgG1 (flow)-FITC conjugated	5.4%
Arber et al,[30] 2001	IHC 1:1000 dilution, Dako, Carpinteria, CA), polyclonal and monoclonal MPO antibody (clone MPO-7;1:100 dilution; Dako)	≥5%
Ahuja et al,[63] 2017, studied patients with AML and their MPO reactivity	IHC: anti–human MPO (Thermo Scientific, United Kingdom) Cytochemistry and flow cytometry: not mentioned	3% for IHC and cytochemistry and 10% flow cytometry
Oberley et al,[64] 2017	Flow cytometry: MPO (clone 8E6; Life Tech, Waltham, MA) IHC (clone 59A5; Leica Biosystems, Newcastle, United Kingdom) plus cytochemistry	>20% for flow 3% cytochemistry
Van den Ancker et al,[29] 2013	Flow cytometry (clone used not reported)	>10%
Guy et al,[28] 2013	Flow cytometry: monoclonal antibody (Dako or Immunotech), FITC	>13% (if using isotype control) >28% (if using internal control: lymphocytes)
Matutes et al,[11] 2011	Flow cytometry: monoclonal MPO (clone used not reported)	>10%

Abbreviations: FITC, fluorescein isothiocyanate; IgG1, immunoglobulin G1; IHC, immunohistochemistry.

MPALs with MPO was superior when treated with an ALL-type therapy.[38] These MPALs expressed CD13, CD33, and CD15 and contained common B-ALL–related cytogenetic abnormalities, such as *ETV6-RUNX1* and trisomy 4 and 10. In summary, definition of isolated MPO expression in B-ALL remains unclear and distinction of this condition from MPAL, especially in pediatric patients, should be addressed in future studies.

ACUTE UNDIFFERENTIATED LEUKEMIA

Acute undifferentiated leukemia is a rare type of acute leukemia that shows no evidence of differentiation along any lineage and is included under MPAL in the WHO classification. In a multi-institutional study, the authors recently showed that patients presented with age, blood counts, and bone marrow cellularity similar to patients with AML with minimal differentiation[24] but showed more frequent mutations in the PHF6 gene and showed more frequent TdT expression. Fourteen acute undifferentiated leukemia cases (58%) had a normal karyotype, and, of the abnormal karyotypes, 5 had trisomy 13. Outcome data showed no difference in overall survival, relapse-free survival, or rates of complete remission between acute undifferentiated leukemia and AML with minimal differentiation groups.

CYTOGENETIC FINDINGS

Most studies describe frequency of an abnormal karyotype in more than 50% of MPAL cases and fewer cases with normal karyotype. Two distinct classes of MPALs are classified based on cytogenetics: MPAL with *BCR-ABL1* and MPAL with *KMT2A* gene rearrangements.[6] MPALs with *KMT2A* are more common in the pediatric age group (infants) and account for about 10% of MPALs, and *BCR-ABL1* in adults accounts for about 20% to 30% of MPALs.[39–41] These conditions are commonly associated with the B/myeloid phenotype.[6] B/myeloid MPALs also frequently show del(1)(p32), trisomy 4, del(6q), 12p11.2 aberrancies, and near-tetraploidy. A recent study reported *ZNF384* rearrangements (with *TCF3*, *EP300*, *TAF15*, and *CREBBP*) in as many as 48% of the pediatric B/myeloid MPALs,[41] although this aberration has not been identified in adult patients.[42] The genomic landscape of B-ALL with *ZNF384*-r and MPALs with *ZNF384*-r was similar, with exception of *KDM6A*, which was observed only in MPALs, and these case showed higher *FLT3* expression.[41] Other gene rearrangements described in a subset of MPALs include those involving *NUP98*[42] and *PICALM* genes.[41] *PICALM* gene rearrangements have been described in association with T-ALL and AMLs in addition to MPALs and occur mostly in young men with extramedullary involvement (**Fig. 3** shows an example).[43]

Complex karyotype with 3 or more aberrations is frequent in MPALs, as are other myelodysplastic syndrome (MDS)-related abnormalities, including monosomy 7.[9,11] At present, there is controversy about whether MPAL cases with complex karyotype should be considered as AML with myelodysplasia-related changes.[36]

MUTATIONAL ANALYSIS

Integrative genomic analysis comparing AML, B-ALL and T-ALL, and MPAL help to further understand the similarities and differences among these groups at the genetic level. Studies show that mutations seen in MPALs have also been documented in both AML and ALL. The number of detected mutations are similar when comparing MPAL with AMLs and T-ALL, with a range of 0 to 7 (median, 2) but significantly more in MPAL compared with B-ALL.[42] B/myeloid MPAL seem to show a different mutational profile compared with T/myeloid MPALs.[42] Other studies show that B/myeloid MPALs harbored fewer mutations compared with T/myeloid MPALs but showed a more frequent rate of complex karyotypes.[44] Other abnormalities found in B/myeloid MPALs include deletions in *IKZF1* (Ikaros), and mutation involving *RUNX1*, *TET2*, *EZH2*, and *ASXL1*.[9] T/myeloid MPALs have mutations in *EZH2*, *PHF6*, *DNMT3A*, *NOTCH1*, *FBXW7*, *IL7R*, and *JAK/STAT* signaling proteins. Other mutations in T/myeloid MPALs include *DNMT3A*, *WT1*, *IDH2*, *FLT3*, *KRAS*, *NRAS*, *CUX1*, *CEBPA*, *CDKN2A/CDKN2B*, *ETV6*, *PHF6*, and *VPREB1*.[41,42,45] Interestingly, early T-cell precursor ALL (ETP-ALL), a subset of T-ALL suggested to have worse outcome, shows a profile that is between T/myeloid MPALs and T-ALL, with frequent mutations in *ETV6*, *WT1*, *EZH2*, and *FLT3*. *NOTCH1* mutations have been identified in T/myeloid MPALs (~10%–15%), although much less frequently than in T-ALL and ETP-ALL. A recent study investigating the mutational profile in a small series of B/T cases identified mutations in *PHF6*, *WT1*, *JAK3*, *MED12*, *CTCF*, *IL7R*, *NOTCH1*, *SF3B1*, *PTPN11*, *EZH2*, *DNMT3A*, and *TP53*.[8]

DIFFERENTIAL DIAGNOSIS OF MIXED-PHENOTYPE ACUTE LEUKEMIA

The challenges faced while making a diagnosis of MPAL can be categorized as technical and interpretive. The technical challenges are encountered when assessing coexpression of markers from different lineages, as described earlier. The interpretive challenges mostly include ruling out other WHO-defined categories that may have MPAL-like immunophenotypes. In addition, as more cytogenetic and molecular data emerge, newer groups of diseases may be better defined by their genetic

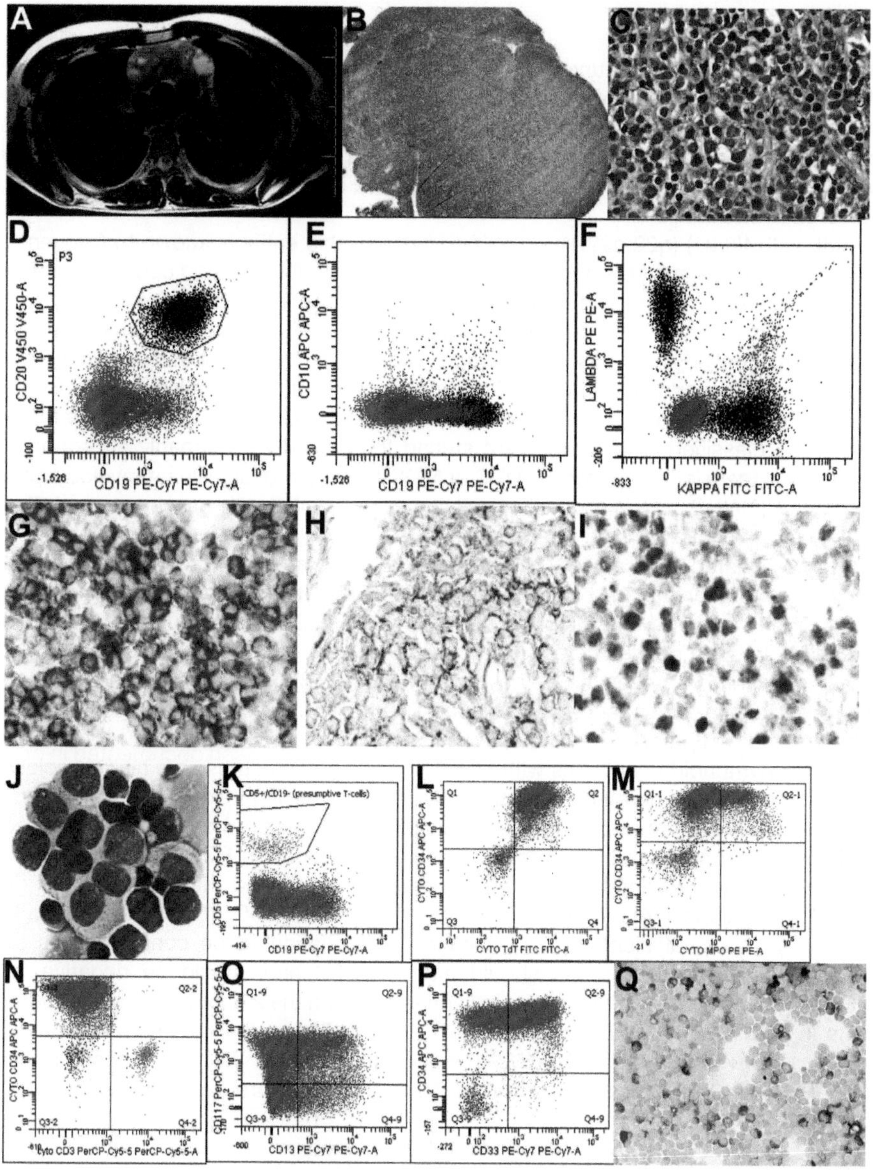

Fig. 3. A 29-year-old man with an anterior mediastinal mass. Acute leukemia with *PICALM* gene rearrangement (highlights differences in immunophenotype in separate locations). (*A*) Computed tomography scan shows heterogeneous partially solid partially cystic enhancing mass lesion measuring 7.6 × 4.2 × 7.2 cm within anterior mediastinum. (*B*) HE (4×) mediastinal mass biopsy. (*C*) High power shows sheets of blasts (hematoxylin-eosin, original magnification ×100). (*D–F*) Flow cytometric studies show (marron population) blasts that are partially CD19+, CD10−, CD20−, and surface immunoglobulin negative with a background of many polytypic B cells and T cells. (*G–I*) IHC staining (original magnification ×100) shows cells are CD79a+, CD34+, and TdT+. MPO was negative on IHC (not shown) and not tested on flow cytometric studies because of lack of cells. (*J*) Cytospin preparation from pleural fluid (Wright Giemas, original magnification ×100). (*K–P*) Flow cytometric studies show cells are CD19 partial+, CD34+, TdT+, MPO partial+, cytoplasmic CD3−, CD117 partial+, and CD33 partial+. (*Q*) Cytochemistry performed for MPO (original magnification ×50) highlights that about 10% of the blasts are positive.

abnormality than the immunophenotype of the blasts (**Fig. 4**). In clinical practice, there is usually a lag before the additional genetic information is received and full classification of acute leukemia can be made. The differential diagnosis and what might be of interest to investigate in a patient that presents with a mixed phenotype are discussed next. The following are well-defined categories described in the 2017 WHO classification.

AML with t(8;21) (q22;q22.1); *RUNX1-RUNX1T1*: this entity is known to frequently express B-lineage markers, including CD19, PAX5, and CD79a, and could be erroneously classified as B/myeloid MPAL based on immunophenotyping alone.

AML with myelodysplasia-related changes (AML-MRC): this diagnosis may be particularly challenging if based on cytogenetics alone, because MPAL can have cytogenetics that overlap the AML-MRC cytogenetics, including 5q deletion, monosomy 7, and complex karyotype.[11,42,46] No definite guidelines exist to determine how these should be classified, and a comment stating the difficulty is probably appropriate. However, if there is prior history of MDS or MDS/MPN and/or significant myelodysplasia, the 2017 WHO criteria suggest classifying as AML-MRC with a secondary notation that the blasts have a mixed phenotype.

Therapy-related AML and CML in blast crisis: these are diagnosed as such with a secondary notation that the blasts have a mixed phenotype (see the example in **Fig. 1**).

Acute leukemias (AML) presenting de novo with t(9;22): if a preceding CML can be excluded, this is a defined category in the 2017 WHO.

Acute leukemias presenting de novo with t(v;11q23.3); KMT2A rearranged: classified based on immunophenotype of blasts. These patients often show mixed lineage markers and can present as infant leukemias.

Myeloid/lymphoid neoplasms with FGFR1 rearrangement: these are hematopoietic neoplasms that can present as acute leukemias expressing mixed lineage markers. Because the FGFR1 rearrangement is definitional, the condition may not be diagnosed as MPAL. Morphologic clues to the possible presence of an *FGFR1* rearrangement include prominent eosinophilia, which is frequently associated with this disease.[6]

ETP-ALL: this is T-ALL characterized by CD1a−, CD8−, $CD5^{weak/-}$ phenotype and frequently show sufficient myeloid lineage differentiation to be considered as an MPAL. However, these cases should express CD3 and should be negative for MPO.[6] Genetic studies show many similarities between the 2 entities, including mutations in *NOTCH1*, *FLT3ITD*, and *N/KRAS* and *KMT2A* and *TLX3* rearrangements, whereas *FBXW7* mutations, *CDKN2AB* deletions, and *STIL-TAL1* are mostly found in T-ALL. This study also showed that *NOTCH1* mutations are associated with better prognosis.[47]

B-ALL with Philadelphia chromosome–like phenotype and B-ALL with isolated MPO, as described earlier, should also be excluded.

CURRENT TREATMENT GUIDELINES

The clinical management of MPAL remains a challenge. There is no real consensus between the therapeutic regimens for the MPALs. This group of acute leukemias should be regarded as high risk and the treatment outcome depends on the patient age and genetics. They carry a prognosis that is usually worse compared with standard-risk ALL or AML.[11,48] There have been controversies over the choice of initial treatment and whether it should be based on immunophenotyping or cytogenetics and so forth. Traditionally, the choice of ALL versus AML or hybrid therapy was more equal.[49] For therapeutic management, most studies suggest starting with ALL therapy with the possibility of bone marrow transplant in the first complete remission. If this approach

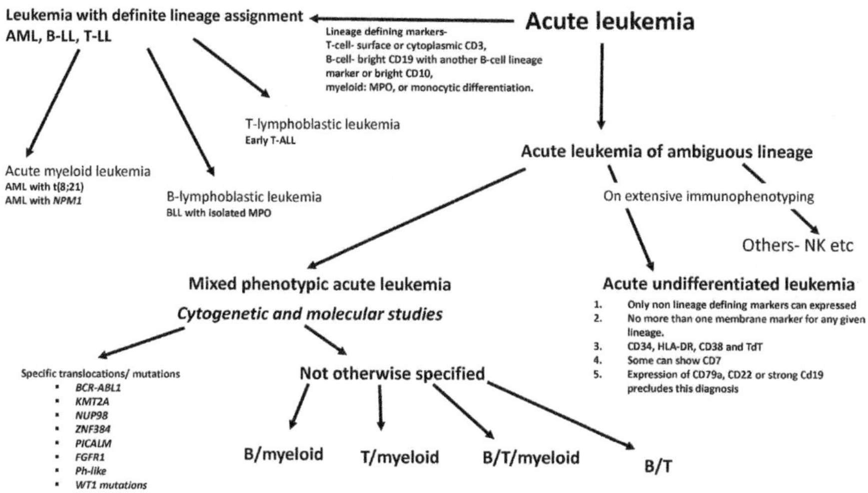

Figure 4- Flow chart in the work up for ALAL including various differential diagnosis to consider

Fig. 4. The work-up for ALAL, including various differential diagnosis to consider.

fails, patients are switched to AML therapy followed by ALL-type therapy or bone marrow transplant in the first complete remission.[38]

More recently, studies recommend starting with an ALL-like approach (plus a tyrosine kinase inhibitor in the case of Philadelphia chromosome–like MPALs) in order to achieve higher remission rates compared with AML or combined therapies,[11,50] and following with allogeneic bone marrow transplant when applicable.[12] In addition, some patients who failed on AML therapy further achieved remission when switched to ALL therapy.[49] In contrast with adults with MPAL, ALL therapy without transplant was adequate to treat most pediatric patients.[51] A retrospective collaborative study evaluating 233 pediatric patients with ALAL identified that most ALALs with expression of CD19 did well on ALL-type therapy and end of induction residual greater than or equal to 5% was associated with a very poor 5-year event-free survival rate (<50%).[52] There are also reports of successfully treating CD19+ MPALs using anti-CD19 therapy (blinatumomab).[53] A recent report describes the use of CAR T-cell therapy in 5 refractory patients with Philadelphia chromosome–positive MPAL with minimal residual disease.[54]

POSTTREATMENT FOLLOW-UP AND MINIMAL RESIDUAL DISEASE TESTING

Role of minimal residual disease (MRD) detection by either flow cytometry or molecular methods in the follow-up and risk of relapse is well established in ALL as well as AML[55–58] but is less clear in MPAL. Besides challenges in making MPAL diagnosis, different therapies used in the clinical setting make comparison with MRD analysis difficult. Oberley and colleagues[51] recently reported on centrally reviewed MPAL cases treated with ALL regiments, but most cases included B/myeloid subtype and therefore results are difficult to extrapolate to other subtypes.[13] They did find that earlier MRD clearance is associated with better treatment success and survival.[51,59] Although the rate of achieving MRD (0.01%) negative at the end of induction varied, it was seen in up to 70% patients in 1 of the studies.[51] End-of-induction MRD positivity was also shown to be predictive of 5-year event-free survival, and patients who cleared MRD by end of consolidation had worse survival compared with those who were MRD negative at end of induction.[51] Posttherapy lineage switch has been described, especially in MPALs with *KMT2A* gene rearrangements.[60–62]

SUMMARY

Diagnosis of MPAL can be challenging. The various studies and review articles uniformly emphasize that an MPAL diagnosis requires a comprehensive approach to immunophenotyping. Multiple methods, including large panels for flow cytometry immunophenotyping, immunohistochemical analysis, and cytochemistry studies for MPO and nonspecific esterase, may be required. It is important to be aware of the pitfalls and caveats of various antibodies and their roles in lineage assignment.

CLINICS CARE POINTS

- Acute leukemias of ambiguous lineage is a heterogeneous group of leukemias which on thorough work-up by immunophenotyping and cytogenetic and molecular studies and can further categorized into more specific diagnoses.
- Work up should include assessment of rearrangements involving KMT2A, BCRABL1, ZNF384, FGFR1, PICALM, BCR-ABL1–like, and WT1 mutations.
- The possibility of a B-lymphoblastic leukemia with isolated MPO staining and Early Precursor T-cell ALL should be considered.
- Treatment approach is not entirely standardized but most prefer ALL-like therapy.
- Follow up with minimal residual disease testing is challengiung and may be aided by knowing the genetic/ molecular signature of the leukemia.
- Post therapy lineage switch could occur.

DISCLOSURE

The authors have nothing to disclose.

REFERENCES

1. Weinberg OK, Seetharam M, Ren L, et al. Mixed phenotype Acute leukemia: a study of 61 cases using World Health Organization and European group for the immunological classification of leukaemias criteria. Am J Clin Pathol 2014;142(6):803–8.
2. Wolach O, Stone RM. Mixed-phenotype acute leukemia: current challenges in diagnosis and therapy. Curr Opin Hematol 2017;24(2):139–45.
3. Patel SS, Weinberg OK. Diagnostic workup of acute leukemias of ambiguous lineage. Am J Hematol 2020;95(6):718–22.
4. Weir EG, Ali Ansari-Lari M, Batista DA, et al. Acute bilineal leukemia: a rare disease with poor outcome. Leukemia 2007;21(11):2264–70.
5. Bene MC, Castoldi G, Knapp W, et al. Proposals for the immunological classification of acute leukemias. European group for the Immunological characterization of leukemias (EGIL). Leukemia 1995;9(10):1783–6.
6. Swerdlow SH, Campo E, Harris NL, et al. WHO classification of tumours of haematopoietic and lymphoid tissues. revised 4th edition ed. Bosman FT, Jaffe ES, Lakhani SR, Ohgaki H, editors: Lyon (France): International Agency for Research on Cancer.2017.pages 71–213.

7. Swerdlow SH, Campo E, Harris NL, et al. WHO Classification of tumor of Haematopoietic and Lymphoid Tissues 4ed. Swerdlow SH, Campo E, Harris NL, et al., editors. Lyon (France): International Agency for Research on Cancer.2008.-page 149.
8. Mi X, Griffin G, Lee W, et al. Genomic and clinical characterization of B/T mixed phenotype acute leukemia reveals recurrent features and T-ALL like mutations. Am J Hematol 2018;93(11):1358–67.
9. Yan L, Ping N, Zhu M, et al. Clinical, immunophenotypic, cytogenetic, and molecular genetic features in 117 adult patients with mixed-phenotype acute leukemia defined by WHO-2008 classification. Haematologica 2012;97(11):1708–12.
10. Weinberg OK, Arber DA. Mixed-phenotype acute leukemia: historical overview and a new definition. Leukemia 2010;24(11):1844–51.
11. Matutes E, Pickl WF, Van't Veer M, et al. Mixed-phenotype acute leukemia: clinical and laboratory features and outcome in 100 patients defined according to the WHO 2008 classification. Blood 2011;117(11):3163–71.
12. Porwit A, Bene MC. Acute leukemias of ambiguous origin. Am J Clin Pathol 2015; 144(3):361–76.
13. Roederer M. Compensation in flow cytometry. Curr Protoc cytometry 2002. https://doi.org/10.1002/0471142956.cy0114s22. Chapter 1:Unit 1 14.
14. Feher K, Kirsch J, Radbruch A, et al. Cell population identification using fluorescence-minus-one controls with a one-class classifying algorithm. Bioinformatics 2014;30(23):3372–8.
15. Ball ED, Davis RB, Griffin JD, et al. Prognostic value of lymphocyte surface markers in acute myeloid leukemia. Blood 1991;77(10):2242–50.
16. Tiacci E, Pileri S, Orleth A, et al. PAX5 expression in acute leukemias: higher B-lineage specificity than CD79a and selective association with t(8;21)-acute myelogenous leukemia. Cancer Res 2004;64(20):7399–404.
17. Bhavsar S, Jain S, Yatsenko S, et al. CD19 expression and its immunophenotypic and molecular cytogenetic associations in acute myeloid leukemia (abs#1332). In (Abstracts from USCAP 2020: Hematopathology). Mod Pathol 2020;33(suppl 2): 1257–8.
18. Rosenthal J, Naqvi AS, Luo M, et al. Heterogeneity of surface CD19 and CD22 expression in B lymphoblastic leukemia. Am J Hematol 2018;93(11):E352–5.
19. Pillai V, Muralidharan K, Meng W, et al. CAR T-cell therapy is effective for CD19-dim B-lymphoblastic leukemia but is impacted by prior blinatumomab therapy. Blood Adv 2019;3(22):3539–49.
20. Hashimoto M, Yamashita Y, Mori N. Immunohistochemical detection of CD79a expression in precursor T cell lymphoblastic lymphoma/leukaemias. J Pathol 2002;197(3):341–7.
21. Arber DA, Jenkins KA, Slovak ML. CD79 alpha expression in acute myeloid leukemia. High frequency of expression in acute promyelocytic leukemia. Am J Pathol 1996;149(4):1105–10.
22. Bhargava P, Kallakury BV, Ross JS, et al. CD79a is heterogeneously expressed in neoplastic and normal myeloid precursors and megakaryocytes in an antibody clone-dependent manner. Am J Clin Pathol 2007;128(2):306–13.
23. Luger D, Yang YA, Raviv A, et al. Expression of the B-cell receptor component CD79a on immature myeloid cells contributes to their tumor promoting effects. PLoS One 2013;8(10):e76115.
24. Weinberg OK, Hasserjian RP, Baraban E, et al. Clinical, immunophenotypic, and genomic findings of acute undifferentiated leukemia and comparison to acute

myeloid leukemia with minimal differentiation: a study from the bone marrow pathology group. Mod Pathol 2019;32(9):1373–85.
25. Janossy G, Coustan-Smith E, Campana D. The reliability of cytoplasmic CD3 and CD22 antigen expression in the immunodiagnosis of acute leukemia: a study of 500 cases. Leukemia 1989;3(3):170–81.
26. Weinberg OK, Chisholm KM, Ok CY, et al. Clinical, immunophenotypic and genomic findings of NK lymphoblastic leukemia: a study from the Bone Marrow Pathology Group. Mod Pathol 2021. https://doi.org/10.1038/s41379-021-00739-4.
27. Manivannan P, Puri V, Somasundaram V, et al. Can threshold for MPO by flow cytometry be reduced in classifying acute leukaemia? A comparison of flow cytometric and cytochemical myeloperoxidase using different flow cytometric cut-offs. Hematology 2015;20(8):455–61.
28. Guy J, Antony-Debre I, Benayoun E, et al. Flow cytometry thresholds of myeloperoxidase detection to discriminate between acute lymphoblastic or myeloblastic leukaemia. Br J Haematol 2013;161(4):551–5.
29. van den Ancker W, Westers TM, de Leeuw DC, et al. A threshold of 10% for myeloperoxidase by flow cytometry is valid to classify acute leukemia of ambiguous and myeloid origin. Cytometry B, Clin Cytom 2013;84(2):114–8.
30. Arber DA, Snyder DS, Fine M, et al. Myeloperoxidase immunoreactivity in adult acute lymphoblastic leukemia. Am J Clin Pathol 2001;116(1):25–33.
31. Alvarado CS, Austin GE, Borowitz MJ, et al. Myeloperoxidase gene expression in infant leukemia: a pediatric Oncology group study. Leuk Lymphoma 1998; 29(1–2):145–60.
32. Crisan D, Topalovski M, O'Malley B. Myeloperoxidase mRNA analysis in acute lymphoblastic leukemia. Diagn Mol Pathol 1996;5(4):236–48.
33. Ferrari S, Mariano MT, Tagliafico E, et al. Myeloperoxidase gene expression in blast cells with a lymphoid phenotype in cases of acute lymphoblastic leukemia. Blood 1988;72(3):873–6.
34. Zhou M, Findley HW, Zaki SR, et al. Expression of myeloperoxidase mRNA by leukemic cells from childhood acute lymphoblastic leukemia. Leukemia 1993; 7(8):1180–3.
35. Zaki SR, Austin GE, Swan D, et al. Human myeloperoxidase gene expression in acute leukemia. Blood 1989;74(6):2096–102.
36. Serrano J, Roman J, Sanchez J, et al. Myeloperoxidase gene expression in acute lymphoblastic leukaemia. Br J Haematol 1997;97(4):841–3.
37. Rytting ME, Kantarjian H, Albitar M. Acute lymphoblastic leukemia with Burkitt-like morphologic features and high myeloperoxidase activity. Am J Clin Pathol 2009; 132(2):182–5 [quiz: 306].
38. Raikar SS, Park SI, Leong T, et al. Isolated myeloperoxidase expression in pediatric B/myeloid mixed phenotype acute leukemia is linked with better survival. Blood 2018;131(5):573–7.
39. Charles NJ, Boyer DF. Mixed-phenotype acute leukemia: diagnostic criteria and pitfalls. Arch Pathol Lab Med 2017;141(11):1462–8.
40. Khan M, Siddiqi R, Naqvi K. An update on classification, genetics, and clinical approach to mixed phenotype acute leukemia (MPAL). Ann Hematol 2018; 97(6):945–53.
41. Alexander TB, Gu Z, Iacobucci I, et al. The genetic basis and cell of origin of mixed phenotype acute leukaemia. Nature 2018;562(7727):373–9.
42. Takahashi K, Wang F, Morita K, et al. Integrative genomic analysis of adult mixed phenotype acute leukemia delineates lineage associated molecular subtypes. Nat Commun 2018;9(1):2670.

43. Huh JY, Chung S, Oh D, et al. Clathrin assembly lymphoid myeloid leukemia-AF10-positive acute leukemias: a report of 2 cases with a review of the literature. Korean J Lab Med 2010;30(2):117–21.
44. Quesada AE, Hu Z, Routbort MJ, et al. Mixed phenotype acute leukemia contains heterogeneous genetic mutations by next-generation sequencing. Oncotarget 2018;9(9):8441–9.
45. Eckstein OS, Wang L, Punia JN, et al. Mixed-phenotype acute leukemia (MPAL) exhibits frequent mutations in DNMT3A and activated signaling genes. Exp Hematol 2016;44(8):740–4.
46. Manola KN, Panitsas F, Polychronopoulou S, et al. Cytogenetic abnormalities and monosomal karyotypes in children and adolescents with acute myeloid leukemia: correlations with clinical characteristics and outcome. Cancer Genet 2013;206(3):63–72.
47. Noronha EP, Marques LVC, Andrade FG, et al. T-lymphoid/myeloid mixed phenotype acute leukemia and early T-cell precursor lymphoblastic leukemia similarities with NOTCH1 mutation as a good prognostic factor. Cancer Manag Res 2019;11:3933–43.
48. Shi R, Munker R. Survival of patients with mixed phenotype acute leukemias: a large population-based study. Leuk Res 2015;39(6):606–16.
49. Rubnitz JE, Onciu M, Pounds S, et al. Acute mixed lineage leukemia in children: the experience of St Jude Children's Research Hospital. Blood 2009;113(21):5083–9.
50. Maruffi M, Sposto R, Oberley MJ, et al. Therapy for children and adults with mixed phenotype acute leukemia: a systematic review and meta-analysis. Leukemia 2018;32(7):1515–28.
51. Oberley MJ, Raikar SS, Wertheim GB, et al. Significance of minimal residual disease in pediatric mixed phenotype acute leukemia: a multicenter cohort study. Leukemia 2020;34(7):1741–50.
52. Hrusak O, de Haas V, Stancikova J, et al. International cooperative study identifies treatment strategy in childhood ambiguous lineage leukemia. Blood 2018;132(3):264–76.
53. El Chaer F, Ali OM, Sausville EA, et al. Treatment of CD19-positive mixed phenotype acute leukemia with blinatumomab. Am J Hematol 2019;94(1):E7–8.
54. Kong D, Qu C, Dai H, et al. CAR-T therapy bridging to allogeneic HSCT provides durable molecular remission of Ph(+) mixed phenotype acute leukaemia with minimal residual disease. Br J Haematol 2020;191(2):e47–9.
55. Ivey A, Hills RK, Simpson MA, et al. Assessment of minimal residual disease in standard-Risk AML. New Engl J Med 2016;374(5):422–33.
56. Gaipa G, Buracchi C, Biondi A. Flow cytometry for minimal residual disease testing in acute leukemia: opportunities and challenges. Expert Rev Mol Diagn 2018;18(9):775–87.
57. Ravandi F, Walter RB, Freeman SD. Evaluating measurable residual disease in acute myeloid leukemia. Blood Adv 2018;2(11):1356–66.
58. Huynh V, Laetsch TW, Schore RJ, et al. Redefining treatment failure for pediatric acute leukemia in the era of minimal residual disease testing. Pediatr Hematol Oncol 2017;34(6–7):395–408.
59. Myint HH, Tandon S, Narula G, et al. Clinicoepidemiologic profile and outcome predicted by minimal residual disease in children with mixed-phenotype Acute leukemia treated on a modified MCP-841 protocol at a tertiary cancer Institute in India. J Pediatr hematology/oncology 2020;42(7):415–9.

60. Rossi JG, Bernasconi AR, Alonso CN, et al. Lineage switch in childhood acute leukemia: an unusual event with poor outcome. Am J Hematol 2012;87(9):890–7.
61. Sakaki H, Kanegane H, Nomura K, et al. Early lineage switch in an infant acute lymphoblastic leukemia. Int J Hematol 2009;90(5):653–5.
62. Rayes A, McMasters RL, O'Brien MM. Lineage switch in MLL-rearranged infant leukemia following CD19-Directed therapy. Pediatr Blood Cancer 2016;63(6): 1113–5.
63. Ahuja A, Tyagi S, Seth T, et al. Comparison of immunohistochemistry, cytochemistry, and flow cytometry in AML for myeloperoxidase detection. Indian J Hematol Blood Transfus 2018;34(2):233–9.
64. Oberley MJ, Li S, Orgel E, et al. Clinical significance of isolated myeloperoxidase expression in pediatric b-lymphoblastic leukemia. Am J Clin Pathol 2017;147(4): 374–81.

Role of Minimal Residual Disease Testing in Acute Myeloid Leukemia

Xueyan Chen, MD, PhD, Sindhu Cherian, MD*

KEYWORDS

- Acute myeloid leukemia • Flow cytometry • Minimal/measurable residual disease

KEY POINTS

- Minimal/measurable residual disease (MRD) testing is an important tool to assess response to therapy and monitor for relapse in pediatric acute myeloid leukemia.
- MRD after therapy provides independent prognostic value for outcome in acute myeloid leukemia.
- Optimal methods to detect MRD depend on the characteristics of the leukemia, the timing of MRD testing, and treatment protocols.

INTRODUCTION

Pediatric acute myeloid leukemia (AML) is a heterogeneous disease with different morphologic, phenotypic, and genetic features, and variable clinical outcomes.[1,2] Over the past few decades, outcomes for pediatric AML have improved substantially, with overall survival reaching 60% to 70% and event-free survival exceeding 50%.[3–7] The improvement in outcomes has been achieved with implementation of risk stratification based on genetic features and response to therapy, intensification of chemotherapy with improved supportive care, and application of hematopoietic stem cell transplant (HCT). Minimal or, more accurately, measurable residual disease (MRD), the presence of persistent leukemic blasts after therapy, represents the integrated effect of leukemia genetics, patient characteristics, and chemotherapy regimens, which together determine a patient's response to therapy. There is growing evidence that MRD is a robust independent prognostic factor in pediatric AML.[8–12] Therefore, MRD has emerged as an essential factor for risk stratification and guiding risk-directed therapy.

Given the independent prognostic value of MRD, it is crucial to develop standardized, sensitive, and accurate methods to detect and monitor MRD. With rapidly

Conflicts of interest: The authors have no conflicts of interest.

Hematopathology, SCCA G7800, 825 Eastlake Ave E., Seattle, WA 98109, USA
* Corresponding author.
E-mail address: cherians@uw.edu

Clin Lab Med 41 (2021) 467–483
https://doi.org/10.1016/j.cll.2021.03.017

improving technology, the assessment of MRD has evolved substantially. At present, MRD in AML is most commonly measured by multiparametric flow cytometry and reverse transcriptase (RT) quantitative polymerase chain reaction (qPCR)–based methods. New molecular methods, such as high-throughput next-generation sequencing (HTS), have evolved into routine laboratory tools for identification of mutations at diagnosis and become promising in MRD detection. Common methods for MRD assessment in AML are compared in **Table 1**.

DEFINITION OF REMISSION AND CONCEPT OF MEASURABLE RESIDUAL DISEASE

In the past, complete remission following therapy in AML was defined by morphologic and clinical criteria as less than 5% blasts in the bone marrow by cytomorphology and peripheral count recovery.[13] However, 20% to 41% of pediatric patients with AML in morphologic remission ultimately relapse,[3,4,6,14–19] indicating that morphology-based methods lack adequate sensitivity and specificity to detect low levels of leukemic blasts responsible for future relapse. Given the inaccuracy in distinguishing leukemic

Table 1
Methods of minimal/measurable residual disease detection in acute myeloid leukemia

	Multiparametric Flow Cytometry	Reverse Transcriptase Quantitative Polymerase Chain Reaction	High-throughput Sequencing
Target	Leukemia-associated immunophenotypes or difference-from-normal approach	Leukemic fusion transcripts	Mutated genes
Sensitivity	3–4 colors: 0.1%–0.01% 6–10 colors: 0.01%–0.001%	0.01%–0.001% —	Up to 0.0001% —
Applicability	All AML	Subset of AML	Most AML
Specimen Requirement	Fresh viable cells	RNA	DNA
Turnaround Time	1–2 d	1–3 d	1–2 wk
Availability	Widely available	Widely available	Limited availability
Cost	Less expensive	More expensive	Most expensive
Advantages	Rapid resulting Direct quantification of leukemic blasts Monitors therapeutic antigen targets Provides information on cellular composition	Rapid resulting Standardized data interpretation Targets remain stable during treatment —	High sensitivity Detects subclones and monitors clonal evolution — —
Disadvantages	Inadequate interlaboratory standardization Requires expert knowledge for data interpretation Reduced sensitivity resulting from immunophenotypic shifts or confounded by regenerating progenitors	Only applicable to AML harboring detectable fusion transcripts Uncertain quantification of leukemic blasts Requires RNA, which is known to be unstable	High cost Time consuming Requires complex bioinformatics Limited clinical validation

blasts from normal blasts and quantification of leukemic blasts by morphology, highly sensitive techniques are needed to measure residual leukemic blasts for better assessment of response to therapy and to identify impending relapse.

The first report of detection of morphologically nonevident residual leukemic blasts in T-lymphoblastic leukemia (T-ALL) using fluorescence microscopy[20] published in 1981 led to the introduction of the fundamental concept of MRD. MRD is used to describe the residual leukemic blasts that persist after therapy at a level below the limit of conventional cytomorphologic detection (<5% blasts).[13] Numerous studies have shown a strong correlation between the presence of MRD and a higher risk of relapse and shorter survival in both childhood and adult AML as well as in patients undergoing allogeneic HCT.[6,10,11,21–33] These data support the rationale to incorporate MRD status into the criteria to establish a more in-depth remission after therapy for better prediction of outcome.[34] However, more data are needed to show that MRD-based complete remission correlates with survival in diverse AML populations undergoing different therapies.

TECHNIQUES TO ASSESS MEASURABLE RESIDUAL DISEASE

The methods to detect and qualify MRD in AML depend on the immunophenotype and genetic abnormalities of the leukemic blasts. Although there are no universal markers for MRD in AML, optimal MRD assays should reliably discriminate leukemic blasts from normal or regenerating progenitors with high sensitivity consistently throughout the course of treatment, and allow wide implementation and standardization across laboratories. Multiparametric flow cytometry to identify leukemic blasts and RT-qPCR–based methods to detect leukemia-specific gene fusion transcripts are the most commonly used methods to monitor MRD in AML.[35] With recent advances in sequencing technology, HTS-based MRD assays to detect gene mutations have been developed and implemented in clinical practice.[36,37]

Multiparametric Flow Cytometry

Distinguishing leukemic blasts from normal or regenerative progenitors relies on the immunophenotypic principle that the antigen expression patterns on the normal myeloid progenitors through maturation are highly reproducible, whereas the leukemic blasts have altered patterns of antigen expression reflecting underlying genetic mutations.[38] Based on this fundamental principle, 2 related methodological approaches have been applied in MRD detection by flow cytometry.[39–43]

The first approach relies on the identification of a combination of antigens expressed on the leukemic blasts and absent on normal progenitors, referred to as leukemia-associated immunophenotypes (LAIPs).[39] The commonly described LAIPs include antigen underexpression/overexpression, asynchronous antigen expression of progenitor markers and differentiation markers, cross-lineage antigen expression, and aberrant light-scatter properties.[39,44] In diagnostic samples, an extensive panel of antibodies is used to identify all LAIPs and define regions in multiparametric space that contain only leukemic blasts but not normal progenitors. Using an informative antibody panel in posttherapy samples, leukemic blasts present in the predefined space are considered as MRD and all of the LAIPs established at diagnosis should be followed to increase sensitivity and specificity of MRD detection. This approach has been successfully used in some studies, but it has some limitations. First, the knowledge of LAIPs identified at diagnosis is required to determine the informative antibody panel that should be used in the subsequent samples to define regions for precise MRD measurement. Second, immunophenotypes of leukemic blasts are unstable and may change during therapy or at relapse because of clonal evolution, tumor heterogeneity with subclonal selection, or progression through cell cycle,[45–48] which can lead to false-negative results if a rigid gating strategy is used to define regions. In addition, similar to leukemic blasts, the immunophenotype of background normal progenitors may be altered in response to therapeutic drugs and appear in regions defined for MRD, causing false-positive results.

An alternative approach, known as difference from normal, recognizes leukemic blasts by their immunophenotypic deviation from normal progenitors of similar lineage and maturation stage.[40,41] A standard antibody panel including antigens commonly seen in LAIPs is used in both diagnostic and posttherapy samples. When performed at diagnosis, this method identifies leukemic blasts similar to the identification of LAIPs, but with no requirement to define regions for LAIPs. Following therapy, all populations are assessed for immunophenotypic deviation from the pattern of normal maturation (**Fig. 1**). Although immunophenotypic aberrancies found at diagnosis can be used as a starting point, a diagnostic immunophenotype is not required for subsequent identification of MRD. In most cases, MRD can be detected even when there are significant immunophenotypic changes on leukemic blasts. The

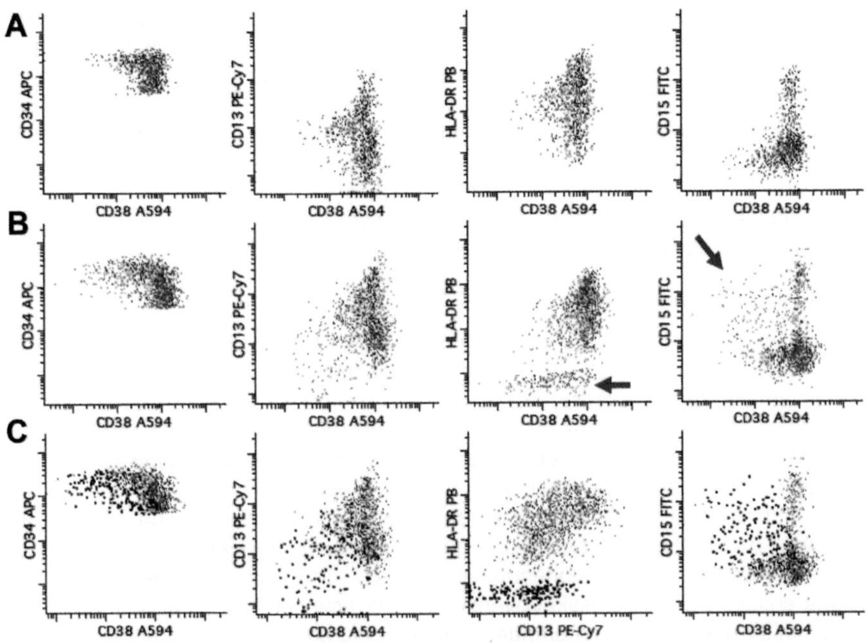

Fig. 1. Example of flow cytometry for AML MRD detection. All plots show CD34-positive blasts. The upper row (*A*) represents a normal sample for comparison, whereas the bottom 2 rows (*B* and *C*) are taken from patient sample submitted for MRD assessment by flow cytometry. When comparing the normal marrow in (*A*) with the patient sample in (*B*), the plots of CD34 versus CD38 and CD13 versus CD38 appear subtly different; however, it is challenging to definitively isolate an abnormal population. The plot of human leukocyte antigen, DR isotype (HLA-DR) versus CD38 allows easier identification of the abnormal population because it lacks expression of HLA-DR and shows variably decreased CD38 expression (*arrow*). On the plot of CD15 versus CD38, the abnormal population can be identified by variable expression of CD15 (*arrow*), an antigen that should be negative on CD34-expressing blasts lacking CD38 expression. In (*C*), the abnormal population is highlighted in dark blue. The abnormal blasts account for 0.15% of the white blood cells.

difference-from-normal approach avoids some of the limitations of LAIPs and allows the implementation of a standard antibody panel; however, this approach requires expert knowledge of antigen expression patterns of progenitors throughout normal maturation and regeneration after therapy, making standardization of data interpretation challenging. In practice, a combined approach with components of both methods is commonly used simultaneously and is recommended by the European LeukemiaNet (ELN) MRD Working Party.[49] In well-controlled studies, the sensitivity of MRD assay by flow cytometry can reach 0.1% to 0.01% in most patients.[50,51] Assay sensitivity may be affected by degree of immunophenotypic deviation of leukemic blasts from normal progenitors and by the abundance of normal progenitors in the background, which may depend on the timing of MRD testing.

MRD assessment by flow cytometry for AML in the pediatric setting poses several challenges that differ from the adult setting because the frequency of different subtypes of AML differs in adult and pediatric settings.[1] AML subtypes that may prove challenging in the MRD setting include AML with monocytic differentiation, acute megakaryoblastic leukemia, and AML with an RAM immunophenotype.[52] Such AML subtypes may lack typical progenitor markers, such as CD34 and/or CD117, which are often used for blast identification, and/or may be outside of typical CD45 versus side scatter–defined blast gates. Because of these features, such blast populations may be overlooked when standard gating strategies are applied. In infants, monocytic leukemia, often associated with rearrangements of *KMT2A*, may be more common. In addition to the challenges noted earlier, monocytic blast equivalents may be difficult to distinguish from normal immature monocytic cells, which may be present in the marrow at low levels. Megakaryoblastic leukemia is more common in children than in adults, in particular in the setting of Down syndrome (DS). Compounding the aforementioned challenges, megakaryoblastic leukemia can be associated with extensive marrow fibrosis, resulting in a so-called dry tap and limiting the sensitivity of MRD detection by flow cytometry. Recognition of such subtypes and their associated immunophenotypic characteristics and related challenges for flow cytometric assessment is critical for accurate identification of AML MRD in the pediatric setting. **Fig. 2** provides several examples of flow cytometric identification of such challenging AML subtypes.

Molecular Methods

The genomic profile in pediatric AML has a different mutational landscape from adult AML and shows significant variability and clonal evolution from diagnosis to relapse.[53,54] qPCR is the mainstay of current molecular MRD testing in AML. The common targets for MRD evaluation are gene fusion transcripts generated by balanced chromosome translocation (ie, *PML-RARA*, *RUNX1-RUNXT1*, *CBFB-MYH11*, and *KMT2A* gene rearrangement) and gene mutations such as *NPM1* and *FLT3*, collectively occurring in ~60% of pediatric AML.[55,56] Europe Against Cancer standardized RT-qPCR assays for clinical implementation more than a decade ago and established common protocols including specific primer-probe sets for each of 9 of the most common fusion genes and reaction conditions for all steps of the procedure through systemic parallel evaluation across 26 international expert laboratories.[57]

The intertumor and intratumor heterogeneity makes it challenging to define specific and stable gene mutations as MRD markers for patients with AML. At present, only the *NPM1* gene is considered as a suitable MRD marker in AML. Using RT-qPCR with a mutation-specific primer, *NPM1*-mutated transcripts have been shown to be stably present at relapse in 99% of cases and persistence of mutated *NPM1* transcripts after the second chemotherapy cycle was associated with greater risk of relapse.[26] Quantification of overexpressed gene transcripts has been attempted as an MRD target in

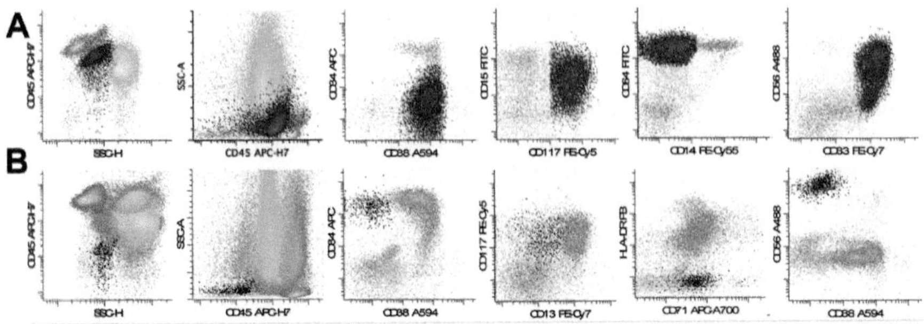

Fig. 2. Examples of challenging immunophenotypes that may be encountered in pediatric AML. (*A* and *B*) The first 2 plots show all viable cells, whereas the remaining plots show all cells in the CD45 versus side scatter–defined blast gate. When present, background mature lymphocytes are shown in blue, monocytic cells in pink, granulocytic cells in green, and CD34-positive normal myeloid progenitors in red. (*A*) This row is taken from a patient with a history of AML with monocytic differentiation and a *KMT2A* mutation. Abnormal blasts/blast equivalents are highlighted in orange and comprise ~5% of the white blood cells. The blast equivalents have a higher CD45 level than typical myeloid blasts and lack CD34, although they express CD117. The blasts show strong expression of CD64 but lack CD14, a characteristic of immature monocytic cells. The blast equivalents also aberrantly express CD56. (*B*) This row is taken from a patient with a reported history of AML with megakaryoblastic differentiation (AML-M7). Abnormal blasts/blast equivalents are highlighted in purple and comprise 0.16% of the white blood cells. The blasts have very low CD45 expression and might be excluded from a traditional CD45 versus side scatter–defined blast gate. In this case, the blasts express both CD34 and CD117 but show low-level CD13, are negative for HLA-DR, and show intermediate intensity of CD71 with bright CD56 expression.

patients lacking leukemia-specific gene fusions or mutations. The best-characterized gene overexpressed in most AML is *WT1*.[58,59] European LeukemiaNet systemically evaluated and standardized qPCR WT1 assay with optimal performance and showed greater reduction in *WT1* transcripts after induction predicted reduced risk of relapse.[58,59]

Compared with flow cytometry, qPCR-based assays have higher analytical sensitivity (often approaching 0.001%) and have been extensively optimized and standardized. Despite the advantages, several concerns have been raised for consideration, including inaccurate enumeration of leukemic blasts, because the number of transcripts per cell may vary; instability of MRD targets (in particular *FLT3* internal tandem duplication), which may become undetectable at relapse[60–62]; and persistence of mutant transcripts in differentiated leukemic blasts with uncertain leukemogenic potential.[63,64]

The development of MRD assays using advanced technology provides a new venue to potentially overcome limitations of flow cytometry and qPCR. The sensitivity of an *NPM1* assay by HTS reached 0.001%, outperforming flow cytometry and comparable with qPCR.[36] Further, HTS could detect *NPM1* mutation in flow cytometry–negative cases and detect alternate *NPM1* mutations in addition to index mutations in one-third of patients. *NPM1* assay by HTS provides increased sensitivity for MRD detection and specificity for MRD quantitation without a requirement for the diagnostic *NPM1* mutation subtype or interpretation of complex flow cytometry data. Theoretically, HTS-based MRD assay can be applied to all genetic mutations in AML. Using a gene panel, this method allows the identification of clonal heterogeneity and evolution. The results may be affected by mutations in preleukemic clones representing clonal hematopoiesis of undetermined potential (CHIP), which may persist even after patients achieve complete remission.[65] Although the presence of such preleukemic clones or CHIP poses a significant consideration in adults,[66] in the pediatric population, such preleukemic clones are rarely detected. Unlike CHIP, germline mutations may be seen with increased frequency in pediatric compared with adult populations, and awareness of whether a mutation may be germline or specific to the leukemic cells is useful in data interpretation.[67] Another novel technology, droplet digital polymerase chain reaction (ddPCR), has been applied in MRD monitoring in *NPM1*-mutated AML.[68] This method enables sensitive detection and specific quantitation of *NPM1* mutation, facilitating testing in patients with unknown diagnostic *NPM1* mutant sequences. Pilot studies using single-molecule molecular inversion probes have shown that this technology offers an ultrasensitive approach to identify gene mutations for MRD detection and has potential utility in clinical practice.[69,70]

APPLICATIONS OF MEASURABLE RESIDUAL DISEASE DATA IN ACUTE MYELOID LEUKEMIA

Although data are limited in pediatric AML compared with ALL, multiple lines of evidence support MRD as an independent predictor for outcome. MRD provides a dynamic assessment of risk of relapse independent of pretreatment prognostic evaluation and may improve outcome using MRD-adapted therapies. Gradually, MRD monitoring has become part of the standard of care for patients with AML across all age groups.

Outcomes and Flow Cytometric Measurable Residual Disease Assessment

In 2003, the Children's Cancer Group reported that flow cytometric evidence of greater than or equal to 0.5% abnormal blasts in bone marrow after induction therapy was the most powerful independent prognostic factor for poor outcome in a prospective study on 252 de novo pediatric patients with AML. The subsequent application of 4-color flow cytometric analysis allowed detection of 0.1% to 0.01% residual leukemic cells in pediatric AML, and showed that detection of MRD by flow cytometry after induction therapy was an independent predictor of outcome.[8] In the multicenter AML02 trial, Inaba and colleagues[25] reported that MRD greater than or equal to 0.1% after induction 1 or 2 by flow cytometry predicted lower event-free survival and higher relapse rate, whereas morphologic findings and molecular MRD results by RT-qPCR on *RUNX1-RUNX1T1* and *CBFbeta-MYH11* did not improve prediction. Risk-stratified therapeutic interventions, specifically the application of targeted therapy or HCT based on MRD levels, improved clinical outcome in this trial.[6] Providing additional supporting data to prior studies, in pediatric patients with AML enrolled into United Kingdom Medical Research Council (MRC) AML12 and Dutch Childhood Oncology Group (DCOG) ANLL97 protocols, MRD greater than or equal to 0.5% by flow cytometry after the first course of chemotherapy was an independent prognostic factor for relapse-free survival and overall survival.[10] Similarly, in patients treated on Children's Oncology Group (COG) AAML03P1, the presence of MRD after induction 1, 2, or consolidation therapy was associated with shorter relapse-free survival and overall survival, and was most predicative of relapse in patients without cytogenetic or molecular risk factors.[11] Recently 2 European studies further showed the prognostic significance of MRD in pediatric AML.[32,71] In the Nordic Society for Pediatric Haematology and Oncology (NOPHO) AML 2004 study, MRD ($\geq$0.1%) before consolidation therapy was the strongest independent prognostic factor for lower event-free survival and had a higher prognostic value than MRD detected at day 15 after induction therapy.[32] In children treated according to the Associazione Italiana di EmatoOncologia Pediatrica (AIEOP) AML

2002/01 study protocol, MRD (≥0.1%) detected by flow cytometry after induction therapy is an independent prognostic factor for lower disease-free survival.[71]

When discussing prognostic impact, it is critical to emphasize that assay quality underlies the predictive value of MRD assessment in AML by flow cytometry. A recent study showed that, when performed in a decentralized and uncontrolled fashion, MRD assessment by flow cytometry may lose predictive value.[72] This study showed that the ability of MRD by flow cytometry to provide useful prognostic data relies, in part, on methodologic differences between assays, including number of parameters evaluated, number of cells collected, and other technical factors. Such observations underscore the crucial importance of the quality of an AML MRD flow cytometric assay.

Outcomes and Molecular Measurable Residual Disease Assessment

Only limited studies have investigated prognostic value of MRD assessment by molecular methods in pediatric AML. In pediatric AML with *RUNX1-RUNX1T1*, MRD detected by RT-qPCR after both induction and consolidation therapy was predictive of relapse.[73] Similarly, Pigazzi and colleagues[74] reported that monitoring of MRD after induction therapy provided a reliable prognostic marker in AML with *RUNX1-RUNX1T1*, whereas early MRD monitoring was not useful for predicting relapse in AML with *CBFB-MYH11*. Interpretation of MRD by molecular methods at a single time point may be confounded by delayed clearance of blasts or persistence/reappearance of low levels of fusion transcripts in bone marrow despite continuous remission.[33,75–77] Therefore, sequential measurements are more informative in guiding future management. A recent study investigated the kinetics and prognostic significance of fusion transcripts (*RUNX1-RUNX1T1*, *CBFB-MYH11*, *KMT2A-MLLT3*, or *KMT2A-ELL*) by RT-qPCR in 75 children with AML on NOPHO-AML 2004, NOPHO-Dutch-Belgian-Holland (DBH) AML 2012, or AML-Berlin-Frankfurt-Münster (BFM) 2012 protocol. In this cohort, MRD monitoring in peripheral blood during consolidation therapy may identify patients with high risk of relapse.[78] In contrast, MRD persistence in bone marrow during consolidation did not increase the risk of relapse, and MRD at completion of therapy did not correlate with outcome. In core-binding factor AML, an increase in MRD greater than 5×10^{-4} in bone marrow inevitably led to overt hematologic relapse.

The predictive value of *WT1* in peripheral blood after chemotherapy has been reported in adult AML.[58,59,79] Recently, Juul-Dam and colleagues[80] established child-specific reference values for *WT1* expression and showed that longitudinal *WT1* measurement in peripheral blood was an informative tool to monitor residual disease in pediatric patients with AML treated according to one of 3 consecutive protocols (NOPHO-AML 93, NOPHO-AML 2004, and NOPHO-DBH AML 2012).

These data provide strong evidence that MRD status after therapy is crucial for prognostication and risk stratification and to determine those patients that may benefit from therapeutic reduction or intensification. However, the methodology, threshold, and optimal timing for MRD testing in pediatric AML remain matters of debate and vary in different trials. Therefore, MRD results cannot be directly compared between studies using different testing methods and threshold and treatment protocols.[56,81,82]

CHALLENGES IN MEASURABLE RESIDUAL DISEASE ASSESSMENT

Clinically Relevant Sensitivity and Optimal Timing for Measurable Residual Disease Testing

Despite unequivocal prognostic significance of MRD in AML, at present, there are no well-established guidelines or recommendations for optimal methods and timing for

MRD testing in AML. The impact of MRD assessment depends in part on characteristics of different patient populations, leukemia-specific factors, and treatment regimens. The ELN MRD Working Party attempted to provide guidelines for the current and future application of MRD in clinical practice.[49] Flow cytometric MRD assessment is intended for use in risk stratification at an early time point before consolidation therapy. Based on most retrospective studies in pediatric and adult AML, the ELN MRD Working Party recommended using 0.1% as the threshold to define MRD-positive patients, although it is noted that MRD less than 0.1% may still represent MRD and has shown prognostic significance in some studies.[21,83] There is no consensus regarding the clinically appropriate intervals for sequential MRD measurement in patients who are in remission and not receiving treatment. For patients with gene fusions, mutated *NPM1*, and other markers during treatment, molecular MRD testing should be performed at diagnosis, after 2 cycles of standard induction/consolidation therapy, and at the end of treatment, and should achieve a sensitivity of at least 1 in 1000 cells (0.1%).[49] Molecular remission is achieved if a patient is in morphologic remission and has 2 successive MRD-negative assessments within an interval of greater than or equal to 4 weeks at a sensitivity level of at least 0.1%. Molecular relapse is defined as an increase of the MRD level of greater than or equal to 1 log10 between 2 positive samples in a patient who was previously MRD negative. After the end of treatment, molecular MRD assessment was recommended every 3 months for a period of 24 months. Further monitoring beyond 2 years should be determined by the risk of relapse. At present, qPCR-based methods are recommended because of high sensitivity and thorough standardization. Other platforms, such as HTS and ddPCR, will likely be widely applicable in routine clinical MRD testing after extensive validation. With development of novel therapeutic interventions, it is necessary to define the most relevant MRD threshold for a novel agent in order to compare it with standard regimens in MRD-guided prospective studies.

Measurable Residual Disease Testing in Acute Myeloid Leukemia Associated with Down Syndrome

Children with DS have increased risk for AML, with ~150-fold increase in children aged less than 5 years and acquired GATA-1 mutations as defining events.[1] Despite the increased risk of developing AML, children with DS tend to have favorable response to therapy and lower cumulative incidence of relapse than patients without DS.[84,85] Collectively, about 80% of patients achieved long-term remission after low-intensity chemotherapy, although the risk of relapse was high in a small subset of patients who did not respond to initial therapy.[86] Given the favorable outcomes and lack of common cytogenetic abnormalities and genetic mutations seen in non-DS AML, the prognostic and prediction models for outcome established for non-DS AML are not suitable to evaluate treatment response in patients with DS. There is a strong need to identify prognostic markers that can accurately predict risk of relapse and guide individualized treatment protocols.

MRD monitoring by flow cytometry has been the primary modality in detecting residual leukemic cells in pediatric AML for more than a decade and has significant prognostic implications.[11] Because of incomplete knowledge on the immunophenotype of normal hematopoietic cells and immunophenotypic alterations during regeneration in patients with DS, MRD detected by flow cytometry in patients with DS did not reach the same level of prognostic significance until recently. For the first time, COG AAML0431 reported MRD by flow cytometry as a new prognostic marker for AML in DS that can be used for risk stratification.[87] MRD greater than 0.01% at day 28 after induction I was the only independent predictor of disease-free survival and overall survival. With these results, an ongoing phase 3 prospective study, AAML1531, was launched by COG to determine the efficacy of risk-stratified therapy based on postinduction MRD status. From a laboratory standpoint, it is important to recognize the unusual immunophenotype of normal and regenerating blasts in DS and develop and validate new algorithms to distinguish leukemic blasts from normal counterparts by both LAIP and difference-from-normal approaches (**Fig. 3**). Given the challenges of MRD detection by flow cytometry and better understanding of the germline and somatic mutations that drive transformation to AML, HTS for GATA1 and other genetic mutations may supplement or eventually replace flow cytometry to monitor MRD in patients with DS with higher sensitivity and specificity.

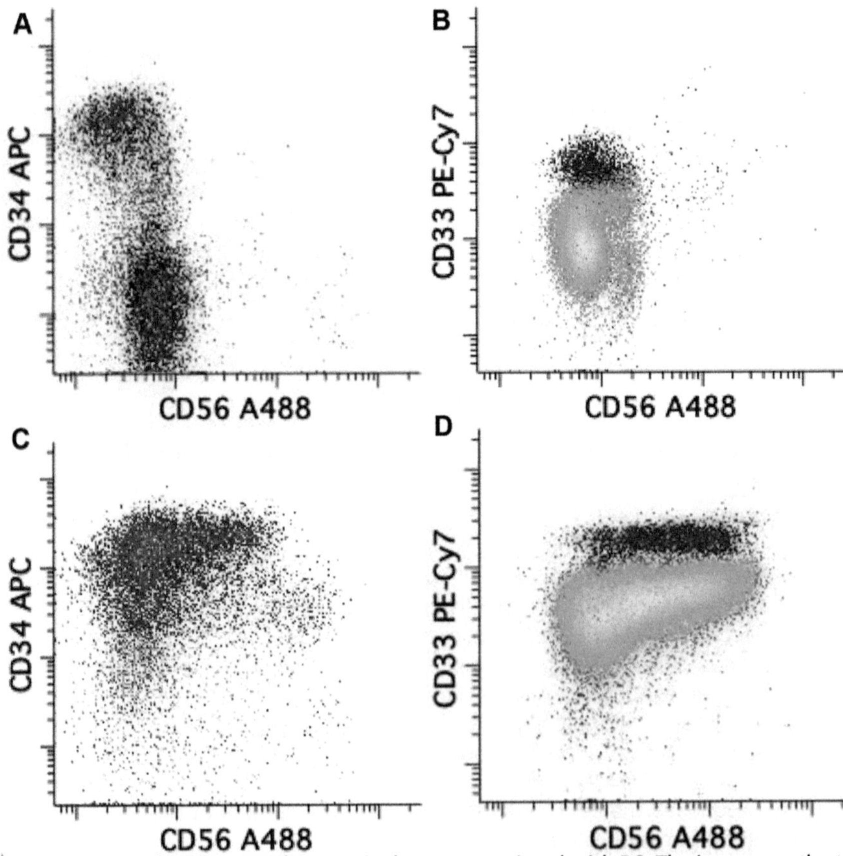

Fig. 3. Regenerative immunophenotypic changes associated with DS. The images on the top row are from healthy resting marrow (*A, B*), whereas the images on the bottom row (*C, D*) are from regenerating marrow (after chemotherapy for acute leukemia) from a patient with DS. Plots (*A*) and (*C*) show cells in the CD45 versus side scatter–defined blast region with CD34-positive blasts highlighted in red, whereas plots (*B*) and (*D*) show myelomonocytic cells with monocytic cells in pink and granulocytic cells in green. Note how CD34-positive blasts, monocytic forms, and granulocytic forms in the patient with DS recovering from chemotherapy show expression of CD56 on subsets. CD56 may be expressed on myelomonocytic cells and progenitors in patients with DS in the setting of marrow regeneration. The intensity of CD56 expression decreases with distance from therapy.

Measurable Residual Disease as a Surrogate End Point for Clinical Outcomes

The conventional end point for proof of clinical benefit in drug approval is survival.[88] The use of survival as an end point requires a long duration to complete follow-up, potentially delaying the assessment of drug efficacy. For this reason, there is a clinical need to identify novel surrogates to survival that can be assessed earlier after therapy to facilitate drug development. A valid surrogate end point must accurately predict changes in outcomes. Although, as a powerful prognostic factor, MRD status could theoretically be considered as a surrogate end point and is available at an early time point, MRD cannot reflect the long-term effects or toxicities of drugs. In addition, because MRD is used for risk stratification in AML, risk-adapted therapy based on MRD itself may attenuate the potential of this variable as a surrogate for survival. Although some studies showed that clinical outcomes with high dosage of daunorubicin[89] or addition of gemtuzumab ozogamicin to standard therapy[90] correlated with MRD status in adult AML, the ability of MRD after induction therapy to predict relapse-free survival and overall survival remains limited.[30] Therefore, a large dataset is required to prove the potential for MRD to serve as a surrogate for survival; that is, confirming MRD correlates with survival regardless of disease state, cytogenetic and molecular features, and intensity of regimens. Accelerated approval of a novel drug using MRD as a primary end point would require establishment of a direct linkage between a change in therapy based on MRD and traditional clinical end points.

SUMMARY

MRD monitoring provides dynamic assessment for risk of relapse and survival in pediatric AML. Apart from serving as a prognostic marker, MRD after therapy integrated with complex genetic information is essential for risk assessment and to guide patient-tailored therapy. Many efforts have been devoted to standardizing current MRD assays to improve accuracy and reproducibility and develop new molecular methods to improve sensitivity and specificity. Prognostication by MRD depends on characteristics of the AML, treatment protocols, and timing of MRD testing. Therefore, future personalized, disease-specific, and treatment-specific protocols should include a schedule for MRD monitoring, methods for MRD detection, and clinically validated threshold for optimal results. In addition, future prospective studies are necessary to prove the efficacy of MRD-adapted treatment protocols.

CLINICS CARE POINTS

- MRD in AML can be assessed by either flow cytometry or molecular studies.
- Performing accurate MRD assessment by flow cytometry requires a multiparametric assay, collection of adequate events, and an experienced analyst with a broad understanding of the immunophenotype of normal and regenerating myeloid progenitors.
- Knowledge of the sensitivity of an MRD assay is critical for determining the predictive value of the assay.

ACKNOWLEDGMENTS

Funding source: None.

REFERENCES

1. Swerdlow SH, Campo E, Harris NL, et al. WHO Classification of Tumours of Haematopoietic and lymphoid Tissues. Revised 4th edition. Lyon: International Agency for Research on Cancer; 2017.
2. Rubnitz JE, Inaba H. Childhood acute myeloid leukaemia. Br J Haematol 2012; 159(3):259–76.
3. Abrahamsson J, Forestier E, Heldrup J, et al. Response-guided induction therapy in pediatric acute myeloid leukemia with excellent remission rate. J Clin Oncol 2011;29(3):310–5.
4. Cooper TM, Franklin J, Gerbing RB, et al. AAML03P1, a pilot study of the safety of gemtuzumab ozogamicin in combination with chemotherapy for newly diagnosed childhood acute myeloid leukemia: a report from the Children's Oncology Group. Cancer 2012;118(3):761–9.
5. Lange BJ, Smith FO, Feusner J, et al. Outcomes in CCG-2961, a children's oncology group phase 3 trial for untreated pediatric acute myeloid leukemia: a report from the children's oncology group. Blood 2008;111(3):1044–53.
6. Rubnitz JE, Inaba H, Dahl G, et al. Minimal residual disease-directed therapy for childhood acute myeloid leukaemia: results of the AML02 multicentre trial. Lancet Oncol 2010;11(6):543–52.
7. Sander A, Zimmermann M, Dworzak M, et al. Consequent and intensified relapse therapy improved survival in pediatric AML: results of relapse treatment in 379 patients of three consecutive AML-BFM trials. Leukemia 2010;24(8):1422–8.
8. Coustan-Smith E, Ribeiro RC, Rubnitz JE, et al. Clinical significance of residual disease during treatment in childhood acute myeloid leukaemia. Br J Haematol 2003;123(2):243–52.
9. Langebrake C, Creutzig U, Dworzak M, et al. Residual disease monitoring in childhood acute myeloid leukemia by multiparameter flow cytometry: the MRD-AML-BFM Study Group. J Clin Oncol 2006;24(22):3686–92.
10. van der Velden VH, van der Sluijs-Geling A, Gibson BE, et al. Clinical significance of flowcytometric minimal residual disease detection in pediatric acute myeloid leukemia patients treated according to the DCOG ANLL97/MRC AML12 protocol. Leukemia 2010;24(9):1599–606.
11. Loken MR, Alonzo TA, Pardo L, et al. Residual disease detected by multidimensional flow cytometry signifies high relapse risk in patients with de novo acute myeloid leukemia: a report from Children's Oncology Group. Blood 2012; 120(8):1581–8.
12. Karol SE, Coustan-Smith E, Cao X, et al. Prognostic factors in children with acute myeloid leukaemia and excellent response to remission induction therapy. Br J Haematol 2015;168(1):94–101.
13. Cheson BD, Bennett JM, Kopecky KJ, et al. Revised recommendations of the international Working group for diagnosis, standardization of response criteria, treatment outcomes, and reporting standards for therapeutic trials in acute myeloid leukemia. J Clin Oncol 2003;21(24):4642–9.
14. Brodersen LE, Gerbing RB, Pardo ML, et al. Morphologic remission status is limited compared to DeltaN flow cytometry: a Children's Oncology Group AAML0531 report. Blood Adv 2020;4(20):5050–61.
15. Creutzig U, Zimmermann M, Bourquin JP, et al. Randomized trial comparing liposomal daunorubicin with idarubicin as induction for pediatric acute myeloid leukemia: results from Study AML-BFM 2004. Blood 2013;122(1):37–43.

16. Gibson BE, Webb DK, Howman AJ, et al. Results of a randomized trial in children with Acute Myeloid Leukaemia: medical research council AML12 trial. Br J Haematol 2011;155(3):366–76.
17. Hasle H, Abrahamsson J, Forestier E, et al. Gemtuzumab ozogamicin as post-consolidation therapy does not prevent relapse in children with AML: results from NOPHO-AML 2004. Blood 2012;120(5):978–84.
18. Pession A, Masetti R, Rizzari C, et al. Results of the AIEOP AML 2002/01 multicenter prospective trial for the treatment of children with acute myeloid leukemia. Blood 2013;122(2):170–8.
19. Tsukimoto I, Tawa A, Horibe K, et al. Risk-stratified therapy and the intensive use of cytarabine improves the outcome in childhood acute myeloid leukemia: the AML99 trial from the Japanese Childhood AML Cooperative Study Group. J Clin Oncol 2009;27(24):4007–13.
20. Bradstock KF, Janossy G, Tidman N, et al. Immunological monitoring of residual disease in treated thymic acute lymphoblastic leukaemia. Leuk Res 1981;5(4–5):301–9.
21. Freeman SD, Virgo P, Couzens S, et al. Prognostic relevance of treatment response measured by flow cytometric residual disease detection in older patients with acute myeloid leukemia. J Clin Oncol 2013;31(32):4123–31.
22. Buccisano F, Maurillo L, Spagnoli A, et al. Cytogenetic and molecular diagnostic characterization combined to postconsolidation minimal residual disease assessment by flow cytometry improves risk stratification in adult acute myeloid leukemia. Blood 2010;116(13):2295–303.
23. Chen X, Xie H, Wood BL, et al. Relation of clinical response and minimal residual disease and their prognostic impact on outcome in acute myeloid leukemia. J Clin Oncol 2015;33(11):1258–64.
24. Goswami M, McGowan KS, Lu K, et al. A multigene array for measurable residual disease detection in AML patients undergoing SCT. Bone Marrow Transplant 2015;50(5):642–51.
25. Inaba H, Coustan-Smith E, Cao X, et al. Comparative analysis of different approaches to measure treatment response in acute myeloid leukemia. J Clin Oncol 2012;30(29):3625–32.
26. Ivey A, Hills RK, Simpson MA, et al. Assessment of minimal residual disease in standard-risk AML. N Engl J Med 2016;374(5):422–33.
27. Jourdan E, Boissel N, Chevret S, et al. Prospective evaluation of gene mutations and minimal residual disease in patients with core binding factor acute myeloid leukemia. Blood 2013;121(12):2213–23.
28. Klco JM, Miller CA, Griffith M, et al. Association between mutation clearance after induction therapy and outcomes in acute myeloid leukemia. JAMA 2015;314(8):811–22.
29. Mule MP, Mannis GN, Wood BL, et al. Multigene measurable residual disease assessment improves acute myeloid leukemia relapse risk stratification in Autologous hematopoietic cell transplantation. Biol Blood Marrow Transplant 2016;22(11):1974–82.
30. Othus M, Wood BL, Stirewalt DL, et al. Effect of measurable ("minimal") residual disease (MRD) information on prediction of relapse and survival in adult acute myeloid leukemia. Leukemia 2016;30(10):2080–3.
31. Terwijn M, van Putten WL, Kelder A, et al. High prognostic impact of flow cytometric minimal residual disease detection in acute myeloid leukemia: data from the HOVON/SAKK AML 42A study. J Clin Oncol 2013;31(31):3889–97.

32. Tierens A, Bjorklund E, Siitonen S, et al. Residual disease detected by flow cytometry is an independent predictor of survival in childhood acute myeloid leukaemia; results of the NOPHO-AML 2004 study. Br J Haematol 2016;174(4):600–9.
33. Yin JA, O'Brien MA, Hills RK, et al. Minimal residual disease monitoring by quantitative RT-PCR in core binding factor AML allows risk stratification and predicts relapse: results of the United Kingdom MRC AML-15 trial. Blood 2012;120(14):2826–35.
34. Dohner H, Estey E, Grimwade D, et al. Diagnosis and management of AML in adults: 2017 ELN recommendations from an international expert panel. Blood 2017;129(4):424–47.
35. Kroger N, Bacher U, Bader P, et al. NCI first international Workshop on the Biology, Prevention, and treatment of relapse after allogeneic hematopoietic stem cell transplantation: report from the Committee on disease-specific methods and strategies for monitoring relapse following allogeneic stem cell transplantation. Part I: methods, acute leukemias, and myelodysplastic syndromes. Biol Blood Marrow Transplant 2010;16(9):1187–211.
36. Salipante SJ, Fromm JR, Shendure J, et al. Detection of minimal residual disease in NPM1-mutated acute myeloid leukemia by next-generation sequencing. Mod Pathol 2014;27(11):1438–46.
37. Kohlmann A, Nadarajah N, Alpermann T, et al. Monitoring of residual disease by next-generation deep-sequencing of RUNX1 mutations can identify acute myeloid leukemia patients with resistant disease. Leukemia 2014;28(1):129–37.
38. Wood BL. Principles of minimal residual disease detection for hematopoietic neoplasms by flow cytometry. Cytometry B Clin Cytom 2016;90(1):47–53.
39. Feller N, van der Velden VH, Brooimans RA, et al. Defining consensus leukemia-associated immunophenotypes for detection of minimal residual disease in acute myeloid leukemia in a multicenter setting. Blood Cancer J 2013;3:e129.
40. Wood B. Multicolor immunophenotyping: human immune system hematopoiesis. Methods Cell Biol 2004;75:559–76.
41. Wood BL. Flow cytometric monitoring of residual disease in acute leukemia. Methods Mol Biol 2013;999:123–36.
42. Xu J, Jorgensen JL, Wang SA. How do We use multicolor flow cytometry to detect minimal residual disease in acute myeloid leukemia? Clin Lab Med 2017;37(4):787–802.
43. Chen X, Cherian S. Acute myeloid leukemia immunophenotyping by flow cytometric analysis. Clin Lab Med 2017;37(4):753–69.
44. Al-Mawali A, Gillis D, Hissaria P, et al. Incidence, sensitivity, and specificity of leukemia-associated phenotypes in acute myeloid leukemia using specific five-color multiparameter flow cytometry. Am J Clin Pathol 2008;129(6):934–45.
45. Quesenberry PJ, Goldberg LR, Dooner MS. Concise reviews: a stem cell apostasy: a tale of four H words. Stem Cells 2015;33(1):15–20.
46. Zeijlemaker W, Gratama JW, Schuurhuis GJ. Tumor heterogeneity makes AML a "moving target" for detection of residual disease. Cytometry B Clin Cytom 2014;86(1):3–14.
47. Baer MR, Stewart CC, Dodge RK, et al. High frequency of immunophenotype changes in acute myeloid leukemia at relapse: implications for residual disease detection (Cancer and Leukemia Group B Study 8361). Blood 2001;97(11):3574–80.

48. Langebrake C, Brinkmann I, Teigler-Schlegel A, et al. Immunophenotypic differences between diagnosis and relapse in childhood AML: implications for MRD monitoring. Cytometry B Clin Cytom 2005;63(1):1–9.
49. Schuurhuis GJ, Heuser M, Freeman S, et al. Minimal/measurable residual disease in AML: a consensus document from the European LeukemiaNet MRD Working Party. Blood 2018;131(12):1275–91.
50. Al-Mawali A, Gillis D, Lewis I. The use of receiver operating characteristic analysis for detection of minimal residual disease using five-color multiparameter flow cytometry in acute myeloid leukemia identifies patients with high risk of relapse. Cytometry B Clin Cytom 2009;76(2):91–101.
51. Buccisano F, Maurillo L, Del Principe MI, et al. Prognostic and therapeutic implications of minimal residual disease detection in acute myeloid leukemia. Blood 2012;119(2):332–41.
52. Eidenschink Brodersen L, Alonzo TA, Menssen AJ, et al. A recurrent immunophenotype at diagnosis independently identifies high-risk pediatric acute myeloid leukemia: a report from Children's Oncology Group. Leukemia 2016;30(10):2077–80.
53. Farrar JE, Schuback HL, Ries RE, et al. Genomic profiling of pediatric acute myeloid leukemia reveals a changing mutational landscape from disease diagnosis to relapse. Cancer Res 2016;76(8):2197–205.
54. Bolouri H, Farrar JE, Triche T Jr, et al. The molecular landscape of pediatric acute myeloid leukemia reveals recurrent structural alterations and age-specific mutational interactions. Nat Med 2018;24(1):103–12.
55. Creutzig U, Zimmermann M, Reinhardt D, et al. Changes in cytogenetics and molecular genetics in acute myeloid leukemia from childhood to adult age groups. Cancer 2016;122(24):3821–30.
56. Grimwade D, Freeman SD. Defining minimal residual disease in acute myeloid leukemia: which platforms are ready for "prime time"? Blood 2014;124(23):3345–55.
57. Gabert J, Beillard E, van der Velden VH, et al. Standardization and quality control studies of 'real-time' quantitative reverse transcriptase polymerase chain reaction of fusion gene transcripts for residual disease detection in leukemia - a Europe against Cancer program. Leukemia 2003;17(12):2318–57.
58. Cilloni D, Renneville A, Hermitte F, et al. Real-time quantitative polymerase chain reaction detection of minimal residual disease by standardized WT1 assay to enhance risk stratification in acute myeloid leukemia: a European LeukemiaNet study. J Clin Oncol 2009;27(31):5195–201.
59. Marani C, Clavio M, Grasso R, et al. Integrating post induction WT1 quantification and flow-cytometry results improves minimal residual disease stratification in acute myeloid leukemia. Leuk Res 2013;37(12):1606–11.
60. Abdelhamid E, Preudhomme C, Helevaut N, et al. Minimal residual disease monitoring based on FLT3 internal tandem duplication in adult acute myeloid leukemia. Leuk Res 2012;36(3):316–23.
61. Chou WC, Hou HA, Liu CY, et al. Sensitive measurement of quantity dynamics of FLT3 internal tandem duplication at early time points provides prognostic information. Ann Oncol 2011;22(3):696–704.
62. Schiller J, Praulich I, Krings Rocha C, et al. Patient-specific analysis of FLT3 internal tandem duplications for the prognostication and monitoring of acute myeloid leukemia. Eur J Haematol 2012;89(1):53–62.
63. Sexauer A, Perl A, Yang X, et al. Terminal myeloid differentiation in vivo is induced by FLT3 inhibition in FLT3/ITD AML. Blood 2012;120(20):4205–14.

64. Tobal K, Liu Yin JA. RT-PCR method with increased sensitivity shows persistence of PML-RARA fusion transcripts in patients in long-term remission of. APL *Leuk* 1998;12(9):1349–54.
65. Voso MT, Ottone T, Lavorgna S, et al. MRD in AML: the role of new techniques. Front Oncol 2019;9:655.
66. Steensma DP, Bejar R, Jaiswal S, et al. Clonal hematopoiesis of indeterminate potential and its distinction from myelodysplastic syndromes. Blood 2015; 126(1):9–16.
67. Porter CC. Germ line mutations associated with leukemias. Hematol Am Soc Hematol Educ Program 2016;2016(1):302–8.
68. Mencia-Trinchant N, Hu Y, Alas MA, et al. Minimal residual disease monitoring of acute myeloid leukemia by massively multiplex digital PCR in patients with NPM1 mutations. J Mol Diagn 2017;19(4):537–48.
69. Hiatt JB, Pritchard CC, Salipante SJ, et al. Single molecule molecular inversion probes for targeted, high-accuracy detection of low-frequency variation. Genome Res 2013;23(5):843–54.
70. Waalkes A, Penewit K, Wood BL, et al. Ultrasensitive detection of acute myeloid leukemia minimal residual disease using single molecule molecular inversion probes. Haematologica 2017;102(9):1549–57.
71. Buldini B, Rizzati F, Masetti R, et al. Prognostic significance of flow-cytometry evaluation of minimal residual disease in children with acute myeloid leukaemia treated according to the AIEOP-AML 2002/01 study protocol. Br J Haematol 2017;177(1):116–26.
72. Paiva B, Vidriales MB, Sempere A, et al. Impact of measurable residual disease by decentralized flow cytometry: a PETHEMA real-world study in 1076 patients with acute myeloid leukemia. Leukemia 2021. https://doi.org/10.1038/s41375-021-01126-3.
73. Zhang L, Cao Z, Ruan M, et al. Monitoring the AML1/ETO fusion transcript to predict outcome in childhood acute myeloid leukemia. Pediatr Blood Cancer 2014; 61(10):1761–6.
74. Pigazzi M, Manara E, Buldini B, et al. Minimal residual disease monitored after induction therapy by RQ-PCR can contribute to tailor treatment of patients with t(8;21) RUNX1-RUNX1T1 rearrangement. Haematologica 2015;100(3):e99–101.
75. Kronke J, Schlenk RF, Jensen KO, et al. Monitoring of minimal residual disease in NPM1-mutated acute myeloid leukemia: a study from the German-Austrian acute myeloid leukemia study group. J Clin Oncol 2011;29(19):2709–16.
76. Ommen HB, Schnittger S, Jovanovic JV, et al. Strikingly different molecular relapse kinetics in NPM1c, PML-RARA, RUNX1-RUNX1T1, and CBFB-MYH11 acute myeloid leukemias. Blood 2010;115(2):198–205.
77. Rucker FG, Agrawal M, Corbacioglu A, et al. Measurable residual disease monitoring in acute myeloid leukemia with t(8;21)(q22;q22.1): results from the AML Study Group. Blood 2019;134(19):1608–18.
78. Juul-Dam KL, Ommen HB, Nyvold CG, et al. Measurable residual disease assessment by qPCR in peripheral blood is an informative tool for disease surveillance in childhood acute myeloid leukaemia. Br J Haematol 2020;190(2): 198–208.
79. Ommen HB, Nyvold CG, Braendstrup K, et al. Relapse prediction in acute myeloid leukaemia patients in complete remission using WT1 as a molecular marker: development of a mathematical model to predict time from molecular to clinical relapse and define optimal sampling intervals. Br J Haematol 2008; 141(6):782–91.

80. Juul-Dam KL, Nyvold CG, Valerhaugen H, et al. Measurable residual disease monitoring using Wilms tumor gene 1 expression in childhood acute myeloid leukemia based on child-specific reference values. Pediatr Blood Cancer 2019; 66(6):e27671.
81. Hokland P, Ommen HB, Mule MP, et al. Advancing the minimal residual disease concept in acute myeloid leukemia. Semin Hematol 2015;52(3):184–92.
82. Hourigan CS, Karp JE. Minimal residual disease in acute myeloid leukaemia. Nat Rev Clin Oncol 2013;10(8):460–71.
83. Walter RB, Buckley SA, Pagel JM, et al. Significance of minimal residual disease before myeloablative allogeneic hematopoietic cell transplantation for AML in first and second complete remission. Blood 2013;122(10):1813–21.
84. Creutzig U, Reinhardt D, Diekamp S, et al. AML patients with Down syndrome have a high cure rate with AML-BFM therapy with reduced dose intensity. Leukemia 2005;19(8):1355–60.
85. Kudo K, Kojima S, Tabuchi K, et al. Prospective study of a pirarubicin, intermediate-dose cytarabine, and etoposide regimen in children with Down syndrome and acute myeloid leukemia: the Japanese Childhood AML Cooperative Study Group. J Clin Oncol 2007;25(34):5442–7.
86. Taga T, Saito AM, Kudo K, et al. Clinical characteristics and outcome of refractory/relapsed myeloid leukemia in children with Down syndrome. Blood 2012; 120(9):1810–5.
87. Taub JW, Berman JN, Hitzler JK, et al. Improved outcomes for myeloid leukemia of Down syndrome: a report from the Children's Oncology Group AAML0431 trial. Blood 2017;129(25):3304–13.
88. Estey E, Othus M, Lee SJ, et al. New drug approvals in acute myeloid leukemia: what's the best end point? Leukemia 2016;30(3):521–5.
89. Prebet T, Bertoli S, Delaunay J, et al. Anthracycline dose intensification improves molecular response and outcome of patients treated for core binding factor acute myeloid leukemia. Haematologica 2014;99(10):e185–7.
90. Lambert J, Lambert J, Nibourel O, et al. MRD assessed by WT1 and NPM1 transcript levels identifies distinct outcomes in AML patients and is influenced by gemtuzumab ozogamicin. Oncotarget 2014;5(15):6280–8.

Laboratory Aspects of Minimal / Measurable Residual Disease Testing in B-Lymphoblastic Leukemia

John Kim Choi, MD, PhD[a,*], Paul E. Mead, PhD, SCYM(ASCP)[b]

KEYWORDS

- Minimal residual disease • MRD • B lymphoblastic leukemia • B-ALL
- Leukemia-associated immunophenotype • LAIP

KEY POINTS

- Minimal residual disease detection provides critical prognostic predictor of treatment outcome and is the standard of care for B lymphoblastic leukemia.
- Flow cytometry–based minimal residual disease detection is the most common test modality and has high sensitivity (0.01%) and rapid turnaround time (24 hours).
- Flow cytometry–based minimal residual disease detection is complicated by variabilities on the antigens examined, combination of antibodies, criteria for the blast numerator, criteria for the cells that defines the denominator, and the approach to flow cytometry data analysis.
- Despite these differences, the final minimal residual disease values show similar clinical outcomes.
- Leukemia-associated immunophenotype analysis is simplified by guide gates that define normal B-cell populations and is more accurate using back-gating to include all B-lymphoblastic leukemia cells and exclude contaminating events.

INTRODUCTION

Detection of minimal residual disease (MRD) is a critical prognostic predictor and has become the standard of care[1] for B-lymphoblastic leukemia (B-ALL) in response to up front chemotherapy and success in bone marrow (BM) transplantation for relapsed and high-risk ALL.[2–6] First shown in the pediatric population, similar usefulness has been shown for the adult population.[7–9] Over time and with the introduction of even

[a] Division of Laboratory Medicine, The University of Alabama at Birmingham, WP P230N, 619 19th Street South, Birmingham, AL 35249-7331, USA; [b] Department of Pathology, St. Jude Children's Research Hospital, 262 Danny Thomas Place, D4026G, Mailstop 342, Memphis, TN 38105, USA
* Corresponding author.
E-mail address: johnchoi@uabmc.edu

Clin Lab Med 41 (2021) 485–495
https://doi.org/10.1016/j.cll.2021.03.013

more sensitive assays, the threshold for minimal is changing and MRD is being redefined as measurable residual disease.

MRD is often defined as disease below the level of reliable detection by morphology or 5% blasts of the total marrow cellularity.[10] Flow cytometry studies have shown that this 5% value is not very sensitive and values as low at 0.01% residual disease during treatment are predictive of relapse.[2–5] In addition, high percentages (>5%) of normal precursor B cells or lymphoblasts can be seen in normal or regenerating marrow without residual leukemia,[11–13] and can complicate disease status determination when using morphology alone or even standard immunophenotyping by flow cytometry. Currently, there is no consensus for the exact MRD percentage for relapse after patient achieve negative MRD. Some institutions use 1% to define relapse, but others such as St. Jude Children's Research Hospital (SJCRH) still use 5%.

CLINICAL MINIMAL RESIDUAL DISEASE TESTING

Currently, flow cytometry is the most common test modality for MRD with a reliable sensitivity of 0.01% and this percentage is used as the threshold for MRD positivity in most clinical treatment strategies. Other modalities with equal to or greater sensitivity include allelic specific quantitative polymerase chain reaction (PCR), using a primer specific for patient leukemic T-cell receptor or B-cell receptor (IgH or IgL) rearrangement[14] or quantitative reverse transcriptase PCR for fusion transcripts in some leukemia with recurrent chromosomal rearrangement,[15,16] both with a sensitivity of 0.001%. More recent approaches have even higher level of sensitivity of 0.0001%. These approaches include next-generation sequencing (NGS) using linear PCR amplification of T-cell receptor or B-cell receptor rearrangements followed by sequencing and comparing the products to the signature leukemic sequences identified at diagnosis.[17] This approach has a sensitivity of 1 cell in 1 million or 0.0001% and, in certain circumstances, residual disease at even less than 0.01% is predictive of outcome.[18,19] Digital droplet PCR, the latest version of quantitative PCR, is being evaluated in small studies with similar sensitivity to NGS.[20,21]

Two studies have examined the clinical significance of MRD detected by flow cytometry compared with allelic-specific quantitative PCR[22] or with NGS.[19] PCR, as expected with its better sensitivity, can detect residual disease in some of the flow MRD negative cases, but missed some detected by flow, possibly because of clonal evolution and sequence drift. NGS using 0.01% positivity cutoff detected all flow positive cases and identified additional cases that were negative by flow. Outcomes for these 2 studies were similar, relapse occurred most frequently when MRD is positive with both test modalities and least frequently when negative for both tests. In patients where the MRD was positive on only 1 testing platform (either flow- or nucleic acid-based MRD methodologies) an intermediate level of relapse (event-free survival) was observed compared with high- or standard-risk patients.

The remainder of this article focuses on the flow cytometry–based MRD detection for B-ALL that is used by many institutions. This modality is the most common method and has advantages of rapid turnaround time (MRD results reported usually within one working day compared with 7–10 days for the other modalities) and its availability in most clinical laboratories. There is no consensus on the timing, preparation, acquisition, and analysis of flow cytometry. Despite all the variability in flow-based assays, MRD findings in multiple published large studies are equivalent with similar levels of sensitivity and correlation to outcome.[2,5,23–25]

Timing for Flow Cytometry Analysis

Flow-based MRD assays are done on peripheral blood or BM aspirate, typically anticoagulated with EDTA or heparin and assayed within 24 hours; but can be assayed as late 72 hours if heparin is used as an anticoagulant. The Children's Oncology Group (COG) typically performed MRD analysis on day 8 peripheral blood and 29 BM of chemotherapy,[2] time points with fewer complicating normal precursor B cells. In contrast, MRD studies for the EuroFlow consortium are done at days 15, 33, and 78,[26,27] whereas for SJCRH, MRD studies are done on day 8 peripheral blood and at every BM aspiration (ie, days 15, 21/22 [if MRD >0.1% at day 15], 43, 49, 119, 296, and 840).[5] MRD at both early and later time points are prognostic indicators.[2,5,28]

Preparation and Acquisition of Sample

Currently, COG, EuroFlow, and SJCRH use a lyse approach to remove the non-nucleated red blood cells, but before 2019 SJCRH used Ficoll gradient to remove the red blood cells. Multiple tubes, each containing 0.5 to 4.0 million cells each are stained with 6 to 10 different antibodies to eventually quantify the residual leukemic cells of interest. A wide variety of different antibodies in different combinations are used by different institutions (see **Table 1** for examples) to distinguish the leukemic cells. In addition to the tubes containing fluorescent molecule conjugated antibodies, COG and SJCRH also have another tube with a nuclear stain (Syto 16 or 13, respectively) to help define the denominator (all nucleated cells). In contrast, EuroFlow and French Consortium use only FSC/SSC exclusion to exclude debris and assume that lysis, or Ficoll separation, has removed all non-nucleated red blood cells.

After staining, a total of 0.5 to 1.0 million, 4.0 million, and all stained cells are acquired on the flow cytometry machine by COG, EuroFlow, and SJCRH, respectively. The large number of total events are collected to reach the sensitivity of 0.01% MRD, a value calculated by the total number of leukemic cells divided by the total number of nucleated cells. The derivation of both the numerator and the denominator varies by institution. In general, the leukemic population is considered real if the population is tightly clustered (a subjective criterion) and is composed of 10 or more events, but other institutions require greater numbers.[29,30] With 10 required leukemic

Table 1
Antibodies and analysis approaches used by different groups

Group[ref]	COG[11]	EuroFlow[26]	French[25]	SJCRH[28]
Antibodies used: In all tubes	*CD45, CD19, CD10,* CD9, CD13/CD33, CD20, CD34, CD38, CD58	*CD45, CD19, CD10, CD20, CD34, CD38, CD81,* CD66c/CD123, CD73/CD304	*CD45, CD19, CD10,* CD2, CD13, CD15, CD20, CD21, CD22, CD24, CD33, CD34, CD38, CD117, CD123	*CD45, CD19, CD10, CD34, CD22,* CD13, CD15, CD20, CD24, CD33, CD38, CD44, CD58, CD66c, CD72, CD73, CD86, CD123, CD133, CD200, NG2 (7.1)
Analysis approach	Different from normal	Different from normal	LAIP	LAIP
Reported MRD % of what cells (denominator)	Mononuclear cells	Total cells	Total cells	Nucleated mononuclear cells

Abbreviation: LAIP, leukemia-associated immunophenotype.

events, a total of 100,000 single, viable, nucleated cell events are needed to reach 0.01% sensitivity; if 50 leukemic events are required to form a positive cluster, then 500,000 gated events are required to reach the 0.01% threshold. The denominator number also varies by institution. EuroFlow uses all nucleated cells (SSC/FSC exclusion of debris) as the denominator, whereas COG and SJCRH use nucleated mononuclear cells (using nucleic acid-binding [Syto] dyes and high SSC exclusion) as the denominator because their initial assays were developed using Ficolled specimens. Upon transition to a bulk-lysis approach, COG uses a digital gate to exclude all the granulocytes to get the mononuclear cell number. SJCRH also uses a digital gate but removes only the granulocytes that have higher SSC than monocytes because this number empirically correlates with the Ficolled sample. An obvious implication is that the EuroFlow denominator better correlates with the denominator used in NGS studies compared with that used by COG and SJCRH.

Analysis Approaches (Different from Normal versus the Leukemia-Associated Immunophenotype)

How the leukemic cells are determined also differs between the groups. Both COG and EuroFlow use a different from normal approach. With experience, leukemic cells (if sufficient in number and tightly clustered) differ from normal precursor B cells maturation pattern by their shape and location on scatter plots (**Fig. 1**). This approach results in variabilities in interlaboratory results.[31] The implementation of a quality assurance program has improved the concordance probably secondary to some guidelines and possibly secondary to decreased number of laboratories performing flow-based MRD.[32,33] Among experts, the concordance of the results is much better. EuroFlow reports 98% concordance in flow-based MRD analysis among 4 centers indicating low, but not absent, variability among experts and 98% concordance with NGS studies.[26] The exact methodology for the different from normal approach is beyond the scope of this article, and its introduction can be found in recent reviews.[30,34]

The other analysis approach, the leukemia-associated immunophenotype, used by St. Jude Children's Research Hospital and the French consortium will be detailed

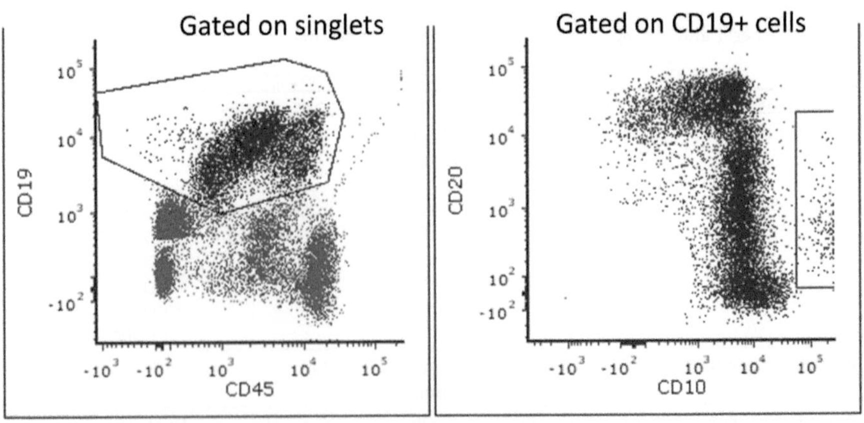

Fig. 1. Normal maturing BM B cells, hematogones (in *blue*), show typical maturation pattern for CD19, CD45, C20, and CD10. Minimal/measurable residual B lymphoblastic leukemia (in *red*) shows aberrant decreased expression of CD45 and increased expression of CD10. Both abnormalities are lost later in treatment.

because of its familiarity to the authors and its easy teachability to others. In the leukemia-associated immunophenotype approach, the leukemic cells are analyzed at diagnosis and a fingerprint of abnormal antigen expression is identified and used to follow the leukemic cells during treatment. In actuality, the leukemia-associated immunophenotype approach is similar to the DNF approach except only the initial abnormality is used as a leukemic marker rather than any abnormality.

SJCRH uses guide gates as an aide for the inexperienced user to distinguish leukemic cells from normal regenerating B-lymphoblasts. Normal regenerating BM (20–25 cases) were used to define the normal pattern of expression for every combination of antibodies used in the B-ALL MRD diagnostic screening panel. A gate was drawn around the normal expression patterns that defines the limits of normal regenerating precursor B cells (frequently referred to as hematogones). Similar normal guide gates have been described by others.[35] Diagnostic marrow is queried with the full panel of potential B-ALL MRD markers, and the best 4 to 6 markers are included for follow-up studies; a Boolean gating scheme is used to define the leukemic population at diagnosis (**Fig. 2**). Although some antigen expressions change during treatment as COG has shown,[36] we find that most abnormal markers remain abnormal. We also find that CD45, CD19, CD10, and CD34 expression are frequently altered in the leukemic cell population, and thus we used these markers as a backbone in each tube of the patient-specific panel and used mainly to identify B cells and their stage of differentiation. The best 4 to 6 antibodies identified at diagnosis, which distinguish leukemic from normal blasts, are used to fill the remaining slots in the follow-up tubes, and this patient-specific panel is run for all subsequent MRD time points. The initial analysis scheme at diagnosis can be modified during treatment to reflect changes in the

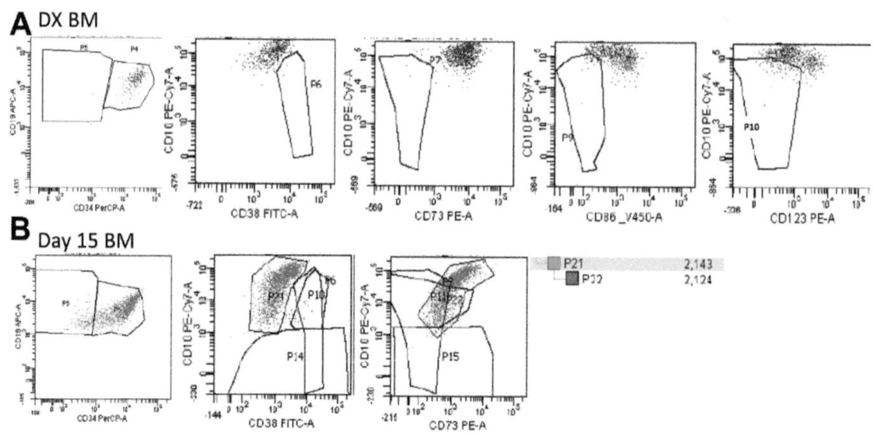

Fig. 2. (*A*) Leukemia-associated immunophenotype (LAIP) is identified at diagnosis. Initial leukemic cells were CD34+, CD10++, and had 4 antigens of varying abnormalities. Gates P4: CD34+CD19+ cells, P5: CD34-CD19+, P6, P7, P9, and P10 represent the boundaries in which hematogones reside for the antigens CD38, CD73, CD86, and CD123, respectively. (*B*) MRD analysis of BM after 15 days of induction shows that the leukemic cells now have variable CD34 and CD10 expression. CD38 decreased further to become a better LAIP marker, whereas CD73 decreased to become a marginal marker. Normal gates for CD34+ and CD34– are superimposed to allow combined analysis of the B-ALL cells and gates P10, 14, P11, P15 represents normal boundaries for the CD34–CD19+ cells. P21 and P22 represent the leukemic cells and Boolean analysis is performed to quantify B-ALL with both abnormalities.

leukemic phenotype in response to treatment. Back-gating is performed on the final leukemic population and is a crucial step to further refine the leukemic gates to include all leukemic blasts and exclude potential noise (**Fig. 3**).

Our approach has the advantage of being simple for new users to learn. Analysis, particularly of regenerating BM at later time points in therapy, can be complicated by the presence of a background of normal precursor B cells (see **Fig. 1**; **Fig. 4**). Our approach is also useful when only 1 population of precursor B cells is observed and the differential includes left-shifted hematogones or leukemic cells (see **Fig. 4**). A disadvantage is that the antibody and instrument setting have to be rigorously controlled to maintain the same level of mean fluorescent intensity on control cells, and ultimately on the leukemic cells; otherwise the guide gates for the normal regenerating B-cell precursors will not be applicable across samples at different time points. This process necessitates retitrating new lots of antibody to give the same mean fluorescent intensity as the previous lot. Another disadvantage is that the normal guide gates are specific to an individual laboratory, must be tediously and manually drawn, and must be determined for any new markers introduced into the diagnostic screening panel. The final disadvantage is that intracellular markers cannot be used as mean fluorescent intensity reproducibility cannot be maintained, at least in our hands.

Minimum Residual Disease of CD19 Negative B-Lymphoblastic Leukemia

B-ALLs are typically distinguished by expression of CD19 and analysis will eventually gate on the CD19-positive population. However, rare B-ALLs have dim to negative CD19 expression. CD19-negative B-ALL is also becoming more frequent with the introduction of anti-CD19 therapy (blinatumomab and CART-19) for high-risk B-ALL. Hence, the analysis must take into account this possibility by either introduction of CD22 as another B-cell marker or use other gating approaches to identify CD19-negative B cells.[37] This process will only get more complicated with the advent of combined anti-CD19 and anti-CD22 therapy, leading to B-ALL that is negative for both markers (**Fig. 5**). In such cases, SJCRH defines CD19–, intracellular CD79a+ as the leukemic population, with trepidation.

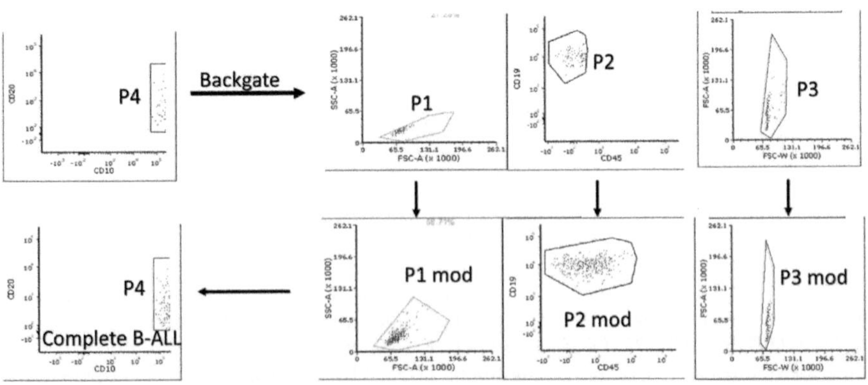

Fig. 3. Back-gate of the initial analysis for B-ALL (P4: CD19+, CD10 bright, CD45 negative). The population in the final leukemic gate is back-gated to all the previous gates. These gates are then modified to include all B-ALL and exclude contaminating cells. In this case, the final population (P4) is back-gated on all the previous gates (P1–3). P1–2 show evidence of exclusion of some B-ALL, whereas P3 shows inclusion of contaminating doublets. P1–3 are modified to include all B-ALL and exclude debris and the new P4 represent all the B-ALL events.

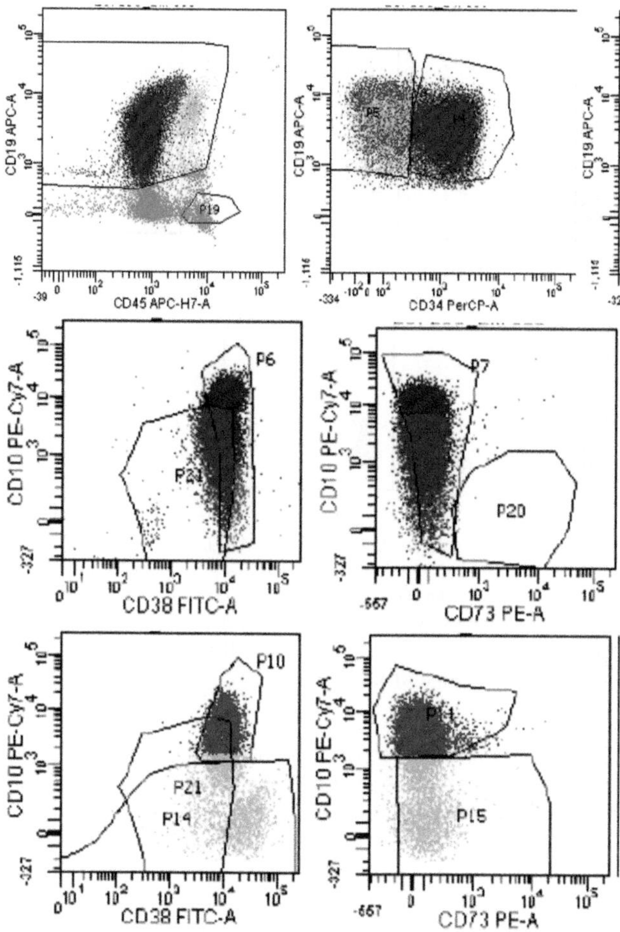

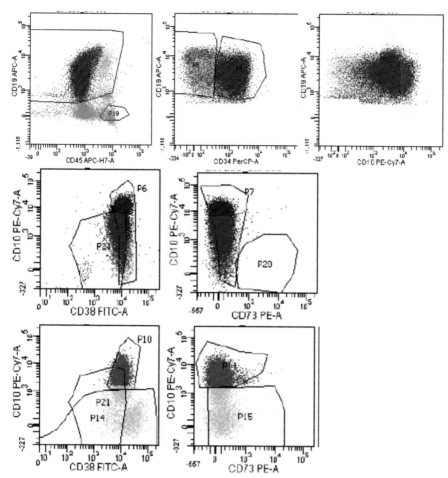

Fig. 4. Left shifted hematogones: Patient with a history of B-ALL, day 43 of treatment. BM with 11% blasts. Analysis shows left shifted hematogones (many at CD34+ and/or CD10+ stage) that lack the aberrant decreased CD38 (P21) or increased CD73 (P20) expression of the B-ALL seen at diagnosis. P6 and 7 represent normal CD34+ B cells. P10, 14, 11, and 15 represent normal CD34- B cells.

Future Advances

More recently, artificial intelligence clustering programs such as tSNE and SPADE have been used to cluster flow data to define and discover normal hematopoietic populations.[38–40] Various laboratories are exploring the possibility of applying these programs to MRD analysis (ie, computer-assisted distinction of leukemic population from normal hematopoietic cells) with promising results.[26,41] These clustering programs are being packaged with current clinical flow cytometry programs, promising that future MRD analysis will become easier and more reproducible.

The current clinical flow cytometry machines are typically limited to 8 to 10 colors. Research-grade flow cytometry can achieve higher numbers,[42] but are impractical in clinical laboratory, mainly owing to technical and regulatory issues. Newer spectral-based flow cytometry instrumentation offers a lot of advantages with many more

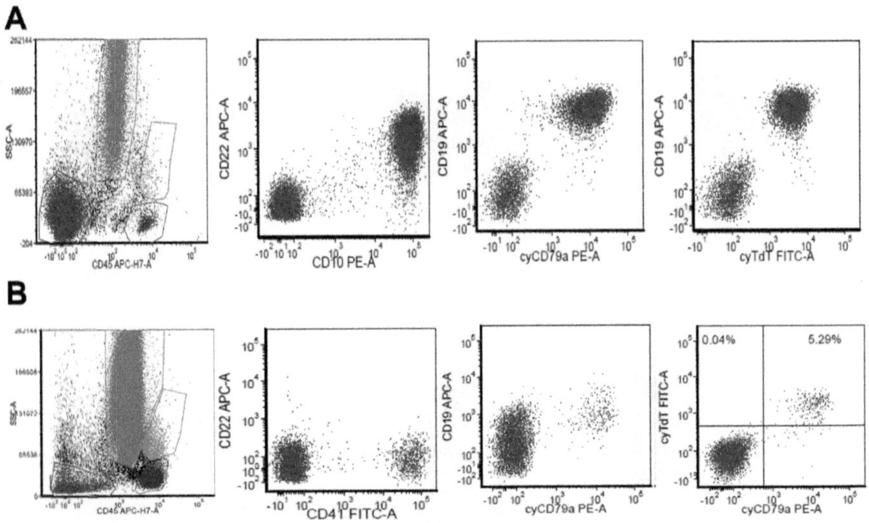

Fig. 5. B-ALL with multiple relapses treated with anti-CD19 and anti-CD22 therapy. (*A*) Initial presentation: B-ALL that is CD45–, CD19+, CD22+, CD10+, CD79a+, and TdT+. (*B*) After anti-CD19 and CD22 therapy. Flow-based MRD is negative, but NGS shows recurrent B-ALL. Peripheral blood immunophenotyping shows abnormal lymphoblasts that are. CD45–, CD19–, CD22–, CD10– (not shown), CD79a+, and TdT+ that was missed on the flow based MRD analysis that gated on CD19+ or CD22+ cells.

colors (>36 markers in a single tube) without need for manual compensation.[43–45] This technology holds promise of a high-parameter single tube analysis, an important benefit when starting with a low cellularity BM sample.

CLINICS CARE POINTS

- Flow based MRD must distinguish residual B lymphoblastic leukemia from normal hematogones.
- In DFN (different from normal) and LAIP (leuekmia associated immunophenotype), the pathologist must have an accurate understanding (often based on years of experience) of normal hematogone flow patterns.
- Analysis can become more objective, and quickly learned by establishing laboratory specific guide gates for normal hematogones.
- Systematic backgating during analysis decreases under and over-estimating MRD.

DISCLOSURE

The authors have no commercial or financial conflicts of interest. This has been funded in part by ALSAC at SJCRH.

REFERENCES

1. Athale UH, Gibson PJ, Bradley NM, et al. Minimal residual disease and childhood leukemia: standard of care recommendations from the Pediatric Oncology Group of Ontario MRD Working Group. Pediatr Blood Cancer 2016;63(6):973–82.

2. Borowitz MJ, Devidas M, Hunger SP, et al. Clinical significance of minimal residual disease in childhood acute lymphoblastic leukemia and its relationship to other prognostic factors: a Children's Oncology Group study. Blood 2008; 111(12):5477–85.
3. Conter V, Bartram CR, Valsecchi MG, et al. Molecular response to treatment redefines all prognostic factors in children and adolescents with B-cell precursor acute lymphoblastic leukemia: results in 3184 patients of the AIEOP-BFM ALL 2000 study. Blood 2010;115(16):3206–14.
4. Vora A, Goulden N, Wade R, et al. Treatment reduction for children and young adults with low-risk acute lymphoblastic leukaemia defined by minimal residual disease (UKALL 2003): a randomised controlled trial. Lancet Oncol 2013;14(3): 199–209.
5. Stow P, Key L, Chen X, et al. Clinical significance of low levels of minimal residual disease at the end of remission induction therapy in childhood acute lymphoblastic leukemia. Blood 2010;115(23):4657–63.
6. Leung W, Pui CH, Coustan-Smith E, et al. Detectable minimal residual disease before hematopoietic cell transplantation is prognostic but does not preclude cure for children with very-high-risk leukemia. Blood 2012;120(2):468–72.
7. Akabane H, Logan A. Clinical significance and management of MRD in adults with acute lymphoblastic leukemia. Clin Adv Hematol Oncol 2020;18(7):413–22.
8. Bruggemann M, Kotrova M. Minimal residual disease in adult ALL: technical aspects and implications for correct clinical interpretation. Blood Adv 2017;1(25): 2456–66.
9. Cassaday RD, Stevenson PA, Wood BL, et al. Description and prognostic significance of the kinetics of minimal residual disease status in adults with acute lymphoblastic leukemia treated with HyperCVAD. Am J Hematol 2018;93(4): 546–52.
10. O'Connor D, Moorman AV, Wade R, et al. Use of minimal residual disease assessment to redefine induction failure in pediatric acute lymphoblastic leukemia. J Clin Oncol 2017;35(6):660–7.
11. Gupta S, Devidas M, Loh ML, et al. Flow-cytometric vs. -morphologic assessment of remission in childhood acute lymphoblastic leukemia: a report from the Children's Oncology Group (COG). Leukemia 2018;32(6):1370–9.
12. Lucio P, Parreira A, van den Beemd MW, et al. Flow cytometric analysis of normal B cell differentiation: a frame of reference for the detection of minimal residual disease in precursor-B-ALL. Leukemia 1999;13(3):419–27.
13. Shalabi H, Yuan CM, Kulshreshtha A, et al. Disease detection methodologies in relapsed B-cell acute lymphoblastic leukemia: opportunities for improvement. Pediatr Blood Cancer 2020;67(4):e28149.
14. Flohr T, Schrauder A, Cazzaniga G, et al. Minimal residual disease-directed risk stratification using real-time quantitative PCR analysis of immunoglobulin and T-cell receptor gene rearrangements in the international multicenter trial AIEOP-BFM ALL 2000 for childhood acute lymphoblastic leukemia. Leukemia 2008; 22(4):771–82.
15. Campana D. Determination of minimal residual disease in leukaemia patients. Br J Haematol 2003;121(6):823–38.
16. Gabert J, Beillard E, van der Velden VH, et al. Standardization and quality control studies of 'real-time' quantitative reverse transcriptase polymerase chain reaction of fusion gene transcripts for residual disease detection in leukemia - a Europe against Cancer program. Leukemia 2003;17(12):2318–57.

17. Faham M, Zheng J, Moorhead M, et al. Deep-sequencing approach for minimal residual disease detection in acute lymphoblastic leukemia. Blood 2012;120(26): 5173–80.
18. Pulsipher MA, Carlson C, Langholz B, et al. IgH-V(D)J NGS-MRD measurement pre- and early post-allotransplant defines very low- and very high-risk ALL patients. Blood 2015;125(22):3501–8.
19. Wood B, Wu D, Crossley B, et al. Measurable residual disease detection by high-throughput sequencing improves risk stratification for pediatric B-ALL. Blood 2018;131(12):1350–9.
20. Della Starza I, De Novi LA, Santoro A, et al. Digital droplet PCR and next-generation sequencing refine minimal residual disease monitoring in acute lymphoblastic leukemia. Leuk Lymphoma 2019;60(11):2838–40.
21. Della Starza I, Chiaretti S, De Propris MS, et al. Minimal residual disease in acute lymphoblastic leukemia: technical and clinical advances. Front Oncol 2019; 9:726.
22. Gaipa G, Cazzaniga G, Valsecchi MG, et al. Time point-dependent concordance of flow cytometry and real-time quantitative polymerase chain reaction for minimal residual disease detection in childhood acute lymphoblastic leukemia. Haematologica 2012;97(10):1582–93.
23. Tembhare PR, Subramanian PG, Ghogale S, et al. A high-sensitivity 10-color flow cytometric minimal residual disease assay in B-lymphoblastic leukemia/lymphoma can easily achieve the sensitivity of 2-in-10(6) and is superior to standard minimal residual disease assay: a study of 622 patients. Cytometry B Clin Cytom 2020;98(1):57–67.
24. Theunissen PMJ, Sedek L, De Haas V, et al. Detailed immunophenotyping of B-cell precursors in regenerating bone marrow of acute lymphoblastic leukaemia patients: implications for minimal residual disease detection. Br J Haematol 2017; 178(2):257–66.
25. Fossat C, Roussel M, Arnoux I, et al. Methodological aspects of minimal residual disease assessment by flow cytometry in acute lymphoblastic leukemia: a French multicenter study. Cytometry B Clin Cytom 2015;88(1):21–9.
26. Theunissen P, Mejstrikova E, Sedek L, et al. Standardized flow cytometry for highly sensitive MRD measurements in B-cell acute lymphoblastic leukemia. Blood 2017;129(3):347–57.
27. Schumich A, Maurer-Granofszky M, Attarbaschi A, et al. Flow-cytometric minimal residual disease monitoring in blood predicts relapse risk in pediatric B-cell precursor acute lymphoblastic leukemia in trial AIEOP-BFM-ALL 2000. Pediatr Blood Cancer 2019;66(5):e27590.
28. Pui CH, Pei D, Raimondi SC, et al. Clinical impact of minimal residual disease in children with different subtypes of acute lymphoblastic leukemia treated with Response-Adapted therapy. Leukemia 2017;31(2):333–9.
29. Chen X, Wood BL. Monitoring minimal residual disease in acute leukemia: technical challenges and interpretive complexities. Blood Rev 2017;31(2):63–75.
30. Shaver AC, Seegmiller AC. B lymphoblastic leukemia minimal residual disease assessment by flow cytometric analysis. Clin Lab Med 2017;37(4):771–85.
31. Keeney M, Halley JG, Rhoads DD, et al. Marked variability in reported minimal residual disease lower level of detection of 4 hematolymphoid neoplasms: a survey of participants in the College of American Pathologists Flow Cytometry Proficiency Testing Program. Arch Pathol Lab Med 2015;139(10):1276–80.

32. Keeney M, Wood BL, Hedley BD, et al. A QA program for MRD testing demonstrates that systematic education can reduce discordance among experienced interpreters. Cytometry B Clin Cytom 2018;94(2):239–49.
33. Hupp MM, Bashleben C, Cardinali JL, et al. Participation in the College of American Pathologists Laboratory accreditation program decreases variability in B-lymphoblastic leukemia and plasma cell myeloma flow cytometric minimal residual disease testing: a follow-up survey. Arch Pathol Lab Med 2021;145(3):336–42.
34. Kroft SH, Harrington AM. Flow cytometry of B-Cell neoplasms. Clin Lab Med 2017;37(4):697–723.
35. Jain S, Mehta A, Kapoor G, et al. Evaluating new markers for minimal residual disease analysis by flow cytometry in precursor B lymphoblastic leukemia. Indian J Hematol Blood Transfus 2018;34(1):48–53.
36. Borowitz MJ, Pullen DJ, Winick N, et al. Comparison of diagnostic and relapse flow cytometry phenotypes in childhood acute lymphoblastic leukemia: implications for residual disease detection: a report from the children's oncology group. Cytometry B Clin Cytom 2005;68(1):18–24.
37. Cherian S, Miller V, McCullouch V, et al. A novel flow cytometric assay for detection of residual disease in patients with B-lymphoblastic leukemia/lymphoma post anti-CD19 therapy. Cytometry B Clin Cytom 2018;94(1):112–20.
38. Belkina AC, Ciccolella CO, Anno R, et al. Automated optimized parameters for T-distributed stochastic neighbor embedding improve visualization and analysis of large datasets. Nat Commun 2019;10(1):5415.
39. Mair F, Hartmann FJ, Mrdjen D, et al. The end of gating? An introduction to automated analysis of high dimensional cytometry data. Eur J Immunol 2016;46(1):34–43.
40. Lucchesi S, Nolfi E, Pettini E, et al. Computational analysis of multiparametric flow cytometric data to dissect B cell subsets in vaccine studies. Cytometry A 2020;97(3):259–67.
41. DiGiuseppe JA, Tadmor MD, Pe'er D. Detection of minimal residual disease in B lymphoblastic leukemia using viSNE. Cytometry B Clin Cytom 2015;88(5):294–304.
42. Perfetto SP, Chattopadhyay PK, Roederer M. Seventeen-colour flow cytometry: unravelling the immune system. Nat Rev Immunol 2004;4(8):648–55.
43. Robinson JP. Spectral flow cytometry-Quo vadimus? Cytometry A 2019;95(8):823–4.
44. Park LM, Lannigan J, Jaimes MC. OMIP-069: forty-color full spectrum flow cytometry panel for deep immunophenotyping of major cell subsets in human peripheral blood. Cytometry A 2020;97(10):1044–51.
45. Latis E, Michonneau D, Leloup C, et al. Cellular and molecular profiling of T-cell subsets at the onset of human acute GVHD. Blood Adv 2020;4(16):3927–42.

Molecular Genetics of Pediatric Acute Myeloid Leukemia

Bryan Krock, PhD, Matthew J. Oberley, MD, PhD*

KEYWORDS

- Acute myeloid leukemia • Pediatric oncology • Molecular genetics • Rearrangement
- Next-generation sequencing

KEY POINTS

- Pediatric acute myeloid leukemia (AML) has drivers that are unique to both infants and children as well as drivers found in common with adult AML.
- Genetic profiling of pediatric acute myeloid leukemia can identify drivers that are diagnostic, prognostic, or predictive in a large majority of patients.
- Profiling of pediatric megakaryoblastic leukemia identifies genetic alterations associated with a wide range of patient outcomes.

INTRODUCTION

Acute myeloid leukemia (AML) is a biologically and genetically heterogeneous malignancy that accounts for approximately 20% of pediatric acute leukemias.[1] With the development of optimized therapeutic regimens and allogeneic hematopoietic stem cell transplantation, overall survival rates of pediatric AML have approached 70% but still significantly lower than that of pediatric acute lymphoblastic leukemia (ALL).[2] As with other hematological malignancies, pediatric AML has been evolving from a morphologic classification scheme to a genetically based one, aided by the rapid progression of molecular detection methods, such as next-generation sequencing (NGS).

The World Health Organization (WHO) currently recognizes several types of AML with recurrent genetic abnormalities, the extent of which is certain to grow with the explosion of genomic profiling studies in recent years. Although many of the recurrent genetic drivers of myeloid leukemia are found in common between pediatric and adult patients, the prevalence and clinical significance of these drivers differ depending on the age of the patient.

Caris Life Sciences, 4610 South 44th Place, Phoenix, AZ, USA
* Corresponding author.
E-mail address: moberley@carisls.com

Clin Lab Med 41 (2021) 497–515
https://doi.org/10.1016/j.cll.2021.03.014
labmed.theclinics.com

AML often is defined by the presence of recurrent chromosomal rearrangements that create chimeric fusion genes that promote AML development and progression. These fusions are diagnostic, prognostic, and, in some cases, predictive biomarkers that drive clinical management. These so-called class II alterations often involve transcription factors that serve to block differentiation of hematopoietic progenitor cells, which subsequently acquire cooperating mutations in other pathways, often tyrosine kinase or RAS, which are progrowth pathway mutations (class I mutations).[3]

This review focuses on genetic variants found in AML that are most germane to clinical management of pediatric patients, while acknowledging that variants found more commonly in adults still can be found in pediatric patients.

DISCUSSION

Classes of Genomic Variation in Pediatric Acute Myeloid Leukemia

NGS has enabled the description of all classes of somatic genomic variation in a single tumor. These studies can reveal the underlying mutational processes that manifest as a particular mutational signature and can facilitate the understanding of the natural history of a given tumor. The Children's Oncology Group–National Cancer Institute Therapeutically Applicable Research to Generate Effective Treatments AML initiative has characterized the genomes of approximately 1000 pediatric AML cases using whole-genome, transcriptome, and epigenetic profiling, providing the most extensive characterization of pediatric AML to date.[4] This study and others have begun to reveal both similarities and differences between adult and pediatric AML.

Although adult AML is defined by a low tumor mutational burden, all subtypes of pediatric AML have an even lower rate of somatic mutations, averaging less than 1 somatic mutation per megabase of genomic sequence.[4–6] Tumor mutational burden is lowest in infants and increases with age of onset.[4] Genes affected by somatic mutations are diverse, but there are few recurrent somatic mutations, with only 5 genes harboring mutations in more than 5% of subjects (FLT3, NPM1, WT1, CEBPA, and KIT).[4] This contrasts with somatic variants in adult AML, where alterations TP53, DNMT3, IDH1, and IDH2 are common, although they are rare in children.[4–6] In contrast to somatic sequence variants, pediatric AML exhibits a higher rate of chromosomal rearrangements than observed in adult AML, with rearrangements involving RUNX1, CBFB, and KMT2A alone found in more than 35% of subjects.[7] The prevalence of structural rearrangements is highest in infants and decreases with age of onset[4] (**Table 1**). Although most recurrent rearrangements are observed in both adult and pediatric AML, there are several that appear with much higher prevalence or are even unique to pediatric subjects, discussed later.

As with sequence variants, copy number variation is low across most subtypes of pediatric AML, with approximately a third of cases exhibiting no identifiable copy number losses or gains.[8] Many of the identified copy number variants are the result of focal microdeletions and amplifications that frequently occur near the breakpoints of chromosomal rearrangements and display a similar age-dependent distribution to structural rearrangements.[4,8–10] Recurrent focal codeletions of MBNL1 and ZEB2 and deletions of ELF1 have been reported, although their clinical significance has yet to be demonstrated.[4] Similarly, copy neutral loss of heterozygosity is identified at a much lower rate in pediatric AML than other malignancies and was identified in 13% of AML cases. Copy neutral loss of heterozygosity typically has been observed in genomic regions with known molecular drivers and tumor suppressors, such as FLT3 internal tandem duplications (FLT3-ITDs) and CDKN2A/B.[8] In contrast to most forms of pediatric AML, acute megakaryoblastic leukemia (AMKL) exhibits a higher rate of copy number variants.[8,11]

Table 1
Common structural rearrangements and sequence variants identified in pediatric acute myeloid leukemia patients

Genetic Alteration	Frequency	Subgroup	Prognostic Implication	Cooperating Mutations
KMT2A rearrangements	20%	Infants (60%)	Neutral; partner imparts influence	NRAS, KRAS, FLT3
RUNX1-RUNX1T1	15%	Children	Favorable	KIT, NRAS, KRAS, FLT3, chromatin modifying genes, cohesins
CBFB-MYH11	10%–15%	Children	Favorable	KIT, NRAS, KRAS, FLT3
NUP98 rearrangements	6%–10%	Children	Poor	FLT3-ITD, WT1
PML-RARA	5%–10%	Older children	Favorable	FLT3-ITD, WT1
DEK-NUP214	<2%	Older children	Poor	FLT3-ITD (70%)
ETS rearrangement	1%	Infants	Poor	Few
CEBPA	4%–9%	Older children	Favorable	GATA2, FLT3, CSF3R
NPM1	4%	Older children	Favorable	FLT3-ITD
FLT3	30%	Children, older children	Poor (FLT3 alone is intermediate among FLT3-ITD group)	NPM1, WT1, NUP98-NSD1
FLT3-ITD, NPM1	—	—	Most favorable among FLT3-ITDs	—
FLT3-ITD, WT1	—	—	Poor among FLT3-ITDs	—
FLT3-ITD, NUP98-NSD1	—	—	Poor among FLT3-ITDs	—
RUNX1 Mutation	3% (AML)	Older children, AMKL (10%)	Poor (AML), excellent (AMKL)	JAK, cohesins (AMKL)
CBFA2T3-GLIS2	15%–20% (AMKL)	AMKL	Poor	Few
HOX gene rearrangement	15% (AMKL)	AMKL	Favorable	MPL
RBM15-MKL1	10% (AMKL)	AMKL	Favorable	Few
NUP98-KDM5A	12% (AMKL)	AMKL	Poor	RB1

World Health Organization Recurrent Genetic Abnormalities in Acute Myeloid Leukemia and Common Co-occurring Mutations

KMT2A rearrangement

KMT2A (also known as mixed lineage leukemia [MLL]) is the most commonly rearranged gene in both adult and pediatric leukemias.[12,13] It is most prevalent in pediatric AML, where it is observed with greatest frequency in infancy.[14,15] The KMT2A gene encodes a lysine methyltransferase that mediates methylation of histone 3 lysine 4. KMT2A translocations involve a large number of partner genes and typically involve the N-terminus of KMT2A fused to the C-terminus of its partner gene, with more than 90 reported to date.[13] Despite the large number of partners, KMT2A partners most commonly are part of the AF4/FMR2 family, which function in the superelongation complex, and KMT2A fusions are thought to drive inappropriate expression of KMT2A target genes, notably HOX genes.[12] Despite this complexity, approximately 70% of pediatric AML KMT2A rearrangements are with 4 partners. The KMT2A-MLLT3 (t[9;11] [p21;q23]) fusion is the most common (43%), followed by KMT2A-MLLT10 (t[10;11]p12;q23); 13%), KMT2A-AFDN (t[6;11] [q27;123]; 5%), and KMT2A- MLLT1(t[11;19] [q23;p13]; 8%).[16]

AML with KMT2A-MLLT3 rearrangement is given its own category in the WHO diagnostic classification system because it is the most clinically homogeneous, whereas other rearrangements of KMT2A are diagnosed as AML, not otherwise specified.[17] The KMT2A fusion partner is relevant for prognosis, because KMT2A-MLLT11 (t[1;11] [q21;q23]) has a better prognosis whereas KMT2A-AFDN, KMT2A-ABI (t[10;11] [p11.2;q23] and KMT2A-AFF1 (t[4;11] [q21;q23]) have a poor prognosis.[18]

Consistent with the typical very young age of onset, pediatric patients with KMT2A fusions had fewer somatic mutations than tumors without these fusions.[4] Cooperating somatic mutations, when present, are recurrent in NRAS, KRAS, and FLT3, whereas GATA2 and CEBPA mutations typically are not found. The identification of cooperating mutations in KMT2A-MLLT3 tumors has been associated with a negative prognostic impact, although further study is needed to confirm this association.[19] In addition, deletion of MBNL1 and ZEB2 show frequent co-occurrence.[4]

Given the significant diversity of KMT2A rearrangement partners, their rarity and the heterogeneous outcomes associated with them, it will continue to be a challenge to integrate risk stratification of these uncommon drivers in clinical practice. When KMT2A rearranged AML is examined morphologically and immunophenotypically, they commonly have a monoblastic phenotype.

Nucleoporin 98kD rearranged

Nucleoporin 98kD (NUP98) rearrangements are relatively common in pediatric AML (6%–10%) and much rarer in adult disease (1%–2%).[20–22] They typically involve the fusion of the NUP98 N-terminus to the C-terminus of at least 31 different partner genes, with the t(5;11) (q35;p15) (NSD1) and t(11;15) (p15;q35) (KMT5A) rearrangements preferentially found in pediatric AML.[23] Most NUP98 rearrangements are not detectible by conventional cytogenetics and require an RNA sequencing approach on a practical basis. NUP98 encodes a structural component of the nuclear pore complex, but more recent data indicate that the N-terminus can act as a transcriptional activator through the recruitment of the chromatin modifying complexes.[24–26] NUP98 rearrangements are associated with a poor prognosis and often are identified with FLT3-ITDs and WT1 cooperating mutations.[20,27] NUP98-KDM5A is preferentially identified in pediatric AMKL, found in approximately 10% of pediatric cases, and characteristically have RB1 mutations that decrease protein expression.[11]

The DEK-NUP214 fusion is the result of t(6;9) (p23;q34.1) and is a relatively rare diagnosis in pediatric AML (<2%).[28,29] This rearrangement typically is associated with older age of onset and basophilia, and outcomes are poor, with high rates of relapse and lower rates of remission.[15,29] FLT3 mutations are common in DEK-NUP214 cases, with FLT3-ITD mutations found in up to 70% of pediatric cases, although the presence of FLT3-ITD mutations do not significantly influence outcomes.[29,30]

ETS rearranged

The recurrent t(7;12) (q36;p13) rearrangement is rare in all pediatric AML cases (approximately 1%) but is more common in infants with AML and is associated with poor clinical outcomes.[4,31] This rearrangement juxtaposes the MNX1 gene with ETV6, but there is debate as to the molecular mechanism by which this alteration drives oncogenesis, because the chimeric MNX1-ETV6 transcript not always is detected in tumors with the chromosomal rearrangement and a fusion protein has not been identified. Oncogenesis likely is mediated, at least in part, by MNX1 overexpression, and a recent study showed MNX1 overexpression could impair hematopoietic differentiation.[32] Genomic landscaping studies have reported only a small number of cases, and recurrent cooperating somatic mutation have not been cataloged. Other rare pediatric rearrangements from the ETS family include ERG rearrangements.[4]

Core binding factor rearranged

Core binding factor (CBF) leukemias drivers fusions include RUNX1-RUNX1T1 t(8;21) (q22;q22) and CBFB-MYH11 inv(16) (p13q22), which commonly are found in pediatric AML cases (20%–30%).[4,15,33] The RUNX1 and CBFB genes are transcription factors that heterodimerize to bind DNA and recruit transcription factors that regulate hematopoiesis.[34] The resulting fusion products block myeloid differentiation through transcriptional repression. These fusions are associated with favorable outcomes, with 90% of patients achieving complete remission with chemotherapy and 70% overall survival, although approximately 30% of patients relapse.[15,33,35,36] The incidence of CBF rearrangements peaks in older children, and when controlled for age, have a higher mutational burden than expected for their age.[4] Often considered similar entities, CBFB-MYH11 and RUNX1-RUNX1T1 rearranged leukemias exhibit divergent patterns of cooperating mutations. Although both commonly exhibit mutations in NRAS, KIT, FLT3, and KRAS, RUNX1-RUNX1T1 cases display a dramatic enhancement of mutations in chromatin modifying genes and the cohesion complex compared with CBFB-MY11 cases.[37] The presence of cooperating mutations does not appear to influence outcomes in CBF rearranged AML.

Somatic mutations in the KIT receptor tyrosine kinase are common alterations in pediatric AML, found in approximately 12% of all pediatric AML cases. They are significantly enriched in CBF-rearranged AML, where they are found in up to 36% of cases.[4] Cooperating KIT mutations are associated with poor outcomes in adult CBF AML, but prognostic significance has been less clear in pediatric patients. Recent studies indicate exon 17, but not exon 8 KIT, mutations may impart a poor prognosis.[38–41] CBFB fusion-positive myeloid blasts often show a myelomonocytic phenotype and marrows of affected patient typically have abnormal eosinophils with basophilic granules.

Other key rearrangements

Acute promyelocytic leukemia (APL) represents approximately 5% to 10% of pediatric AML cases and is defined by the PML-RARA fusion, typically through the balanced translocation t(15;17) (q24.1;q21.2).[14] Rare cases, however, exhibit the clinical and morphologic features of APL without t(15;17), and these patients may have a cryptic PML-RARA rearrangement or a rare variant RARA translocations.[42] Importantly, the variants ZBTB16-RARA and STAT5B-RARA exhibit resistance to all-trans retinoic acid.[42] The incidence of this diagnosis is low in infants, increases in childhood, and peaks in adolescents and young adults. Morphologically, both hypergranular and hypogranular variants exist without apparent correlation to the underlying RARA fusion variant.

CBFA2T3-GLIS2. CBFA2T3-GLIS2 rearrangements, typically the result of a cryptic inversion inv(16) (p13.3q24.3), are identified nearly exclusively in pediatric patients less than 3 years of age.[43] They originally were identified in AMKL, where it is found in 20% to 30% of pediatric AMKL and associated with a dismal outcome.[44]

Subsequently, this fusion has been shown to be enriched in AML with normal cytogenetics but also has been detected as a rare rearrangement in AML with other cytogenetic findings; regardless of the morphologic subtype, this fusion has been associated with adverse outcomes.[11,43,45] Few cooperating mutations are identified in CBFA2T3-GLIS2–positive malignancies, and, interestingly, forced expression of this fusion in cord blood stem cells was sufficient to drive malignant transformation.[45] Importantly, conventional cytogenetics often fails to identify this rearrangement, placing patients in a standard risk category, so appropriate molecular methods are essential to identify this important lesion. CBFA2T3-GLIS2 leukemias have a distinct immunophenotype, known as the RAM phenotype, with high expression of CD56 with absent to dim expression of HLA-DR, CD38, and CD45. Recent data suggest this phenotype alone may be sufficient to identify CBFA2T3-GLIS2–positive cases.[45]

RBM15-MKL1. The RBM15-MKL1 fusion caused by t(1;22) (p13.3;q13.1) typically is identified in young children and is the second most common structural rearrangement in neonatal leukemias.[46] This leukemia commonly has a megakaryoblastic phenotype, accounting for 10% of pediatric AMKL, and can present as a myeloid sarcoma that is CD45 and CD34 negative, which can make diagnosis difficult and easy to mistake for a poorly differentiated tumor of another lineage. RBM15-MKL1 is associated with a favorable prognosis among pediatric AMKL cases.[11,46]

KAT6A-CREBBP. The KAT6A-CREBB fusion caused by t(8;16) (p11.2;p13.3) is a rare finding in pediatric AML, occurring in less than 1% of cases. This leukemia generally has a monocytic or myelomonocytic phenotype. It occurs most commonly in infants and is congenital in approximately 25% of cases.[47] This diagnosis generally is associated with poor outcome, although paradoxically, some neonatal patients experience spontaneous remission.[47–50]

Acute Myeloid Leukemia with Normal Cytogenetics

Cytogenetically normal AML is significantly less common in pediatric AML (15%–25%) compared with adult AML (40%–47%) and is associated with an intermediate prognosis.[51,52] Significant heterogeneity has been noted within this group, likely due to the diversity of subtypes represented herein, and prognosis is altered with identification of cryptic rearrangements, such as NUP98-NSD1, NUP98-KDM5A, or specific somatic mutations, such as variants in NPM1, CEBPA, RUNX1, FLT3, and RAS pathway genes. Those without FLT3-ITDs have favorable prognosis. Younger patients with a normal karyotype and no FLT3-ITDs have a prognosis comparable to that of patients with CBF AML.[53]

NPM1 mutations

Somatic mutations in the last exon of the NPM1 gene are found in 2% to 8% of pediatric AML, significantly rarer than adult AML.[54,55] These mutations, often frameshift insertions and deletions at the far C-terminus, result in NPM1 mislocalization through the removal of 1 or 2 nuclear localization sequences and the creation of a nuclear export signal.[56,57] Patients with NPM1 mutations have a favorable prognosis and typically have a normal karyotype.[54] Coexistent FLT3-ITD mutations are frequent, although patients with both mutations exhibit outcomes similar to NPM1 mutation alone.[4,54]

Biallelic CEBPA

Approximately 4% to 9% of children and young adults with AML carry mutations in the single-exon gene CEBPA, of which there are 2 distinct groups of mutations.[58,59] Truncating mutations in the N-terminal region of CEBPA are located between the primary translation start site and a second alternative site, which abrogates expression of the longer p42 isoform while preserving translation of the p30 isoform. This p30 isoform has been shown to act in a dominant negative manner, inhibiting activity of p42.[60–62] The second class of CEBPA mutations typically are in-frame deletions and insertions that disrupt the C-terminal basic leucine zipper (bZIP) region and are thought to impair DNA binding and/or homodimerization.[63] Biallelic CEBPA–mutated AML typically exhibits a combination of a truncating N-terminal mutation with a mutation altering the bZIP region.

Data primarily from adult AML indicate that biallelic mutations are associated with favorable outcomes, and the recent WHO classification of AML creates a distinct provisional category for such occurrences in AML.[64–67] A recent study of pediatric CEBPA-mutated AML found no difference in outcomes between monoallelic and biallelic CEBPA mutations; instead, it was the presence of a bZIP mutation alone that was associated with improved event-free survival and overall survival.[68] Whether this association is unique to pediatric AML or extends to adult AML has yet to be determined, although previous studies indicate that monoallelic and biallelic CEBPA–mutated AML exhibit distinct transcriptional profiles and may be distinct entities.[69,70]

Patients with CEBPA-mutated AML typically have a normal karyotype. Cooperating mutations often are detected in GATA2, FLT3, and CSF3R.[71,72] Although GATA2 mutations did not influence outcomes, biallelic CEBPA–mutated pediatric AML with co-occurring CSF3R mutations exhibited significantly inferior event free survival due to high rates of relapse. Approximately 10% of individuals with biallelic CEBPA mutations carry a germline pathogenic variant in CEPBA that is, associated with a hereditary predisposition to AML.[63,69]

RUNX1

Pediatric AML cases carry somatic mutations in RUNX1 much less frequently (3%) than is observed in adult patients (15%), although there is an increased prevalence of RUNX1 mutations in pediatric AMKL (10%).[11,73,74] AML with mutated RUNX1 is associated with inferior outcomes and older age in pediatric cases.[4,75] Although most cases have a normal karyotype, they also can be identified with complex karyotypes, and 1 study found RUNX1-RUNX1T1 rearrangements in 22% of cases harboring a RUNX1 mutation.[75]

FLT3

FLT3 is a receptor tyrosine kinase that is essential for normal hematopoietic development. Somatic activating mutations in FLT3 are among the most common somatic alterations in pediatric AML, found in approximately 30% of cases, and are associated with a normal karyotype.[4,76] The most common activating FLT3 mutation is an internal-tandem duplication in the juxtamembrane domain, which is observed in 10% to 15% of pediatric cases.[4] Point mutations in the activation loop domain, most commonly at codons Asp835/I836, are found in approximately 10% of pediatric AML, and recent evidence suggests that there are pediatric-specific activating mutations in the transmembrane domain and juxtamembrane domain found in 7% of cases and are associated with poor responses to standard therapy.[4,77] Importantly, FLT3-ITD mutations with a high allelic ratio (>0.5) are predictive of adverse outcomes in pediatric AML,[78–80] and patients are directed to consider HSCT at first complete remission. Mutations In the activation loop, however, do not confer the same poor prognosis.[78]

The outcomes of pediatric patients with FLT3-ITD mutations are influenced by cooperating mutations; NPM1 comutations are associated with the best outcomes. In contrast, the presence of a WT1 mutation or NUP98-NSD1 fusion imparted worse outcomes compared with FLT3-ITDs alone.[4] Importantly, FLT3 is a molecular lesion in AML for which there is a targeted therapy, as the FLT3 tyrosine kinase inhibitors midostaurin and gilteritinib both have been approved for FLT3-mutated adult AML, and trials for FLT3 inhibitors are under way in pediatric AML.[81]

Acute megakaryoblastic leukemia

AMKL is genetically unique in pediatric patients. Individuals with constitutional trisomy 21 have a greatly increased chance of developing lymphoblastic and myeloid leukemia in general, and, when myeloid leukemia occurs, it often has a megakaryoblastic phenotype. The distinction between AMKL occurring in the setting of Down syndrome (DS), versus AMKL occurring in non-DS patients, is important because DS patients with AMKL have a good prognosis.[82] In contrast, non-DS AMKL have a variety of outcomes influenced by the underlying molecular driver.

Non–DS AMKL has a high rate of structural variation, with 72% of cases carrying a recurrent chromosomal translocation resulting in a gene fusion, including CBFA2T3-GLIS (18%), NUP98-KDM5A (11.5%), RBM15-MKL1 (10%), and KMT2A fusions (17%) and a new collection of rearrangements involving HOX genes (15%).[11] In cases without a recurrent chromosomal translocation, truncating mutations in exons 2 and 3 of GATA1 were identified in 9% of cases.[11]

Gene expression and clustering analysis indicate these recurrent genomic alterations represent distinct subtypes of non–DS AMKL. Cooperating mutations also were identified in JAK/STAT genes (17%), cohesion or CTCF genes (18%), and RAS pathway genes (18%) and focal deletions/loss of heterozygosity in RB1 (14%) and gains of chromosomes 19 and 21.[11] KMT2A fusions often were associated with mutations in the RAS pathway, whereas GATA1 mutations had coexistent JAK and cohesin mutations. Cases of HOX gene rearrangements are enriched significantly in activating MPL mutations and NUP98-KDM5A cases carried RB1 mutations in nearly all samples.[11]

Clinical outcomes appear to be highly correlated with the genetic subtype of non–DS AMKL, with CBFA2T3-GLIS representing the subtype with the worst survival.[11] KMT2A-rearrangenments and NUP98-KDM5A also represented high-risk subtypes. Patients with GATA1 mutations had excellent outcomes, similar to those with DS AMKL, potentially indicating these represent similar entities. HOX gene rearrangements, RBM15-MKL1, and cases without a recurrent genomic alteration all showed a favorable prognosis.[11]

These recurrent rearrangements are not found commonly in adult AMKL and highlight the need for appropriate molecular testing to triage non-DS AMKL patients to risk-adapted therapy. Both DNA and RNA sequencing with appropriate panels represents the best current method to distinguish among these genetic groups.

Germline Predisposition to Acute Myeloid Leukemia

The WHO recently has included germline variant driven AML as separate disease entities, which becomes important to identify for patient management and family counseling. Recent germline testing studies have demonstrated at least 10% of children with cancer harbored a germline mutation in a cancer predisposition gene, although rates in pediatric hematologic malignancies are lower.[83–85]

Although it long has been recognized that bone marrow failure disorders, such as Shwachman-Diamond syndrome or Diamond-Blackfan anemia, have an increased predisposition to AML, it now is recognized that there are a significant number of other pathogenic germline variants that are associated with hematologic abnormalities, such as thrombocytopenia and predisposition to AML. Although discussion of bone marrow failure disorders is beyond the scope of this article, germline predisposition due to pathogenic variants in CEBPA, DDX41, RUNX1, ANKRD26, and ETV6 is discussed.

Germline pathogenic variants in CEBPA are associated with a highly penetrant autosomal dominant predisposition to AML.[86] Patients generally present with AML as children or young adults; the diagnosis can be challenging, because no preceding clinical phenotypes are reported and usually is considered upon tumor sequencing when biallelic CEBPA mutations are identified in the tumor.

Among all patients with biallelic CEBPA mutations in AML, it is estimated that approximately 10% carry a germline CEBPA mutation.[63,69] Pathogenic germline CEBPA variants generally are truncating variants located at the N-terminus of the gene, with somatic inactivation of the second allele the result of a truncating or in-frame deletion mutation in the C-terminal region.[60] Prognosis for patients with pathogenic germline CEBPA variants typically is very good, similar to that for sporadic AML with biallelic somatic CEBPA mutations; however, those with pathogenic germline CEBPA variants are at a higher risk of recurrence/relapse.[87] The second somatic CEBPA mutation usually is different upon recurrence, indicating the primary malignancy was cured and that recurrence is due to a new tumor clone and represents a new leukemic episode.[87]

Pathogenic germline DDX41 variants are associated with an autosomal dominant form of hereditary predisposition to AML without additional clinical features, similar to CEBPA.[88] Affected individuals often develop a second mutation on the other DDX41 allele, consistent with its proposed function as a tumor suppressor. Age of onset, however, highly overlaps with sporadic adult disease and has not been reported in children to date.[89,90] Recent data suggest it is fairly common in sporadic adult AML, where a pathogenic germline variant in DDX41 was identified in 2.4% of cases.[90] Although still a newly described entity, DDX41-associated predisposition to AML may not be a pediatric-onset condition; further investigation is needed to understand this condition fully.

Pathogenic germline variants in RUNX1 are causal for familial platelet disorder with predisposition to AML.[91] It is a rare diagnosis, with only 130 reported families to date, despite its first report more than 20 years ago. Affected individuals report mild to moderate thrombocytopenia, platelet dysfunction, although many do not exhibit a clear bleeding history.[92] Approximately 35% of patients develop myelodysplastic syndrome (MDS), and/or AML occurs at an average age of 33 but has been reported in children as young as 6.[93] This disorder is inherited in an autosomal dominant manner, with most reported and de novo germline RUNX1 mutations reported in patients without a family history.[94,95] Clinical presentation can be variable, even within the same family, and some patients initially can present with AML.[93] Prognosis for affected individuals who progress to AML is poor, and allogenic stem cell transplantation typically is recommended in pediatric patients. Asymptomatic RUNX1 mutation carriers develop a clonal hematopoiesis of indeterminate potential with a cumulative risk of greater than 80% by age 50, demonstrating there are additional clinical features in carriers.[96]

Germline RUNX1 mutations are are truncating variants that are distributed throughout the coding region of the gene and missense mutations that are enriched in the RUNT domain.

AML samples from affected individuals often show somatic mutations affecting the second RUNX1 allele but otherwise show few additional somatic mutations. When they are identified, ASXL1, PTPN11, STAG2, BCOR, DNMT3A, and GATA2 have been reported.[93,96]

ANKRD26 is associated with one of the most common inherited thrombocytopenias, with patients exhibiting lifelong mild to moderate thrombocytopenia, normal platelet size, and a mild bleeding phenotype, although some may present initially with a myeloid malignancy.[97,98] Studies demonstrate an increased risk for developing acute leukemias (4.9%), MDS (2.2%), and chronic myeloid leukemia (CML) (1.3%).[99] Pathogenic ANKRD26 variants primarily are substitutions located within a discrete region of the 5′ UTR of ANKRD26, and additional studies indicate these variants result in upregulation and persistent expression of ANKRD26 through a loss of the repressive binding of RUNX1 and FLI1.[97] Penetrance for thrombocytopenia is nearly complete and diagnosed in adulthood, and transformation to myeloid malignancies has been reported as early as 30 years, suggesting this may not be a pediatric-onset malignancy; however, with only 230 affected individuals reported to date, pediatric onset cannot be excluded.[98,100]

ETV6 is associated with an autosomal dominant inherited thrombocytopenia in which affected individuals display an increased risk for a variety of hematological malignancies, including ALL, CML, and MDS/AML.[101,102] Thrombocytopenias in affected individuals are highly variable, although bleeding symptoms typically are mild and accompanied by either normal or large platelets.[103] Pathogenic variants typically are missense or frameshift alterations in the C-terminal ETS domain that confer a dominant negative effect through binding and mislocalization of wild-type ETV6.[101,102] Among the germline mutation carriers published, ALL, typically pre–B-cell leukemia, is the most common malignancy identified, followed by myeloid malignancies. Age of presentation for malignancies ranges from 2 years to 82 years, demonstrating this is a pediatric-relevant cancer predisposition syndrome.[103]

Finally, patients with pathogenic germline variants in GATA2 have variable syndromic presentations characterized by immunodeficiency, bone marrow failure, and an autosomal dominant predisposition to development of MDS/AML.[104–107] Affected individuals typically exhibit B-cytopenia, DC-cytopenia, NK-cytopenia, and monocytopenia and show susceptibility to nontuberculosis mycobacterial, fungal, and viral (in particular, Epstein-Barr virus and human papillomavirus) infections. Presentations are highly variable in terms of age of onset and disease severity and also can include additional phenotypes, such as primary lymphedema, deafness, and aplastic anemia.[104,108] Pathogenic loss of function variants typically are truncating alterations upstream of zinc finger 2, missense variants within zinc finger 2, or noncoding variants within intron 4 that disrupts a transcriptional enhancer.[104]

Myeloid neoplasms develop in up to 75% of patients with an age of onset ranging from 3 years to 78 years with a median of 20 years.[109] Because a majority of pathogenic germline variants are de novo, most patients do not have a suggestive family history. Furthermore, myeloid malignancies can present in the absence of preceding hematological phenotypes, demonstrating the utility of genomic testing for this diagnosis.

Clinical Genomic Testing

Advances in genomic technologies have altered the landscape of clinical genetic testing for hematological malignancies dramatically. The diversity and prominence of chromosomal rearrangements and cooperating somatic sequence variants in pediatric AML necessitate the diagnostic testing for both types of genomic variants.

Structural variants historically have been evaluated by traditional cytogenetics, including karyotype and fluorescence in situ hybridization. These approaches later were augmented with targeted polymerase chain reaction (PCR)-based molecular methods, including quantitative real-time PCR and qualitative PCR, which can query a small number of known rearrangement partners, often with superior sensitivity.

NGS-based methodologies have the advantage of assessing many or even all genomic regions for structural variation simultaneously. NGS-based methods for the detected of chromosomal rearrangements can query DNA or RNA. DNA-based methods typically rely on the enrichment of known breakpoint regions through either hybrid capture or amplicon-based methods. This approach has the advantage that it can be added to a gene panel for the detection of somatic sequence variants, enabling the detection of both variant types in 1 assay. DNA-based fusion detection requires prior knowledge of the DNA breakpoints, which typically reside within intronic regions, are highly variable, and can be composed of repetitive or nonunique sequences that are challenging to specifically capture, sequence, and bioinformatically map to the appropriate genomic region. Thus, DNA panel–based methods typically exhibit lower sensitivity for known fusions and offer limited ability to identify novel rearrangements. Additionally, this approach cannot determine whether the identified fusion is transcribed or whether it is likely to result in a functional protein, because novel or unexpected patterns of RNA splicing often are observed. Whole-genome sequencing theoretically can identify any known or novel structural variant, but its clinical utility is limited by the high cost, lower depth of sequence recovered, and computational burden related to the large amount of data generated by this method.

RNA-based fusion detection methods rely on an initial reverse transcription step to produce a cDNA library, and can use an upstream enrichment for known fusion partners through hybrid capture or anchored multiplex PCR.[110–112] Because these enrichment approaches generally target exonic regions, they are able to reduce the burden of sequencing per sample while retaining high sensitivity and the ability to identify novel rearrangement partners. A recent study revealed RNA-based approach exhibited superior performance to DNA, identifying fusions in 15% of lung cancer cases without a significant oncogenic driver.[113] A more unbiased approach, whole transcriptome sequencing, retains sensitivity of other RNA-based approaches but offers the ability to identify completely novel and unanticipated fusion genes. The main limitation of RNA-based methods is that they rely on the production of a chimeric transcript, which is not produced by some rearrangements that rely on the association of an oncogene with a strong promoter element, such as the immunoglobulin rearrangements common in lymphomas. With respect to pediatric AML, most reference laboratories offer assays designed for adult malignancies, with a few academic laboratories offering diagnostics designed for pediatric patients.[114–116] Although there is significant overlap between adult and pediatric AML, there are several pediatric specific and rare rearrangements that may not be assayed by targeted approaches. Thus, nonpediatric specific reference tests that utilize transcriptome sequencing may represent a superior approach.

Molecular genetic testing for somatic mutations has similarly progressed from the targeted analysis of a small number of genomic regions through targeted molecular methods and Sanger sequencing, to the simultaneous sequencing of many genes via NGS. NGS-based diagnostics are able to detect single nucleotide variants and small insertions/deletions (<20 bp) with high sensitivity. The sensitivity for insertions/deletions greater than 20 bp diminishes with increasing length of the variant also can be negatively influenced by homologous sequences elsewhere in the genome or low sequence complexity (repetitive elements). This is an important consideration for somatic mutations that involve tandem duplications, such as FLT3-ITDs, for which custom bioinformatics approaches are needed to specifically identify this mutation and may not match the sensitivity of targeted molecular methods at this time. Larger exon and gene level copy number changes also can be detected by NGS, with greater sensitivity for larger genomic copy number changes and gene amplifications.

Clinical DNA sequencing typically relies on the enrichment for coding exons and other clinically relevant genomic regions by hybrid capture or amplicon-based approaches and can vary significantly in the number of genes assayed. Targeted panels ranging from 10 genes to 100 genes, and in some cases focusing only on mutation hotspots and/or actionable genomic findings may be offered to reduce costs while maintaining clinical sensitivity. The rapid evolution of targeted therapies, however, necessitates frequent content updates that require revalidation of the assay and may mitigate some benefits of focused assays. Many commercial panels use a pan-cancer approach that targets most clinically relevant genes across all cancer types and also can offer reporting of genomic signatures, such as microsatellite instability, tumor mutational burden, and a variety of mutational signatures that are associated with clinical benefit to targeted therapies. It is common practice for diagnostic laboratories to offer solid tumor and hematological tests as separate tests, which can be based on the same wet bench procedure with different bioinformatic/interpretive processes or completely separate wet bench processes. Exome sequencing for oncology diagnostics now is clinically available, providing a more complete mutational landscape for oncology patients, and offers the advantage of being able to identify new and emerging biomarkers.

SUMMARY

Although there likely are additional rare driver genetic lesions to be identified in pediatric AML, the field going forward will focus more on optimizing prognosis for pediatric AML subtypes based on coexistent mutations. The possibility of a germline predisposition to AML always should be considered, particularly when genomic testing of malignancies reveals a suggestive mutation. The development of emerging precision therapies will serve only to increase the utility of genomic testing for this patient population.

CLINICS CARE POINTS

- Given the remarkable heterogeneity of chromosomal and molecular alterations that drive pediatric AML, broad testing methodologies, such as NGS-based panels and exome/genome sequencing, and RNA-based fusion detection should be employed to augment conventional cytogenetics for optimal sensitivity.
- Detection of a diverse set of driver mutations in pediatric AMKL has high prognostic significance.
- Hereditary predisposition to AML, although rare, should be considered when interpreting somatic genomic testing.

DISCLOSURE

The authors are both employees of Caris Life Sciences.

REFERENCES

1. Steliarova-Foucher E, Colombet M, Ries LAG, et al. International incidence of childhood cancer, 2001-10: a population-based registry study. Lancet Oncol 2017;18(6):719–31.
2. Zwaan CM, Kolb EA, Reinhardt D, et al. Collaborative efforts driving progress in pediatric acute myeloid leukemia. J Clin Oncol 2015;33(27):2949–62.

3. Gilliland DG, Griffin JD. The roles of FLT3 in hematopoiesis and leukemia. Blood 2002;100(5):1532–42.
4. Bolouri H, Farrar JE, Triche T Jr, et al. The molecular landscape of pediatric acute myeloid leukemia reveals recurrent structural alterations and age-specific mutational interactions. Nat Med 2018;24(1):103–12.
5. Papaemmanuil E, Gerstung M, Bullinger L, et al. Genomic classification and prognosis in acute myeloid leukemia. N Engl J Med 2016;374(23):2209–21.
6. Cancer Genome Atlas Research N, Ley TJ, Miller C, et al. Genomic and epigenomic landscapes of adult de novo acute myeloid leukemia. N Engl J Med 2013; 368(22):2059–74.
7. Rubnitz JE, Inaba H. Childhood acute myeloid leukaemia. Br J Haematol 2012; 159(3):259–76.
8. Radtke I, Mullighan CG, Ishii M, et al. Genomic analysis reveals few genetic alterations in pediatric acute myeloid leukemia. Proc Natl Acad Sci U S A 2009; 106(31):12944–9.
9. Mullighan CG, Goorha S, Radtke I, et al. Genome-wide analysis of genetic alterations in acute lymphoblastic leukaemia. Nature 2007;446(7137):758–64.
10. Zhang Y, Rowley JD. Chromatin structural elements and chromosomal translocations in leukemia. DNA Repair (Amst) 2006;5(9–10):1282–97.
11. de Rooij JD, Branstetter C, Ma J, et al. Pediatric non-down syndrome acute megakaryoblastic leukemia is characterized by distinct genomic subsets with varying outcomes. Nat Genet 2017;49(3):451–6.
12. Winters AC, Bernt KM. MLL-rearranged leukemias-an update on science and clinical approaches. Front Pediatr 2017;5:4.
13. Meyer C, Burmeister T, Groger D, et al. The MLL recombinome of acute leukemias in 2017. Leukemia 2018;32(2):273–84.
14. Creutzig U, Zimmermann M, Reinhardt D, et al. Changes in cytogenetics and molecular genetics in acute myeloid leukemia from childhood to adult age groups. Cancer 2016;122(24):3821–30.
15. Harrison CJ, Hills RK, Moorman AV, et al. Cytogenetics of childhood acute myeloid leukemia: United Kingdom Medical Research Council Treatment trials AML 10 and 12. J Clin Oncol 2010;28(16):2674–81.
16. Balgobind BV, Zwaan CM, Pieters R, et al. The heterogeneity of pediatric MLL-rearranged acute myeloid leukemia. Leukemia 2011;25(8):1239–48.
17. Arber DA, Orazi A, Hasserjian R, et al. The 2016 revision to the World Health Organization classification of myeloid neoplasms and acute leukemia. Blood 2016; 127(20):2391–405.
18. Balgobind BV, Raimondi SC, Harbott J, et al. Novel prognostic subgroups in childhood 11q23/MLL-rearranged acute myeloid leukemia: results of an international retrospective study. Blood 2009;114(12):2489–96.
19. Matsuo H, Yoshida K, Fukumura K, et al. Recurrent CCND3 mutations in MLL-rearranged acute myeloid leukemia. Blood Adv 2018;2(21):2879–89.
20. Struski S, Lagarde S, Bories P, et al. NUP98 is rearranged in 3.8% of pediatric AML forming a clinical and molecular homogenous group with a poor prognosis. Leukemia 2017;31(3):565–72.
21. Shiba N, Yoshida K, Hara Y, et al. Transcriptome analysis offers a comprehensive illustration of the genetic background of pediatric acute myeloid leukemia. Blood Adv 2019;3(20):3157–69.
22. Bisio V, Zampini M, Tregnago C, et al. NUP98-fusion transcripts characterize different biological entities within acute myeloid leukemia: a report from the AIEOP-AML group. Leukemia 2017;31(4):974–7.

23. Gough SM, Slape CI, Aplan PD. NUP98 gene fusions and hematopoietic malignancies: common themes and new biologic insights. Blood 2011;118(24):6247–57.
24. Franks TM, McCloskey A, Shokirev MN, et al. Nup98 recruits the Wdr82-Set1A/COMPASS complex to promoters to regulate H3K4 trimethylation in hematopoietic progenitor cells. Genes Dev 2017;31(22):2222–34.
25. Light WH, Freaney J, Sood V, et al. A conserved role for human Nup98 in altering chromatin structure and promoting epigenetic transcriptional memory. PLoS Biol 2013;11(3):e1001524.
26. Fontoura BM, Blobel G, Matunis MJ. A conserved biogenesis pathway for nucleoporins: proteolytic processing of a 186-kilodalton precursor generates Nup98 and the novel nucleoporin, Nup96. J Cell Biol 1999;144(6):1097–112.
27. Ostronoff F, Othus M, Gerbing RB, et al. NUP98/NSD1 and FLT3/ITD coexpression is more prevalent in younger AML patients and leads to induction failure: a COG and SWOG report. Blood 2014;124(15):2400–7.
28. Sandahl JD, Coenen EA, Forestier E, et al. t(6;9)(p22;q34)/DEK-NUP214-rearranged pediatric myeloid leukemia: an international study of 62 patients. Haematologica 2014;99(5):865–72.
29. Tarlock K, Alonzo TA, Moraleda PP, et al. Acute myeloid leukaemia (AML) with t(6;9)(p23;q34) is associated with poor outcome in childhood AML regardless of FLT3-ITD status: a report from the Children's Oncology Group. Br J Haematol 2014;166(2):254–9.
30. Slovak ML, Gundacker H, Bloomfield CD, et al. A retrospective study of 69 patients with t(6;9)(p23;q34) AML emphasizes the need for a prospective, multicenter initiative for rare 'poor prognosis' myeloid malignancies. Leukemia 2006;20(7):1295–7.
31. Tosi S, Mostafa Kamel Y, Owoka T, et al. Paediatric acute myeloid leukaemia with the t(7;12)(q36;p13) rearrangement: a review of the biological and clinical management aspects. Biomark Res 2015;3:21.
32. Ingenhag D, Reister S, Auer F, et al. The homeobox transcription factor HB9 induces senescence and blocks differentiation in hematopoietic stem and progenitor cells. Haematologica 2019;104(1):35–46.
33. von Neuhoff C, Reinhardt D, Sander A, et al. Prognostic impact of specific chromosomal aberrations in a large group of pediatric patients with acute myeloid leukemia treated uniformly according to trial AML-BFM 98. J Clin Oncol 2010;28(16):2682–9.
34. Downing JR. The AML1-ETO chimaeric transcription factor in acute myeloid leukaemia: biology and clinical significance. Br J Haematol 1999;106(2):296–308.
35. Pession A, Masetti R, Rizzari C, et al. Results of the AIEOP AML 2002/01 multicenter prospective trial for the treatment of children with acute myeloid leukemia. Blood 2013;122(2):170–8.
36. Gibson BE, Webb DK, Howman AJ, et al. Results of a randomized trial in children with Acute Myeloid Leukaemia: medical research council AML12 trial. Br J Haematol 2011;155(3):366–76.
37. Faber ZJ, Chen X, Gedman AL, et al. The genomic landscape of core-binding factor acute myeloid leukemias. Nat Genet 2016;48(12):1551–6.
38. Paschka P, Marcucci G, Ruppert AS, et al. Adverse prognostic significance of KIT mutations in adult acute myeloid leukemia with inv(16) and t(8;21): a Cancer and Leukemia Group B Study. J Clin Oncol 2006;24(24):3904–11.

39. Shimada A, Taki T, Tabuchi K, et al. KIT mutations, and not FLT3 internal tandem duplication, are strongly associated with a poor prognosis in pediatric acute myeloid leukemia with t(8;21): a study of the Japanese Childhood AML Cooperative Study Group. Blood 2006;107(5):1806–9.
40. Nanri T, Matsuno N, Kawakita T, et al. Mutations in the receptor tyrosine kinase pathway are associated with clinical outcome in patients with acute myeloblastic leukemia harboring t(8;21)(q22;q22). Leukemia 2005;19(8):1361–6.
41. Pollard JA, Alonzo TA, Gerbing RB, et al. Prevalence and prognostic significance of KIT mutations in pediatric patients with core binding factor AML enrolled on serial pediatric cooperative trials for de novo AML. Blood 2010; 115(12):2372–9.
42. Adams J, Nassiri M. Acute promyelocytic leukemia: a review and discussion of variant translocations. Arch Pathol Lab Med 2015;139(10):1308–13.
43. Masetti R, Pigazzi M, Togni M, et al. CBFA2T3-GLIS2 fusion transcript is a novel common feature in pediatric, cytogenetically normal AML, not restricted to FAB M7 subtype. Blood 2013;121(17):3469–72.
44. Gruber TA, Larson Gedman A, Zhang J, et al. An Inv(16)(p13.3q24.3)-encoded CBFA2T3-GLIS2 fusion protein defines an aggressive subtype of pediatric acute megakaryoblastic leukemia. Cancer Cell 2012;22(5):683–97.
45. Smith JL, Ries RE, Hylkema T, et al. Comprehensive transcriptome profiling of cryptic CBFA2T3-GLIS2 fusion-positive AML defines novel therapeutic Options: a COG and target pediatric AML study. Clin Cancer Res 2020;26(3):726–37.
46. Roberts I, Fordham NJ, Rao A, et al. Neonatal leukaemia. Br J Haematol 2018; 182(2):170–84.
47. Coenen EA, Zwaan CM, Reinhardt D, et al. Pediatric acute myeloid leukemia with t(8;16)(p11;p13), a distinct clinical and biological entity: a collaborative study by the International-Berlin-Frankfurt-Munster AML-study group. Blood 2013;122(15):2704–13.
48. Wu X, Sulavik D, Roulston D, et al. Spontaneous remission of congenital acute myeloid leukemia with t(8;16)(p11;13). Pediatr Blood Cancer 2011;56(2):331–2.
49. Diab A, Zickl L, Abdel-Wahab O, et al. Acute myeloid leukemia with translocation t(8;16) presents with features which mimic acute promyelocytic leukemia and is associated with poor prognosis. Leuk Res 2013;37(1):32–6.
50. Sainati L, Bolcato S, Cocito MG, et al. Transient acute monoblastic leukemia with reciprocal (8;16)(p11;p13) translocation. Pediatr Hematol Oncol 1996;13(2): 151–7.
51. Balgobind BV, Hollink IH, Arentsen-Peters ST, et al. Integrative analysis of type-I and type-II aberrations underscores the genetic heterogeneity of pediatric acute myeloid leukemia. Haematologica 2011;96(10):1478–87.
52. Marcucci G, Haferlach T, Dohner H. Molecular genetics of adult acute myeloid leukemia: prognostic and therapeutic implications. J Clin Oncol 2011;29(5): 475–86.
53. Dohner K, Schlenk RF, Habdank M, et al. Mutant nucleophosmin (NPM1) predicts favorable prognosis in younger adults with acute myeloid leukemia and normal cytogenetics: interaction with other gene mutations. Blood 2005; 106(12):3740–6.
54. Hollink IH, Zwaan CM, Zimmermann M, et al. Favorable prognostic impact of NPM1 gene mutations in childhood acute myeloid leukemia, with emphasis on cytogenetically normal AML. Leukemia 2009;23(2):262–70.
55. Brown P, McIntyre E, Rau R, et al. The incidence and clinical significance of nucleophosmin mutations in childhood AML. Blood 2007;110(3):979–85.

56. Nishimura Y, Ohkubo T, Furuichi Y, et al. Tryptophans 286 and 288 in the C-terminal region of protein B23.1 are important for its nucleolar localization. Biosci Biotechnol Biochem 2002;66(10):2239–42.
57. Falini B, Bolli N, Liso A, et al. Altered nucleophosmin transport in acute myeloid leukaemia with mutated NPM1: molecular basis and clinical implications. Leukemia 2009;23(10):1731–43.
58. Ho PA, Alonzo TA, Gerbing RB, et al. Prevalence and prognostic implications of CEBPA mutations in pediatric acute myeloid leukemia (AML): a report from the Children's Oncology Group. Blood 2009;113(26):6558–66.
59. Matsuo H, Kajihara M, Tomizawa D, et al. Prognostic implications of CEBPA mutations in pediatric acute myeloid leukemia: a report from the Japanese Pediatric Leukemia/Lymphoma Study Group. Blood Cancer J 2014;4:e226.
60. Leroy H, Roumier C, Huyghe P, et al. CEBPA point mutations in hematological malignancies. Leukemia 2005;19(3):329–34.
61. Kirstetter P, Schuster MB, Bereshchenko O, et al. Modeling of C/EBPalpha mutant acute myeloid leukemia reveals a common expression signature of committed myeloid leukemia-initiating cells. Cancer Cell 2008;13(4):299–310.
62. Lin FT, MacDougald OA, Diehl AM, et al. A 30-kDa alternative translation product of the CCAAT/enhancer binding protein alpha message: transcriptional activator lacking antimitotic activity. Proc Natl Acad Sci U S A 1993;90(20):9606–10.
63. Pabst T, Eyholzer M, Haefliger S, et al. Somatic CEBPA mutations are a frequent second event in families with germline CEBPA mutations and familial acute myeloid leukemia. J Clin Oncol 2008;26(31):5088–93.
64. Green CL, Koo KK, Hills RK, et al. Prognostic significance of CEBPA mutations in a large cohort of younger adult patients with acute myeloid leukemia: impact of double CEBPA mutations and the interaction with FLT3 and NPM1 mutations. J Clin Oncol 2010;28(16):2739–47.
65. Hollink IH, van den Heuvel-Eibrink MM, Arentsen-Peters ST, et al. Characterization of CEBPA mutations and promoter hypermethylation in pediatric acute myeloid leukemia. Haematologica 2011;96(3):384–92.
66. Hou HA, Lin LI, Chen CY, et al. Reply to 'Heterogeneity within AML with CEBPA mutations; only CEBPA double mutations, but not single CEBPA mutations are associated with favorable prognosis. Br J Cancer 2009;101(4):738–40.
67. Pabst T, Eyholzer M, Fos J, et al. Heterogeneity within AML with CEBPA mutations; only CEBPA double mutations, but not single CEBPA mutations are associated with favourable prognosis. Br J Cancer 2009;100(8):1343–6.
68. Tarlock KAT, Wang YC, Gerbing RB, et al. Somatic Bzip mutations of CEBPA are associated with favorable outcome regardless of presence as single Vs. Double mutation. Blood 2019;134(1):181.
69. Taskesen E, Bullinger L, Corbacioglu A, et al. Prognostic impact, concurrent genetic mutations, and gene expression features of AML with CEBPA mutations in a cohort of 1182 cytogenetically normal AML patients: further evidence for CEBPA double mutant AML as a distinctive disease entity. Blood 2011;117(8):2469–75.
70. Wouters BJ, Lowenberg B, Erpelinck-Verschueren CA, et al. Double CEBPA mutations, but not single CEBPA mutations, define a subgroup of acute myeloid leukemia with a distinctive gene expression profile that is uniquely associated with a favorable outcome. Blood 2009;113(13):3088–91.
71. Maxson JE, Ries RE, Wang YC, et al. CSF3R mutations have a high degree of overlap with CEBPA mutations in pediatric AML. Blood 2016;127(24):3094–8.

72. Tarlock K, Alonzo T, Wang YC, et al. Prognostic impact of CSF3R mutations in favorable risk childhood acute myeloid leukemia. Blood 2020;135(18):1603–6.
73. Tang JL, Hou HA, Chen CY, et al. AML1/RUNX1 mutations in 470 adult patients with de novo acute myeloid leukemia: prognostic implication and interaction with other gene alterations. Blood 2009;114(26):5352–61.
74. Mendler JH, Maharry K, Radmacher MD, et al. RUNX1 mutations are associated with poor outcome in younger and older patients with cytogenetically normal acute myeloid leukemia and with distinct gene and MicroRNA expression signatures. J Clin Oncol 2012;30(25):3109–18.
75. Yamato G, Shiba N, Yoshida K, et al. RUNX1 mutations in pediatric acute myeloid leukemia are associated with distinct genetic features and an inferior prognosis. Blood 2018;131(20):2266–70.
76. Tarlock K, Alonzo TA, Loken MR, et al. Disease characteristics and prognostic implications of cell-surface FLT3 receptor (CD135) expression in pediatric acute myeloid leukemia: a report from the Children's oncology group. Clin Cancer Res 2017;23(14):3649–56.
77. Katherine Tarlock MM, Hansen E, Hylkema T, et al. Discovery and functional validation of novel pediatric specific FLT3 activating mutations in acute myeloid leukemia: results from the COG/NCI target initiative. Blood 2015;126(23):87.
78. Meshinchi S, Alonzo TA, Stirewalt DL, et al. Clinical implications of FLT3 mutations in pediatric AML. Blood 2006;108(12):3654–61.
79. Staffas A, Kanduri M, Hovland R, et al. Presence of FLT3-ITD and high BAALC expression are independent prognostic markers in childhood acute myeloid leukemia. Blood 2011;118(22):5905–13.
80. Manara E, Basso G, Zampini M, et al. Characterization of children with FLT3-ITD acute myeloid leukemia: a report from the AIEOP AML-2002 study group. Leukemia 2017;31(1):18–25.
81. Lonetti A, Pession A, Masetti R. Targeted therapies for pediatric AML: gaps and perspective. Front Pediatr 2019;7:463.
82. Gruber TA, Downing JR. The biology of pediatric acute megakaryoblastic leukemia. Blood 2015;126(8):943–9.
83. Zhang J, Walsh MF, Wu G, et al. Germline mutations in predisposition genes in pediatric cancer. N Engl J Med 2015;373(24):2336–46.
84. Mody RJ, Wu YM, Lonigro RJ, et al. Integrative clinical sequencing in the management of refractory or relapsed cancer in youth. JAMA 2015;314(9):913–25.
85. Parsons DW, Roy A, Yang Y, et al. Diagnostic yield of clinical tumor and germline whole-exome sequencing for children with solid tumors. JAMA Oncol 2016;2(5): 616–24.
86. Smith ML, Cavenagh JD, Lister TA, et al. Mutation of CEBPA in familial acute myeloid leukemia. N Engl J Med 2004;351(23):2403–7.
87. Tawana K, Wang J, Renneville A, et al. Disease evolution and outcomes in familial AML with germline CEBPA mutations. Blood 2015;126(10):1214–23.
88. Polprasert C, Schulze I, Sekeres MA, et al. Inherited and somatic Defects in DDX41 in myeloid neoplasms. Cancer Cell 2015;27(5):658–70.
89. Lewinsohn M, Brown AL, Weinel LM, et al. Novel germ line DDX41 mutations define families with a lower age of MDS/AML onset and lymphoid malignancies. Blood 2016;127(8):1017–23.
90. Sebert M, Passet M, Raimbault A, et al. Germline DDX41 mutations define a significant entity within adult MDS/AML patients. Blood 2019;134(17):1441–4.

91. Song WJ, Sullivan MG, Legare RD, et al. Haploinsufficiency of CBFA2 causes familial thrombocytopenia with propensity to develop acute myelogenous leukaemia. Nat Genet 1999;23(2):166–75.
92. Schlegelberger B, Heller PG. RUNX1 deficiency (familial platelet disorder with predisposition to myeloid leukemia, FPDMM). Semin Hematol 2017;54(2):75–80.
93. Brown AL, Arts P, Carmichael CL, et al. RUNX1-mutated families show phenotype heterogeneity and a somatic mutation profile unique to germline predisposed AML. Blood Adv 2020;4(6):1131–44.
94. Ouchi-Uchiyama M, Sasahara Y, Kikuchi A, et al. Analyses of genetic and clinical parameters for screening patients with inherited thrombocytopenia with small or normal-sized platelets. Pediatr Blood Cancer 2015;62(12):2082–8.
95. Schmit JM, Turner DJ, Hromas RA, et al. Two novel RUNX1 mutations in a patient with congenital thrombocytopenia that evolved into a high grade myelodysplastic syndrome. Leuk Res Rep 2015;4(1):24–7.
96. Churpek JE, Pyrtel K, Kanchi KL, et al. Genomic analysis of germ line and somatic variants in familial myelodysplasia/acute myeloid leukemia. Blood 2015; 126(22):2484–90.
97. Pippucci T, Savoia A, Perrotta S, et al. Mutations in the 5' UTR of ANKRD26, the ankirin repeat domain 26 gene, cause an autosomal-dominant form of inherited thrombocytopenia, THC2. Am J Hum Genet 2011;88(1):115–20.
98. Noris P, Perrotta S, Seri M, et al. Mutations in ANKRD26 are responsible for a frequent form of inherited thrombocytopenia: analysis of 78 patients from 21 families. Blood 2011;117(24):6673–80.
99. Noris P, Favier R, Alessi MC, et al. ANKRD26-related thrombocytopenia and myeloid malignancies. Blood 2013;122(11):1987–9.
100. Perez Botero J, Dugan SN, Anderson MW. ANKRD26-related thrombocytopenia. In: Adam MP, Ardinger HH, Pagon RA, et al, editors. GeneReviews((R)). 1993. Available at: https://www.ncbi.nlm.nih.gov/books/NBK507664/.
101. Noetzli L, Lo RW, Lee-Sherick AB, et al. Germline mutations in ETV6 are associated with thrombocytopenia, red cell macrocytosis and predisposition to lymphoblastic leukemia. Nat Genet 2015;47(5):535–8.
102. Zhang MY, Churpek JE, Keel SB, et al. Germline ETV6 mutations in familial thrombocytopenia and hematologic malignancy. Nat Genet 2015;47(2):180–5.
103. Hock H, Shimamura A. ETV6 in hematopoiesis and leukemia predisposition. Semin Hematol 2017;54(2):98–104.
104. Hsu AP, McReynolds LJ, Holland SM. GATA2 deficiency. Curr Opin Allergy Clin Immunol 2015;15(1):104–9.
105. Hsu AP, Sampaio EP, Khan J, et al. Mutations in GATA2 are associated with the autosomal dominant and sporadic monocytopenia and mycobacterial infection (MonoMAC) syndrome. Blood 2011;118(10):2653–5.
106. Dickinson RE, Griffin H, Bigley V, et al. Exome sequencing identifies GATA-2 mutation as the cause of dendritic cell, monocyte, B and NK lymphoid deficiency. Blood 2011;118(10):2656–8.
107. Hahn CN, Chong CE, Carmichael CL, et al. Heritable GATA2 mutations associated with familial myelodysplastic syndrome and acute myeloid leukemia. Nat Genet 2011;43(10):1012–7.
108. Ostergaard P, Simpson MA, Connell FC, et al. Mutations in GATA2 cause primary lymphedema associated with a predisposition to acute myeloid leukemia (Emberger syndrome). Nat Genet 2011;43(10):929–31.
109. Wlodarski MW, Collin M, Horwitz MS. GATA2 deficiency and related myeloid neoplasms. Semin Hematol 2017;54(2):81–6.

110. Zheng Z, Liebers M, Zhelyazkova B, et al. Anchored multiplex PCR for targeted next-generation sequencing. Nat Med 2014;20(12):1479–84.
111. Levin JZ, Berger MF, Adiconis X, et al. Targeted next-generation sequencing of a cancer transcriptome enhances detection of sequence variants and novel fusion transcripts. Genome Biol 2009;10(10):R115.
112. Mercer TR, Gerhardt DJ, Dinger ME, et al. Targeted RNA sequencing reveals the deep complexity of the human transcriptome. Nat Biotechnol 2011;30(1): 99–104.
113. Benayed R, Offin M, Mullaney K, et al. High yield of RNA sequencing for targetable kinase fusions in lung Adenocarcinomas with No Mitogenic driver alteration detected by DNA sequencing and low tumor mutation burden. Clin Cancer Res 2019;25(15):4712–22.
114. Surrey LF, MacFarland SP, Chang F, et al. Clinical utility of custom-designed NGS panel testing in pediatric tumors. Genome Med 2019;11(1):32.
115. Hiemenz MC, Ostrow DG, Busse TM, et al. OncoKids: a comprehensive next-generation sequencing panel for pediatric malignancies. J Mol Diagn 2018; 20(6):765–76.
116. Hiemenz MC, Oberley MJ, Doan A, et al. A multimodal genomics approach to diagnostic evaluation of pediatric hematologic malignancies. Cancer Genet 2021;254-255:25–33.

Pediatric Myelodysplastic Syndromes

Sanjay S. Patel, MD, MPH

KEYWORDS

• Myelodysplastic syndrome • MDS • Dysplasia • Inherited bone marrow failure
• Stem cell transplant

KEY POINTS

- Pediatric myelodysplastic syndrome (MDS) is rare and often develops in the setting of an underlying inherited bone marrow failure syndrome.
- Refractory cytopenia of childhood and MDS with excess blasts comprise most cases.
- Definitive diagnosis frequently requires repeat marrow sampling and correlation with ancillary laboratory testing.
- Allogeneic hematopoietic stem cell transplant represents the only curative intervention, and should be considered in all patients based on clinical and genetic features.
- Comprehensive next-generation sequencing–based studies are starting to reveal novel and unique aspects of biology in pediatric MDS.

CLINICAL AND LABORATORY PARAMETERS

Approximately 20% of pediatric myelodysplastic syndrome (MDS) cases are detected incidentally on routine laboratory investigation, or during the work-up for a suspected inherited bone marrow failure (IBMF) syndrome.[1–9] More frequently, patients present with symptoms related to occult cytopenias, including fatigue, fever, infection, and/or bleeding.[9] In contrast with adults, pediatric patients with MDS more often present with bicytopenias, rather than isolated anemia. Given the association with IBMF syndromes in many cases, physical examination findings may be particularly informative, and may reveal skeletal, cutaneous, genitourinary, cardiovascular, and/or gastrointestinal anomalies. The combination of cytopenias and a hypocellular bone marrow is alone nonspecific, and therefore the following differential diagnostic considerations warrant exclusion: vitamin and/or mineral deficiencies and zinc toxicity[10], viral infections; toxin or drug exposures[11]; autoimmune and other rheumatologic disorders, such as juvenile rheumatoid arthritis; mitochondrial disorders (eg, Pearson syndrome); various metabolic disorders; inherited anemias; and IBMF syndromes.

Conflict of interest: The author has no conflict of interest with respect to the subject matter discussed in this article.
Division of Hematopathology, Weill Cornell Medical College/NewYork-Presbyterian Hospital, 525 East 68th Street, Starr 711A, New York, NY 10065, USA
E-mail address: sap9151@med.cornell.edu

Clin Lab Med 41 (2021) 517–528
https://doi.org/10.1016/j.cll.2021.03.015

In a recent retrospective review of laboratory data collected from 246 patients suspected of presenting with either an IBMF or MDS, the investigators analyzed morphologic, flow cytometric, karyotypic, and fluorescence in situ hybridization (FISH) data from 595 specimens (246 total patients) to evaluate their potential diagnostic utility.[12] The number of bone marrow biopsy samples examined per patient ranged from 1 to 24 (median, 1). Interestingly, of the 595 total cases evaluated, 506 (85.0%) were associated with completely normal bone marrow examinations (ie, dysplasia <10%, normal flow cytometry results, normal karyotype, no aberrations by MDS-specific FISH studies). Out of all patients in the study, 194 (78.9%) had normal results for all of their bone marrow samples examined during the study period. Approximately 30% of the total cases ultimately had no diagnostic evidence of an IBMF syndrome, germline mutation-related syndrome, or myeloid neoplasm.

Peripheral Blood Values

White blood cell (WBC) count, hemoglobin level, mean corpuscular volume (MCV), and absolute neutrophil count (ANC) at the time of marrow evaluation were scored as either low, high, or normal per the established age-specific ranges. There were no identifiable correlations between the presence of abnormal ancillary test results (eg, definite flow cytometric evidence of a myeloid stem cell disorder, karyotypic abnormalities, and/or abnormal FISH studies) and abnormal peripheral blood values, including decreased WBC count, decreased hemoglobin level, increased MCV, or decreased ANC. However, cases with abnormal ancillary test results were enriched for concomitant thrombocytopenia; notably, of 511 cases with normal ancillary test results and known platelet values, thrombocytopenia was present in 311, indicating that an absence of thrombocytopenia was highly predictive of normal ancillary test results. In addition, the absence of thrombocytopenia was highly predictive of an absence of significant dysplasia in any single lineage. Out of the 246 patients in the study, only 4 showed blasts in the peripheral blood.

Histomorphologic Findings

The original bone marrow reports from all cases in the study were reviewed, and the presence of dysplasia, the specific lineages involved, and increased blasts, were noted. Given the retrospective nature of the study, any samples associated with an original observation of dysplasia (n = 117) were rereviewed by a single hematopathologist and ascribed a quantification component, with dysplasia involving less than 10% or greater than or equal to 10% per lineage. Representative examples of lineage dysplasia that may be encountered during diagnostic evaluation are shown in **Fig. 1**. Iron stains were additionally performed to interrogate for the presence of ring sideroblasts. All cases were also evaluated for marrow cellularity using the core biopsy specimen.

Of the 595 samples examined for morphologic dysplasia, 543 (91.3%) were associated with relatively normal morphology (ie, <10% dysplastic features); 52 (8.7%, n = 31 patients) had greater than or equal to 10% dysplasia in at least 1 lineage and/or greater than or equal to 5% blasts. Of the 52 samples, 38 showed unilineage dysplasia: dyserythropoiesis (n = 6, 1%), dysmyelopoiesis (n = 14, 2.4%), or dysmegakaryopoiesis (n = 18, 3.0%). Bilineage dysplasia was present in 13 samples (2.2%), including erythroid/myeloid dysplasia (n = 4, 0.7%), myeloid/megakaryocytic dysplasia (n = 8, 1.3%), or erythroid/megakaryocytic dysplasia (n = 1, <0.1%). Blasts greater than or equal to 5% was identified in 7 cases (1.2%); 6 of these cases had at least unilineage dysplasia. An increase in ring sideroblasts was not identified in any

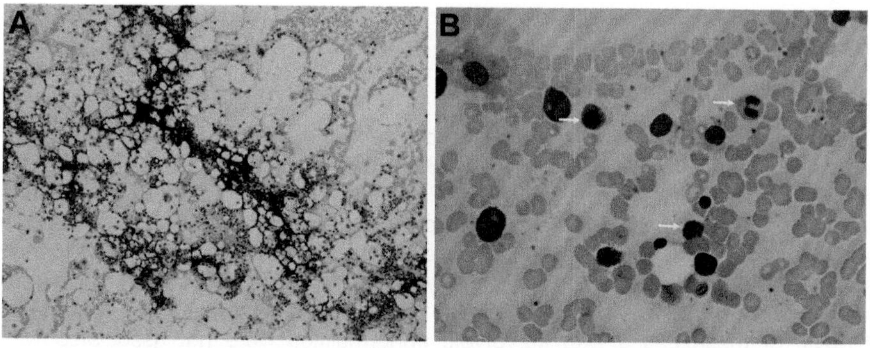

Fig. 1. Bone marrow evaluation in a 6-year-old patient ultimately diagnosed with MIRAGE (myelodysplasia, infection, growth restriction, adrenal hypoplasia, genital phenotypes, and enteropathy) syndrome. (*A*) Representative low-power image of an aspirate smear, showing marrow hypocellularity (Wright-Giemsa, original magnification ×100). (*B*) Representative field of an aspirate smear showing examples of dysplastic changes in multiple lineages (*yellow arrows*), including myeloid (pseudo–Pelger-Huët form) and erythroid (nuclear irregularity/budding, nuclear-cytoplasmic dyssynchrony) precursors (Wright-Giemsa, original magnification ×1000 (Oil)). (Images courtesy of Dr Vinodh Pillai, MD PhD, Children's Hospital of Pennsylvania, Perelman School of Medicine, University of Pennsylvania, Philadelphia, PA).

sample. Of the 52 samples associated with either dysplasia and/or an increase in blasts, additional ancillary data were available for 21 (40.4%, n = 13 patients).

Flow Cytometric Immunophenotyping

Flow cytometric immunophenotyping was performed and reviewed by expert hematopathologists at the University of Washington Hematopathology Laboratory.[12] Available samples (n = 360, 60.5%) were evaluated using a combinatorial approach, including the following parameters: (1) difference from normal based on known normal patterns for myeloid progenitor, granulocyte, and monocyte maturation; (2) aberrant antigen expression (eg, lymphoid antigens on myeloid cells); (3) increased or decreased normal antigen intensity; (4) homogeneous antigen expression; and (5) asynchronous expression of 2 antigens.[13–15]

Only 42 of the 360 cases analyzed (11.7%) had identifiable phenotypic abnormalities, 3 of which had abnormal B-cell or T-cell populations, of uncertain significance. In 39 cases (n = 27 patients) there were abnormal myeloid progenitors, granulocyte maturation, and/or monocyte maturation; in only 10 of these cases were the data considered definitively diagnostic of a myeloid stem cell disorder, all of which were additionally associated with morphologic dysplasia and/or increased marrow blasts, and 7 of which also had abnormal cytogenetics. In the remaining 29 cases the phenotypic abnormalities were considered to be insufficient evidence to render a definitive diagnosis of a myeloid stem cell neoplasm; instead, a reactive/regenerative process was favored in most cases. Notably, only 7 of these cases were associated with morphologic dysplasia in the corresponding smear preparations.

In cases with abnormal flow cytometric findings, the following changes were noted: (1) maturing granulocytes with increased cluster of differentiation (CD) 14/CD64 expression (n = 14) and/or abnormal CD13/CD16 pattern (n = 5); and (2) myeloid progenitor abnormalities, including decreased CD13 expression (n = 4), decreased/absent human leukocyte antigen HLA-DR expression (n = 3), increased CD117 (n = 4), and/or CD33 expression (n = 3). Monocytes in 1 case showed aberrant CD56 expression.

Cytogenetic Features

Data from concurrent conventional karyotyping (n = 586, 98.5%) and FISH studies using an MDS-specific probe panel (n = 477, 80.2%) were reviewed, and 586 karyotypes were successfully performed, of which 523 (89.2%) had normal results. Of the 63 cases (10.8%) with karyotypic abnormalities, 18 (3.1%) were constitutional in origin (eg, trisomy 21), and 42 (7.2%, n = 16 patients) were somatic; these latter abnormalities included del(20q) (n = 14), monosomy/del(7q) (n = 12), trisomy 8 (n = 4), monosomy 7 plus trisomy 8 (n = 2), del(5q) (n = 3), and several others (n = 7). Notably, 26 (61.9%) of these cases with karyotypic abnormalities were not associated with dysplastic changes in greater than or equal to 10% of any 1 lineage, whereas the significant dysplasia observed in 16 cases (38.1%) was most commonly restricted to a single lineage. All 25 cases with abnormal karyotypes and no significant dysplasia or increase in blasts were in patients with underlying constitutional disorders, including Schachman-Diamond syndrome, dyskeratosis congenita, and germline *RUNX1* or *GATA2* mutations, or in patients diagnosed with juvenile myelomonocytic leukemia (JMML) or aplastic anemia.

FISH data were available for 477 cases, of which 437 (91.6%) were not associated with any abnormalities. Thirty-eight (8%) cases, from 14 total patients, were associated with acquired abnormalities: −7/del(7q) (n = 17), del(20q) (n = 14), del(5q) (n = 2), monosomy 7 and trisomy 8 (n = 2), trisomy 8 (n = 1), i7q (n = 1), and del(5q) and del(7q) (n = 1). In line with the karyotypic data, 27 patients with abnormalities detected by FISH were not associated with evidence of morphologic dysplasia in greater than or equal to 10% of a single lineage.

Overall, of 451 cases with both karyotypic and FISH data available, the results from the 2 methods were concordant in 443 (98.2%).

CLASSIFICATION SCHEMA

Pediatric MDS cases are broadly subclassified into 2 major categories, based on the stratification of peripheral blood (≥2%) and/or bone marrow (≥5% and <20%) blasts: refractory cytopenia of childhood (RCC) and advanced MDS. Additional considerations, including MDS with excess blasts in transformation (MDS-EB-t) and therapy-related MDS are also briefly discussed.

Refractory Cytopenia of Childhood

RCC is the most common MDS variant in children.[4,16] The median age at presentation with RCC is 7 to 8 years, although the diagnosis can be rendered in children of any age.[9,17] In contrast with adult patients with MDS, who often present with anemia, pediatric patients have been noted to more frequently present with thrombocytopenia and/or neutropenia, in addition to anemia, all of which result from ineffective hematopoiesis.[3,4,9] In such studies, an age-adjusted increase in MCV and/or moderate increases in the percentage of hemoglobin F have also been observed in a large proportion of patients.

By definition, a diagnosis of RCC requires less than 2% blasts in the peripheral blood and less than 5% in the bone marrow. Notably, in contrast with adults with MDS, RCC is often associated with marked marrow hypocellularity in up to 80% of patients.[4,18] Dysplastic changes must also be documented, and most frequently involve the erythroid and/or megakaryocytic lineages.[3,18,19] The peculiar finding of islands of erythroid elements accompanied by sparsely distributed granulocytes has also been reported. Megakaryocytes are either decreased in number or absent, and, as in adult patients, micromegakaryocytes are occasionally present and are most easily identified by immunoperoxidase studies. CD42b is a useful marker in addition to CD41 and CD61. GATA1 is also a useful nuclear marker of early erythroids and megakaryocytes.[20] A representative example of RCC in evolution to an accelerated phase of MDS with excess blasts is shown in **Fig. 2**.

Cytogenetic abnormalities are detected in ~30% of patients, with an enrichment for monosomy 7, which has been reported in ~11% of patients, with an increased incidence in patients with either normocellular or hypercellular marrows.[4,9]

Differential diagnostic considerations most importantly include aplastic anemia (AA) and IBMF syndromes. Although AA can be reliably distinguished based on morphologic features (eg, absence of lineage dysplasia), IBMF syndromes, and in particular Fanconi anemia (FA), can exhibit significant clinical and histologic overlap with RCC; FA is typically considered indistinguishable from RCC by light microscopy

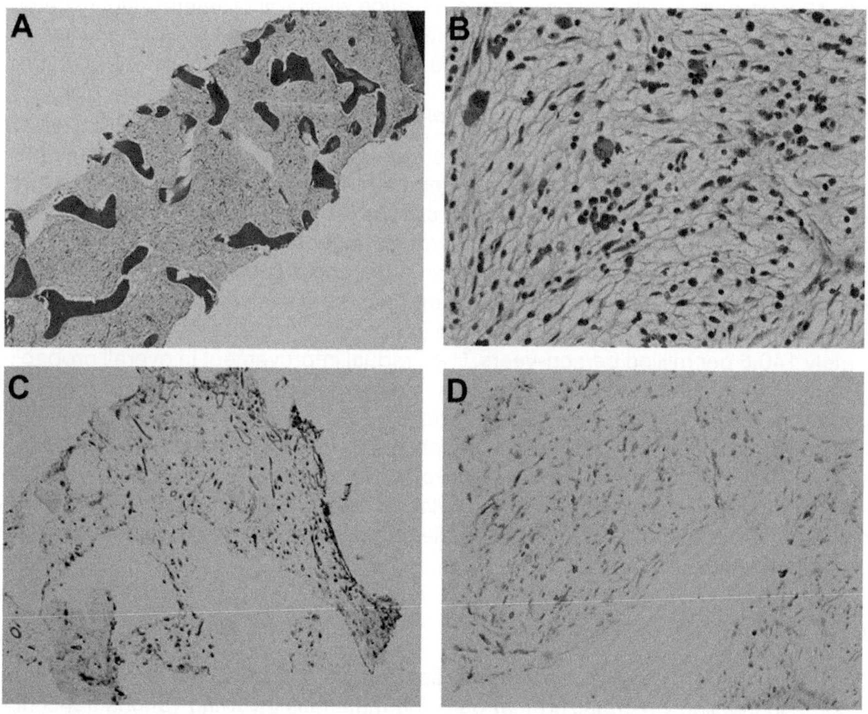

Fig. 2. Bone marrow evaluation in a 7-year-old patient with a history of presumed RCC in evolution to MDS with excess blasts-2. (*A*) Representative low-power image of the core biopsy specimen, showing marrow hypocellularity (hematoxylin-eosin, original magnification ×100). (*B*) Representative high-power field of the core biopsy specimen showing conspicuous atypical megakaryocytes (hematoxylin-eosin, original magnification ×400). Immunohistochemical evaluation including CD34 (Immunohistochemistry using DAB chromogen, original magnification ×200) (*C*) and CD42b (*D*) reveals increased blasts and frequent atypical megakaryocytes, respectively (Immunohistochemistry using DAB chromogen, original magnification ×200). (Images courtesy of Dr Elizabeth Margolskee, MD, Children's Hospital of Pennsylvania, Perelman School of Medicine, University of Pennsylvania, Philadelphia, PA).

evaluation alone. Of note, select studies have revealed that ~30% of patients ultimately diagnosed with FA, and other IBMF syndromes, may present with no obvious physical abnormalities.[21,22] Thus, a thorough medical history and clinical examination is required, in conjunction with specific ancillary/functional studies (as discussed elsewhere in this chapter), to investigate for chromosomal breakage, G2 cell-cycle arrest, western blot or mutational analyses for FA-associated genes, and assessment of telomere length, before rendering a definitive diagnosis of RCC.

Advanced Myelodysplastic Syndrome

Advanced MDSs are typically associated with an increase in blasts, greater than or equal to 2% in the peripheral blood and/or greater than or equal to 5% in the bone marrow. Most of these cases are categorized as MDS with excess blasts (MDS-EB).[3] MDS-EB-t, previously known as refractory anemia with excess blasts in transformation, is defined by the presence of 20% to 29% bone marrow blasts. In contrast with secondary acute myeloid leukemia (AML) arising out of an antecedent MDS in adults, pediatric MDS and AML are no longer reliably distinguished based on the marrow blast percentage alone. An extensive work-up is required, including cytogenetic studies, immunophenotyping, and correlation with clinical features (eg, hepatosplenomegaly). In many cases, a repeat bone marrow evaluation at ~4-week intervals is necessary to establish an AML diagnosis.

Therapy-related and Secondary Myelodysplastic Syndrome

Therapy-related (t-MDS) in children is rare but has increasingly gained attention as therapies for other childhood malignancies have evolved and become more successful, increasing the total population of children at risk. A representative example of *MLL*-rearranged therapy-related acute megakaryoblastic leukemia (t-AMKL) in a patient after intensive chemotherapy for an antecedent B-cell acute lymphoblastic leukemia (B-ALL) is shown in **Fig. 3**. Recent data have shown that the global world standard population of registered cancers in children aged 0 to 14 years is approximately 140.6 per million person-years.[23] A gradual improvement in overall probability of long-term survival has been reported in recent years, and is now estimated at greater than 80% in the United States and Europe.[24] The cumulative incidence of therapy-related myeloid neoplasms in children, including t-MDS and therapy-related AML, ranges from 5% to 11% for children treated with standard solid-tumor protocols, including high-dose alkylating agents and topoisomerase II inhibitors, and from less than 1% to 5% for patients previously treated for acute lymphoblastic leukemias.[25–27]

MOLECULAR GENETIC FEATURES

As comprehensive, large-scale genetic sequencing studies have evolved, it has become increasingly recognized that germline mutations involving various transcription factors, including *GATA2*, *RUNX1*, *ETV6*, *CEBPA*, *ANKRD26*, and *SRP72*, can lead to familial MDS/AML.[28–33] Of these, *GATA2* deficiency, or germline mutations, represent the most frequent germline genetic predisposition in childhood MDS, occurring in approximately 7% of patients.[33] *GATA2* lesions are more frequently encountered in adolescents (>4 years old) with advanced MDS and in patients with monosomy 7.[33,34] More recently, comprehensive gene sequencing studies have focused on elucidating the landscape of both germline and somatic mutations in pediatric MDS.[35–37] Notably, genes frequently found to be mutated in adult MDS (eg, *TET2*, *DNMT3A*, *TP53*, spliceosome machinery genes)[38–42] are not involved in the

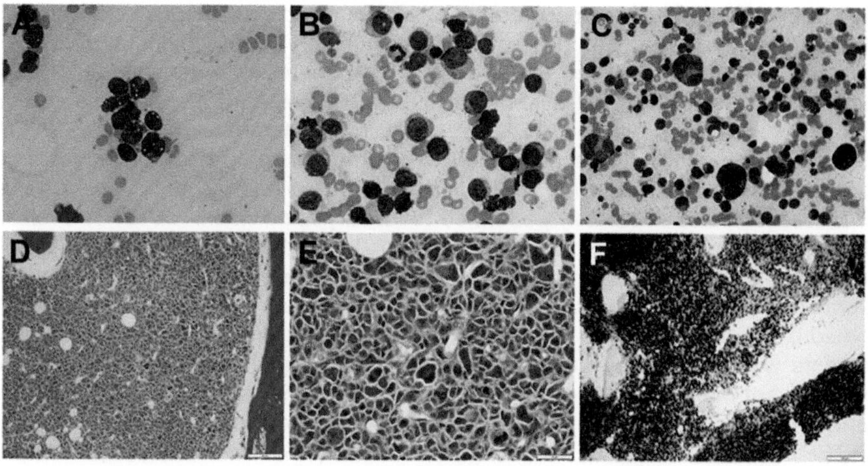

Fig. 3. Histomorphologic and immunophenotypic findings in a patient with *MLL*-rearranged t-AMKL, after chemotherapy for B-ALL. (*A*) Representative image of a Wright-Giemsa–stained aspirate smear, showing B lymphoblasts at the time of the patient's original B-ALL diagnosis (Wright-Giemsa, original magnification ×1000(Oil)). Representative images of Wright-Giemsa–stained aspirate smears, abnormal blasts (Wright-Giemsa, original magnification ×1000(Oil)) (*B*) and dysplastic megakaryocytes (Wright-Giemsa, original magnification ×600(Oil)) (*C*) at repeat presentation (t-AMKL). Representative hematoxylin-eosin–stained sections of the bone marrow core biopsy tissue at repeat presentation (t-AMKL), showing a hypercellular marrow (hematoxylin-eosin, original magnification ×100) (*D*) with increased numbers of blasts and dysplastic megakaryocytes (hematoxylin-eosin, original magnification ×400) (*E*). (*F*) GATA-1 immunohistochemistry highlights most of the marrow cells, indicating erythroid-megakaryocytic derivation (Immunohistochemistry using DAB chromogen, original magnification ×200). These cells were also positive for the megakaryocytic antigen CD42b (not shown). (Images courtesy of Dr Vinodh Pillai, MD PhD, Children's Hospital of Pennsylvania, Perelman School of Medicine, University of Pennsylvania, Philadelphia, PA).

pathogenesis of pediatric disease.[35,36,43,44] Schwartz and colleagues[36] performed tumor and normal whole-exome sequencing on 32 pediatric patients with primary MDS and targeted sequencing on an additional 14 patients (n = 46, total); these data were compared with those derived from patients with overlapping myelodysplastic/myeloproliferative (MDS/MPN) features, including JMML, and 8 patients with AML with myelodysplasia-related changes (AML-MRC). In addition, RNA sequencing was performed on 43 samples with available material. Of the patients with primary MDS, 50% were classified as RCC, and 50% as refractory anemia with excess blasts (now known as MDS-EB). In both subgroups of pediatric MDS, mutations involving genes important in the Ras/mitogen-activated protein kinase (MAPK) pathway (eg, *PTPN11*, *NRAS*, *SETBP1*, *CBL*, *PHF6*), including both germline and somatic variants, were most common (43% of the primary MDS cases), whereas RNA splicing factor gene variants were rare, and *DNMT3A/ASXL1/TET2* mutations were absent. Notably, *PTPN11* (15 mutations in 14 patients) and *NRAS* (10 mutations in 9 patients) were most common. Interestingly, 8 patients (17%) within the primary MDS cohort were also found to have presumed *SAMD9* or *SAMD9L* germline variants. Using RNA sequencing, Schwartz and colleagues[36] also interrogated for gene fusion events, and identified only 2 fusions (*RUNX1-MECOM* and *CSNK1A1-LECT2*) in 25 patients with primary MDS patients.

In a separate study, Pastor and colleagues[35] examined a cohort of 50 children and adolescents diagnosed with primary MDS, intentionally biasing their cohort toward patients with more advanced disease (eg, 48% patients with monosomy 7, 38% diagnosed as MDS-EB). One-third of the cohort (18 cases) harbored known germline mutations involving either *GATA2* or *RUNX1*. Capture-based targeted next-generation sequencing was performed to interrogate for variants in 104 genes known to be associated with myeloid neoplasia, and allele-specific polymerase chain reaction was separately performed to identify mutations in *SETBP1*. Overall, 64 total mutations were identified across 36 (72%) of the patients, involving 25 of the 105 analyzed genes. Through paired normal sequencing, 24 somatic mutations were confirmed in 17 patients (34%) and 35 germline variants in 25 (50%). As anticipated by the investigators, somatic mutations were significantly more common in patients with MDS-EB versus RCC (68% vs 13%, *P*<.001), and in patients with concomitant monosomy 7 versus other karyotypes (56% vs 18%, *P*<.001). Recurrent somatic mutations were most frequently identified in the following genes: *SETBP1* (18%), *ASXL1* (8%), *RUNX1* (6%), *PTPN11* (6%), and *NRAS* (4%). Interestingly, the top 3 mutated genes (*SETBP1*, *ASXL1*, *RUNX1*) were only identified in patients with concomitant monosomy 7; given the contrast of these findings with the data reported by Schwartz and colleagues,[36] it seems likely that mutations involving genes such as *ASXL1* may represent a progression event most frequently, or only, encountered in cases of incipient AML. As found by other groups, mutations commonly encountered in adult MDS and/or in age-related clonal hematopoiesis of indeterminate potential (CHIP), namely those involving *TET2*, *DNMT3A*, *TP53*, and spliceosome machinery genes, were not detected in this cohort. These CHIP mutations have also been shown to be of low prevalence in survivors of childhood cancer.[45]

CLINICAL MANAGEMENT

Management for Refractory Cytopenia of Childhood

The therapeutic approach to patients with RCC is often challenging, and must take into account all clinical, histomorphologic, and cytogenetic data in each case. In the absence of cytogenetic abnormalities, transfusion dependency, and/or severe neutropenia (ie, <1000/μL or even <500/μL), a careful wait-and-watch approach is often warranted.[1,9,17] In contrast, treatment is typically reserved and indicated for patients with persistent neutropenia and regular transfusion dependency. Given the high risk of progression to MDS-EB in patients with RCC with monosomy 7 and/or a complex karyotype, more aggressive management may be pursued in such cases, even in the absence of the aforementioned clinical indications for intervention.

Hematopoietic stem cell transplant (SCT) is considered for every child with MDS in need of treatment and, therefore, HLA typing of patient and family members as soon as MDS diagnosis is confirmed is recommended[46]; in the absence of an available HLA-identical related or unrelated donor, unrelated cord blood transplant warrants consideration.[47] Historically, SCT using a myeloablative regimen has resulted in a probability of event-free survival of 75%, with transplant-related mortality being the major cause of treatment failure.[48] Reduced-intensity conditioning may be considered in patients with a hypocellular marrow and/or normal karyotype who still require intervention based on other parameters (eg, transfusion dependency).[46,49] Data for haploidentical SCT in pediatric patients with RCC remain limited, and thus this approach may be best reserved for patients enrolled in clinical trials and/or being managed at major centers with extensive experience in pediatric SCT.

Treatment of Advanced Myelodysplastic Syndrome

Allogeneic SCT remains the only curative treatment of patients with advanced pediatric MDS, although the selection of an appropriate pretransplant conditioning regimen is also a matter of ongoing debate. Although blast count reduction before SCT is desirable, chemotherapy is associated with significant toxicity.[1] Of note, conventional AML-type chemotherapy, without SCT, has been reported to have an associated survival rate of less than 30%.[50] Some studies have suggested that there may be no added value associated with the use of AML-type pre-SCT conditioning regimens in pediatric patients with MDS.[51] An increased risk of relapse post-SCT has been observed in patients with monosomal or complex karyotypes, as well as in patients with secondary AML arising out of an antecedent MDS, compared with those with MDS-EB or MDS-EB-t.[52]

SUMMARY

Pediatric MDS is a rare and challenging diagnosis. A definitive diagnosis frequently requires comprehensive ancillary testing and potentially repeat marrow sampling to exclude competing causes for persistent cytopenia in a pediatric patient, including several constitutional disorders that may be associated with similar clinicopathologic features. Although not diagnostic, targeted next-generation sequencing studies can often be helpful to interrogate for germline variants and somatic mutations, the latter of which have recently been found to constitute a profile that seems distinct from clonal hematopoiesis and MDS encountered in adults. Therapeutic decision making for pediatric patients with MDS can be equally challenging, and necessitates a multifactorial assessment of clinical and genetic status to balance the benefits of potentially curative interventions, such as allogeneic hematopoietic SCT, with their associated morbidity. Ongoing and future studies around pediatric MDS are likely to further explore the unique biological features of this class of diseases using cutting-edge molecular diagnostic techniques.

CLINICS CARE POINTS

- The most common causes of cytopenias in the pediatric age group include autoimmune syndromes, drug toxicities, and infectious causes.
- Pediatric MDS warrants consideration in patients presenting with cytopenias who have a known underlying genetic predisposition syndrome (eg, inherited bone marrow failure syndromes) or a history of antecedent chemotherapy for an unrelated malignancy.
- A bone marrow biopsy evaluation, and in many cases serial evaluations, may be required to render a definitive diagnosis.
- Comprehensive genetic testing is required for a definitive diagnosis, including conventional karyotyping and/or targeted FISH testing using an MDS-specific probe set.
- Targeted next-generation sequencing studies may be helpful to interrogate for the presence of germline mutations in key transcription factors (eg, *GATA2*) or somatic mutations in recurrently implicated genes (eg, RAS pathway).

REFERENCES

1. Locatelli F, Strahm B. How I treat myelodysplastic syndromes of childhood. Blood 2018;131(13):1406–14.

2. Glaubach T, Robinson LJ, Corey SJ. Pediatric myelodysplastic syndromes: they do exist! J Pediatr Hematol Oncol 2014;36(1):1–7.
3. Hasle H, Kerndrup G, Jacobsen BB. Childhood myelodysplastic syndrome in Denmark: incidence and predisposing conditions. Leukemia 1995;9(9):1569–72.
4. Niemeyer CM, Baumann I. Classification of childhood aplastic anemia and myelodysplastic syndrome. Hematol Am Soc Hematol Educ Program 2011; 2011:84–9.
5. Bader-Meunier B, Miélot F, Tchernia G, et al. Myelodysplastic syndromes in childhood: report of 49 patients from a French multicentre study. French Society of Paediatric Haematology and Immunology. Br J Haematol 1996;92(2):344–50.
6. Luna-Fineman S, Shannon KM, Atwater SK, et al. Myelodysplastic and myeloproliferative disorders of childhood: a study of 167 patients. Blood 1999;93(2): 459–66.
7. Mandel K, Dror Y, Poon A, et al. A practical, comprehensive classification for pediatric myelodysplastic syndromes: the CCC system. J Pediatr Hematol Oncol 2002;24(7):596–605.
8. Cada M, Segbefia CI, Klaassen R, et al. The impact of category, cytopathology and cytogenetics on development and progression of clonal and malignant myeloid transformation in inherited bone marrow failure syndromes. Haematologica 2015;100(5):633–42.
9. Kardos G, Baumann I, Passmore SJ, et al. Refractory anemia in childhood: a retrospective analysis of 67 patients with particular reference to monosomy 7. Blood 2003;102(6):1997–2003.
10. Gabreyes AA, Abbasi HN, Forbes KP, et al. Hypocupremia associated cytopenia and myelopathy: a national retrospective review. Eur J Haematol 2013;90(1):1–9.
11. Bowen DT. Occupational and environmental etiology of MDS. Best Pract Res Clin Haematol 2013;26(4):319–26.
12. Chisholm KM, Xu M, Davis B, et al. Evaluation of the utility of bone marrow morphology and ancillary studies in pediatric patients under surveillance for myelodysplastic syndrome. Am J Clin Pathol 2018;149(6):499–513.
13. Kussick SJ, Fromm JR, Rossini A, et al. Four-color flow cytometry shows strong concordance with bone marrow morphology and cytogenetics in the evaluation for myelodysplasia. Am J Clin Pathol 2005;124(2):170–81.
14. Kussick SJ, Wood BL. Using 4-color flow cytometry to identify abnormal myeloid populations. Arch Pathol Lab Med 2003;127(9):1140–7.
15. Wood BL. Myeloid malignancies: myelodysplastic syndromes, myeloproliferative disorders, and acute myeloid leukemia. Clin Lab Med 2007;27(3):551–75, vii.
16. Passmore SJ, Chessells JM, Kempski H, et al. Paediatric myelodysplastic syndromes and juvenile myelomonocytic leukaemia in the UK: a population-based study of incidence and survival. Br J Haematol 2003;121(5):758–67.
17. Hasegawa D, Chen X, Hirabayashi S, et al. Clinical characteristics and treatment outcome in 65 cases with refractory cytopenia of childhood defined according to the WHO 2008 classification. Br J Haematol 2014;166(5):758–66.
18. Baumann I, Führer M, Behrendt S, et al. Morphological differentiation of severe aplastic anaemia from hypocellular refractory cytopenia of childhood: reproducibility of histopathological diagnostic criteria. Histopathology 2012;61(1):10–7.
19. Swerdlow SH, Campo E, Harris NL, et al. WHO Classification of Tumours of haematopoietic and lymphoid tissues. Lyon: IARC. 2016.
20. Lee WY, Weinberg OK, Pinkus GS. GATA1 is a sensitive and specific nuclear marker for erythroid and megakaryocytic lineages. Am J Clin Pathol 2017; 147(4):420–6.

21. Shimamura A, Alter BP. Pathophysiology and management of inherited bone marrow failure syndromes. Blood Rev 2010;24(3):101–22.
22. Yoshimi A, Niemeyer C, Baumann I, et al. High incidence of Fanconi anaemia in patients with a morphological picture consistent with refractory cytopenia of childhood. Br J Haematol 2013;160(1):109–11.
23. Steliarova-Foucher E, Colombet M, Ries LAG, et al. International incidence of childhood cancer, 2001-10: a population-based registry study. Lancet Oncol 2017;18(6):719–31.
24. Kaatsch P. Epidemiology of childhood cancer. Cancer Treat Rev 2010;36(4): 277–85.
25. Schmiegelow K, Al-Modhwahi I, Andersen MK, et al. Methotrexate/6-mercaptopurine maintenance therapy influences the risk of a second malignant neoplasm after childhood acute lymphoblastic leukemia: results from the NOPHO ALL-92 study. Blood 2009;113(24):6077–84.
26. Le Deley M-C, Leblanc T, Shamsaldin A, et al. Risk of secondary leukemia after a solid tumor in childhood according to the dose of epipodophyllotoxins and anthracyclines: a case-control study by the Société Française d'Oncologie Pédiatrique. J Clin Oncol 2003;21(6):1074–81.
27. Pui CH, Ribeiro RC, Hancock ML, et al. Acute myeloid leukemia in children treated with epipodophyllotoxins for acute lymphoblastic leukemia. N Engl J Med 1991;325(24):1682–7.
28. Zhang MY, Churpek JE, Keel SB, et al. Germline ETV6 mutations in familial thrombocytopenia and hematologic malignancy. Nat Genet 2015;47(2):180–5.
29. Babushok DV, Bessler M, Olson TS. Genetic predisposition to myelodysplastic syndrome and acute myeloid leukemia in children and young adults. Leuk Lymphoma 2016;57(3):520–36.
30. Song WJ, Sullivan MG, Legare RD, et al. Haploinsufficiency of CBFA2 causes familial thrombocytopenia with propensity to develop acute myelogenous leukaemia. Nat Genet 1999;23(2):166–75.
31. Smith ML, Cavenagh JD, Lister TA, et al. Mutation of CEBPA in familial acute myeloid leukemia. N Engl J Med 2004;351(23):2403–7.
32. Noris P, Favier R, Alessi M-C, et al. ANKRD26-related thrombocytopenia and myeloid malignancies. Blood 2013;122(11):1987–9.
33. Wlodarski MW, Hirabayashi S, Pastor V, et al. Prevalence, clinical characteristics, and prognosis of GATA2-related myelodysplastic syndromes in children and adolescents. Blood 2016;127(11):1387–97 [quiz 1518].
34. Collin M, Dickinson R, Bigley V. Haematopoietic and immune defects associated with GATA2 mutation. Br J Haematol 2015;169(2):173–87.
35. Pastor V, Hirabayashi S, Karow A, et al. Mutational landscape in children with myelodysplastic syndromes is distinct from adults: specific somatic drivers and novel germline variants. Leukemia 2017;31(3):759–62.
36. Schwartz JR, Ma J, Lamprecht T, et al. The genomic landscape of pediatric myelodysplastic syndromes. Nat Commun 2017;8(1):1557.
37. Keel SB, Scott A, Sanchez-Bonilla M, et al. Genetic features of myelodysplastic syndrome and aplastic anemia in pediatric and young adult patients. Haematologica 2016;101(11):1343–50.
38. Papaemmanuil E, Cazzola M, Boultwood J, et al. Somatic SF3B1 mutation in myelodysplasia with ring sideroblasts. N Engl J Med 2011;365(15):1384–95.
39. Graubert TA, Shen D, Ding L, et al. Recurrent mutations in the U2AF1 splicing factor in myelodysplastic syndromes. Nat Genet 2011;44(1):53–7.

40. Haferlach T, Nagata Y, Grossmann V, et al. Landscape of genetic lesions in 944 patients with myelodysplastic syndromes. Leukemia 2014;28(2):241–7.
41. Yoshida K, Sanada M, Shiraishi Y, et al. Frequent pathway mutations of splicing machinery in myelodysplasia. Nature 2011;478(7367):64–9.
42. Makishima H, Yoshizato T, Yoshida K, et al. Dynamics of clonal evolution in myelodysplastic syndromes. Nat Genet 2017;49(2):204–12.
43. Hirabayashi S, Flotho C, Moetter J, et al. Spliceosomal gene aberrations are rare, coexist with oncogenic mutations, and are unlikely to exert a driver effect in childhood MDS and JMML. Blood 2012;119(11):e96–9.
44. Malcovati L, Papaemmanuil E, Ambaglio I, et al. Driver somatic mutations identify distinct disease entities within myeloid neoplasms with myelodysplasia. Blood 2014;124(9):1513–21.
45. Collord G, Park N, Podestà M, et al. Clonal haematopoiesis is not prevalent in survivors of childhood cancer. Br J Haematol 2018;181(4):537–9.
46. Strahm B, Locatelli F, Bader P, et al. Reduced intensity conditioning in unrelated donor transplantation for refractory cytopenia in childhood. Bone Marrow Transpl 2007;40(4):329–33.
47. Madureira ABM, Eapen M, Locatelli F, et al. Analysis of risk factors influencing outcome in children with myelodysplastic syndrome after unrelated cord blood transplantation. Leukemia 2011;25(3):449–54.
48. Starý J, Locatelli F, Niemeyer CM. European working group on myelodysplastic syndrome (EWOG-MDS) and pediatric diseases working party of the EBMT. Stem cell transplantation for aplastic anemia and myelodysplastic syndrome. Bone Marrow Transpl 2005;35(Suppl 1):S13–6.
49. Inagaki J, Fukano R, Kurauchi K, et al. Hematopoietic stem cell transplantation in children with refractory cytopenia of childhood: single-center experience using high-dose cytarabine containing myeloablative and aplastic anemia oriented reduced-intensity conditioning regimens. Biol Blood Marrow Transpl 2015;21(3):565–9.
50. Woods WG, Barnard DR, Alonzo TA, et al. Prospective study of 90 children requiring treatment for juvenile myelomonocytic leukemia or myelodysplastic syndrome: a report from the Children's Cancer Group. J Clin Oncol 2002;20(2):434–40.
51. Strahm B, Nöllke P, Zecca M, et al. Hematopoietic stem cell transplantation for advanced myelodysplastic syndrome in children: results of the EWOG-MDS 98 study. Leukemia 2011;25(3):455–62.
52. Göhring G, Michalova K, Beverloo HB, et al. Complex karyotype newly defined: the strongest prognostic factor in advanced childhood myelodysplastic syndrome. Blood 2010;116(19):3766–9.

Pediatric Myeloproliferative Neoplasms

Farah El-Sharkawy, MD[a], Elizabeth Margolskee, MD, MPH[a,b,*]

KEYWORDS

- Myeloproliferative neoplasms • Pediatrics • Polycythemia vera
- Essential thrombocythemia • Primary myelofibrosis • Chronic myeloid leukemia

KEY POINTS

- Although rare, myeloproliferative neoplasms can affect young children and present unique diagnostic and therapeutic challenges.
- The criteria used to establish a diagnosis of myeloproliferative neoplasm were established in adults and thus it is unclear how to apply them in the pediatric setting.
- In young patients, the differential diagnosis may include familial or germline disorders, which may not be a consideration in older individuals with a history of normal complete blood counts.

Myeloproliferative neoplasms (MPNs) are clonal hematopoietic stem cell disorders characterized by hyperproliferation of the myeloid lineages. The annual incidence in adults is low, with approximately 6 per 100,000 individuals. Typically, the onset of MPN is in the fifth to seventh decade of life, but, rarely, these diseases can occur in the pediatric setting. Because of the rarity of pediatric MPNs, little is known about the natural history, pathology, and molecular features of these cases. Depending on the practice setting, pediatric hematologists may not be familiar with the diagnosis of pediatric MPNs according to current World Health Organization (WHO) criteria; in these situations, hematopathologists can be a useful resource for their clinical colleagues.

In the 1950s, William Dameshek[1] described 4 myeloproliferative disorders based primarily on their clinical presentation and bone marrow morphology: chronic myeloid leukemia, polycythemia vera (PV), essential thrombocythemia (ET), and primary myelofibrosis (PMF).[1,2] Over the ensuing decades, a proliferation of molecular data showed the clonal nature of these MPNs and transformed classification of these

The authors have nothing to disclose.

[a] Department of Pathology and Laboratory Medicine, Hospital of the University of Pennsylvania, Philadelphia, PA, USA; [b] Department of Pathology and Laboratory Medicine, Children's Hospital of Philadelphia, Philadelphia, PA, USA

* Corresponding author. Department of Pathology and Laboratory Medicine, Hospital of the University of Pennsylvania, Philadelphia, PA.

E-mail address: margolskee@chop.edu

Twitter: @bethmcm (E.M.)

Clin Lab Med 41 (2021) 529–540

https://doi.org/10.1016/j.cll.2021.04.010

neoplasms into an integrated process incorporating clinical, laboratory, morphologic, and molecular findings. In the 1960s and 1970s, the Philadelphia (Ph) chromosome with fusion of BCR and ABL1 was identified as the driver of chronic myeloid leukemia (CML).[3,4] At the turn of the twenty-first century, imatinib was developed as a targeted therapeutic for patients with CML. The *JAK2* V617F mutation was identified as a driver mutation in MPN in 2005, followed subsequently by the discovery of *MPL* and *CALR* mutations.[5–7] These driver mutations now play a critical role in the diagnosis and classification of MPN; in patients with CML, BCR-ABL1 transcripts are used as a marker of disease burden.

This article reviews the 4 major myeloproliferative neoplasms using the diagnostic criteria published in the 2016 WHO update, with attention to unique considerations for pediatric patients. Pediatricians are fond of saying that children are not just tiny adults. Therefore, is it appropriate to apply the diagnostic criteria used in adults to pediatric MPN? Is the natural history of pediatric MPN identical to adult MPN? Can the same therapeutic modalities be used in a growing young person? Data on pediatric MPN are limited. They consist primarily of large decentralized meta-analyses and small case reports. Thus, it is possible that this article raises as many questions about the diagnosis of pediatric MPN as it answers.

ESSENTIAL THROMBOCYTHEMIA

ET is a megakaryocytic proliferation that results in sustained thrombocytosis. The WHO lists a series of major and minor criteria; establishing the diagnosis requires the presence of either all 4 major criteria or the first 3 major criteria plus the 2 minor criteria (**Table 1**). ET is the second most common MPN in adults, with a median age at diagnosis of 60 years and an incidence of 0.5 to 2 cases per 100,000 individuals. The annual incidence of ET among children is low, approximately 1 case in 10 million.[8] Adults typically present when thrombocytosis is noted on routine blood work, but, if symptomatic, they may have headache or splenomegaly. Rarely, thromboembolic or hemorrhagic events may be a heralding event in adults with ET; however, this is virtually never seen in children. For children with ET, 50% are asymptomatic at the time of presentation. Headache, bone pain, and splenomegaly are the most common symptoms for children.[9]

In general, reactive processes are the most common cause of thrombocytosis in both adults and children. Iron deficiency, hemolysis, infection, inflammation, and malignancy can all cause the platelet count to increase. However, if primary thrombocytosis is suspected, the differential diagnosis for adults and children is different. In adults, ET or another myeloid neoplasm would be the most likely diagnosis. In children

Table 1
Diagnostic criteria for essential thrombocythemia

Major Criteria	Minor Criteria
Platelet count > 450 × 10^9/L	Presence of a clonal marker
Biopsy showing proliferation of megakaryocytes that appear enlarged with hyperlobulated nuclei. No significant increase in granulopoiesis or erythropoiesis	Exclusion of a reactive thrombocytosis
Exclusion of other myeloid neoplasms	—
Presence of a *JAK2*, *CALR*, or *MPL* mutation	—

Table 2
Genes implicated in familial thrombocytosis

Gene	Mutation	
THPO	5′ untranslated region or splice sites	Increased thrombopoietin production
MPL	S505N, K39N, P106L	Constitutive activation of thrombopoietin receptor[50]
JAK2	Non-V617F mutation	—

and infants, familial thrombocytosis is much more common than acquisition of a sporadic thrombocytosis. The most commonly mutated genes are listed in **Table 2**.

In patients with ET, the bone marrow is typically normocellular for the patient's age, although it may be slightly hypercellular. There is typically a proliferation of megakaryocytes with atypical morphology. They may appear large with abundant cytoplasm and hypersegmented or stag-horn nuclei. Loose clusters may be seen (**Fig. 1**). The myeloid/erythroid (M/E) ratio is normal, with absence of dysplasia. Fibrosis is minimal. Stainable iron is present.[10] In the pediatric setting, distinguishing normocellular marrow from hypercellular can be difficult; at baseline, children typically have greater than 80% cellularity.

To complete the diagnostic work-up, genetic testing is strongly recommended. Because the differential diagnosis may include CML, fluorescence in situ hybridization for *BCR-ABL1* rearrangement must be performed. Next-generation sequencing to identify a driver mutation in *JAK2*, *CALR*, or *MPL* is helpful to establish clonality. In adults, driver mutations are found in 90% of cases of ET; the remaining 10% (so-called triple-negative ET) are associated with a favorable prognosis.[9] In pediatric ET, 57% of cases are triple negative. Mutations in *JAK2*, *CALR*, and *MPL* are seen in 31%, 10%, and 2% of cases, respectively. The genetic landscape of adult ET includes mutations in genes associated with epigenetic regulation, such as *ASXL1*, *TET2*, *DNMT3a*, and *EZH2*, but these mutations are rare in the pediatric setting.[11]

As in the adult setting, the long-term outlook for children diagnosed with ET is favorable. In the pediatric setting, the 10-year risk of thrombotic events or myelofibrosis was less than 10%.[9] No children progressed to blast phase. The risk of miscarriage was equivalent to the general population.

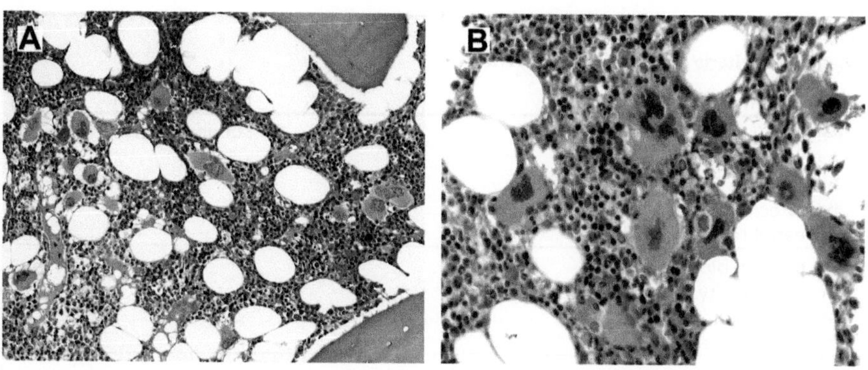

Fig. 1. Bone marrow of patients with ET.

POLYCYTHEMIA VERA

PV is characterized by increased, uncontrolled red blood cell production. Among patients diagnosed with PV, 0.1% are less than 20 years old.[12] Among children, the most common presentation is headache, although a substantial number are diagnosed after experiencing thrombotic complications (e.g. Budd-Chiari syndrome), which can be seen up to 20% of children with PV. Stroke and bleeding complications can also be seen.[13]

According to the WHO, the diagnosis requires 3 major criteria or the first 2 major criteria plus the minor criterion (**Table 3**). The WHO criteria were developed with adults in mind, not children, leading some investigators to question the applicability to pediatrics.[14,15] The cutoffs for erythrocytosis in men and women were originally derived using normal reference ranges for hemoglobin, with those beyond the 99th percentile being worrisome for PV. The identification of masked PV recently led the WHO to lower hemoglobin thresholds further to 16.5 and 16 g/dL.[16] However, applying the same logic to pediatrics suggests an even lower threshold is appropriate for this age group, because the normal hemoglobin range for children less than 12 years old is 10.5 to 13.5 g/dL. Use of red blood cell mass testing in children is infrequent. The value of erythropoietin (EPO) levels in establishing a diagnosis of pediatric PV is also unclear, because normal EPO levels can be seen in this setting.[13] *JAK2* mutations are also less common in children with polycythemia vera, seen in 25% to 37% of cases.[15]

Bone marrow biopsy typically shows a hypercellular marrow with increased trilineage hematopoiesis (panmyelosis) (**Fig. 2**). The megakaryocytes are increased and appear pleomorphic. Iron stains show absence of storage iron. Although it is easy to assess hypercellularity in older adults, who are expected to have cellularity of less than 50% depending on age, in a child less than 20 years of age, a marrow is expected to be 80% to 90% cellular. Thus, applying the morphologic criteria in children relies much more heavily on megakaryocytic morphology than assessment of marrow cellularity.

As in ET, the differential diagnosis of polycythemia in children includes congenital disorders. Congenital polycythemia is typically identified on routine bloodwork; these patients do not have organomegaly, thrombosis, and hemorrhage as can be seen in PV. Primary familial and congenital polycythemia are associated with highly variable mutations in *EPOR*, the EPO receptor, which may be intronic or exonic.[17,18] Congenital causes of secondary polycythemia can be divided into variants causing high oxygen affinity of hemoglobin and variants affecting oxygen-sensing pathway proteins.

Table 3
Diagnostic criteria for polycythemia vera

Major Criteria	Minor Criterion
Hemoglobin >16.5 g/dL or hematocrit >49% (men), hemoglobin >16 g/dL or hematocrit >48% (women), or increased red blood cell mass	Subnormal erythropoietin level
Bone marrow biopsy showing hypercellularity with panmyelosis and increased, pleomorphic megakaryocytes	—
Presence of JAK2 mutation	—

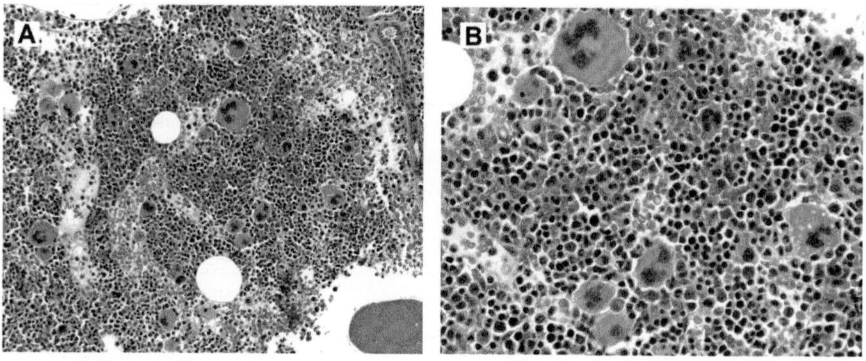

Fig. 2. Bone marrow biopsy typically shows a hypercellular marrow with increased trilineage hematopoiesis (panmyelosis).

The first group includes high-affinity hemoglobin variants, congenital methemoglobinemia, and mutations in 2,3-bisphosphoglyceric acid (2,3-BPG).[19] The second includes mutations in *VHL* (Chuvash polycythemia) and *PHD2*.[20,21]

For adults, the median overall survival for patients with PV is 13 years. Patients may experience thrombotic complications, second malignancies, or progression of disease to myelofibrosis or acute myeloid leukemia (AML). In children, the long-term life expectancy is essentially unknown. One recent series showed that the 10-year risk of complications is low, with only 5% of patients developing thrombosis and none having progression of PV.[22] A meta-analysis of European patients found a mortality of 0.65%, but the sample size was small.[9] Treatment options include phlebotomy and hydroxyurea. Pegylated interferon, which is widely used in adults, may also be an option for young patients.[23]

PRIMARY MYELOFIBROSIS

PMF is a proliferation of megakaryocytes and granulocytes in the bone marrow associated with the deposition of fibrous connective tissue. To establish the diagnosis of PMF, a patient must fulfill all major and 1 minor criterion, as specified by the WHO (**Table 4**). Of the 3 MPNs discussed in this article, PMF is the least common among adults and it is vanishingly rare in children. The median age at presentation is 70 years, with only 10% of cases presenting before age 45 years.[24] Almost all information about pediatric PMF derives from a few case series and case reports. The 3 largest case series are described later; all looked at clinical and pathologic characteristics but only 1 study used more extensive sequencing to show clonality.[25]

In 1 case series, DeLario and colleagues[26] described 19 children with PMF with a median age of 14 months. These children typically presented with hepatosplenomegaly and anemia. Biopsy showed hypercellular marrow with frequent dysmegakaryopoiesis, eosinophilia, and MF2 to MF3 fibrosis. All were negative for *JAK2* and *MPL* mutations, and several families in the study were consanguineous, raising the possibility of an unidentified autosomal recessive genetic disorder. Interestingly, 5 children with normal karyotype had a spontaneous resolution, which is distinct from adult PMF, where fibrosis is typically stable. A subsequent study from a Chinese group described 14 patients (median age, 13.5 years) who presented with anemia and thrombocytopenia, and who were diagnosed with PMF.[25] Bone marrow examination showed megakaryocytic hyperplasia and MF2 to MF3 fibrosis.[27] Similar to the prior study,

Table 4
Diagnostic criteria for primary myelofibrosis

Major Criteria	Minor Criteria
Megakaryocytic proliferation and atypia and/or grade 2+ fibrosis	Anemia
Exclusion of other myeloid neoplasms	Leukocytosis
Presence of *JAK2, CALR,* or *MPL* mutation; evidence of clonality; or absence of reactive myelofibrosis	Splenomegaly Leukoerythroblastosis
—	Increased lactate dehydrogenase level

the megakaryocytes appeared small and hypolobated. Hypocellular marrows were seen in 8 of their patients. Six of these patients progressed to AML and the remaining 9 have stable or improving disease. Because type II *CALR* mutations (5-base-pair TTGC insertion) were identified in 7 patients and 7 had no evidence of clonality, they stratified the patients by *CALR* mutation status and found no statistically significant differences in patient characteristics, survival, or leukemia-free survival.

In a recent study of 15 cases of pediatric myelofibrosis from 2020, the median age was 6 years.[28] Symptomatic anemia was seen in 14, and thrombocytopenia in 10. Bone marrow biopsy typically showed hypercellularity, granulocytic predominance, and MF2 to MF3 fibrosis. Small, dysplastic megakaryocytes were seen in 8 of the 15 patients. Three patients showed megakaryocytic clustering. The typical morphologic features seen in adult PMF (hyperchromasia, dense clusters) were notably absent. Only 1 patient had evidence of clonality (trisomy 8 and JAK2 V617F mutation), but only karyotype and selected sequencing studies were performed on these patients. Follow-up was limited, but 1 child received a hematopoietic stem cell transplant and 1 patient had spontaneous resolution of disease. The remaining 13 received supportive care.

Most cases of myelofibrosis in children are secondary. In a study of 214 children with secondary myelofibrosis, oncologic causes were identified in 147 patients. Other underlying diseases identified in this study included aplastic anemia, hemophagocytic lymphohistiocytosis, autoimmune disorders, and common variable immunodeficiency.[29] With respect to primary bone marrow disorders, the differential diagnosis could include other myeloid neoplasms associated with fibrosis, particularly myelodysplastic syndrome with fibrosis (MDS-F). The megakaryocytes in MDS-F are typically small with nuclear hypolobation. The bone marrow typically shows erythroid predominance, in contrast with the increased granulopoiesis seen in PMF. In very young children, germline disorders resulting in myelofibrosis must be excluded. Case reports describing a PMF-like picture have been linked to mutations in *CDC42* and *VPS45*, but this list will almost certainly grow as next-generation sequencing studies become standard of care.[30,31]

To summarize the 3 case series described earlier, pediatric PMF typically presents with symptomatic anemia and thrombocytopenia. Leukoerythroblastosis is rare, but splenomegaly is seen in more than half of cases. On bone marrow examination, megakaryocytic hyperplasia, increased M/E ratio, hypercellularity, and MF2 to MF3 fibrosis are seen. The megakaryocytes are typically small and hypolobated, not clustered with nuclear hyperchromasia and bare nuclei (**Fig. 3**). To date, type II *CALR* mutation and *JAK2* V617F mutations have been identified, but typically *JAK2*, *MPL*, and *CALR* are

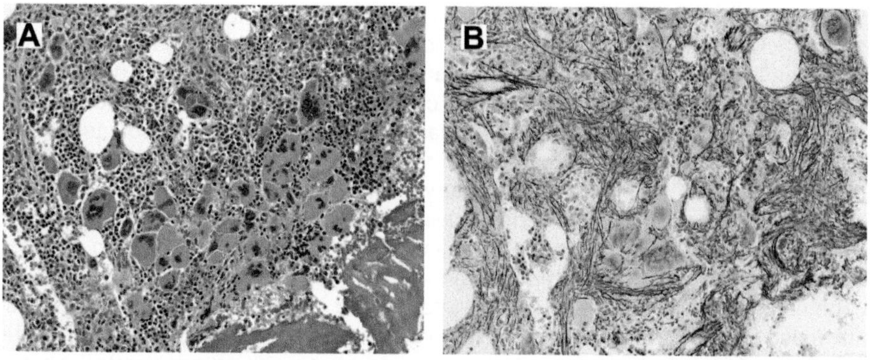

Fig. 3. Bone marrow examination showing megakaryocytic hyperplasia, increased M/E ratio, hypercellularity, and MF2 to MF3 fibrosis.

wild-type in this setting. Progression to AML is rare, and occasionally patients have spontaneous resolution of disease.

Clearly, pediatric and adult PMF differ with respect to genetic background, morphologic features, and clinical course, raising the question of whether and how the criteria used to define disease in adults ought to be applied in the pediatric setting. For example, reference ranges for lactate dehydrogenase vary by age and sex (**Table 5**); values that are increased in adults may be age appropriate in children. Thus, it is important that a laboratory uses age-specific and sex-specific reference ranges. In addition, given the overall low prevalence of *JAK2*, *MPL*, and *CALR* mutation in pediatric PMF, next-generation sequencing panels are more likely to be informative than sequencing studies of specific genes.

CHRONIC MYELOID LEUKEMIA

CML is a myeloproliferative neoplasm characterized by increased proliferation of the granulocytic cell line. It is defined by the presence of the chromosomal translocation

Table 5
Reference ranges for lactate dehydrogenase

Age (y)	Male/Female (U/L)	—
4–6	470–900	—
7–9	420–750	—
Age (y)	**Male**	**Female**
10–11	432–700	380–770
12–13	470–750	380–640
14–15	360–730	390–580
16–18	340–670	340–670
>19 y	313–618	313–618

Adapted from Gregory, G. A., & Andropoulos, D. B. (2012). Gregory's Pediatric Anesthesia. In G. A. Gregory & D. B. Andropoulos (Eds.), *Gregory's Pediatric Anesthesia: Fifth Edition*. Wiley-Blackwell. https://doi.org/10.1002/9781444345186.[49]

t(9;22)(q34.1;q11.2), which gives rise to the Ph chromosome and the BCR-ABL1 fusion gene.[32,33] The annual incidence of CML increases with age, ranging from 1.4 cases per million in children younger than 15 years, to 2.1 cases per million in adolescents 15 to 19 years of age, and greater than 25 cases per million in elderly individuals.[33,34] Similarly, CML constitutes 15% of leukemias in adults,[35] whereas it accounts for only 2% to 3% of leukemias in children younger than 15 years and 9% in adolescents 15 to 19 years of age.[34,36] An international registry (I-CML-Ped [International CML Pediatric] Study) that included 351 children and adolescents less than 18 years of age with newly diagnosed CML showed that the median age at diagnosis in pediatric CML is 12.4 years with a slight male preponderance.[37]

The natural history of CML is divided into chronic, accelerated, and blast phases, with most patients presenting in the chronic phase.[33,37] According to the I-CML-Ped Study, 92% of children present in chronic phase, 8% in accelerated phase, and 1% in blast phase.[37] In the chronic phase of CML, there is expansion of the myeloid cell line without dysplasia in the peripheral blood (leukocytosis) and the bone marrow. Granulocytes in various stages of maturation are seen, especially myelocytes (so-called myelocyte bulge) and segmented neutrophils. Absolute basophilia and eosinophilia are common. Monocyte levels can also be increased. By definition, blasts are less than 10%. Megakaryocytes in the bone marrow may be normal or increased in number; they are small and display hypolobated nuclei (dwarf megakaryocytes).[33]

The accelerated phase of CML is defined by the presence of any of the following parameters: 10% to 19% blasts in the peripheral blood or bone marrow, persistent or increasing white blood cell (WBC) count ($>10 \times 10^9$/L), persistent or increasing splenomegaly, basophils greater than or equal to 20% in peripheral blood, persistent thrombocytosis ($>1000 \times 10^9$/L), unresponsive to therapy, persistent thrombocytopenia ($<100 \times 10^9$/L) unrelated to therapy, any new clonal abnormality, or additional clonal abnormalities in Ph+ cells. In addition, the bone marrow can show clusters of small megakaryocytes associated with significant fibrosis.[33,38]

The blast phase of CML is defined by greater than or equal to 20% blasts in the peripheral blood or bone marrow, or by the presence of an extramedullary blast proliferation.[33] The most common extramedullary sites are the lymph nodes, spleen, skin, bone, and central nervous system. In adults, blasts are most commonly of the myeloid lineage (60%–80% of cases).[39] In contrast, most pediatric patients who progress to blast phase (62%), or present in de novo blast phase (76%), have lymphoid blasts.[40,41] Therefore, the *de novo* lymphoid blast phase of CML can be difficult to distinguish from Ph+ acute lymphoblastic leukemia (ALL).

The differential diagnosis of CML in children includes leukemoid reaction, juvenile myelomonocytic leukemia (JMML), and other myeloproliferative neoplasms. Leukemoid reaction is a benign acute response to an underlying disorder, usually infectious, and is defined as WBC count greater than 30×10^9/L in some studies or greater than 50×10^9/L in others.[42,43] In children, the most common cause of leukemoid reaction is pneumonia.[42] Leukemoid reaction differs from CML by the absence of basophilia, eosinophilia, and the myelocyte bulge, and by the presence of toxic granulations and Döhle bodies in granulocytes.[44] JMML is most commonly diagnosed in infants and children younger than 6 years. It is characterized by a proliferation of the granulocytic and monocytic lineages. Blasts (including promonocytes) are less than 20%. Common symptoms include fever, rash, hepatosplenomegaly, lymphadenopathy, and cough. Genetic alterations in the RAS signaling pathway (in particular *PTPN11*, *NRAS*, *KRAS*, *CBL*, and *NF1*), are identified in up to 85% of children with JMML, whereas the t(9;22) chromosomal translocation is always absent.[33,45]

Recent studies have found several differences between pediatric and adult CML. Similar to adults, most pediatric patients are diagnosed in the chronic phase. However, the proportion of pediatric patients that present with advanced-stage disease (accelerated or blast phases) is overall higher than for adults.[33,34] Common findings at presentation both in children and adults include fatigue, splenomegaly, weight loss, anemia, and leukocytosis.[33,46] However, children tend to present with a higher leukocyte count (median, 242 $\times$ 10^9/L) than adults (median, 12–174 $\times$ 10^9/L)[33] and have a proportionally larger spleen (median, 11 cm).[37] Taken together, these findings suggest that pediatric patients tend to present with more aggressive disease. On the genetic level, studies have shown that breakpoint distribution in the *BCR* gene is different in pediatric CML compared with adult CML, and is similar to the pattern observed in adult ALL with BCR-ABL1 rearrangement.[33,34,47] In addition, the frequency of *ASXL1* mutations is significantly higher in pediatric patients than in adults.[48]

SUMMARY

In this article, the clinicopathologic features of childhood ET, PV, PMF, and CML are reviewed. MPNs are rare in the pediatric population; pediatric hematologists and hematopathologists only rarely encounter these patients. When evaluating these patients, it is important to keep in mind that the data in this area remain limited. Should clinicians apply the same diagnostic criteria developed in adults? Can they use the same drugs on these patients? Should they assume the same long-term prognosis? Close collaboration with clinicians and molecular pathologists is critical for these patients. Some experts have recommended using the diagnosis of MPN, unclassified, for a subset of young patients with MPN where there is clear evidence of neoplasm but subclassification remains difficult.[14] It is hoped that future studies will aid in the diagnosis and treatment of these patients.

REFERENCES

1. Dameshek W. Editorial some speculations on the myeloproliferative syndromes. Blood 1951;6(4):372–5.
2. Tefferi A. The history of myeloproliferative disorders: before and after dameshek. Leukemia 2008;22(1):3–13.
3. Rowley JD. A new consistent chromosomal abnormality in chronic myelogenous leukaemia identified by quinacrine fluorescence and Giemsa staining. Nature 1973;243(5405):290–3.
4. Shtivelman E, Lifshitz B, Gale RP, et al. Fused transcript of ABL and BCR genes in chronic myelogenous leukaemia. Nature 1985;315(6020):550–4.
5. Kralovics R, Passamonti F, Buser AS, et al. A gain-of-function mutation of JAK2 in myeloproliferative disorders. N Engl J Med 2005;352(17):1779–90.
6. Milosevic Feenstra JD, Nivarthi H, Gisslinger H, et al. Whole-exome sequencing identifies novel MPL and JAK2 mutations in triple-negative myeloproliferative neoplasms. Blood 2016;127(3):325–32.
7. Nangalia J, Massie CE, Baxter EJ, et al. Somatic CALR Mutations in myeloproliferative neoplasms with nonmutated JAK2. N Engl J Med 2013;369(25):2391–405.
8. Hasle H. Incidence of essential thrombocythaemia in children. Br J Haematol 2000;110(3):751.

9. Ianotto JC, Curto-Garcia N, Lauermanova M, et al. Characteristics and outcomes of patients with essential thrombocythemia or polycythemia vera diagnosed before 20 years of age: a systematic review. Haematologica 2019;104(8):1580–8.
10. Putti MC, Pizzi M, Bertozzi I, et al. Bone marrow histology for the diagnosis of essential thrombocythemia in children: a multicenter Italian study. Blood 2017; 129(22):3040–2.
11. Randi ML, Geranio G, Bertozzi I, et al. Are all cases of paediatric essential thrombocythaemia really myeloproliferative neoplasms? Analysis of a large cohort. Br J Haematol 2015;169(4):584–9.
12. Osgood E. Polycythemia vera: age relationship and survival. Blood 1965;26: 243–56.
13. Cario H, McMullin MF, Pahl HL. Clinical and hematological presentation of children and adolescents with polycythemia vera. Ann Hematol 2009;88(8):713–9.
14. Kucine N, Al-Kawaaz M, Hajje D, et al. Difficulty distinguishing essential thrombocythaemia from polycythaemia vera in children with JAK2 V617F-positive myeloproliferative neoplasms. Br J Haematol 2019a;185(1):136–9.
15. Teofili L, Giona F, Martini M, et al. The revised WHO diagnostic criteria for Ph-negative myeloproliferative diseases are not appropriate for the diagnostic screening of childhood polycythemia vera and essential thrombocythemia. Blood 2007;110(9):3384–6.
16. Barbui T, Thiele J, Gisslinger H, et al. Masked polycythemia vera (mPV): results of an international study. Am J Hematol 2014;89(1):52–4.
17. Al-Sheikh M, Mazurier E, Gardie B, et al. A study of 36 unrelated cases with pure erythrocytosis revealed three new mutations in the erythropoietin receptor gene. Haematologica 2008;93(7):1072–5.
18. Rives S, Pahl HL, Florensa L, et al. Molecular genetic analyses in familial and sporadic congenital primary erythrocytosis. Haematologica 2007;92(5):674–7.
19. Soliman DS, Yassin M. Congenital methemoglobinemia misdiagnosed as polycythemia vera: case report and review of literature. Hematol Rep 2018;10(1):7–10.
20. Lanikova L, Lorenzo F, Yang C, et al. Novel homozygous VHL mutation in exon 2 is associated with congenital polycythemia but not with cancer. Blood 2013; 121(19):3918–24.
21. Percy MJ, Furlow PW, Beer PA, et al. A novel erythrocytosis-associated PHD2 mutation suggests the location of a HIF binding groove. Blood 2007;110(6):2193–6.
22. Giona F, Teofili L, Moleti ML, et al. Thrombocythemia and polycythemia in patients younger than 20 years at diagnosis: clinical and biologic features, treatment, and long-term outcome. Blood 2012;119(10):2219–27.
23. Kucine N, Bergmann S, Krichevsky S, et al. Use of pegylated interferon in six pediatric patients with myeloproliferative neoplasms. Blood 2019b; 134(Supplement_1):4194.
24. Hofmann I. Myeloproliferative neoplasms in children. J Hematopathol 2015;8(3): 143–57.
25. An W, Wan Y, Guo Y, et al. CALR mutation screening in pediatric primary myelofibrosis. Pediatr Blood Cancer 2014;61(12):2256–62.
26. Delario MR, Sheehan AM, Ataya R, et al. Clinical, histopathologic, and genetic features of pediatric primary myelofibrosis-an entity different from adults. Am J Hematol 2012;87(5):461–4.
27. Thiele J, Kvasnicka HM, Facchetti F, et al. European consensus on grading bone marrow fibrosis and assessment of cellularity. Haematologica 2005;90(8): 1128–32.

28. Mishra P, Halder R, Aggarwal M, et al. Pediatric myelofibrosis: WHO 2024 update on myeloproliferative neoplasms calling? Pediatr Blood Cancer 2020;67(5): e28232.
29. Soundar EP, Berger D, Marcogliese A, et al. Secondary bone marrow fibrosis in children and young adults: an institutional experience. J Pediatr Hematol Oncol 2016;38(2):97–101.
30. Verboon JM, Mahmut D, Kim AR, et al. Infantile myelofibrosis and myeloproliferation with CDC42 dysfunction. J Clin Immunol 2020;40(4):554–66.
31. Vilboux T, Lev A, Malicdan MCV, et al. A congenital neutrophil defect syndrome associated with mutations in VPS45. N Engl J Med 2013;369(1):54–65.
32. Nowell C. The minute chromosome (Ph1) in chronic granulocytic leukemia. Blut 1962;8(2):65–6.
33. Swerdlow SH, Campo E, Harris NL, et al. WHO classification of tumours of haematopoietic and lymphoid tissues. Revised 4th Edition. International Agency for Research on Cancer; 2017.
34. Hijiya N, Schultz KR, Metzler M, et al. Pediatric chronic myeloid leukemia is a unique disease that requires a different approach. Blood 2016;127(4):392–9.
35. Deininger MW, Shah NP, Altman JK, et al. Chronic myeloid leukemia, version 2.2021. J Natl Compr Canc Netw 2020;18(10):1385–415.
36. Madabhavi I, Patel A, Modi G, et al. Pediatric chronic myeloid leukemia: a single-center experience. J Cancer Res Ther 2020;16(1):110.
37. Millot F, Guilhot J, Suttorp M, et al. The experience of the international registry for chronic myeloid leukemia (CML) in children and adolescents (I-CML-Ped Study): pronostic consideration. Blood 2014;124(21):521.
38. Athale U, Hijiya N, Patterson BC, et al. Management of chronic myeloid leukemia in children and adolescents: recommendations from the children's oncology group CML working group. Pediatr Blood Cancer 2019;66(9):1–23.
39. Silver RT. The blast phase of chronic myeloid leukaemia. Best Pract Res Clin Haematol 2009;22(3):387–94.
40. Meyran D, Petit A, Guilhot J, et al. Description and management of accelerated phase and blast crisis in 21 cml pediatric patients. Blood 2015;126(23):2789.
41. Millot F, Maledon N, Guilhot J, et al. Favourable outcome of de novo advanced phases of childhood chronic myeloid leukaemia. Eur J Cancer 2019;115:17–23.
42. Hoofien A, Yarden-Bilavski H, Ashkenazi S, et al. Leukemoid reaction in the pediatric population: etiologies, outcome, and implications. Eur J Pediatr 2018;177(7): 1029–36.
43. Potasman I, Grupper M. Leukemoid reaction: spectrum and prognosis of 173 adult patients. Clin Infect Dis 2013;57(11):e177–81.
44. Marionneaux S. Nonmalignant leukocyte disorders. In: Rodak's hematology. Elsevier; 2020. p. 445–65. https://doi.org/10.1016/B978-0-323-53045-3.00035-0.
45. Emanuel PD. Juvenile myelomonocytic leukemia and chronic myelomonocytic leukemia. Leukemia 2008;22(7):1335–42.
46. Millot F, Traore P, Guilhot J, et al. Clinical and biological features at diagnosis in 40 children with chronic myeloid leukemia. Pediatrics 2005;116(1):140–3.
47. Krumbholz M, Karl M, Tauer JT, et al. Genomic BCR-ABL1 breakpoints in pediatric chronic myeloid leukemia. Genes Chromosomes Cancer 2012;51(11): 1045–53.
48. Ernst T, Busch M, Rinke J, et al. Frequent ASXL1 mutations in children and young adults with chronic myeloid leukemia. Leukemia 2018;32(9):2046–9.

49. Gregory GA, Andropoulos DB. Gregory's pediatric anesthesia. In: Gregory GA, Andropoulos DB, editors. Gregory's pediatric anesthesia. Fifth Edition. Wiley-Blackwell; 2012. https://doi.org/10.1002/9781444345186.
50. Plo I, Bellanne-Chantelot C, Mosca M, et al. Genetic Alterations of the Thrombepoietic/MPL/JAK2 Axis Impacting Megakaryopoiesis. Front Endocrinol (Lausanne) 2017;8:234.

Infant Acute Leukemia

Gerald Wertheim, MD, PhD

KEYWORDS

• Acute leukemia • Infants • Transient myelopoiesis of Down syndrome
• Acute megakaryoblastic leukemia

KEY POINTS

- Infant acute leukemia is a rare yet aggressive disease
- Rearrangements in KMT2A are the most common genetic abnormality in infant leukemia
- Megakaryoblastic differentiation is common in infant AML
- Treatment of infant acute leukemia is challenging, and protocols are specifically tailored for these patients
- Transient abnormal myelopoiesis frequently occurs in neonates with Down syndrome, universally harbors a truncating *GATA1* mutation, and is cytologically indistinguishable from AML.

Leukemia arising in the first year of life is generally referred to as infant leukemia.[1] Although these age-defined malignancies are rare, infant leukemias are distinct from their counterparts arising in older children both in clinical characteristics and in the underlying biology that drives tumorigenesis.[2] As with all leukemia, those that arise in infants are subdivided into those that exhibit a hematopoietic maturation arrest and an expansion of blasts (ie, acute leukemia) and those characterized by an expansion of mature elements. Of the infant leukemias in the latter subcategory, juvenile myelomonocytic leukemia (JMML) and the related myeloproliferations associated with congenital syndromes are the most notable; mature lymphoid neoplasms and other chronic myeloid neoplasms are almost nonexistent.[3] These chronic processes, including JMML, are covered elsewhere in this issue. Acute leukemias are by far more common in infants than their chronic counterparts. Although classifying acute leukemia as acute lymphoblastic leukemia (ALL) or acute myeloblastic leukemia (AML) is currently used for treatment and as a criterion for clinical trial enrollment, this distinction may not be as biologically relevant for infants as it is for older patients. Many infant acute leukemias show similar genetic alterations with either lymphoid or myeloid differentiation, frequently undergo a phenotypic switch upon treatment and often arise as either a mixed phenotype acute leukemia or an acute undifferentiated leukemia.[1,2,4] These features point to an underlying pathologic mechanism in infant leukemia in which

Dr G. Wertheim has no relevant commercial or financial conflicts of interest.

Children's Hospital of Philadelphia, Perelman School of Medicine at the University of Pennsylvania, 5199b Main Building, 3401 Civic Center Boulevard, Philadelphia, PA 19104-4399, USA
E-mail address: wertheimg@email.chop.edu

Clin Lab Med 41 (2021) 541–550
https://doi.org/10.1016/j.cll.2021.04.002
labmed.theclinics.com
0272-2712/21/

the inciting genetic lesion occurs in an early hematopoietic progenitor capable of either lymphoid or myeloid lineage commitment.

As expected, given both the limited age range and the limited time frame in which individuals must acquire oncogenic lesions, infant acute leukemia is quite rare, with an annual incidence of 3 to 4 cases per 100,000 individuals.[5] As opposed to acute leukemia in older children, which shows a slight male predominance and a distinct predominance of lymphoid over myeloid differentiation, infant leukemia affects females slightly more frequently than males, and the incidence of lymphoid and myeloid lesions is relatively equal. The relatively high incidence of myeloid differentiation is particularly striking in infants younger than 1 month, in which ~70% of acute leukemia cases are AML, whereas 20% are ALL, and the remaining 10% of cases are either undifferentiated or mixed phenotype. Of the lymphoblastic malignancies, B cell ALL (B-ALL) is significantly more frequent than T cell ALL.[6]

The distinction of acute leukemia in infants from that in older children is quite relevant in terms of clinical characteristics. Overall, infant acute leukemia displays a more aggressive phenotype than acute leukemia in older children, and treatment algorithms that extrapolate pediatric therapeutics to infants have been suboptimal.[7] Infants with ALL frequently present with peripheral blood hyperleukocytosis (more than 100,000/mL), and up to one-third of cases have initial white blood cell (WBC) counts greater than 200,000/mL. Hepatosplenomegaly and central nervous system involvement are common. Similarly, infants with AML have significantly higher peripheral WBC counts at diagnosis than older children with AML.[8] The blasts frequently display monocytic or megakaryoblastic differentiation and often involve extramedullary sites. In particular, leukemic involvement of skin (leukemia cutis), typically presenting as nonblanching macules or nodules, frequently occurs in the absence of blood or marrow findings (**Fig. 1**).

The relatively rapid postnatal onset of infant acute leukemia suggests that the causative genetic events actually occur prenatally and manifest as leukemia at or soon after birth. Indirect evidence to support this hypothesis was provided by studies of monozygotic twins with acute leukemia. Monozygotic twins essentially share a hematopoietic system in utero through vascular anastomoses, and they show a concordance rate approaching 100% for infant acute leukemia.[9] Also consistent with the prenatal hypothesis, the same pathogenic genetic lesion can be identified in both twins. As expected, dizygotic twins who have entirely separate vascular systems do not show this extreme concordance. Direct evidence of in utero acquisition of leukemogenic mutations was demonstrated by work led by Mel Greaves. These studies examined the *preleukemic* Guthrie spots of cord blood from infants who subsequently developed acute leukemia.[10] Polymerase chain reaction assessment of the DNA from the Guthrie spots

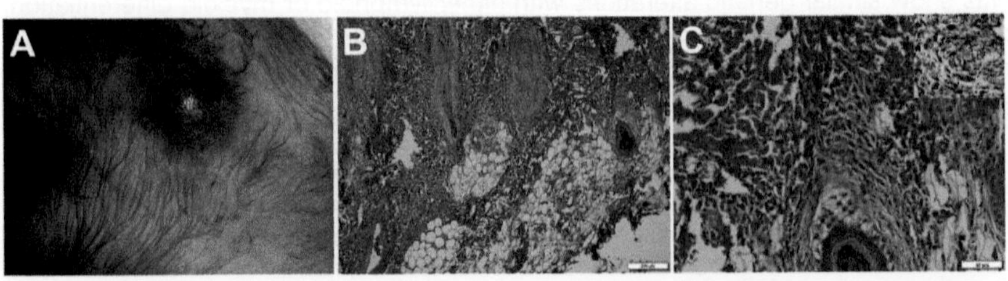

Fig. 1. Leukemia cutis in an infant. (*A*) Nodule on the scalp of an infant with AML involving the skin. (*B* and *C*) Histologic images of a skin biopsy from an infant with AML. The images show a dermal and subcutaneous infiltrate with cells that are positive for myeloperoxidase (*inset*).

identified the same recurrent somatic genetic lesions that were present in the leukemic blasts. As a negative control, these lesions were not detected in Guthrie spots from infants who did not develop leukemia. The acquisition of mutations in utero suggests that maternal risk factors may increase the likelihood of infant acute leukemia. Some of these factors, such as maternal diet and flavonoid intake, have been modestly corroborated by epidemiologic and in vitro studies, although strong maternal risk factors have not been definitively identified.[11,12]

As a severely restricted tumor latency is a logical extension from the definition of infant acute leukemia, the genomic profile of infant leukemia would be expected to remain devoid of extensive mutations. Similarly, the leukemogenic mutations associated with infant leukemia would be expected to encompass a restricted set of highly potent oncogenes. Studies examining both the genomic landscape of infant leukemia and the spectrum of leukemogenic drivers confirm both these hypotheses. Whole-genome sequencing of infant *KMT2A*-rearranged B-ALL identified an average of 1.3 nonsilent mutations, which is among the lowest number of total mutations across all human cancer types.[13] The recurrent mutations seen in infant leukemia are indeed quite restricted and many are unique to infants or young children.

By far the most common genetic lesion observed in infant leukemia with either myeloid or lymphoid differentiation is a translocation involving the epigenetic modifier lysine methyltransferase 2A or KMT2A (previously termed the mixed lineage leukemia gene [MLL]). *KMT2A* translocations occur in 70% to 80% of infant ALL and approximately half of infant AML.[6,8] Although upward of 100 distinct *KMT2A* translocation partners have been identified,[14] the vast majority of infant leukemia is associated with a small subset of these. *KMT2A* in infant AML predominantly associates with *MLLT3* (previously AF9), *MLLT10* (previously *AF10*), and *ELL*, whereas in ALL, *KMT2A* associates with *AFF1* (pervious *AF4*), *MLLT1* (previously *ENL*), and *MLLT3*. As indicated in earlier discussion, multiple additional mutations are infrequent in these tumors, yet about one-half of *KMT2A*-rearranged infant ALL has additional activating mutations in the RAS or phosphoinositide 3-kinase pathway.[13,15] In addition, most *KMT2A*-rearranged infant leukemia overexpress FLT3.[16]

Wild-type KMT2A, as its name implies, methylates histone H3 at lysine-4 (H3K4) and activates gene transcription, particularly of HOX cluster genes that are important in hematopoiesis.[17] Translocated KMT2A, however, associates with noncanonical factors such as DOT1L to promote the methylation of lysine-79 (H3K79) and the superelongation complex to promote RNA polymerase II transcription.[18,19] In addition, DNA CpG islands are hypermethylated in *KMT2A*-rearranged ALL relative to both non-*KMT2A*-rearranged infant ALL and normal marrow.[20] Thus, multiple aspects of the epigenome are uniquely dysregulated in *KMT2A*-rearranged acute leukemia and likely involve the dysregulation of multiple factors that drive oncogenesis.

Although *KMT2A*-rearranged leukemia encompasses most acute leukemia cases in infants, there is a significant subset of cases that are germline for *KMT2A*. Many of these latter cases share several features with *KMT2A*-rearranged leukemia, suggesting that cases of infant AML may be interrelated and that features of *KMT2A*-rearranged leukemia may be extrapolated to other cases of infant acute leukemia. In terms of infant ALL, global gene expression profiling and principal component analysis of pediatric cases (including infant and noninfant ALL) demonstrated that *KMT2A* wild-type infant leukemia are more closely related to *KMT2A*-rearranged infant leukemia than they are to *KMT2A* wild-type leukemia arising in older children.[21] Whether this gene expression similarity among all infant cases, regardless of *KMT2A* status, represents similarities in pathogenesis or simply reflects age-associated gene expression is uncertain.

The comparison among *KMT2A*-rearranged and nonrearranged cases is perhaps more interesting among patients with AML, because differentiation patterns and the types of genetic alterations are similar between the 2 subcategories of infant AML. Although *KMT2A*-rearranged AML shows monocytic differentiation in older children and adults, a *KMT2A* rearrangement in infant AML is frequently associated with megakaryoblastic differentiation.[8] Acute megakaryoblastic leukemia (AMKL) is actually quite frequent among infant AML cases and is associated with other chromosomal translocations. One of these translocations is t(1;22)(p13;q13), which fuses *RBM15* to *MKL1* and actually defines a World Health Organization-described subclass of AML.[22] Both the genes in this fusion influence myeloid maturation, and *MKL1* is specifically required for megakaryocytic differentiation.[23,24] Although rare cases of AMKL with this translocation are seen in older children, it is almost exclusively present in infants younger than 4 months.[25] Despite the significant association of *RBM15-MKL1* with young infants, a relatively recent study that assessed outcomes across multiple trials suggested that this translocation confers a relatively favorable prognosis.[26]

A second chromosomal alteration associated with infant AMKL is inv(16)(p13.3q24.3), resulting in a fusion of the genes *CBFA2T3* and *GLIS2*.[27] This inversion is molecularly distinct from and should not be confused with the well-described inv(16) (p13q22) involving *CBFB* and *MYH11*. Both *CBFA2T3* and *GLIS2* are transcription factors and both are required for the leukemogenic phenotype. Like *KMT2A*-rearranged AML, the leukemic cells show widespread epigenetic alterations, with decreased H3K27 methylation and increased H3K4 methylation and H3K27 acetylation.[28] Furthermore, the blasts harboring this translocation frequently display a characteristic immunophenotype (termed the RAM phenotype) with little to no CD45 expression, lack of CD38 and HLA-DR expression, and bright expression of CD56[29] (**Fig. 2**). The translocation is associated with a poor prognosis.[26]

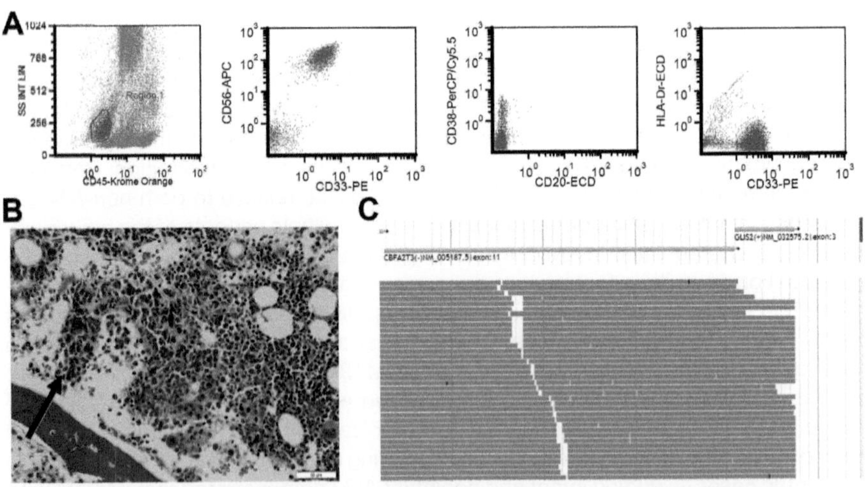

Fig. 2. Diagnostic studies from patient with AML harboring a *CBFA2T3-GLIS2* fusion. (*A*) Flow cytometry of the bone marrow shows a small atypical population of cells within a background of normal hematopoiesis. These cells are positive for CD33 and CD56(bright) while negative for CD45, CD38 and HLA-DR. (*B*) Histologic sections of bone marrow show clusters of atypical large mononuclear cells (arrow) in the background of normal hematopoiesis. (*C*) Sequencing studies identify the *CBFA2T3-GLIS2* fusion.

Two additional genes involved in recurrent translocations found in infant AML are, like *KMT2A* itself, genes involved directly in histone modifications. One of these is *KDM5A* (also known as *JARID1A*), which demethylates histone H3 at lysine-4 and is involved in an oncogenic fusion with the fusion-promiscuous gene *NUP98* that is observed cytogenetically as t(11;12)(p15;p13).[30,31] Similar to *KMT2A*-rearranged leukemia, *NUP98-KDM5A* fusion AML shows frequent megakaryocytic differentiation (along with monocytic and erythroid differentiation, **Fig. 3**) and dysregulation of multiple HOX genes, although the overall gene expression profile appears distinct from *KMT2A*-rearranged leukemia.[32] Outcomes of infants with this translocation are poor.[26] The other histone modifier involved in infant leukemia is *KAT6A*, which is fused with *CREBBP* in leukemia with t(8;16)(p11;p13). KAT6A activity leads to acetylation on histone H3 at lysine-9, but it can also acetylate other proteins such as TP53.[33] Cases with infant AML with the *KAT6A-CREBBP* fusion display myelomonocytic or monocytic differentiation, frequently involve the skin, and display prominent erythrophagocytosis by the leukemic blasts[34] (**Fig. 4**). Infant *KAT6A-CREBBP* fusion leukemia may actually spontaneously regress, yet disease re-emergence almost invariably results, and the prognosis is poor. This subset of AML is clearly biologically related to *KMT2A*-rearranged infant leukemia, as both have dysregulated HOX gene expression, and both subclasses have remarkably similar gene expression profiles.[35] Moreover, both fusions are not only frequently seen in infant AML but also associated with AML that arises after cytotoxic chemotherapy.[36]

Treatment of infant acute leukemia presents numerous challenges.[1,37] Infants not only frequently harbor mutations that are associated with aggressive disease but also are more susceptible to chemotherapeutic toxicities and posttherapy sequelae. Initial studies into therapy for infant leukemia grouped infants into trials evaluating all pediatric patients. The poor outcomes of infants in these studies led to risk classification refinement that categorized infants as high-risk patients. Further recognition of the unique features of infant leukemia resulted in trials specifically geared to infant leukemia, which currently must be done within large consortia, given the relative rarity of infant acute leukemia. Large trials conducted by the United States Children's Oncology Group, the Japanese Pediatric Leukemia/Lymphoma Study Group, and the large international Interfant consortium form the basis of the current treatment recommendations and important prognostic features for infants with acute leukemia.

Current National Comprehensive Cancer Network (NCCN) guidelines for infants with ALL recommend that all should be placed on an open study, or if this is not possible, they should receive standard Interfant-based induction, consisting of a prednisone prophase, followed by combination chemotherapy consisting of cytarabine,

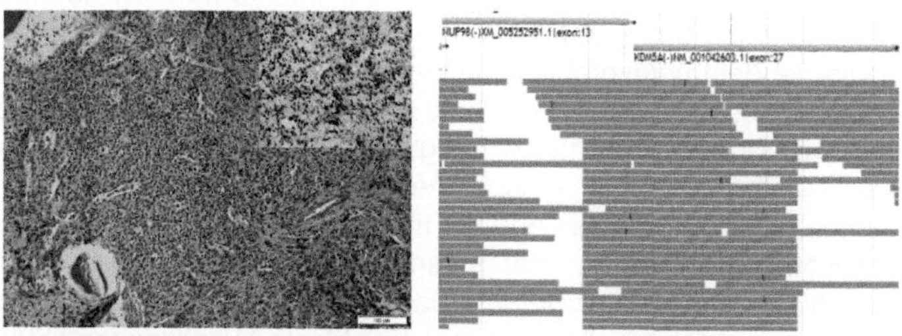

Fig. 3. *NUP98-KDM5A* fusion AML. Histologic sections show marrow replaced by sheets of mononuclear cells with GATA1 expression (*insert*). B Sequencing studies identify the *NUP98-KDM5A* fusion.

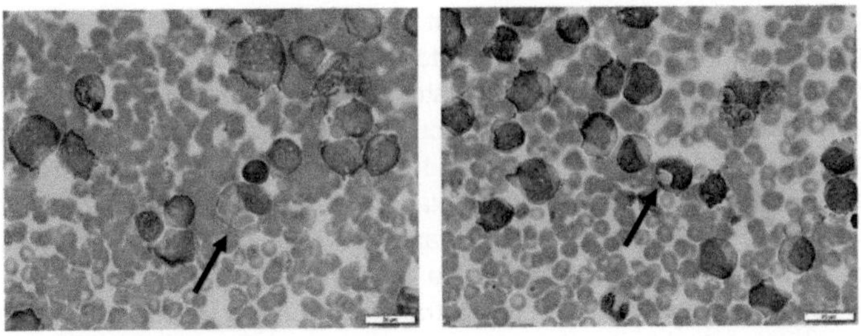

Fig. 4. Wright-Giemsa-stained bone marrow aspirate smears for an infant with AML harboring a *KAT6A-CREBBP* fusion. Arrows show cells with characteristic erythrophagocytosis.

vincristine, dexamethasone, daunorubicin, and L-asparaginase, along with intrathecal methotrexate and prednisone.[38] Further therapy depends largely on *KMT2A* status. Treatment of infant AML does not significantly differ from that of older children, with induction based on a combination of cytarabine and an anthracycline, and consolidation using high-dose cytarabine. Perhaps the most controversial aspect regarding therapy for infants with acute leukemia is the role of allogeneic hematopoietic stem cell transplant (HSCT) as consolidation. For both AML and ALL, the outcomes vary across trials, and a clear benefit of HSCT for infants is lacking. Recent trials have, however, shown improved survival for defined restricted subsets of patients with either AML or ALL.[39,40]

As previously mentioned, infant leukemias are relatively aggressive diseases. This is particularly true with infant ALL. The most recent Interfant-06 study,[40] which assessed 651 infants with ALL, showed 6-year event-free survival (EFS) of ~46% and an overall survival (OS) of 58%, both well below the survival rates of older children with ALL. As with numerous previous studies, *KMT2A* status had the most robust influence on prognosis, with infants harboring a KMT2A rearrangements faring significantly worse than those with germline *KMT2A* (median 6-year EFS of 36% and 74%, respectively). In addition, age at diagnosis (older infants have a better prognosis than younger ones), white blood cell count, and initial response to prednisone were also independently prognostic. These factors were also recognized in the previous Interfant-99 study and were used to stratify patients in Interfant-06.[7,40] Furthermore, similar to results with older pediatric patients, the Japanese consortium identified the presence of minimal residual disease after therapy as a strong independent prognostic variable in infant ALL. In contrast to ALL, prognosis of infants with AML (5-year EFS and OS of 40%–50% and 60%–75%, respectively) is not significantly worse than that in older children and does not seem to be independently associated with a *KMT2A* rearrangement.[39,41] The most important factor in prognosis of infants with AML is the presence of blasts after induction therapy. In addition, the presence of the *CBFA2T3-GLIS2* fusion is an independent unfavorable prognostic variable.

The description of acute leukemia in infants is certainly incomplete without a discussion of infants with Down syndrome. Although children with Down syndrome have a high risk of developing either AML or ALL, these leukemias are most frequently diagnosed in children older than 2 years and are thus outside the scope of this review. Infants with trisomy 21 are by no means without hematologic dysfunction. Approximately 80% of syndromic infants have neutrophilia, up to two-thirds have thrombocytopenia, and almost all have circulating blasts.[42] Approximately 10% of infants with Down syndrome develop a clonal hematopoietic proliferation that resembles AMKL both morphologically and immunophenotypically.[43] This proliferation, however, invariably spontaneously resolves and is, therefore, termed transient abnormal myelopoiesis (TAM) of Down syndrome. TAM usually presents within days of birth and is almost never seen after age 2 months. Resolution of the blast proliferation occurs by 3 months, and any leukemic process in infants with Down syndrome older than 3 months should be considered bona fide acute myeloid leukemia. Although transient, TAM is not an entirely benign condition, and a significant subset of patients with a severe increase in blasts can develop liver failure, coagulopathies, and cardiac dysfunction.[44] TAM is actually fatal in approximately 10% of cases.

The underlying genetic lesion in TAM is a mutation in the N-terminal region of the erythroid/megakaryocytic transcription factor *GATA1* that leads to a truncated protein (GATA1s).[45,46] The mutation is thought to arise in fetal liver hematopoietic stem cells[47,48]; these do not have sustained viability during postnatal hematopoiesis, leading to the regression of TAM. About 20% of infants with clinically recognized TAM subsequently develop AML with megakaryoblastic differentiation.[49] The blasts from these patients with post-TAM AML harbor the same *GATA1* mutation identified in the TAM blasts, indicating that TAM is actually a preleukemic condition. Additionally, the AML blasts harbor secondary pathogenic mutations, many of which are in genes commonly mutated in myeloid malignancies including cohesin complex genes, both *JAK* and *RAS* family members, *CKIT*, and epigenetic modifiers.[50]

In summary, infant leukemia is rare, yet poses several clinical challenges given the aggressiveness of the diseases and the unique physiology of newborns. Despite rather intensive chemotherapy, mortality rates of infants with acute leukemia remain high. The paucity of mutational events in infant leukemia hinders the development of target therapy. Current directed therapy focused on features that are not restricted to tumor cells, such as CD19- or CD33-directed agents may provide improved outcomes for these patients.

CLINICS CARE POINTS

- Infant leukemia should be considered in infants with non-blanching skin lesions or skin biopsies with malignant cells.
- Megakaryocytic markers should be included in the pathologic workup of infant leukemia.
- Specific genetic lesions should be tested for in infants with acute leukemia, as a subset have distinct prognostic implications.
- As some genetic alterations are associated with spontaneous regression of leukemic cells (e.g. constitution trisomy 22 and somatic CREBB-KAT6A fusions), these entities should be recognized and treated accordingly.

REFERENCES

1. Brown P, Pieters R, Biondi A. How I treat infant leukemia. Blood 2019;133(3):205–14.
2. Biondi A, Cimino G, Pieters R, et al. Biological and therapeutic aspects of infant leukemia. Blood 2000;96(1):24–33.
3. Strullu M, Caye A, Lachenaud J, et al. Juvenile myelomonocytic leukaemia and Noonan syndrome. J Med Genet 2014;51(10):689.
4. Rossi JG, Bernasconi AR, Alonso CN, et al. Lineage switch in childhood acute leukemia: an unusual event with poor outcome. Am J Hematol 2012;87(9):890–7.
5. Howlander N, Noone AM, Krapcho M, et al. SEER cancer statistics review, 1975-2017. Bethesda, MD: National Cancer Institute; 2020.

6. Silverman LB. Acute lymphoblastic leukemia in infancy. Pediatr Blood Cancer 2007;49(S7):1070–3.
7. Pieters R, Schrappe M, Lorenzo PD, et al. A treatment protocol for infants younger than 1 year with acute lymphoblastic leukaemia (Interfant-99): an observational study and a multicentre randomised trial. Lancet 2007;370(9583):240–50.
8. Masetti R, Vendemini F, Zama D, et al. Acute myeloid leukemia in infants: biology and treatment. Front Pediatr 2015;3:37.
9. Greaves MF, Maia AT, Wiemels JL, et al. Leukemia in twins: lessons in natural history. Blood 2003;102(7):2321–33.
10. Gale KB, Ford AM, Repp R, et al. Backtracking leukemia to birth: identification of clonotypic gene fusion sequences in neonatal blood spots. Proc Natl Acad Sci U S A 1997;94(25):13950–4.
11. Strick R, Strissel PL, Borgers S, et al. Dietary bioflavonoids induce cleavage in the MLL gene and may contribute to infant leukemia. Proc Natl Acad Sci U S A 2000; 97(9):4790–5.
12. Spector LG, Xie Y, Robison LL, et al. Maternal diet and infant leukemia: the DNA topoisomerase II inhibitor hypothesis: a report from the Children's Oncology group. Cancer Epidemiol Prev Biomarkers 2005;14(3):651–5.
13. Andersson AK, Ma J, Wang J, et al. The landscape of somatic mutations in infant MLL-rearranged acute lymphoblastic leukemias. Nat Genet 2015;47(4):330–7.
14. Meyer C, Burmeister T, Gröger D, et al. The MLL recombinome of acute leukemias in 2017. Leukemia 2018;32(2):273–84.
15. Driessen EMC, van Roon EHJ, Spijkers-Hagelstein JAP, et al. Frequencies and prognostic impact of RAS mutations in MLL-rearranged acute lymphoblastic leukemia in infants. Haematologica 2013;98(6):937–44.
16. Brown P, Levis M, Shurtleff S, et al. FLT3 inhibition selectively kills childhood acute lymphoblastic leukemia cells with high levels of FLT3 expression. Blood 2005; 105(2):812–20.
17. Winters AC, Bernt KM. MLL-rearranged leukemias—an update on science and clinical approaches. Front Pediatr 2017;5:4.
18. Bernt KM, Zhu N, Sinha AU, et al. MLL-rearranged leukemia is dependent on aberrant H3K79 methylation by DOT1L. Cancer Cell 2011;20(1):66–78.
19. Liang K, Volk AG, Haug JS, et al. Therapeutic targeting of MLL degradation pathways in MLL-rearranged leukemia. Cell 2017;168(1–2):59–72.e13.
20. Schafer E, Irizarry R, Negi S, et al. Promoter hypermethylation in MLL-r infant acute lymphoblastic leukemia: biology and therapeutic targeting. Blood 2010; 115(23):4798–809.
21. Stam RW, Schneider P, Hagelstein JAP, et al. Gene expression profiling–based dissection of MLL translocated and MLL germline acute lymphoblastic leukemia in infants. Blood 2010;115(14):2835–44.
22. Arber DA, Orazi A, Hasserjian R, et al. The 2016 revision to the World Health Organization classification of myeloid neoplasms and acute leukemia. Blood 2016; 127(20):2391–405.
23. Ma X, Renda MJ, Wang L, et al. Rbm15 modulates notch-induced transcriptional activation and affects myeloid dfferentiation ▽ †. Mol Cell Biol 2007;27(8): 3056–64.
24. Cheng E, Luo Q, Bruscia EM, et al. Role for MKL1 in megakaryocytic maturation. Blood 2009;113(12):2826–34.
25. Bernstein J, Dastugue N, Haas O, et al. Nineteen cases of the t(1;22)(p13;q13) acute megakaryblastic leukaemia of infants/children and a review of 39 cases: report from a t(1;22) study group. Leukemia 2000;14(1):216–8.

26. Rooij JDE de, Masetti R, van den Heuvel-Eibrink MM, et al. Recurrent abnormalities can be used for risk group stratification in pediatric AMKL: a retrospective intergroup study. Blood 2016;127(26):3424–30.
27. Gruber TA, Larson Gedman A, Zhang J, et al. An inv(16)(p13.3q24.3)-encoded CBFA2T3-GLIS2 fusion protein defines an aggressive subtype of pediatric acute megakaryoblastic leukemia. Cancer Cell 2012;22(5):683–97.
28. Thirant C, Ignacimouttou C, Lopez CK, et al. ETO2-GLIS2 hijacks transcriptional complexes to drive cellular identity and self-renewal in pediatric acute megakaryoblastic leukemia. Cancer Cell 2017;31(3):452–65.
29. Brodersen LE, Alonzo TA, Menssen AJ, et al. A recurrent immunophenotype at diagnosis independently identifies high-risk pediatric acute myeloid leukemia: a report from Children's Oncology Group. Leukemia 2016;30(10):2077–80.
30. Klose RJ, Yan Q, Tothova Z, et al. The retinoblastoma binding protein RBP2 is an H3K4 demethylase. Cell 2007;128(5):889–900.
31. van Zutven LJCM, Önen E, Velthuizen SCJM, et al. Identification of NUP98 abnormalities in acute leukemia: JARID1A (12p13) as a new partner gene. Genes Chromosomes Cancer 2006;45(5):437–46.
32. Noort S, Wander P, Alonzo TA, et al. The clinical and biological characteristics of NUP98-KDM5A in pediatric acute myeloid leukemia. Haematologica 2020; 106(2):630–4.
33. Arboleda VA, Lee H, Dorrani N, et al. De novo nonsense mutations in KAT6A, a lysine acetyl-transferase gene, cause a syndrome including microcephaly and global developmental delay. Am J Hum Genet 2015;96(3):498–506.
34. Montewis A, Eveillard M. Acute myeloid leukemia with erythrophagocytosis indicative of KAT6A rearrangement. Blood 2016;128(2):314.
35. Coenen EA, Zwaan CM, Reinhardt D, et al. Pediatric acute myeloid leukemia with t(8;16)(p11;p13), a distinct clinical and biological entity: a collaborative study by the International-Berlin-Frankfurt-Münster AML-study group. Blood 2013;122(15): 2704–13.
36. Block AW, Carroll AJ, Hagemeijer A, et al. Rare recurring balanced chromosome abnormalities in therapy-related myelodysplastic syndromes and acute leukemia: report from an International Workshop†. Genes Chromosomes Cancer 2002; 33(4):401–12.
37. Brown P. Treatment of infant leukemias: challenge and promise. Hematology 2013;2013(1):596–600.
38. Brown P, Inaba H, Annesley C, et al. Pediatric acute lymphoblastic leukemia, version 2.2020, NCCN clinical practice guidelines in oncology. J Natl Compr Canc Netw 2020;18(1):81–112.
39. Creutzig U, Zimmermann M, Bourquin J-P, et al. Favorable outcome in infants with AML after intensive first- and second-line treatment: an AML-BFM study group report. Leukemia 2012;26(4):654–61.
40. Pieters R, Lorenzo PD, Ancliffe P, et al. Outcome of infants younger than 1 year with acute lymphoblastic leukemia treated with the interfant-06 protocol: results from an international phase III randomized study. J Clin Oncol 2019;37(25): 2246–56.
41. Masetti R, Rondelli R, Fagioli F, et al. Infants with acute myeloid leukemia treated according to the Associazione Italiana di Ematologia e Oncologia Pediatrica 2002/01 protocol have an outcome comparable to that of older children. Haematologica 2014;99(8):e127–9.

42. Roberts I, Alford K, Hall G, et al. GATA1-mutant clones are frequent and often unsuspected in babies with Down syndrome: identification of a population at risk of leukemia. Blood 2013;122(24):3908–17.
43. Bhatnagar N, Nizery L, Tunstall O, et al. Transient abnormal myelopoiesis and AML in Down syndrome: an update. Curr Hematol Malig Rep 2016;11(5):333–41.
44. Gamis AS, Alonzo TA, Gerbing RB, et al. Natural history of transient myeloproliferative disorder clinically diagnosed in Down syndrome neonates: a report from the Children's Oncology Group Study A2971. Blood 2011;118(26):6752–9.
45. Wechsler J, Greene M, McDevitt MA, et al. Acquired mutations in GATA1 in the megakaryoblastic leukemia of Down syndrome. Nat Genet 2002;32(1):148–52.
46. Kanezaki R, Toki T, Terui K, et al. Down syndrome and GATA1 mutations in transient abnormal myeloproliferative disorder: mutation classes correlate with progression to myeloid leukemia. Blood 2010;116(22):4631–8.
47. Taub JW, Mundschau G, Ge Y, et al. Prenatal origin of GATA1 mutations may be an initiating step in the development of megakaryocytic leukemia in Down syndrome. Blood 2004;104(5):1588–9.
48. Tunstall-Pedoe O, Roy A, Karadimitris A, et al. Abnormalities in the myeloid progenitor compartment in Down syndrome fetal liver precede acquisition of GATA1 mutations. Blood 2008;112(12):4507–11.
49. Shimizu R, Engel JD, Yamamoto M. GATA1-related leukaemias. Nat Rev Cancer 2008;8(4):279–87.
50. Yoshida K, Toki T, Okuno Y, et al. The landscape of somatic mutations in Down syndrome–related myeloid disorders. Nat Genet 2013;45(11):1293–9.

Gene Rearrangement Detection in Pediatric Leukemia

Marian H. Harris, MD, PhD

KEYWORDS

- Pediatric leukemia • Gene rearrangements • Fusions • Karyotype • FISH • RT-PCR
- Next-generation sequencing (NGS)

KEY POINTS

- Gene rearrangements are prevalent in pediatric leukemias.
- The detection of gene rearrangements is essential for diagnostic, prognostic, and therapeutic decision making.
- Many assays are available to detect gene rearrangements, with different strengths and weaknesses, including karyotype, fluorescence in situ hybridization, reverse transcription polymerase chain reaction, DNA sequencing, and RNA sequencing.

INTRODUCTION

Cancer is understood to be a genetic disease. In pediatric leukemias, as in other cancer types, genetic alterations lead to dysregulation of cellular processes and, ultimately, to malignancy. There are many types of clinically significant genetic alterations. General categories of alterations include sequence mutations, such as single nucleotide changes (single nucleotide variants [SNVs]) and small insertions and deletions (indels), and structural mutations, such as copy number changes (copy number variants [CNVs]) and chromosomal rearrangements. Structural mutations gain significance when they result in oncogenic gene fusions or gene dysregulation. Pediatric tumors in particular, which generally have a low overall mutation rate compared with adult tumors, have a high frequency of tumors where a gene rearrangement is the oncogenic driver.[1,2] This article provides an overview of different methods to detect these gene rearrangements.

The author has nothing to disclose.
Department of Pathology, Boston Children's Hospital, 300 Longwood Avenue, Boston, MA 02115, USA
E-mail address: marian.harris@childrens.harvard.edu

Clin Lab Med 41 (2021) 551–561
https://doi.org/10.1016/j.cll.2021.04.012
labmed.theclinics.com

CLINICAL SIGNIFICANCE OF GENE REARRANGEMENTS

Pediatric leukemias comprise a diverse group of diseases, including acute lymphoblastic leukemia (ALL), acute myeloid leukemia (AML), mixed-phenotype acute leukemia (MPAL), chronic myeloid leukemia (CML), and juvenile myelomonocytic leukemia (JMML). The prevalence of oncogenic gene rearrangements in pediatric leukemias means that it is imperative to test for these changes at the time of diagnosis. Clinical guidelines recommend assays capable of detecting gene rearrangements as part of the work-up for new acute leukemias,[3,4] and the latest revision of the World Health Organization (WHO) classification includes many leukemia subtypes defined by gene rearrangements.[5] The detection of gene rearrangements may have diagnostic, prognostic, and/or therapeutic significance.[6]

Diagnostic Significance

Rearrangements are an integral part of the WHO classification of leukemias. In ALL, the WHO categorization includes several B-cell ALL (B-ALL) subtypes defined by gene rearrangements, including *BCR-ABL1*, *KMT2A* rearrangement, *ETV6-RUNX1*, *IL3-IGH*, and *TCF3-PBX1*. In addition, the provisional entity of B-ALL, *BCR-ALB1*–like, which is a subtype of B-ALL with an expression profile similar to B-ALL with *BCR-ABL1*, includes several typical gene rearrangements.[5,7] New subtypes of B-ALL that are defined by rearrangements but not yet included in the WHO categorization include *TCF3-HLF*, *DUX4* rearranged, *MEF2D* rearranged, and *ZNF384* rearranged.[8–13] Characteristic gene rearrangements are also found in T-cell ALL, including *STIL-TAL* and rearrangements with T-cell receptor genes, although these rearrangements do not define specific subgroups in the WHO classification.

The WHO classification of AML also includes many subtypes defined by gene rearrangements, including *RUNX1-RUNX1T1*, *CBFB-MYH11*, *PML-RARA*, *MLLT3-KMT2A*, *DEK-NUP214*, *RBM15-MKL1*, and AML with deregulated *MECOM* and *GATA2* expression, and the provisional entity AML with *BCL-ABL1*.[5] Additional gene rearrangements known to be recurrent in pediatric AML include *ETV6* rearrangements, *KAT6A* rearrangements with *CREBBP* or *EP300*, other *KMT2A* rearrangements, other *RUNX1* rearrangements, *NUP98-NSD1* and other *NUP98* fusions, *CBFA2T3-GLIS2*, and *FUS-ERG*.[5,14,15]

MPAL has also been shown to have recurrent rearrangements, including *BCR-ABL1* and *KMT2A* rearrangements, both of which define specific subtypes of MPAL in the WHO classification.[5,16]

Other pediatric leukemias that may carry diagnostically significant gene rearrangements include CML with *BCR-ABL1*, JMML (rearrangements are rare),[17,18] and a category of malignancy with the descriptive name of myeloid/lymphoid neoplasms with eosinophilia and rearrangement of *PDGFRA*, *PDGFRB*, or *FGFR1*, or with *PCM1-JAK2*.[19]

Prognostic Significance

The detection of a gene rearrangement often carries prognostic significance, especially in pediatric ALL and AML, where risk-adapted therapy is considered standard of care.[20,21] Risk stratification for both ALL and AML relies on the presence or absence of specific gene fusions. Although specific risk group definitions vary from protocol to protocol, some commonalities in ALL include placing patients with *KMT2A* rearrangement or *TCF3-HLF* into higher risk groups, whereas patients without these fusions may be eligible for less intense therapy (depending on other features). In AML as in ALL, risk group definitions vary by protocol but, for example, patients with *RUNX1-RUNX1T1* or *CBFB-MYH11* are typically treated in lower risk groups.

Therapeutic Significance

Several targeted therapies are now available for which a gene fusion event is the relevant biomarker. Imatinib is the prototypical example, which is a tyrosine kinase inhibitor (TKI) originally developed to target the BCR-ABL1 oncoprotein in CML.[22] Imatinib and related TKIs have also been used in pediatric *BCR-ABL1*–positive B lymphoblastic leukemia,[23] in a subset of *BCR-ABL1*–like B-ALL,[24] in the provisional category of AML with *BCR-ABL1*,[25] and in MPAL with *BCR-ABL1*.[26] Other targeted therapies for which the presence of a specific fusion may suggest sensitivity include all-transretinoic acid (ATRA) in *PML-RARA* and other *RARA* rearrangements,[27] Janus kinase (JAK) inhibitors in a subset of *BCR-ABL1*–like B-ALL,[28] and tropomyosin receptor kinase (TRK) inhibitors in TRK-fusion positive B-ALL.[29–31]

METHODS TO DETECT GENE REARRANGEMENTS

Many different modalities are available to test for gene rearrangements, so consideration must be given to selecting the most appropriate assay. Factors to consider include the alterations that each assay is capable of identifying, the acceptable sample type for each technique, turnaround time, cost, and the potential for multiplexing (**Table 1**). Many of the most commonly used clinical assay for the detection of genetic rearrangements are discussed here, including some illustrative examples.

Karyotype

Nowell and Hungerford[32] used karyotyping to discover the first recurrent structural chromosomal change in oncology when they described the Philadelphia chromosome in CML, and karyotypes are still part of the routine leukemia work-up.[3,4] Karyotyping can identify several well-known, recurrent rearrangements, although some common rearrangements are typically cryptic by karyotype, such as *ETV6-RUNX1* in pediatric B-ALL. Each metaphase analyzed in a karyotype represents an unbiased overview of the genetics of a single cell, which may also facilitate the identification of subclonal populations. In addition to well-known rearrangements, novel changes may also be found by this technique, but the specific genes involved cannot be identified. The genetic resolution is at the cytoband level, which typically contains several megabases of DNA and hundreds of genes. Karyotyping requires the successful culture of cells from a viable sample in order to capture cells in metaphase; therefore, a fresh sample is required and results may take anywhere from a few days to a week or more. Typically, 20 cells are analyzed, so detection of rare and/or subclonal events is limited.

Fluorescence In Situ Hybridization

Fluorescence in situ hybridization (FISH) uses fluorescently labeled, sequence-specific DNA probes to map genomic structure. FISH began to be used in leukemia in the 1990s.[33] Two different types of FISH techniques are now commonly used to detect rearrangements: break-apart and dual-color dual-fusion techniques. Break-apart FISH assays are composed of 2 probes complementary to sequences proximal and distal to the breakpoint of interest, each labeled with a different color. For example, a FISH assay to detect a *KMT2A* rearrangement might include a red probe on one side of the breakpoint region and a green probe on the other. When the gene is intact, the red and green probes are so close together they appear as a single, fused signal. However, when there is a *KMT2A* rearrangement, the 2 sides of *KMT2A* are separated and appear as 2 distinct signals, 1 red and 1 green. Break-apart probes are particularly useful for detecting rearrangements of genes such as *KMT2A* that have many possible fusion partners, such that setting up individual assays for each

Table 1
Common methods used for clinical gene rearrangement detection

Method	Sensitivity	Turnaround Time	Sample Requirements	Scope of Detection	Detection of Novel Fusions
Karyotype	+	Days to weeks	Fresh samples only	Unbiased detection of rearrangements (although some rearrangements are cryptic)	Yes, but specific genes not identified
FISH	++	Days	Fresh or archival	One gene or gene pair per assay	No
RT-PCR	+++	Days	Fresh or archival	One gene pair per assay; limited multiplexing possible	No
DNA panel	+++	Days to weeks	Fresh or archival	Multiplex detection of targeted rearrangements	Possible, depending on assay
Whole-genome sequencing	++ (depending on depth)	Weeks	Fresh preferred	Unbiased detection of rearrangements	Yes
RNA panel	+++	Days to weeks	Fresh or archival, although sensitive to sample degradation	Multiplex detection of targeted rearrangements	Possible, depending on assay
Whole-transcriptome sequencing	+++	Weeks	Fresh preferred	Unbiased detection of rearrangements	Yes

Abbreviations: FISH, fluorescence in situ hybridization; RT-PCR, reverse transcription polymerase chain reaction.

potential pair of partners would be impractical. Dual-color, dual-fusion FISH is another common strategy used to identify specific fusion pairs, with each partner labeled in a different color. For example, a FISH assay to detect an *ETV6-RUNX1* rearrangement would include a probe to the 5′ end of *ETV6* labeled green, and another probe to the 3′ end of *RUNX1* labeled red. In a normal cell, without a rearrangement, a pattern of 2 green signals and 2 red signals would be observed. However, in a cell with an *ETV6-RUNX1* rearrangement, 1 of the 5′ *ETV6* signals and 1 of the *3′RUNX1* signals would be close enough together in each cell to appear fused, yielding an expected pattern of 1 red, 1 green, and 2 fused signals per cell (1 fused signal for *ETV6-RUNX1* and 1 for its reciprocal rearrangement *RUNX1-ETV6*; variant patterns may occur).

FISH has the advantage of being able to detect clinically significant rearrangements, such as *ETV6-RUNX1*, that are cryptic by karyotype. FISH can also detect a variety of genetic changes beyond gene rearrangements, including the gain or loss of whole regions or chromosomes, and copy number changes of targeted genes. For example, FISH for *ETV6-RUNX1* also detects multiple copies of *RUNX1*, as found in trisomy 21 or B-ALL with iAMP21. Rarely, a gene fusion may be difficult to detect by FISH. For example, in the *NUP214-ABL1* fusion, the genes are so close together on chromosome 9 in a normal genome that the alteration caused by the fusion is difficult to discern with *ABL1* break-apart FISH.[34] Some fusions that are routinely detected by FISH may also be cryptic in specific cases because of rare breakpoints and/or probe-specific factors. For example, in cases of acute promyelocytic leukemia with *PML-RARA* in which *RARA* has inserted into the *PML* locus, the fusion may be hard to detect with certain probe sets.[35]

For all FISH assays, background thresholds need to be defined on an assay-by-assay basis, yielding variable sensitivity that is typically greater than that of karyotyping. FISH can be performed on metaphase chromosomes such as those used for karyotyping, but can also be used on cells in interphase, in which case cell culture is not required. In addition to fresh blood or tissue samples, interphase FISH can be performed on archival sample types, including air-dried touch preparations or smears and formalin-fixed paraffin-embedded tissue (FFPE). Unlike karyotyping, which provides an unbiased look at the entire genome of a cell, FISH assays can only detect changes in the specific targets tested. Thus, a complete FISH-based work-up for a newly diagnosed leukemia might include multiple FISH assays.

Reverse Transcription Polymerase Chain Reaction

Reverse transcription polymerase chain reaction (RT-PCR) is an RNA-based technique that can be used to detect fusions. RNA is a useful substrate for fusion detection compared with DNA because introns are spliced out in RNA, leaving only exons. The breakpoints for gene rearrangements usually occur in introns, which are often many kilobases long. By using RNA, RT-PCR for fusions does not need to amplify these long introns. The forward primer usually targets the 5′ gene partner in the exon preceding the breakpoint of interest, and the reverse primer targets the 3′ gene partner in the exon following the breakpoint of interest. These targets are adjacent and amplifiable from RNA only if a rearrangement is present. RT-PCR may be used with fresh or archival specimens. However, RNA is susceptible to degradation, especially in FFPE or other stored specimens, and, even in fresh samples, pre-analytical factors such as time to RNA extraction and temperature can affect RNA quality. Consequently, controls must be included to confirm sufficient RNA quality in each sample. Because RT-PCR primers are targeted to specific exons, gene fusions that are known to have varying exonic breakpoints may require multiple primer sets, such as the p190, p210, and p230 isoforms of *BCR-ABL1*. Many other fusions with recurrent gene pairs are amenable to detection by RT-PCR, and RT-PCR can be multiplexed to detect multiple rearrangements in the same assay.[36,37] However, rearrangement detection for a gene that can have multiple different partners is less well suited to RT-PCR, because each partner gene would require a distinct assay. For example, *KMT2A* can rearrange with more than 100 different partners in AML and ALL, which would be challenging to target in a single assay.[38] RT-PCR is extremely sensitive, and, in addition to being used qualitatively, may also be run quantitatively. Quantitative RT-PCR for *BCR-ABL1* is routinely used to follow response to therapy in CML.[39] RT-PCR typically has a quick turnaround time of 1 to 2 days.

Next-Generation Sequencing–Based Methods

Next-generation sequencing (NGS)–based approaches to fusion detection in leukemia have become increasingly available. NGS assays can be designed to use either DNA or RNA, and may target specific regions of the genome or may offer coverage of the whole exome, genome, or transcriptome; these different approaches are discussed later. NGS-based approaches are attractive in that they can test for many different fusions simultaneously, potentially increasing testing efficiency. NGS-based assays also have the advantage of being able to identify exonic and/or genomic breakpoints, and some assays are able to identify new fusion partners to recurrently rearranged genes, or even novel fusion pairs. Both fresh and archival specimens may be used for NGS, but specific assay requirements vary. Fresh blood and bone marrow are acceptable samples for most NGS assays. Air-dried bone marrow aspirate smears or peripheral blood smears are acceptable for some assays. FFPE may be acceptable, although most decalcified samples are not suitable for NGS, which means that FFPE from most bone marrow core biopsies is not acceptable (samples decalcified with ethylenediaminetetraacetic acid [EDTA] rather than acid may be useable). Bone marrow clot preparations are not decalcified, so FFPE from these specimens is another potential source of testable material. Turnaround time for a targeted NGS-based assay is often around 2 weeks; whole-exome/genome/transcriptome assays may take longer.

Next-Generation Sequencing–Based DNA Sequencing

Targeted DNA sequencing assays sequence-specific preselected regions of the genome, which are usually a subset of gene-coding exons. Therefore, using targeted DNA sequencing panels for fusion detection faces the challenge described in the discussion of RT-PCR (ie, that fusion breakpoints are variable and typically occur in introns): a large amount of DNA must be sequenced in order to detect a fusion. For example, in order to detect a *RUNX1-RUNX1T1* fusion in AML, an assay needs to cover intron 6 of *RUNX1*, ~25 kb, where breaks most often occur for this leukemia. The need to cover many such large spans of DNA at high depth (appropriate for somatic alterations), has limited the use of targeted DNA sequencing panels for multiplex fusion detection. In addition, introns may also contain repetitive regions that are difficult to target, further limiting the practicality of sequencing introns for fusion detection.[40] Nevertheless, some DNA panels have been designed and validated to detect specific fusions this way, although these are primarily in the solid tumor setting.[41,42] Two general methods may be used: the hybrid capture-based method, in which probes to targeted regions of the genome are used to enrich for areas of interest, and the amplicon-based method, in which PCR primers are used to amplify areas of interest. In general, the hybrid capture approach is more amenable to detection of gene fusions, and may also be able to detect novel, untargeted partners to targeted genes.[42] One advantage of DNA sequencing for fusion detection is the identification of the exact genomic breakpoint in DNA, which is sometimes clinically significant and could theoretically be used for patient-specific measurable residual disease testing. In addition, DNA sequencing permits simultaneous detection of other variant types, such as SNVs, indels, and CNVs, along with any targeted fusions in a single assay.

DNA sequencing assays that are more broad than the targeted panels described earlier include whole-exome sequencing (WES) and whole-genome sequencing (WGS). WES is like a very large panel, but does not typically cover introns and is not designed to detect fusions. WGS is, as the name suggests, unbiased sequencing of the DNA of the entire genome. In theory, WGS is able to capture any fusion, whether novel or recurrent, as well as other DNA changes such as SNVs, indels, and even copy number changes. However, at present the wide breadth of WGS means that it usually offers less depth than is desired for somatic analysis, and also requires significant informatics resources to analyze such that WGS for leukemia diagnostics is not widely available.

Next-Generation Sequencing–Based RNA Sequencing

The challenges associated with fusion detection using DNA-based strategies have led to the development of RNA-based approaches, both targeted RNA sequencing and whole-transcriptome RNA sequencing. The same principle that underlies RT-PCR also applies to RNA sequencing for fusion detection: the absence of introns in RNA means that fusions may be sensitively detected while sequencing much less genomic territory per fusion than in DNA sequencing. The detection of a fusion by RNA sequencing can confirm that the fusion is both in frame and expressed, and RNA sequencing has the potential to detect expression of aberrantly spliced isoforms such as ERGalt in DUX4-rearranged B-ALL.[9,10] RNA sequencing also provides data about gene expression levels, and larger RNA panels, particularly whole-transcriptome sequencing, have been used for expression profile–based leukemia subtyping. In contrast, rearrangements that are not highly transcribed or that do not result in a chimeric transcript may be difficult to detect. For example, the *IGH-CRLF2* fusion leads to high expression of *CRLF2* driven by the *IGH* promoter, but does not result in a chimeric transcript detectable by a fusion analysis pipeline. The same problem applies to other rearrangements between *IGH*, *IGK*, *IGL*, or a T-cell receptor and a target gene, although some of these rearrangements may be detectable by RNA sequencing because of aberrantly high expression of the target gene.[43]

Targeted RNA sequencing requires less input material, has a shorter turnaround time, and may even be more sensitive for targeted fusions than whole-transcriptome sequencing or DNA sequencing,[44,45] and is thus increasingly widely used for clinical testing.[43,46–48] Similar to targeted DNA sequencing, targeted RNA sequencing may be performed using hybrid capture–based or amplicon-based approaches. Some targeted assays allow open-ended sequencing from 1 partner in a gene pair, which avoids the need to target every known partner of promiscuous genes such as *KMT2A* and allows the identification of novel partners.[49]

Whole-transcriptome RNA sequencing has been instrumental in mapping the genomic landscape of pediatric leukemias.[7,14,15,50–53] However, the expense, turnaround time, and analytical requirements have limited clinical use thus far, although it is available in some laboratories.[54,55] No doubt the future will see improvements in these factors and more widespread adoption.

Other Techniques

Other techniques that may also be used to detect gene rearrangements include mate pair sequencing (DNA-based NGS using long circularized fragments, used for unbiased detection of structural abnormalities),[56] NanoString (RNA-based, targeting of both fusion partners required),[57] droplet digital PCR (ddPCR; RNA-based, highly sensitive, used for measurable residual disease),[58] and antibody-based methods such as flow cytometry and immunohistochemistry (only useful in specific applications, such as overexpression of CRLF2 in *CRLF2*-rearranged B-ALL).[59]

SUMMARY

Gene rearrangements are common driver events in pediatric leukemia, with diagnostic, prognostic, and/or therapeutic significance. There are an ever-increasing number of approaches available to detect these rearrangements, from karyotyping to WGS. The selection of the most appropriate assay or assays depends on the type of sample available to test, the rearrangements that need to be detected, assay availability, turnaround time, and cost. Current practice often requires multiple assays to be combined in a diagnostic algorithm, either sequentially or in parallel. Future advances will certainly bring further changes, and may allow welcome consolidation in testing, but the detection of these events will remain crucial to the clinical care of patients.

CLINICS CARE POINTS

- Many different types of assays may be used to detect gene rearrangements in pediatric leukemia.
- Diagnostic algorithms may require the use of more than one type of assay to detect gene rearrangements at the time of diagnosis.
- High-throughput sequencing assays to detect gene fusions are becoming more widely available and can query for multiple fusions at once.

REFERENCES

1. Grobner SN, Worst BC, Weischenfeldt J, et al. The landscape of genomic alterations across childhood cancers. Nature 2018;555(7696):321–7.
2. Vellichirammal NN, Chaturvedi NK, Joshi SS, et al. Fusion genes as biomarkers in pediatric cancers: a review of the current state and applicability in diagnostics and personalized therapy. Cancer Lett 2021;499:24–38.
3. Arber DA, Borowitz MJ, Cessna M, et al. Initial diagnostic workup of acute leukemia: guideline from the College of American Pathologists and the American Society of Hematology. Arch Pathol Lab Med 2017;141(10):1342–93.
4. de Haas V, Ismaila N, Advani A, et al. Initial diagnostic work-up of acute leukemia: ASCO clinical practice guideline endorsement of the College of American Pathologists and American Society of Hematology Guideline. J Clin Oncol 2019;37(3):239–53.
5. Swerdlow SH, Campo E, Harris NL, et al. WHO classification of tumours of haematopoietic and lymphoid tissues. 4th edition ed. Lyon, France: International Agency for Research on Cancer; 2017.
6. Harris MH, Czuchlewski DR, Arber DA, et al. Genetic testing in the diagnosis and biology of acute leukemia. Am J Clin Pathol 2019;152(3):322–46.
7. Roberts KG, Li Y, Payne-Turner D, et al. Targetable kinase-activating lesions in Ph-like acute lymphoblastic leukemia. N Engl J Med 2014;371(11):1005–15.
8. Fischer U, Forster M, Rinaldi A, et al. Genomics and drug profiling of fatal TCF3-HLF-positive acute lymphoblastic leukemia identifies recurrent mutation patterns and therapeutic options. Nat Genet 2015;47(9):1020–9.

9. Yasuda T, Tsuzuki S, Kawazu M, et al. Recurrent DUX4 fusions in B cell acute lymphoblastic leukemia of adolescents and young adults. Nat Genet 2016; 48(5):569–74.
10. Zhang J, McCastlain K, Yoshihara H, et al. Deregulation of DUX4 and ERG in acute lymphoblastic leukemia. Nat Genet 2016;48(12):1481–9.
11. Gu Z, Churchman M, Roberts K, et al. Genomic analyses identify recurrent MEF2D fusions in acute lymphoblastic leukaemia. Nat Commun 2016;7:13331.
12. Suzuki K, Okuno Y, Kawashima N, et al. MEF2D-BCL9 fusion gene is associated with high-risk acute B-cell precursor lymphoblastic leukemia in adolescents. J Clin Oncol 2016;34(28):3451–9.
13. Hirabayashi S, Ohki K, Nakabayashi K, et al. ZNF384-related fusion genes define a subgroup of childhood B-cell precursor acute lymphoblastic leukemia with a characteristic immunotype. Haematologica 2017;102(1):118–29.
14. Bolouri H, Farrar JE, Triche T Jr, et al. The molecular landscape of pediatric acute myeloid leukemia reveals recurrent structural alterations and age-specific mutational interactions. Nat Med 2018;24(1):103–12.
15. Shiba N, Yoshida K, Hara Y, et al. Transcriptome analysis offers a comprehensive illustration of the genetic background of pediatric acute myeloid leukemia. Blood Adv 2019;3(20):3157–69.
16. Alexander TB, Gu Z, Iacobucci I, et al. The genetic basis and cell of origin of mixed phenotype acute leukaemia. Nature 2018;562(7727):373–9.
17. Murakami N, Okuno Y, Yoshida K, et al. Integrated molecular profiling of juvenile myelomonocytic leukemia. Blood 2018;131(14):1576–86.
18. Chao AK, Meyer JA, Lee AG, et al. Fusion driven JMML: a novel CCDC88C-FLT3 fusion responsive to sorafenib identified by RNA sequencing. Leukemia 2020; 34(2):662–6.
19. Pozdnyakova O, Orazi A, Kelemen K, et al. Myeloid/lymphoid neoplasms associated with eosinophilia and rearrangements of PDGFRA, PDGFRB, or FGFR1 or with PCM1-JAK2. Am J Clin Pathol 2021;155(2):160–78.
20. Childhood Acute Lymphoblastic Leukemia Treatment (PDQ(R)): Health Professional Version. PDQ cancer information summaries. Available at: https://www.ncbi.nlm.nih.gov/pubmed/26389206. Accessed May 01, 2021.
21. Childhood Acute Myeloid Leukemia/Other Myeloid Malignancies Treatment (PDQ(R)): Health Professional Version. PDQ cancer information summaries. Available at: https://www.ncbi.nlm.nih.gov/pubmed/26389454. Accessed May 01, 2021.
22. Druker BJ, Sawyers CL, Kantarjian H, et al. Activity of a specific inhibitor of the BCR-ABL tyrosine kinase in the blast crisis of chronic myeloid leukemia and acute lymphoblastic leukemia with the Philadelphia chromosome. N Engl J Med 2001; 344(14):1038–42.
23. Slayton WB, Schultz KR, Kairalla JA, et al. Dasatinib plus intensive chemotherapy in children, adolescents, and young adults with Philadelphia chromosome-positive acute lymphoblastic leukemia: results of children's oncology group trial AALL0622. J Clin Oncol 2018;36(22):2306–14.
24. Tanasi I, Ba I, Sirvent N, et al. Efficacy of tyrosine kinase inhibitors in Ph-like acute lymphoblastic leukemia harboring ABL-class rearrangements. Blood 2019; 134(16):1351–5.
25. Megias-Vericat JE, Ballesta-Lopez O, Barragan E, et al. Tyrosine kinase inhibitors for acute myeloid leukemia: a step toward disease control? Blood Rev 2020;44: 100675.

26. Maruffi M, Sposto R, Oberley MJ, et al. Therapy for children and adults with mixed phenotype acute leukemia: a systematic review and meta-analysis. Leukemia 2018;32(7):1515–28.
27. Fenaux P, Chastang C, Chevret S, et al. A randomized comparison of all transretinoic acid (ATRA) followed by chemotherapy and ATRA plus chemotherapy and the role of maintenance therapy in newly diagnosed acute promyelocytic leukemia. The European APL Group. Blood 1999;94(4):1192–200.
28. Cario G, Leoni V, Conter V, et al. BCR-ABL1-like acute lymphoblastic leukemia in childhood and targeted therapy. Haematologica 2020;105(9):2200–4.
29. Nardi V, Ku N, Frigault MJ, et al. Clinical response to larotrectinib in adult Philadelphia chromosome-like ALL with cryptic ETV6-NTRK3 rearrangement. Blood Adv 2020;4(1):106–11.
30. Schewe DM, Lenk L, Vogiatzi F, et al. Larotrectinib in TRK fusion-positive pediatric B-cell acute lymphoblastic leukemia. Blood Adv 2019;3(22):3499–502.
31. Taylor J, Pavlick D, Yoshimi A, et al. Oncogenic TRK fusions are amenable to inhibition in hematologic malignancies. J Clin Invest 2018;128(9):3819–25.
32. Nowell PC, Hungerford DA. A minute chromosome in human chronic granulocytic leukemia. Science 1960;142:1497.
33. Tkachuk DC, Westbrook CA, Andreeff M, et al. Detection of BCR-ABL fusion in chronic myelogeneous leukemia by in situ hybridization. Science 1990; 250(4980):559–62.
34. Peterson JF, Pitel BA, Smoley SA, et al. Detection of a cryptic NUP214/ABL1 gene fusion by mate-pair sequencing (MPseq) in a newly diagnosed case of pediatric T-lymphoblastic leukemia. Cold Spring Harb Mol Case Stud 2019;5(2):a003533.
35. Campbell LJ, Oei P, Brookwell R, et al. FISH detection of PML-RARA fusion in ins(15;17) acute promyelocytic leukaemia depends on probe size. Biomed Res Int 2013;2013:164501.
36. Salto-Tellez M, Shelat SG, Benoit B, et al. Multiplex RT-PCR for the detection of leukemia-associated translocations: validation and application to routine molecular diagnostic practice. J Mol Diagn 2003;5(4):231–6.
37. Olesen LH, Clausen N, Dimitrijevic A, et al. Prospective application of a multiplex reverse transcription-polymerase chain reaction assay for the detection of balanced translocations in leukaemia: a single-laboratory study of 390 paediatric and adult patients. Br J Haematol 2004;127(1):59–66.
38. Meyer C, Burmeister T, Groger D, et al. The MLL recombinome of acute leukemias in 2017. Leukemia 2018;32(2):273–84.
39. Press RD, Kamel-Reid S, Ang D. BCR-ABL1 RT-qPCR for monitoring the molecular response to tyrosine kinase inhibitors in chronic myeloid leukemia. J Mol Diagn 2013;15(5):565–76.
40. Krook MA, Reeser JW, Ernst G, et al. Fibroblast growth factor receptors in cancer: genetic alterations, diagnostics, therapeutic targets and mechanisms of resistance. Br J Cancer 2021;124(5):880–92.
41. Cheng DT, Mitchell TN, Zehir A, et al. Memorial sloan kettering-integrated mutation profiling of actionable cancer targets (MSK-IMPACT): a hybridization capture-based next-generation sequencing clinical assay for solid tumor molecular oncology. J Mol Diagn 2015;17(3):251–64.
42. Garcia EP, Minkovsky A, Jia Y, et al. Validation of oncopanel: a targeted next-generation sequencing assay for the detection of somatic variants in cancer. Arch Pathol Lab Med 2017;141(6):751–8.
43. Chang F, Lin F, Cao K, et al. Development and clinical validation of a large fusion gene panel for pediatric cancers. J Mol Diagn 2019;21(5):873–83.

44. Beg S, Bareja R, Ohara K, et al. Integration of whole-exome and anchored PCR-based next generation sequencing significantly increases detection of actionable alterations in precision oncology. Transl Oncol 2021;14(1):100944.
45. Benayed R, Offin M, Mullaney K, et al. High yield of RNA sequencing for targetable kinase fusions in lung adenocarcinomas with no mitogenic driver alteration detected by DNA sequencing and low tumor mutation burden. Clin Cancer Res 2019;25(15):4712–22.
46. Hiemenz MC, Ostrow DG, Busse TM, et al. OncoKids: a comprehensive next-generation sequencing panel for pediatric malignancies. J Mol Diagn 2018; 20(6):765–76.
47. Engvall M, Cahill N, Jonsson BI, et al. Detection of leukemia gene fusions by targeted RNA-sequencing in routine diagnostics. BMC Med Genomics 2020; 13(1):106.
48. Kim B, Lee H, Shin S, et al. Clinical evaluation of massively parallel RNA sequencing for detecting recurrent gene fusions in hematologic malignancies. J Mol Diagn 2019;21(1):163–70.
49. Zheng Z, Liebers M, Zhelyazkova B, et al. Anchored multiplex PCR for targeted next-generation sequencing. Nat Med 2014;20(12):1479–84.
50. Liu Y, Easton J, Shao Y, et al. The genomic landscape of pediatric and young adult T-lineage acute lymphoblastic leukemia. Nat Genet 2017;49(8):1211–8.
51. Liu YF, Wang BY, Zhang WN, et al. Genomic profiling of adult and pediatric B-cell acute lymphoblastic leukemia. EBioMedicine 2016;8:173–83.
52. Ma X, Liu Y, Liu Y, et al. Pan-cancer genome and transcriptome analyses of 1,699 paediatric leukaemias and solid tumours. Nature 2018;555(7696):371–6.
53. Gu Z, Churchman ML, Roberts KG, et al. PAX5-driven subtypes of B-progenitor acute lymphoblastic leukemia. Nat Genet 2019;51(2):296–307.
54. Beaubier N, Tell R, Lau D, et al. Clinical validation of the tempus xT next-generation targeted oncology sequencing assay. Oncotarget 2019;10(24): 2384–96.
55. Rusch M, Nakitandwe J, Shurtleff S, et al. Clinical cancer genomic profiling by three-platform sequencing of whole genome, whole exome and transcriptome. Nat Commun 2018;9(1):3962.
56. Aypar U, Smoley SA, Pitel BA, et al. Mate pair sequencing improves detection of genomic abnormalities in acute myeloid leukemia. Eur J Haematol 2019;102(1): 87–96.
57. Zhong Y, Beimnet K, Alli Z, et al. Multiplexed digital detection of B-cell acute lymphoblastic leukemia fusion transcripts using the NanoString nCounter system. J Mol Diagn 2020;22(1):72–80.
58. Brunetti C, Anelli L, Zagaria A, et al. Droplet digital PCR is a reliable tool for monitoring minimal residual disease in acute promyelocytic leukemia. J Mol Diagn 2017;19(3):437–44.
59. Ohki K, Takahashi H, Fukushima T, et al. Impact of immunophenotypic characteristics on genetic subgrouping in childhood acute lymphoblastic leukemia: Tokyo Children's Cancer Study Group (TCCSG) study L04-16. Genes Chromosomes Cancer 2020;59(10):551–61.

Printed and bound by CPI Group (UK) Ltd, Croydon, CR0 4YY
03/10/2024
01040479-0009

Atrial Fibrillation and Heart Failure

Editors

ANDREW A. GRACE
SANJIV M. NARAYAN
MARK D. O'NEILL

HEART FAILURE CLINICS

www.heartfailure.theclinics.com

Consulting Editors
MANDEEP R. MEHRA
JAVED BUTLER

Founding Editor
JAGAT NARULA

October 2013 • Volume 9 • Number 4

ELSEVIER

1600 John F. Kennedy Boulevard • Suite 1800 • Philadelphia, Pennsylvania, 19103-2899

http://www.theclinics.com

HEART FAILURE CLINICS Volume 9, Number 4
October 2013 ISSN 1551-7136, ISBN-13: 978-0-323-22720-9

Editor: Barbara Cohen-Kligerman
Developmental Editor: Susan Showalter

Heart Failure Clinics (ISSN 1551-7136) is published quarterly by Elsevier Inc., 360 Park Avenue South, New York, NY 10010-1710. Months of publication are January, April, July, and October. Business and editorial offices: 1600 John F. Kennedy Boulevard, Suite 1800, Philadelphia, PA 19103-2899. Periodicals postage paid at New York, NY, and additional mailing offices. Subscription prices are USD 235.00 per year for US individuals, USD 386.00 per year for US institutions, USD 80.00 per year for US students and residents, USD 280.00 per year for Canadian individuals, USD 442.00 per year for Canadian institutions, USD 300.00 per year for international individuals, USD 442.00 per year for international institutions, and USD 100.00 per year for Canadian and foreign students/residents. To receive student and resident rate, orders must be accompanied by name of affiliated institution, date of term, and the *signature* of program/residency coordinator on institution letterhead. Orders will be billed at individual rate until proof of status is received. Foreign air speed delivery is included in all *Clinics* subscription prices. All prices are subject to change without notice. **POSTMASTER:** Send address changes to *Heart Failure Clinics*, Elsevier Health Sciences Division, Subscription Customer Service, 3251 Riverport Lane, Maryland Heights, MO 63043. **Customer Service: 1-800-654-2452 (US and Canada). From outside of the US and Canada, call 314-447-8871. Fax: 314-447-8029. For print support, e-mail: JournalsCustomerService-usa@elsevier.com. For online support, e-mail: JournalsOnlineSupport-usa@elsevier.com.**

Reprints. For copies of 100 or more of articles in this publication, please contact the Commercial Reprints Department, Elsevier Inc., 360 Park Avenue South, New York, NY 10010-1710. Tel.: 212-633-3874; Fax: 212-633-3820; E-mail: reprints@elsevier.com.

Heart Failure Clinics is covered in *MEDLINE/PubMed (Index Medicus).*

Printed and bound by CPI Group (UK) Ltd, Croydon, CR0 4YY

Transferred to digital print 2012

Contributors

CONSULTING EDITORS

MANDEEP R. MEHRA, MD
Professor of Medicine, Harvard Medical School; Co-Director, BWH Cardiovascular; and Executive Director, Center for Advanced Heart Disease, Brigham and Women's Hospital, Boston, Massachusetts

JAVED BUTLER, MD, MPH
Professor of Medicine; Director, Heart Failure Research, Emory University, Atlanta, Georgia

EDITORS

ANDREW A. GRACE, MB, PhD, FRCP
Department of Biochemistry, University of Cambridge; Papworth Hospital, Cambridge, United Kingdom

SANJIV M. NARAYAN, MD, PhD, FRCP, FHRS
Professor of Medicine, Director of Electrophysiology, San Diego VA Healthcare System, University of California, San Diego, San Diego, California

MARK D. O'NEILL, DPhil, FRCP, FHRS
Consultant Cardiologist and Reader in Clinical Cardiac Electrophysiology, Divisions of Imaging Sciences and Biomedical Engineering and Cardiovascular Medicine, Medical Engineering Centre, St. Thomas' Hospital, London, United Kingdom

AUTHORS

ISSAM H. ABU-TAHA, PhD
Faculty of Medicine, Institute of Pharmacology, University Duisburg-Essen, Essen, Germany

AYOTUNDE BAMIMORE, MB, ChB
Electrophysiology Fellow/Clinical Instructor, Division of Cardiology, University of North Carolina, Chapel Hill, Chapel Hill, North Carolina

S. SERGE BAROLD, MD, FACC, FAHA, FHRS
Clinical Professor of Medicine Emeritus, University of Rochester School of Medicine and Dentistry, Rochester, New York

JOHN G.F. CLELAND, MD, FRCP, FACC, FESC
Department of Cardiology, Castle Hill Hospital, Hull York Medical School, University of Hull, Kingston-upon-Hull, United Kingdom

EUGENE C. DEPASQUALE, MD
Clinical Instructor, Ahmanson-UCLA Cardiomyopathy Center, David Geffen School of Medicine, Los Angeles, California

BENJAMIN DICKEN, MBBS, MRCP
Department of Cardiology, Castle Hill Hospital, Hull York Medical School, University of Hull, Kingston-upon-Hull, United Kingdom

DOBROMIR DOBREV, MD
Faculty of Medicine, Institute of Pharmacology, University Duisburg-Essen, Essen; Division of Experimental Cardiology, Medical Faculty Mannheim, Heidelberg University; DZHK (German Centre for Cardiovascular Research) partner site Mannheim/Heidelberg, Mannheim, Germany

GREGG C. FONAROW, MD
Eliot Corday Professor of Cardiovascular Medicine and Science, Co-Chief of Clinical Cardiology, UCLA Division of Cardiology, Director, Ahmanson-UCLA Cardiomyopathy Center, David Geffen School of Medicine, Los Angeles, California

DARREL P. FRANCIS, FRCP, MD
International Centre for Circulatory Health, National Heart and Lung Institute, Imperial College London, London, United Kingdom

ANDREAS GOETTE, MD
Department of Cardiology and Intensive Care Medicine, St. Vincenz Hospital Paderborn GmbH, EUTRAF Working Group, University Hospital Magdeburg, Paderborn, Germany

ANDREW A. GRACE, MB, PhD, FRCP
Department of Biochemistry, University of Cambridge; Papworth Hospital, Cambridge, United Kingdom

PATRICK M. HECK, BM BCh
Department of Cardiology, Papworth Hospital, Papworth Everard, Cambridge, United Kingdom

JORDI HEIJMAN, PhD
Faculty of Medicine, Institute of Pharmacology, University Duisburg-Essen, Essen, Germany

BENGT HERWEG, MD, FACC, FHRS
Associate Professor of Medicine, Director, Electrophysiology and Arrhythmia Services, Department of Cardiovascular Disease, University of South Florida Morsani College of Medicine, Tampa, Florida

FREIDOON KESHAVARZI, MD, MRCP
Department of Cardiology, Castle Hill Hospital, Hull York Medical School, University of Hull, Kingston-upon-Hull, United Kingdom

SENTHIL KIRUBAKARAN, MRCP, MD
Cardiothoracic Department, Guy's and St Thomas' NHS Trust, London, United Kingdom

PETER M. KISTLER, MBBS, PhD
Associate Professor, Department of Cardiology, Baker IDI, Melbourne; Department of Cardiovascular Medicine, Alfred Heart Centre, Alfred Hospital, Baker IDI Heart and Diabetes Institute, University of Melbourne, Victoria, Australia

STEPHEN R. LARGE, MA, MS, FRCS, FRCP, MBA
Papworth Hospital, Cambridge, United Kingdom

JUSTIN M.S. LEE, BM BCh
Department of Cardiology, Papworth Hospital, Papworth Everard, Cambridge, United Kingdom

GREGORY Y.H. LIP, MD
Professor of Cardiovascular Medicine, University of Birmingham Centre for Cardiovascular Sciences, City Hospital, Birmingham, West Midlands, United Kingdom

PAUL MOUNSEY, BSc, BM BCh, PhD, MRCP, FACC
Chief of Electrophysiology and Professor of Medicine, Division of Cardiology, University of North Carolina, Chapel Hill, Chapel Hill, North Carolina

SANJIV M. NARAYAN, MD, PhD
Professor of Medicine, Director of Electrophysiology, San Diego VA Healthcare System, University of California, San Diego, San Diego, California

SAMER A.M. NASHEF, MB ChB, FRCS, PhD
Papworth Hospital, Cambridge, United Kingdom

MARK D. O'NEILL, DPhil, FRCP, FHRS
Consultant Cardiologist and Reader in Clinical Cardiac Electrophysiology, Divisions of Imaging Sciences and Biomedical Engineering and Cardiovascular Medicine, Medical Engineering Centre, St. Thomas' Hospital, London, United Kingdom

PIERPAOLO PELLICORI, MD
Department of Cardiology, Castle Hill Hospital, Hull York Medical School, University of Hull, Kingston-upon-Hull, United Kingdom

MICHIEL RIENSTRA, MD, PhD
Department of Cardiology, University Medical Center Groningen, University of Groningen, Groningen, The Netherlands

EDUARD SHANTSILA, PhD
Research Fellow, University of Birmingham Centre for Cardiovascular Sciences, City Hospital, Birmingham, West Midlands, United Kingdom

JAGMEET P. SINGH, MD, PhD, DPhil
Cardiac Arrhythmia Service, Massachusetts General Hospital, Associate Professor of Medicine, Harvard Medical School, Boston, Massachusetts

NITESH SOOD, MD
Division of Cardiology, Lahey Clinic, Tufts University, Burlington, Massachusetts

JONATHAN S. STEINBERG, MD, FACC, FHRS
Director, Arrhythmia Institute, Valley Health System, Ridgewood, New Jersey; Professor of Medicine, Columbia University College of Physicians and Surgeons, New York, New York

ISABELLE C. VAN GELDER, MD, PhD
Department of Cardiology, University Medical Center Groningen, University of Groningen, Groningen, The Netherlands

ESZTER M. VEGH, MD
Cardiac Arrhythmia Service, Massachusetts General Hospital, Harvard Medical School, Boston, Massachusetts

NIELS VOIGT, MD
Faculty of Medicine, Institute of Pharmacology, University Duisburg-Essen, Essen; Division of Experimental Cardiology, Medical Faculty Mannheim, Heidelberg University, Mannheim, Germany

ZACHARY I. WHINNETT, BMedSci, BMBS, MRCP, PhD
International Centre for Circulatory Health, National Heart and Lung Institute, Imperial College London, London, United Kingdom

Contents

Foreword: Atrial Fibrillation and Heart Failure: It Takes Two to Tango **xiii**

Mandeep R. Mehra and Javed Butler

Preface: Atrial Fibrillation and Heart Failure **xv**

Andrew A. Grace, Sanjiv M. Narayan, and Mark D. O'Neill

Common Threads in Atrial Fibrillation and Heart Failure **373**

Andrew A. Grace and Sanjiv M. Narayan

The prevalence of both chronic heart failure and atrial fibrillation is increasing as a result of systemic multimorbid risk and improved therapy of acute heart disease. Current treatment options are unsatisfactory especially regarding antiarrhythmic drugs. We propose that a systems biology approach to increase understanding of cardiac arrhythmias offers the best immediate way forward. Such an approach would be based on an accumulation of large clinical datasets, and application of next-generation sequencing in conjunction with selected experimental and computer-based models. Such an approach would in turn facilitate the development and targeted application of currently available and novel therapeutic approaches.

Continuous Monitoring of Atrial Fibrillation in Heart Failure **385**

Bengt Herweg, S. Serge Barold, and Jonathan S. Steinberg

In patients with atrial fibrillation (AF) undergoing cardiac resynchronization therapy (CRT) for heart failure, continuous monitoring of the percentage of biventricular (BiV%) pacing has shown that the greatest improvement and reduction in mortality occur with a BiV pacing greater than 98%. Continuous monitoring of BiV pacing has improved the CRT management of patients with AF. Continuous monitoring has generated important new questions about anticoagulant therapy, which require randomized trials. Anticoagulant therapy should probably be considered in patients who have a high risk of thromboembolism according to standard scoring systems.

Ventricular Rate Control of Atrial Fibrillation in Heart Failure **397**

Michiel Rienstra and Isabelle C. Van Gelder

In the last few years, there has been a major shift in the treatment of atrial fibrillation (AF) in the setting of hear failure (HF), from rhythm to ventricular rate control in most patients with both conditions. In this article, the authors focus on ventricular rate control and discuss the indications; the optimal ventricular rate-control target, including detailed results of the Rate Control Efficacy in Permanent Atrial Fibrillation: a Comparison Between Lenient versus Strict Rate Control II (RACE II) study; and the pharmacologic and nonpharmacologic options to control the ventricular rate during AF in the setting of HF.

Rhythm Control of Atrial Fibrillation in Heart Failure **407**

Jordi Heijman, Niels Voigt, Issam H. Abu-Taha, and Dobromir Dobrev

Atrial fibrillation (AF) and heart failure (HF) are common cardiovascular pathologies with severe prognostic implications that show bidirectional interactions. Rate and rhythm control are the main therapeutic strategies for patients with AF and HF. There is a paucity of safe and effective antiarrhythmic drugs for rhythm control of AF in HF, with amiodarone and (in the United States) dofetilide as the only imperfect options. The basic mechanisms of AF are discussed and the evidence and limitations of AF rhythm control options for patients with HF are reviewed. In addition, novel potential antiarrhythmic strategies for rhythm control of AF are highlighted.

Upstream Therapy for Atrial Fibrillation in Heart Failure **417**

Andreas Goette

Atrial fibrillation (AF) is a common arrhythmia that occurs as the result of various pathophysiologic processes. Heart failure increases the likelihood of AF. Several aspects of the morphologic and electrophysiologic alterations promoting AF in heart failure (congestive heart failure [CHF]) have been studied in animal models and patients with CHF. Under these conditions, ectopic activity originating from the pulmonary veins or other sites is more likely to occur and trigger longer episodes of AF. This article summarizes the impact of angiotensin-converting enzyme inhibitors, angiotensin II receptor blockers and statins, so-called upstream therapy, in patients who have CHF with AF.

Stroke Prevention in Atrial Fibrillation in Heart Failure **427**

Eduard Shantsila and Gregory Y.H. Lip

Heart failure and atrial fibrillation are major problems of modern cardiology with important clinical, prognostic, and socioeconomic implications. The risks are high morbidity, impaired quality of life, poor outcome, and increased risk of stroke. Oral anticoagulation with vitamin K antagonists or novel licensed medicines should be considered unless contraindicated. Possible benefits of sinus rhythm maintenance are not entirely clear and need to be explored further. Relatively scarce data are available on stroke prevention in atrial fibrillation in heart failure with preserved ejection fraction; this requires further research.

Impact of Atrial Fibrillation on Outcomes in Heart Failure **437**

Eugene C. DePasquale and Gregg C. Fonarow

The prevalence of atrial fibrillation (AF) and heart failure increases with advancing age. It is estimated that the annual incidence of AF in the general heart failure population is approximately 5%, whereas as many as 40% of patients with advanced heart failure have AF. The goals of therapy in patients with heart failure and AF are symptom control and prevention of arterial thromboembolism. The adverse hemodynamic events of AF may lead to symptom deterioration and reduced exercise capacity. This review addresses the impact of AF on heart failure outcomes as they pertain to prognosis and management.

Atrial Fibrillation in Heart Failure in the Older Population **451**

Patrick M. Heck, Justin M.S. Lee, and Peter M. Kistler

Atrial fibrillation (AF) is an important and often-underrecognized cause of cardiovascular morbidity and mortality. It is an arrhythmia that is commonly seen in the older patient; the median age of patients with AF in early studies was 75 years. Heart failure (HF) is also more frequently seen in the older patient with an approximate doubling of HF prevalence with each decade of life. There is clear interaction between

AF and HF, with evidence that HF can lead to AF and AF exacerbates HF. This review focuses on the specific aspect of AF management in elderly patients with HF.

Case Selection for Cardiac Resynchronization in Atrial Fibrillation **461**

John G.F. Cleland, Freidoon Keshavarzi, Pierpaolo Pellicori, and Benjamin Dicken

Remarkably little evidence exists that cardiac resynchronization therapy (CRT) is effective in patients who have atrial fibrillation (AF) but who otherwise seem suitable for this treatment. The landmark trials of CRT generally excluded patients with AF because atrioventricular (AV) resynchronization was considered a possibly important mechanism by which CRT might deliver its benefits. The only landmark trial that included many patients with AF confirmed marked benefit among patients in sinus rhythm but no benefit among those with AF. Evidence is lacking that biventricular rather than AV resynchronization is an important mechanism for delivering the benefits of CRT.

Cardiac Resynchronization Therapy Mechanisms in Atrial Fibrillation **475**

Zachary I. Whinnett and Darrel P. Francis

This article examines how to assess the reliability of potential techniques for performing optimization of biventricular pacemakers in patients with atrial fibrillation. It explores the magnitude of improvement that is likely to be obtained with the optimization of biventricular pacing in this clinical setting and discusses the lessons that can be learned with regard to the mechanisms of action of biventricular pacing in the general heart failure population.

The Role of Ablation of the Atrioventricular Junction in Patients with Heart Failure and Atrial Fibrillation **489**

Eszter M. Vegh, Nitesh Sood, and Jagmeet P. Singh

Ablation of the atrioventricular junction (AVJ) is a technically easy procedure that is safe and has a high success rate as an intervention for effective ventricular rate control in patients in symptomatic atrial fibrillation. AVJ ablation has been reported to improve quality of life, left ventricular ejection fraction, and exercise duration in these patients and minimize the incidence of inappropriate shocks. Because right ventricular pacing after AVJ ablation may result in decrease in left ventricular function and worsening of heart failure symptoms, there is increasing evidence to support the effectiveness of cardiac resynchronization therapy in atrial fibrillation populations.

Ablation of Atrial Tachycardia and Atrial Flutter in Heart Failure **501**

Ayotunde Bamimore and Paul Mounsey

Atrial tachycardia and atrial flutter are common tachyarrhythmias in the heart failure population. They commonly lead to, exacerbate, and increase the morbidity and mortality associated with heart failure and, thereby, warrant urgent and early definitive therapy in the form of catheter ablation. Catheter ablation requires careful patient stabilization and extensive preprocedural planning, particularly with regards to anesthesia, strategy, catheter choice, mapping system, and fluid balance, to increase efficacy and limit adverse effects. Heart failure may limit the success of catheter ablation with higher reported recurrence rates, and in selected patients, a hybrid epicardial-endocardial ablation can be considered.

Catheter Ablation of Atrial Fibrillation in Heart Failure 515

Senthil Kirubakaran and Mark D. O'Neill

Atrial fibrillation in the presence of heart failure is an independent predictor of mortality and is associated with increased hospitalizations and worsening New York Heart Association functional class. Despite these associations, large-scale trials have not shown a benefit in rhythm restoration. However, further analysis of these trials showed that patients who remained in sinus rhythm did have improved survival rates. Studies to examine the efficacy of catheter ablation of atrial fibrillation were therefore conducted and reported efficacy rates ranging from 50% to 92% at maintaining sinus rhythm with associated improvements in left ventricular ejection fraction, quality of life, and New York Heart Association functional class.

Surgical Treatment of Atrial Fibrillation in the Heart Failure Population 533

Stephen R. Large and Samer A.M. Nashef

Surgery to correct a structural heart valve problem can restore sinus rhythm in approximately one-fifth of patients with atrial fibrillation (AF), and the addition of a maze procedure will increase this proportion. Evidence shows that the maze procedure may restore atrial function in some patients and may have beneficial effects on functional symptoms and prognosis. The role of the maze procedure as an isolated treatment for lone AF in the context of heart failure with no structurally correctable cause is unknown. Future progress will determine the appropriate indications for treatment and the risks and benefits of any intervention.

Index 541

HEART FAILURE CLINICS

FORTHCOMING ISSUES

January 2014
Heart Failure in Adult Congenital Heart Disease
Alexander R. Opotowsky and Michael Job Landzberg, *Editors*

April 2014
Co-morbidities in Patients with Heart Failure
Faiez Zannad and Hector Ventura, *Editors*

July 2014
Heart Failure with Preserved Ejection Fraction
Carolyn Lam Su Ping and Burkert Pieske, *Editors*

RECENT ISSUES

July 2013
Hospitalization For Heart Failure
Mihai Gheorghiade and Savina Nodari, *Editors*

April 2013
Takotsubo (Stress) Cardiomyopathy
Eduardo Bossone and Raimund Erbel, *Editors*

January 2013
Comparative-Effectiveness Research in Heart Failure
Mark Hlatky, *Editor*

ISSUES OF RELATED INTEREST

Cardiac Electrophysiology Clinics June 2013 (Vol. 5, No. 2)
Mapping of Atrial Tachycardias Post-Atrial Fibrillation Ablation
Ashok J. Shah, Michel Haissaguerre, and Shinsuke Miyazaki, *Editors*
Available at: http://www.cardiacep.theclinics.com

Interventional Cardiology Clinics July 2013 (Vol. 2, No. 3)
Percutaneous Ventricular Support
Howard A. Cohen and Jose P.S. Henriques, *Editors*
Available at: http://www.cardiacep.theclinics.com

Foreword

Atrial Fibrillation and Heart Failure: It Takes Two to Tango

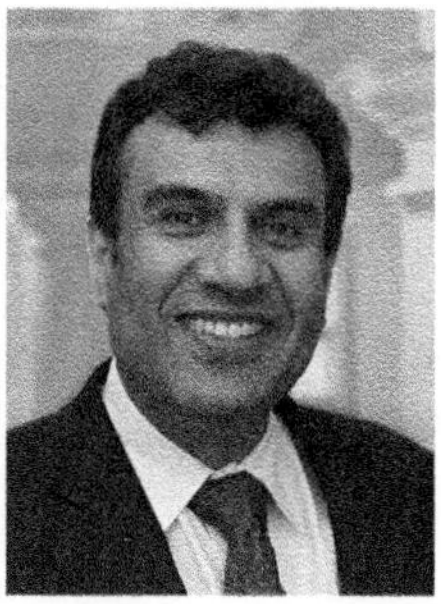

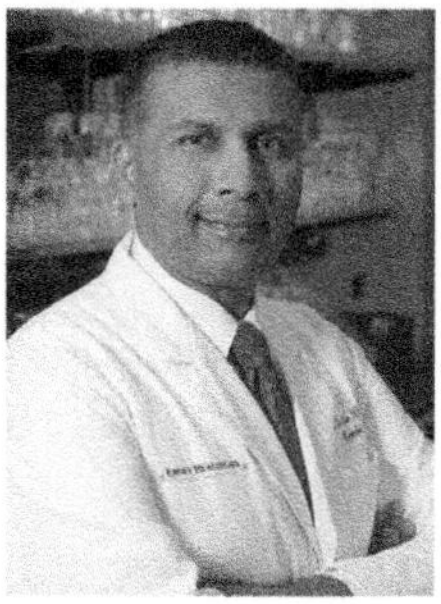

Mandeep R. Mehra, MD Javed Butler, MD, MPH
Consulting Editors

Even as we celebrate control of preclinical risk markers such as hypertension, endorse campaigns to reduce adverse cardiovascular consequences of tobacco, and gain comfort in strategies to target episodes of crises such as sudden death and acute coronary syndromes, the growing combined burden of atrial fibrillation and heart failure remains a gnawing sore. It is estimated that unless tackled meticulously by 2050, the epidemics of atrial fibrillation and heart failure will gulp down the cardiovascular economic resources and create a frightening combined morbidity.

Atrial fibrillation can cause heart failure by reducing atrial contribution to cardiac output and decreasing diastolic filling time (including influencing myocardial coronary blood flow). This may be of particular importance among patients with heart failure and preserved ejection fraction. If the rapid heart rates are left unchecked, tachycardia-induced cardiomyopathy can result. Heart failure can raise intra-atrial filling pressures, stimulate stretch-induced fibrosis, and promote aberrant cellular signaling that can perpetuate atrial fibrillation even further, rendering it difficult to treat. The neurohormonal milieu activated in heart failure has been shown to induce these very structural cellular and tissue changes in the atria that set up the nidus for a complex interplay between these two syndromes.

Thus, it is not at all surprising that the onset of atrial fibrillation in the journey of heart failure syndromes signals an adverse prognosis and decreases the quality of life for our patients. Therapy targeted as an anti-arrhythmic can often destabilize the heart failure syndrome by promoting pro-arrhythmia and negative myocardial effects. Similarly, the presence of heart failure reduces the effectiveness of such therapy and the ability to optimally titrate treatment to control the arrhythmia. Complex therapeutics and smaller gains have propelled the scientific community to seek mechanical treatment options using ablative techniques with variable success.

Heart Failure Clin 9 (2013) xiii–xiv
http://dx.doi.org/10.1016/j.hfc.2013.08.001
1551-7136/13/$ – see front matter

Also, considering the increased risk of stroke in these patients, recent research has also focused on developing novel drugs and devices that are more effective or have a better safety profile for stroke prevention in atrial fibrillation.

In this timely issue of *Heart Failure Clinics*, the combined editorial force of Drs Andrew A. Grace, Sanjiv M. Narayan, and Mark D. O'Neill bring to our readers an extraordinary compilation of articles that outline the current and future challenges in this arena. We invite you to review their thoughtful coverage of this issue in a "one-stop shop" of the state of art in this evolving important field.

Mandeep R. Mehra, MD
Center for Advanced Heart Disease
Brigham and Women's Hospital
75 Francis Street
A Building, 3rd Floor, Room AB324
Boston, MA 02115, USA

Javed Butler, MD, MPH
Emory Clinical Cardiovascular Research Institute
1462 Clifton Road NE, Suite 504
Atlanta, GA 30322, USA

E-mail addresses:
MMEHRA@partners.org (M.R. Mehra)
javed.butler@emory.edu (J. Butler)

Preface
Atrial Fibrillation and Heart Failure

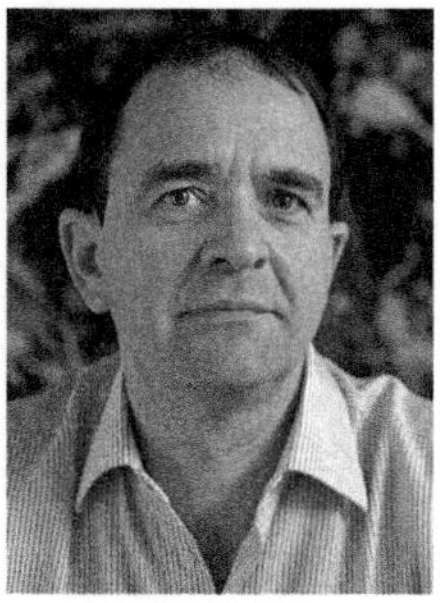

Andrew A. Grace, MB, PhD, FRCP

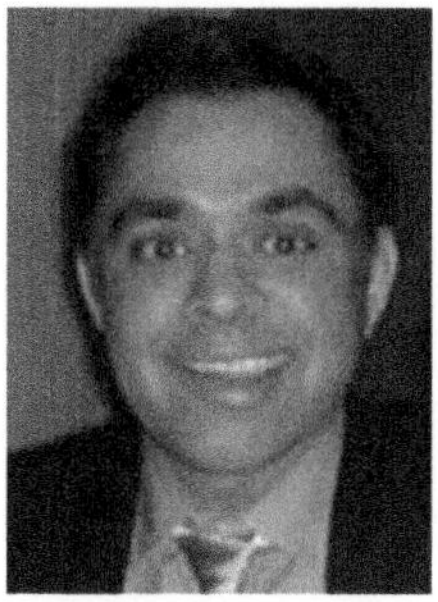

Sanjiv M. Narayan, MD, PhD, FRCP, FHRS

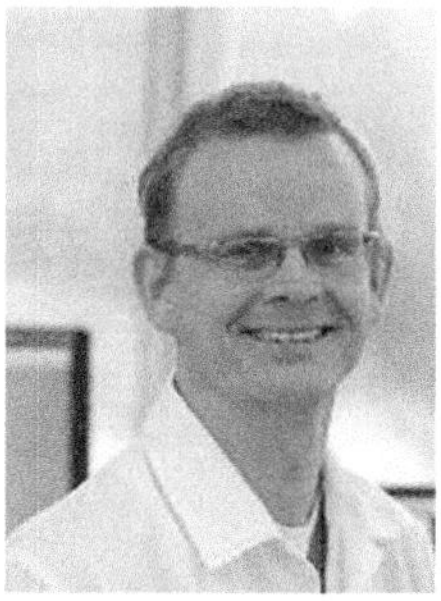

Mark D. O'Neill, DPhil, FRCP, FHRS

Editors

Atrial fibrillation and heart failure each have major medical impact. The substantial scale of their independent influence on morbidity, mortality, and public health has however only been appreciated recently. This realization has already had population benefit with improved early detection and prophylaxis against stroke and progressive pump failure.

Their frequent coexistence, while long recognized, adds new layers to management decisions and the situations that can then arise are addressed in this volume. Our target audience are the subscribers to the *Heart Failure Clinics* series and the objective has been to enhance patient care. The authors of individual articles, while mostly having as their primary interest cardiac arrhythmia, actually represent a broad diversity of interests and talents and present contrasting but complementary perspectives.

The prevalence of atrial fibrillation and heart failure will continue to rise and treatment options are set to expand. Accordingly, the complexity of the decisions for this group is set to increase. It is hoped that the perspectives in this issue will assist the broader community in making the smartest, most effective choices to achieve the very best in patient care.

Andrew A. Grace, MB, PhD, FRCP
Department of Biochemistry
University of Cambridge
Hopkins Building, Tennis Court Road
CB2 1QW, UK
Papworth Hospital
Cambridge CB23 3RE, UK

Sanjiv M. Narayan, MD, PhD, FRCP, FHRS
San Diego VA Healthcare System
University of California, San Diego
3350 La Jolla Village Drive
San Diego, CA 92161, USA

Mark D. O'Neill, DPhil, FRCP, FHRS
Divisions of Imaging Sciences & Biomedical
Engineering & Cardiovascular Medicine
Medical Engineering Centre
3rd Floor, Lambeth Wing
St. Thomas' Hospital
London SE1 7EH, UK

E-mail addresses:
aag1000@cam.ac.uk (A.A. Grace)
snarayan@ucsd.edu (S.M. Narayan)
mark.oneill@kcl.ac.uk (M.D. O'Neill)

Heart Failure Clin 9 (2013) xv
http://dx.doi.org/10.1016/j.hfc.2013.08.002
1551-7136/13/$ – see front matter

Common Threads in Atrial Fibrillation and Heart Failure

Andrew A. Grace, MB, PhD, FRCP[a,b,*],
Sanjiv M. Narayan, MD, PhD[c]

KEYWORDS

• Chronic heart failure • Atrial fibrillation • Systems biology • Genetics • Genomics • Remodeling

KEY POINTS

- The prevalence of both chronic heart failure and atrial fibrillation is increasing as a result of systemic *multimorbid* risk and improved therapy of acute heart disease.
- Atrial and ventricular tissues are exposed to the same toxicities but the time-dependent responses of different chambers in individuals while apparently idiosyncratic are likely to have an intrinsic/genetic determination.
- Current treatment options are unsatisfactory, especially regarding the availability of effective and safe antiarrhythmic drugs.
- The proposal is that a *systems biology* approach to increase understanding of cardiac arrhythmias offers the best immediate way forward. Such an approach would be based on an accumulation of large clinical datasets, and application of next-generation sequencing in conjunction with selected experimental and computer-based models. Such an approach would in turn facilitate the development and targeted application of currently available and novel therapeutic approaches.

INTRODUCTION

Chronic heart failure (CHF) and atrial fibrillation (AF) are inextricably linked and usually the phenotypic outcome of an exposure to common risks.[1–4] Accordingly, a principal thread is that they each represent chamber-specific expressions of a more global disease of cardiac muscle. The relative contribution of atrial versus ventricular manifestations in an individual is then founded on a combination of intrinsic genetic and acquired/epigenetic influences.[5–8]

When primary clinical expression of disease affects the ventricles, symptoms are likely to be those of pump failure.[9–11] Alternatively, if the primary expression is atrial, then rhythm disturbance will probably be the first thing that brings an individual to the physician's attention.[1,12] Of course it has been recognized for some time that the first presentation in 30% to 35% of patients with CHF may also include explicit clinical evidence of AF.[13,14] Nevertheless, whatever the primary clinical evidence, we propose that this will be only the most obvious expression of disease and

The British Heart Foundation, the Medical Research Council, the Wellcome Trust, and the Biotechnology and Biological Research Council, UK supports A.A. Grace. S.M. Narayan is supported by grants from the National Institutes of Health (R01 HL83359, K24 HL103800).
Commercial and Funding Relationships: A.A. Grace is Founder and equity holder in Electus Medical Inc, Consultant to Medtronic Inc and Xention Ltd. S.M. Narayan is equity holder in Topera Medical Inc, and reports having received honoraria from Medtronic, St. Jude Medical, and Biotronik.
[a] Department of Biochemistry, University of Cambridge, Hopkins Building, Tennis Court Road, Cambridge CB2 1QW, UK; [b] Papworth Hospital, Cambridge CB23 3RE, UK; [c] San Diego VA Healthcare System, University of California, San Diego, 3350 La Jolla Village Drive, San Diego, CA 92161, USA
* Corresponding author. Department of Biochemistry, University of Cambridge, Hopkins Building, Tennis Court Road, Cambridge CB2 1QW, UK.
E-mail address: aag1000@cam.ac.uk

Heart Failure Clin 9 (2013) 373–383
http://dx.doi.org/10.1016/j.hfc.2013.07.011
1551-7136/13/$ – see front matter

in fact contractile and electrical reserve will likely be compromised across all compartments essentially from the outset. Of course when electrical failure (fibrillation) is the first expression of ventricular disease (which most likely will arise at some point in the natural history in fully 50% of patients with CHF), then survival is unlikely unless prompt defibrillation is applied.[10]

After initial presentation, the clinical picture evolves over time based on differential and/or specific chamber remodeling that varies widely among individuals.[15–18] Of course, once patients present with symptoms, drugs will be prescribed that again interface with underlying disease processes to modify progression and the consequences for atrial versus ventricular clinical expression.[1] Disease progress will also be based on the presence and continuing activity of risk factors.[5,19,20]

In this article, we introduce this issue by concentrating on those clinically relevant overlapping mechanisms of disease common to both AF and CHF. The mechanisms more apposite to CHF alone have been covered previously in other contributions in this series and elsewhere.[16]

COEXISTENCE AND RISING PREVALENCE

Approximately 40% of individuals presenting with either CHF or AF will develop clinical evidence of the other condition during further periods of observation.[13] The prevalence of the 2 conditions is rising,[21] but although the incidence of AF continues to rise, CHF incidence may be starting to plateau.[10,21]

Heart failure as a primary diagnosis tends to present in the older population and affects in broad terms 10% of men and 8% of women older than 60 years,[10] with the prevalence of CHF likely to rise to more than 750,000 in the United States over the next 4 decades.[21] AF has a prevalence again in the United States that is currently estimated in the range of 2.7 to 6.1 million, and is anticipated to rise inexorably, with estimates reaching 16 million by 2050.[22] This upward trend is also consistently seen in Europe and elsewhere.[23,24] In the prospective Framingham Heart Study, 1470 participants developed either new AF or new CHF, with 383 (26%) developing both.[13] What is clear is that the more advanced the clinical CHF, the greater is its association with AF (**Fig. 1**).[25] The overall prevalence of AF in CHF is in the range of 13% to 27%.[1,12]

The nature of the relationship between AF and CHF, however, is complex and case specific.[1,4,12] On occasion there will be a common setting for both, such as the individual with dilated cardiomyopathy who presents with AF.[12] In other cases, CHF, for example due to an ST elevation myocardial infarction, may lead secondarily to AF. From the practical clinical standpoint, it is prudent to assume that all patients will have the potential to develop the other condition given time.[1]

COINCIDENT RISK FACTORS

The common etiologic thread linking the coincidence of AF and CHF is that each arises in response to an accumulated exposure of cardiac muscle to a common set of "cardiovascular" risk factors.[5,8,26] These comorbid risks tend to increase with age, thereby explaining the age-related increase in prevalence of each phenotype.[19,27] The simple proposition is that "acquired" conditions,

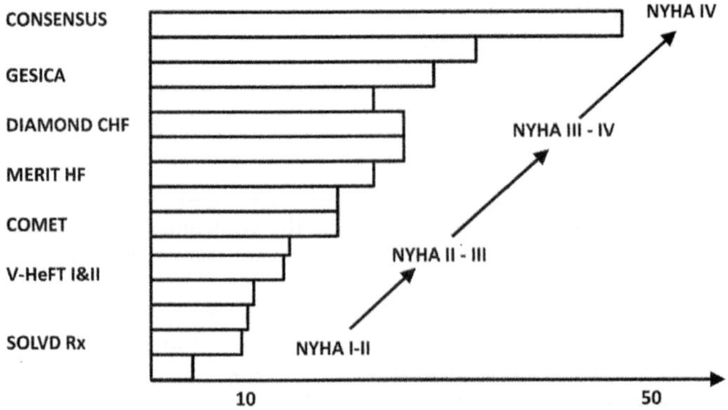

Fig. 1. Atrial fibrillation in patients with symptomatic heart failure: prevalence of atrial fibrillation related to New York Heart Association symptomatic classification in various clinical studies. These relationships highlight the relationship but raise issues of causality and mechanism. (*Adapted from* Savelieva I, John Camm A. Atrial fibrillation and heart failure: natural history and pharmacologic treatment. Europace 2004;5(Suppl 1):S5–19; with permission.)

including hypertension, diabetes, and chronic renal disease, interact with an underlying genetic susceptibility of the individual cardiac chambers, leading to disease expression.[8] The general background risk is therefore set by the increasingly prevalent chronic disease state of *multimorbidity* exposing vulnerable individuals to the development of a disease complex affecting all the cardiac chambers, albeit to a variable clinically explicit extent.[20]

Genetic Variants

Some well-described *monogenic* variants can result in both AF and CHF.[8,12] These include familial cardiomyopathies,[12] laminopathies[28] and some ion channel variants (eg, mutations in the *cardiac* sodium channel gene, *SCN5A*), that can result in both a cardiomyopathic phenotype and AF.[29,30] Although these combinations are relatively rare, they provide insights into "common" CHF by demonstrating the sheer impact of genetic variants on disease expression.[8,19,31]

There are a number of well-described genetic determinants of AF.[7,8,19,30] In this context, the familial occurrence of AF is clear and having an affected parent leads to a doubling of risks in offspring.[8] Ion channel genes are strongly implicated in some families with AF, and patients with ion channel diseases have an increased risk of AF.[8,19] Although there have been practical difficulties in the genetic elucidation of AF, a number of susceptibility alleles have been identified.[7,8,19] Genetic sequence variants at chromosomal location 4q25, representing a noncoding region with the nearest candidate gene being *Pitx2c*, have been strongly associated with AF.[7,32] The relative importance of the interaction between such variants and CHF phenotypes remains the subject of intense study.

Conversely, genetic influences on "common" CHF have been somewhat elusive.[33] Candidate gene studies have identified polymorphic variants that modify risk and are associated with disease progression.[33] Many of these variants encode receptors or the postreceptor cell-signaling machinery of the sympathetic and renin-angiotensin pathways.[33]

It seems highly likely that the capacity to develop either ventricular pump disease or AF in the face of a range of insults will be essentially person specific and determined by the carriage of genetic modifiers.[8,19,31,33] We would therefore anticipate that next-generation sequencing applied to large, well-phenotyped populations will provide genetic/genomic insights of practical value to personalized disease management.[19,31]

Coronary Heart Disease

The direct association of coronary disease with AF is modest,[8] with much of the association being indirect following, for example, myocardial infarction.[12] Coronary disease is, however, the main cause of CHF through both direct and rather more indirect routes.[10] Indeed, substantially improved management of acute coronary disease is a major driver of the current prevalence of CHF,[9,10] with individuals receiving effective immediate coronary intervention likely for all practical purposes to remain at risk of subsequent cardiac muscle attrition and possible CHF.[10] In the wake of an acute coronary event, other manifestations of heart disease dependent on intrinsic susceptibility to, respectively, AF, pump failure, and ventricular fibrillation are all possible.[19]

Obesity and Other Metabolic Factors

Metabolic disease represents a clear and present threat to worldwide public health.[34] Accordingly, whereas hypertension remains a prominent risk factor for CHF and AF, obesity is now also a clearly proven important risk for the development of both.[35,36] In a large community-based sample, obese subjects had an approximately doubling of the risk of CHF.[35] Similarly, for AF, the Framingham Heart Study estimated that obesity was associated with a 50% increase in the risk of AF,[36] further supported from Olmsted County where obesity accounted for 60% of the enhanced age-adjusted and sex-adjusted increase in AF incidence.[22] Furthermore, the Women's Health Study documented both a linear association between body mass index (BMI) and AF, and also that short-term changes in BMI were associated with AF risk.[37] Although some of the influences of obesity may be hemodynamic, such as through impaired ventricular relaxation or atrial stretch, more direct metabolic effects also seem likely (see later in this article).[19]

CONVENTIONAL INTERPRETATIONS OF MECHANISM

Widely diverse presentations and patterns of disease development are well-recognized features of both AF and CHF.[1,4,12] Unsurprisingly, the range of behaviors, emerging clinical scenarios, and complexity expands considerably when both conditions coexist.[1] These characteristics of heterogeneity have served to limit recruitment to clinical studies and thus slowed the acquisition of robust practically useful clinical trial–based data.[1,8]

Initial presentations of combined AF and CHF, although usually occurring against a background of a systemic predisposition, can have a more cardiac-specific trigger, such as acute myocardial infarction or myocarditis.[4,12] In patients presenting with rapidly conducted AF, if the rate remains uncontrolled, then an undefined proportion may go on to develop CHF through the well-recognized clinical progression that defines tachycardiopathy.[12] Conversely, in those with severe pump failure, AF may well supervene, although similarly this is not always the case.[13] These variations in the clinical course support an intrinsic susceptibility in the different chambers.[15,19,26]

Impact of Rate, Rhythm, and Stretch

The intuitive view is that AF can damage the ventricles through junctional transmission of rapid irregular impulses,[12] with the reaction appearing idiosyncratic with no obvious threshold/cutoff in terms of rates/durations.[4,12] Conversely, if the ventricles are failing, then they, in their turn, can negatively influence the atria through their failure to empty and reduced diastolic filling times (**Fig. 2**).[12,38] The evidence to support these various views comes from a range of clinical observations and experimental models.[12,15,16,39,40] This bidirectional clinical interaction will be further influenced through systemic effects arising as a result of the circulation being compromised in the face of rapid rates and/or impaired hemodynamics.

Atrial damage in response to a loss of normal ventricular function is generally thought to arise fundamentally through the actions of atrial "stretch."[1,12,26,39,40] The most prevalent idea is that stretch-activated channels, usually membrane bound, play a key role with downstream alterations in calcium signaling, action potential shortening, and an increased dispersion of refractoriness.[1,26,40] In addition, at the physically observable level, atrial chamber dilatation increases the endocardial surface area (critical mass) that may further facilitate both the initiation and perpetuation of fibrillation.[41] In rabbit hearts, gadolinium and tarantula toxin extract have been shown to inhibit some of these processes.[42] In sheep atria, stretch increased both the rate of AF and facilitated the conduction of rapid activity from the pulmonary veins to the left atrial body,[43] with reversal of stretch being potentially antiarrhythmic.[44]

Systemic Influences

The interest in metabolic determinants of arrhythmias is increasing.[19,45,46] The common cumulative exposure of atria and ventricles to metabolic risks activate highly promiscuous biologic pathways.[17,19] Indeed, inflammatory pathways invoked in vascular and ventricular disease have significant importance for AF.[47,48] Oxidative stress has been strongly implicated as a mechanism for human AF,[47,49,50] with transcriptomes/metabolomes showing coordinated downregulation of enzymes controlling fatty acid oxidation.[16,45] In addition, the propensity to canine AF directly correlates to cellular bioenergetic status[26] and mice with cardiac-specific *Rac1*GTPase overexpression and AF have activated nicotinamide adenine dinucleotide phosphate (NADPH) oxidase.[51] Furthermore, it has now been shown that DNA from degraded mitochondria promotes inflammation, leading to myocellular damage and CHF, with likely implications for the pathogenesis

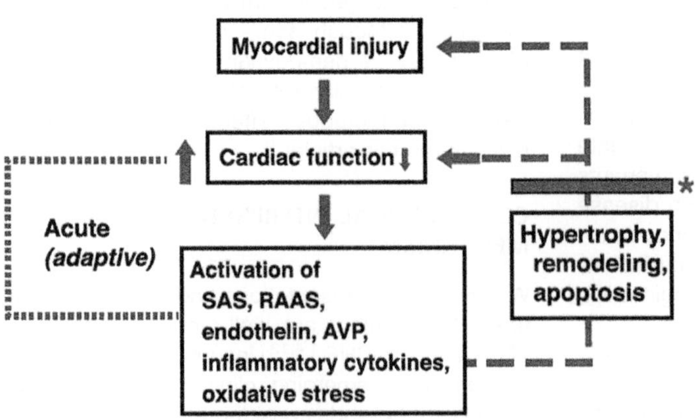

Fig. 2. Interplay between cardiac function and neurohumoral and cytokine systems. Myocardial injury, which may have any of a number of causes, might depress cardiac function, which in turn may cause activation of the sympathoadrenal system (SAS) and the renin-angiotensin-aldosterone system (RAAS) and the elaboration of endothelin, arginine vasopressin (AVP), and cytokines, such as tumor necrosis factor-α. In acute heart failure (*left*), these are adaptive and tend to maintain arterial pressure and cardiac function. In chronic heart failure (*right*), they cause maladaptive hypertrophic remodeling and apoptosis, which cause further atrial and ventricular injury and impairment of cardiac function with electrophysiological consequences. The horizontal line on the right shows that chronic maladaptive influences can be inhibited by angiotensin-converting enzyme inhibitors, β-adrenergic blockers, angiotensin II type 1 receptor blockers, and/or aldosterone antagonists. *, one proposed area of intervention to block remodeling. (*From* Braunwald E. Heart failure. JACC Heart Fail 2013;1:1–20; with permission.)

of AF (**Fig. 3**).[52,53] Additionally, mitochondria have been proposed as an appropriate target for drug intervention in CHF.[54] In sum, the body of biologic evidence supporting the importance of metabolism linking epidemiologic observations through mechanisms to clinical outcomes is now substantial.[19,36,46]

Structural and Electrical Remodeling

At a multicellular tissue level, physiologic substrates for pump failure and arrhythmogenesis evolve over time.[15,16,39] Several components of electrical remodeling are analogous between atria and ventricles: for instance, the calcium overload that characterizes ventricular phenotypes has also been described in the atria.[15,55] Although it was originally thought that functional substrates for AF were defined simply by shortened action potentials and hence abbreviated refractoriness,[39,56] it has since been recognized that structural changes ensue with scarring and fibrosis.[57] Temporal evolution of these derangements is collectively termed "remodeling," during which the relative contributions of functional and anatomic aspects of the substrate to AF change.[15,26] Remodeling shows wide interindividual variation governed by many factors (eg, genetic, individual behavior, epigenetic, and the responses to administered treatment).[19,26,40] Rapid rates undoubtedly promote remodeling in both atria and ventricles, and indeed have been used to generate animals prone to both CHF and AF.[16,40]

Although clinicians clearly recognize remodeling in their patients, the underlying biology remains poorly understood.[15,58] Some patients progress from relatively infrequent runs of self-terminating AF to more persistent patterns over relatively short time frames, whereas in others, clinical evidence of arrhythmia may even regress.[59] Similarly, as presented previously, the ventricle in some patients may be compromised quickly, whereas others may sustain exposure to rapid rates with no obvious sequelae for long periods.[1,12]

Atrial Structural and Functional Remodeling

Structural abnormalities of the atria may be linked even more tightly with atrial fibrillation than previously recognized.[4,16,40,57,60] One recent notable histologic study in humans indicated, for example, that the extent of atrial fibrosis was not directly associated with age, as previously highlighted,[61–63] but instead with the presence and severity of AF.[64] During AF in failing hearts, there is a heterogeneous distribution of fibrosis at the posterior left atrial wall that likely influences dynamic pattern of AF activation and signal complexity.[65] However, although a clear relationship has been identified between the presence of late gadolinium enhancement in the atrium and responses to AF therapy,[66] the relationship between structural remodeling of the atrium and left ventricular function has yet to be established.[66] Intriguingly, transcriptomic studies indicate a

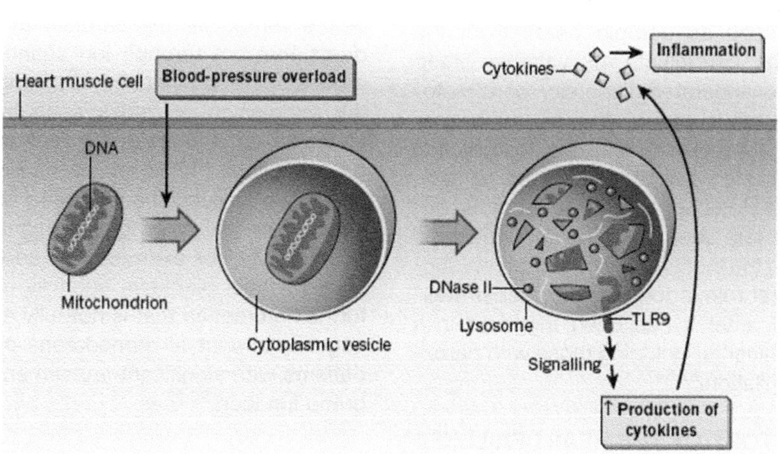

Fig. 3. Mitochodrial DNA induces inflammation and heart failure: Oka and colleagues[52] carried out experiments in mice that suggest a possible mechanism contributing to heart failure. Various processes that put stress on the heart, such as blood-pressure overload, may damage mitochondria in heart muscle cells. These mitochondria are engulfed into cytoplasmic vesicles and transported to lysosomes (intracellular organelles in which mitochondrial components are digested by various enzymes, such as DNase II, which degrades DNA). If mitochondrial DNA accumulates, then the protein TLR9 is activated. Signals from TLR9 induce the production of cytokine proteins, which are then secreted from the cell and act on the same and other heart cells to induce inflammation and contribute over time to adverse organ remodeling. (*From* Konstantinidis K, Kitsis RN. Cardiovascular biology: escaped DNA inflames the heart. Nature 2012;485(7397):179–80; with permission.)

ventricularization of atrial gene expression during AF.[26,67]

Fibrillation Mechanisms

Common themes are emerging that link preclinical and clinical observations, and are helping to rationalize our understanding of the initiation and perpetuation of fibrillation.[68,69] In preclinical models, there is considerable evidence that fibrillation in both atrial and ventricular compartments are sustained by stable localized sources[68,70,71] formed, in turn, by the interaction of action potential duration alternans and conduction velocity slowing to create localized electrical spiral waves (reentry) or regions of triggered focal activity.[68,70,72]

The clinical relevance of the initiation and perpetuation of fibrillation has attracted considerable attention.[39,68] Two principal hypotheses have been advanced to explain the "substrates" (mechanisms that sustain) of human AF.[19,39] The multiple wavelet hypothesis is based on mapping in dogs and humans and proposes that multiple nonlocalized interacting circuits meander around the atria.[73] The alternative localized source hypothesis proposes that rapidly conducted impulses (eg, from focal delayed afterdepolarization-mediated sources or electrical spiral waves [rotors]) result in complex fibrillatory activity.[68,74–76]

With the increasing application and positive results of ablation therapy, the perceived importance of localized sources for atrial fibrillation has gained ground.[76,77] There is general acceptance that triggers, such as ectopic beats from the pulmonary veins, can initiate AF, whereas steep restitution and exaggerated dispersion of refractoriness observed around those pulmonary veins[62,78–82] and patterns of left atrial ion channel expression facilitate wave break and the initiation of reentry.[18,19,26] Recent clinical work now describes atrial rotors seemingly directly amenable to ablation, with the most recent observations suggesting a central role in forming the "substrates" that sustain AF after it has been triggered in a wide range of patients, including those with paroxysmal atrial fibrillation.[83,84]

NATURAL HISTORY OF THE HEART FAILURE/ATRIAL FIBRILLATION RELATIONSHIP

Structural Clinical Phenotypes

The proportion of patients presenting with heart failure with preserved ejection fraction (HF*p*EF) is increasing in proportion to those with heart failure with reduced ejection fraction (HF*r*EF),[85] and is of particular relevance due to an association of HF*p*EF with AF.[6,11,14,21,86] The presence and severity of diastolic dysfunction is independently predictive of AF,[6,38] with these patients having distinct associated cellular phenotypes supporting separation and possible association with AF.[87] The loss of effective atrial contractile function is possibly more important to those with HF*p*EF rather than those with HF*r*EF. In addition, left atrial functional impairment that limits exercise capacity may have an impact on prognosis.[88]

Influence of Atrial Fibrillation on Heart Failure Outcomes

The prognostic significance of AF on CHF is becoming clearer, and new-onset AF may provide a grave indicator in patients with CHF.[1,12,89] This risk may be intrinsic or may arise following initiation of antiarrhythmic therapy.[89,90] In a recent study in which AF was present in a third of CHF cases, use of antiarrhythmic medications was associated with adverse hospital outcomes, longer hospital stay, and higher risks of in-hospital death.[91] This has also been reported in patients without CHF in a substudy of the Atrial Fibrillation Follow-Up Investigation of Rhythm Management (AFFIRM) trial.[92] Notably, in a propensity-matched study, AF actually had no intrinsic association with mortality, although it was associated with an increased risk of CHF hospitalization.[93]

Drug Interactions with Substrate

One major practical issue in the management of patients with AF and CHF is that the responses of the ventricular myocardium to antiarrhythmic drugs that act through ion channel blockade is modified.[16,89,90,94] Indeed, transcriptional shifts in the expression of genes encoding cardiac ion channels may increase susceptibility to adverse drug reactions.[16,89] Most specifically, downregulation of potassium channel gene expression with action potential prolongation might increase susceptibility to, for example, the addition of potassium channel blockers, such as D-sotalol.[16,95] A further interaction that is not fully explained is the negative impact of dronedarone on prognosis in patients with significant impairment of ventricular pump function.[96,97]

SYSTEMATIC APPROACHES TO COMPLEX CARDIAC DISEASE

To integrate and make sense of the enormous amount of accumulating biologic and clinical information relevant to the conditions discussed here, a *systems biology* approach to disease analysis seems appropriate.[19,98] Although semantics remain contentious for our practical purposes,

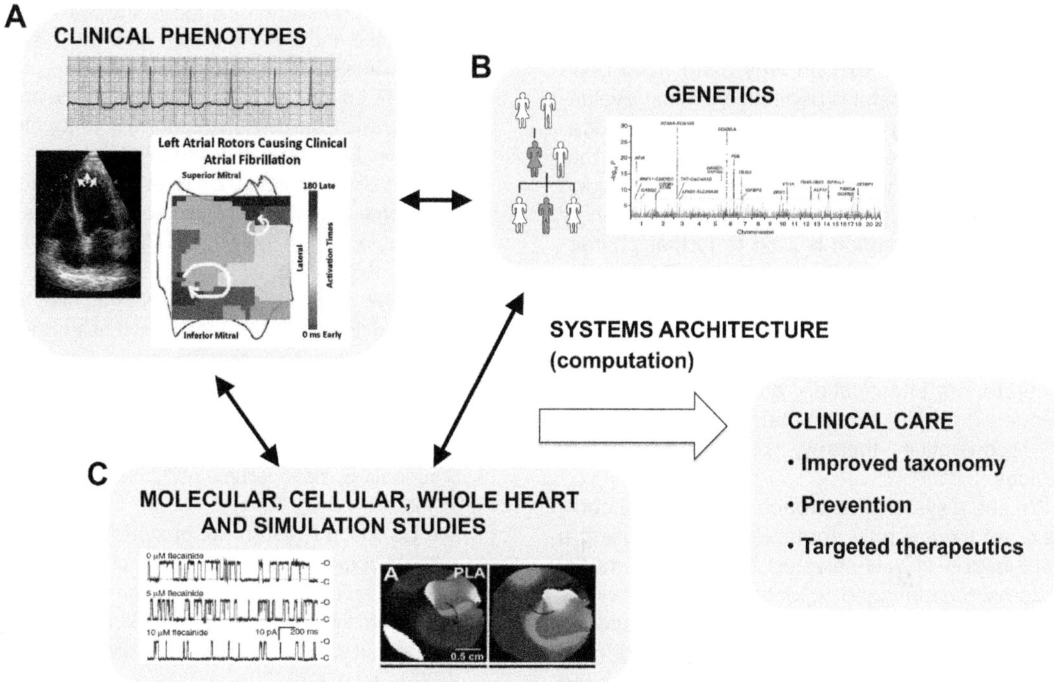

Fig. 4. A systems approach to an analysis of atrial fibrillation and heart failure: the final objective is a new taxonomy of disease susceptibility of clinical utility that integrates multiparameter data. Accordingly, clinical (*A*) and genetic (*B*) inputs are used in conjunction with appropriately designed mechanistic studies (*C*) in clinical and model systems. Iterative computer-based modeling provides an architectural framework leading to improved taxonomy, allowing for tailoring of medical treatment (precision medicine). *Arrows* show defined patient-specific abnormalities in cardiac function (in this case, apical hypertrophy).

we can define a *systems* approach as an analytic framework characterized by integrated descriptions of multiple biologic processes based on systematic measurement (**Fig. 4**).[19] Such a strategy requires as a starting point large high-quality data sets describing the phenotypes and natural history of disease. Once appropriate populations of patients are identified, then genetic and genomic analysis can ideally be complemented by the use of experimental systems to model functional consequences. For overlapping phenotypes, in this case AF and CHF, this is a substantial problem, with the situation for CHF further complicated by limitations to the quantification of the phenotype. Technical advances in relevant genomic technologies and the acquisition of target populations are particularly valuable, although the absence of genetically manipulable model systems relevant to CHF provide some limitations.[19,99]

We do, however, think it likely that, over time, relationships between atrial and ventricular biology, even in such complex settings, will become tractable.[19,98] This may be most amenable initially through unpicking electrophysiological phenotypes in which the prospects for quantification seem higher.[19,99] In view of the sheer volume of information obtained from such systems approaches, computational models to elaborate underlying network architecture will almost certainly be of value.[99] There are already examples of the use of computerized models to analyze the generation of fibrillation within the context of CHF.[69,99–101] The important goal when developing disease models is to allow the responses to therapeutic interventions to be assessed.[19]

SUMMARY

Atrial fibrillation and heart failure have much in common and tend to occur in the same vulnerable populations.[1,9,10,12] Affected individuals are often older and frequently have underlying systemic *multimorbidity*.[20] Although the initial manifestation of atrial disease is through arrhythmia, there are also significant issues with contractile performance.[88] The first manifestation of ventricular disease is most usually contractile, but those chambers also remain electrically sensitive with a risk of fibrillation and sudden cardiac death.[10]

The complex clinical settings caused by the interaction of 2 independently highly heterogeneous disorders explain why there have been few practically useful prospective clinical evaluations addressing the combined clinical scenario.[92,102,103] We are, however, optimistic that significant advances will be made, although necessarily in a stepwise fashion. We strongly advocate that attention is paid to further characterization of the myocardial substrates for disease. We believe such an approach will lead to opportunities for a greater understanding of the underlying biology, greater opportunities for accurate risk stratification, and the possibility of rescue via pharmacologic therapy, tissue ablation or regenerative therapy, or by appropriate devices.[76,84,104,105]

We see a systems approach to this highly complex, yet increasingly tractable, problem, using a combination of well-selected translational model systems, the managed collection of large amounts of data and computerized modeling, as offering the best hope in achieving medium-term to long-term advances.[19] In the interim, we will also need a community-wide effort to more vigorous multifaceted approaches to prevention, which will be reliant also on the identification of novel risk factors plus early disease detection.[5] The fact that populations of patients with both AF and CHF continue to increase should motivate funding agencies to make targeted research in this area a priority.

REFERENCES

1. Anter E, Jessup M, Callans DJ. Atrial fibrillation and heart failure: treatment considerations for a dual epidemic. Circulation 2009;119(18): 2516–25.
2. Carson PE, Johnson GR, Dunkman WB, et al. The influence of atrial fibrillation on prognosis in mild to moderate heart failure. The V-HeFT Studies. The V-HeFT VA Cooperative Studies Group. Circulation 1993;87(Suppl 6):VI102–10.
3. Stevenson WG, Stevenson LW. Atrial fibrillation in heart failure. N Engl J Med 1999;341(12): 910–1.
4. Ben Morrison T, Jared Bunch T, Gersh BJ. Pathophysiology of concomitant atrial fibrillation and heart failure: implications for management. Nat Clin Pract Cardiovasc Med 2009;6(1):46–56.
5. Benjamin EJ, Chen PS, Bild DE, et al. Prevention of atrial fibrillation: report from a National Heart, Lung, and Blood Institute workshop. Circulation 2009; 119(4):606–18.
6. Tsang TS, Gersh BJ, Appleton CP, et al. Left ventricular diastolic dysfunction as a predictor of the first diagnosed nonvalvular atrial fibrillation in 840 elderly men and women. J Am Coll Cardiol 2002; 40(9):1636–44.
7. Ellinor PT, Lunetta KL, Albert CM, et al. Meta-analysis identifies six new susceptibility loci for atrial fibrillation. Nat Genet 2012;44(6):670–5.
8. Magnani JW, Rienstra M, Lin H, et al. Atrial fibrillation: current knowledge and future directions in epidemiology and genomics. Circulation 2011; 124(18):1982–93.
9. Yancy CW, Jessup M, Bozkurt B, et al. 2013 ACCF/AHA guideline for the management of heart failure: a report of the American College of Cardiology Foundation/American Heart Association Task Force on practice guidelines. J Am Coll Cardiol 2013. [Epub ahead of print].
10. Braunwald E. Heart failure. JACC Heart Fail 2013; 1:1–20.
11. Lee DS, Gona P, Vasan RS, et al. Relation of disease pathogenesis and risk factors to heart failure with preserved or reduced ejection fraction: insights from the Framingham Heart Study of the National Heart, Lung, and Blood Institute. Circulation 2009;119(24):3070–7.
12. Darby AE, Dimarco JP. Management of atrial fibrillation in patients with structural heart disease. Circulation 2012;125(7):945–57.
13. Wang TJ, Larson MG, Levy D, et al. Temporal relations of atrial fibrillation and congestive heart failure and their joint influence on mortality: the Framingham Heart Study. Circulation 2003; 107(23):2920–5.
14. Olsson LG, Swedberg K, Ducharme A, et al. Atrial fibrillation and risk of clinical events in chronic heart failure with and without left ventricular systolic dysfunction: results from the Candesartan in Heart Failure–Assessment of Reduction in Mortality and morbidity (CHARM) program. J Am Coll Cardiol 2006;47(10):1997–2004.
15. Nattel S, Maguy A, Le Bouter S, et al. Arrhythmogenic ion-channel remodeling in the heart: heart failure, myocardial infarction, and atrial fibrillation. Physiol Rev 2007;87(2):425–56.
16. Aiba T, Tomaselli GF. Electrical remodeling in the failing heart. Curr Opin Cardiol 2010;25(1):29–36.
17. Barth AS, Kumordzie A, Frangakis C, et al. Reciprocal transcriptional regulation of metabolic and signaling pathways correlates with disease severity in heart failure. Circ Cardiovasc Genet 2011;4(5): 475–83.
18. Michael G, Xiao L, Qi XY, et al. Remodelling of cardiac repolarization: how homeostatic responses can lead to arrhythmogenesis. Cardiovasc Res 2009;81(3):491–9.
19. Grace AA, Roden DM. Systems biology and cardiac arrhythmias. Lancet 2012;380(9852): 1498–508.

20. Tinetti ME, Fried TR, Boyd CM. Designing health care for the most common chronic condition—multimorbidity. JAMA 2012;307(23):2493–4.
21. Go AS, Mozaffarian D, Roger VL, et al. Heart disease and stroke statistics—2013 update: a report from the American Heart Association. Circulation 2013;127(1):e6–245.
22. Miyasaka Y, Barnes ME, Gersh BJ, et al. Secular trends in incidence of atrial fibrillation in Olmsted County, Minnesota, 1980 to 2000, and implications on the projections for future prevalence. Circulation 2006;114(2):119–25.
23. Miyasaka Y, Barnes ME, Gersh BJ, et al. Incidence and mortality risk of congestive heart failure in atrial fibrillation patients: a community-based study over two decades. Eur Heart J 2006;27(8):936–41.
24. Stefansdottir H, Aspelund T, Gudnason V, et al. Trends in the incidence and prevalence of atrial fibrillation in Iceland and future projections. Europace 2011;13(8):1110–7.
25. Savelieva I, John Camm A. Atrial fibrillation and heart failure: natural history and pharmacological treatment. Europace 2004;5(Suppl 1):S5–19.
26. Wakili R, Voigt N, Kaab S, et al. Recent advances in the molecular pathophysiology of atrial fibrillation. J Clin Invest 2011;121(8):2955–68.
27. Lopez-Otin C, Blasco MA, Partridge L, et al. The hallmarks of aging. Cell 2013;153(6):1194–217.
28. Fatkin D, MacRae C, Sasaki T, et al. Missense mutations in the rod domain of the lamin A/C gene as causes of dilated cardiomyopathy and conduction-system disease. N Engl J Med 1999;341(23):1715–24.
29. Olson TM, Michels VV, Ballew JD, et al. Sodium channel mutations and susceptibility to heart failure and atrial fibrillation. JAMA 2005;293(4):447–54.
30. Darbar D, Kannankeril PJ, Donahue BS, et al. Cardiac sodium channel (SCN5A) variants associated with atrial fibrillation. Circulation 2008;117(15):1927–35.
31. Kathiresan S, Srivastava D. Genetics of human cardiovascular disease. Cell 2012;148:1242–57.
32. Gudbjartsson DF, Arnar DO, Helgadottir A, et al. Variants conferring risk of atrial fibrillation on chromosome 4q25. Nature 2007;448(7151):353–7.
33. Cappola TP, Dorn GW 2nd. Clinical considerations of heritable factors in common heart failure. Circ Cardiovasc Genet 2011;4(6):701–9.
34. O'Rahilly S. Human genetics illuminates the paths to metabolic disease. Nature 2009;462(7271):307–14.
35. Kenchaiah S, Evans JC, Levy D, et al. Obesity and the risk of heart failure. N Engl J Med 2002;347(5):305–13.
36. Wang TJ, Parise H, Levy D, et al. Obesity and the risk of new-onset atrial fibrillation. JAMA 2004;292(20):2471–7.
37. Tedrow UB, Conen D, Ridker PM, et al. The long- and short-term impact of elevated body mass index on the risk of new atrial fibrillation: the WHS (Women's Health Study). J Am Coll Cardiol 2010;55(21):2319–27.
38. Rosenberg MA, Gottdiener JS, Heckbert SR, et al. Echocardiographic diastolic parameters and risk of atrial fibrillation: the Cardiovascular Health Study. Eur Heart J 2012;33(7):904–12.
39. Nattel S. New ideas about atrial fibrillation 50 years on. Nature 2002;415(6868):219–26.
40. Schotten U, Verheule S, Kirchhof P, et al. Pathophysiological mechanisms of atrial fibrillation: a translational appraisal. Physiol Rev 2011;91(1):265–325.
41. Byrd GD, Prasad SM, Ripplinger CM, et al. Importance of geometry and refractory period in sustaining atrial fibrillation: testing the critical mass hypothesis. Circulation 2005;112(Suppl 9):I7–13.
42. Bode F, Sachs F, Franz MR. Tarantula peptide inhibits atrial fibrillation. Nature 2001;409(6816):35–6.
43. Kalifa J, Jalife J, Zaitsev AV, et al. Intra-atrial pressure increases rate and organization of waves emanating from the superior pulmonary veins during atrial fibrillation. Circulation 2003;108(6):668–71.
44. John B, Stiles MK, Kuklik P, et al. Reverse remodeling of the atria after treatment of chronic stretch in humans: implications for the atrial fibrillation substrate. J Am Coll Cardiol 2010;55(12):1217–26.
45. Mayr M, Yusuf S, Weir G, et al. Combined metabolomic and proteomic analysis of human atrial fibrillation. J Am Coll Cardiol 2008;51(5):585–94.
46. Barth AS, Tomaselli GF. Cardiac metabolism and arrhythmias. Circ Arrhythm Electrophysiol 2009;2(3):327–35.
47. Reilly SN, Jayaram R, Nahar K, et al. Atrial sources of reactive oxygen species vary with the duration and substrate of atrial fibrillation: implications for the antiarrhythmic effect of statins. Circulation 2011;124(10):1107–17.
48. Friedrichs K, Klinke A, Baldus S. Inflammatory pathways underlying atrial fibrillation. Trends Mol Med 2011;17(10):556–63.
49. Li J, Solus J, Chen Q, et al. Role of inflammation and oxidative stress in atrial fibrillation. Heart Rhythm 2010;7(4):438–44.
50. Mihm MJ, Yu F, Carnes CA, et al. Impaired myofibrillar energetics and oxidative injury during human atrial fibrillation. Circulation 2001;104(2):174–80.
51. Adam O, Frost G, Custodis F, et al. Role of Rac1 GTPase activation in atrial fibrillation. J Am Coll Cardiol 2007;50(4):359–67.
52. Oka T, Hikoso S, Yamaguchi O, et al. Mitochondrial DNA that escapes from autophagy causes inflammation and heart failure. Nature 2012;485(7397):251–5.
53. Konstantinidis K, Kitsis RN. Cardiovascular biology: escaped DNA inflames the heart. Nature 2012;485(7397):179–80.

54. Bayeva M, Gheorghiade M, Ardehali H. Mitochondria as a therapeutic target in heart failure. J Am Coll Cardiol 2013;61(6):599–610.
55. El-Armouche A, Boknik P, Eschenhagen T, et al. Molecular determinants of altered Ca2+ handling in human chronic atrial fibrillation. Circulation 2006;114(7):670–80.
56. Wijffels MC, Kirchhof CJ, Dorland R, et al. Atrial fibrillation begets atrial fibrillation. A study in awake chronically instrumented goats. Circulation 1995; 92(7):1954–68.
57. Ausma J, Wijffels M, Thone F, et al. Structural changes of atrial myocardium due to sustained atrial fibrillation in the goat. Circulation 1997; 96(9):3157–63.
58. Du J, Xie J, Zhang Z, et al. TRPM7-mediated Ca2+ signals confer fibrogenesis in human atrial fibrillation. Circ Res 2010;106(5):992–1003.
59. Jahangir A, Lee V, Friedman PA, et al. Long-term progression and outcomes with aging in patients with lone atrial fibrillation: a 30-year follow-up study. Circulation 2007;115(24):3050–6.
60. Spach MS. Mounting evidence that fibrosis generates a major mechanism for atrial fibrillation. Circ Res 2007;101(8):743–5.
61. Kistler PM, Sanders P, Fynn SP, et al. Electrophysiologic and electroanatomic changes in the human atrium associated with age. J Am Coll Cardiol 2004;44(1):109–16.
62. Stiles MK, John B, Wong CX, et al. Paroxysmal lone atrial fibrillation is associated with an abnormal atrial substrate: characterizing the "second factor." J Am Coll Cardiol 2009;53(14):1182–91.
63. Roberts-Thomson KC, Stevenson IH, Kistler PM, et al. Anatomically determined functional conduction delay in the posterior left atrium relationship to structural heart disease. J Am Coll Cardiol 2008;51(8):856–62.
64. Platonov PG, Mitrofanova LB, Orshanskaya V, et al. Structural abnormalities in atrial walls are associated with presence and persistency of atrial fibrillation but not with age. J Am Coll Cardiol 2011; 58(21):2225–32.
65. Tanaka K, Zlochiver S, Vikstrom KL, et al. Spatial distribution of fibrosis governs fibrillation wave dynamics in the posterior left atrium during heart failure. Circ Res 2007;101(8):839–47.
66. Higuchi K, Akkaya M, Akoum N, et al. Cardiac MRI assessment of atrial fibrosis in atrial fibrillation: implications for diagnosis and therapy. Heart 2013. [Epub ahead of print].
67. Barth AS, Merk S, Arnoldi E, et al. Reprogramming of the human atrial transcriptome in permanent atrial fibrillation: expression of a ventricular-like genomic signature. Circ Res 2005;96(9):1022–9.
68. Pandit SV, Jalife J. Rotors and the dynamics of cardiac fibrillation. Circ Res 2013;112(5):849–62.
69. Rappel WJ, Narayan SM. Theoretical considerations for mapping activation in human cardiac fibrillation. Chaos 2013;23(2):023113.
70. Davidenko JM, Pertsov AV, Salomonsz R, et al. Stationary and drifting spiral waves of excitation in isolated cardiac muscle. Nature 1992; 355(6358):349–51.
71. Mandapati R, Skanes A, Chen J, et al. Stable microreentrant sources as a mechanism of atrial fibrillation in the isolated sheep heart. Circulation 2000;101(2):194–9.
72. Klos M, Calvo D, Yamazaki M, et al. Atrial septopulmonary bundle of the posterior left atrium provides a substrate for atrial fibrillation initiation in a model of vagally mediated pulmonary vein tachycardia of the structurally normal heart. Circ Arrhythm Electrophysiol 2008;1(3):175–83.
73. Moe GK, Rheinboldt WC, Abildskov JA. A computer model of atrial fibrillation. Am Heart J 1964;67:200–20.
74. Mines GR. On dynamic equilibrium in the heart. J Physiol 1913;46(4–5):349–83.
75. Lewis T. Oliver-Sharpey Lectures on the nature of flutter and fibrillation of the auricle. Br Med J 1921;1(3146):551–5.
76. Narayan SM, Krummen DE, Shivkumar K, et al. Treatment of atrial fibrillation by the ablation of localized sources: CONFIRM (Conventional Ablation for Atrial Fibrillation With or Without Focal Impulse and Rotor Modulation) trial. J Am Coll Cardiol 2012;60:628–36.
77. Haissaguerre M, Jais P, Shah DC, et al. Spontaneous initiation of atrial fibrillation by ectopic beats originating in the pulmonary veins. N Engl J Med 1998;339(10):659–66.
78. Narayan SM, Bayer JD, Lalani G, et al. Action potential dynamics explain arrhythmic vulnerability in human heart failure: a clinical and modeling study implicating abnormal calcium handling. J Am Coll Cardiol 2008;52(22):1782–92.
79. Rostock T, Steven D, Lutomsky B, et al. Atrial fibrillation begets atrial fibrillation in the pulmonary veins on the impact of atrial fibrillation on the electrophysiological properties of the pulmonary veins in humans. J Am Coll Cardiol 2008; 51(22):2153–60.
80. Narayan SM, Franz MR, Clopton P, et al. Repolarization alternans reveals vulnerability to human atrial fibrillation. Circulation 2011;123(25):2922–30.
81. Markides V, Schilling RJ, Ho SY, et al. Characterization of left atrial activation in the intact human heart. Circulation 2003;107(5):733–9.
82. Lalani GG, Schricker A, Gibson M, et al. Atrial conduction slows immediately before the onset of human atrial fibrillation: a bi-atrial contact mapping study of transitions to atrial fibrillation. J Am Coll Cardiol 2012;59(6):595–606.

83. Shivkumar K, Ellenbogen KA, Hummel JD, et al. Acute termination of human atrial fibrillation by identification and catheter ablation of localized rotors and sources: first multicenter experience of focal impulse and rotor modulation (FIRM) ablation. J Cardiovasc Electrophysiol 2012;23(12):1277–85.
84. Narayan SM, Krummen DE, Clopton P, et al. Direct or coincidental elimination of stable rotors or focal sources may explain successful atrial fibrillation ablation: on-treatment analysis of the CONFIRM trial (Conventional Ablation for AF With or Without Focal Impulse and Rotor Modulation). J Am Coll Cardiol 2013;62(2):138–47.
85. Owan TE, Hodge DO, Herges RM, et al. Trends in prevalence and outcome of heart failure with preserved ejection fraction. N Engl J Med 2006;355(3):251–9.
86. Bhatia RS, Tu JV, Lee DS, et al. Outcome of heart failure with preserved ejection fraction in a population-based study. N Engl J Med 2006;355(3):260–9.
87. van Heerebeek L, Borbely A, Niessen HW, et al. Myocardial structure and function differ in systolic and diastolic heart failure. Circulation 2006;113(16):1966–73.
88. Kusunose K, Motoki H, Popovic ZB, et al. Independent association of left atrial function with exercise capacity in patients with preserved ejection fraction. Heart 2012;98(17):1311–7.
89. Grace AA, Camm AJ. Quinidine. N Engl J Med 1998;338(1):35–45.
90. Kannankeril P, Roden DM, Darbar D. Drug-induced long QT syndrome. Pharmacol Rev 2010;62(4):760–81.
91. Mountantonakis SE, Grau-Sepulveda MV, Bhatt DL, et al. Presence of atrial fibrillation is independently associated with adverse outcomes in patients hospitalized with heart failure: an analysis of get with the guidelines–heart failure. Circ Heart Fail 2012;5(2):191–201.
92. Saksena S, Slee A, Waldo AL, et al. Cardiovascular outcomes in the AFFIRM trial (Atrial Fibrillation Follow-Up Investigation of Rhythm Management). An assessment of individual antiarrhythmic drug therapies compared with rate control with propensity score–matched analyses. J Am Coll Cardiol 2011;58(19):1975–85.
93. Ahmed MI, White M, Ekundayo OJ, et al. A history of atrial fibrillation and outcomes in chronic advanced systolic heart failure: a propensity-matched study. Eur Heart J 2009;30(16):2029–37.
94. Dobrev D, Carlsson L, Nattel S. Novel molecular targets for atrial fibrillation therapy. Nat Rev Drug Discov 2012;11(4):275–91.
95. Waldo AL, Camm AJ, deRuyter H, et al. Effect of d-sotalol on mortality in patients with left ventricular dysfunction after recent and remote myocardial infarction. The SWORD Investigators. Survival With Oral d-Sotalol. Lancet 1996;348(9019):7–12.
96. Kober L, Torp-Pedersen C, McMurray JJ, et al. Increased mortality after dronedarone therapy for severe heart failure. N Engl J Med 2008;358(25):2678–87.
97. Connolly SJ, Camm AJ, Halperin JL, et al. Dronedarone in high-risk permanent atrial fibrillation. N Engl J Med 2011;365(24):2268–76.
98. Rudy Y, Ackerman MJ, Bers DM, et al. Systems approach to understanding electromechanical activity in the human heart: a National Heart, Lung, and Blood Institute workshop summary. Circulation 2008;118(11):1202–11.
99. Trayanova NA. Whole-heart modeling: applications to cardiac electrophysiology and electromechanics. Circ Res 2011;108(1):113–28.
100. Thul R, Coombes S, Roderick HL, et al. Subcellular calcium dynamics in a whole-cell model of an atrial myocyte. Proc Natl Acad Sci U S A 2012;109(6):2150–5.
101. Comtois P, Nattel S. Impact of tissue geometry on simulated cholinergic atrial fibrillation: a modeling study. Chaos 2011;21(1):013108.
102. Roy D, Talajic M, Nattel S, et al. Rhythm control versus rate control for atrial fibrillation and heart failure. N Engl J Med 2008;358(25):2667–77.
103. Talajic M, Khairy P, Levesque S, et al. Maintenance of sinus rhythm and survival in patients with heart failure and atrial fibrillation. J Am Coll Cardiol 2010;55(17):1796–802.
104. Saumarez RC, Chojnowska L, Derksen R, et al. Sudden death in noncoronary heart disease is associated with delayed paced ventricular activation. Circulation 2003;107(20):2595–600.
105. Saumarez RC, Pytkowski M, Sterlinski M, et al. Paced ventricular electrogram fractionation predicts sudden cardiac death in hypertrophic cardiomyopathy. Eur Heart J 2008;29(13):1653–61.

Continuous Monitoring of Atrial Fibrillation in Heart Failure

Bengt Herweg, MD, FHRS[a,*], S. Serge Barold, MD, FHRS[b], Jonathan S. Steinberg, MD, FHRS[c,d]

KEYWORDS

- Atrial fibrillation • Heart failure • Cardiac resynchronization • Dual-chamber pacemaker
- Continuous cardiac monitoring • Stroke • Thromboembolism

KEY POINTS

- Knowledge of atrial fibrillation (AF) in heart failure has increased dramatically because of the widespread use of continuous monitoring provided by implanted cardiac rhythm devices.
- Continuous monitoring has improved cardiac resynchronization therapy (CRT) management of patients with AF.
- Data from continuous monitoring have generated new questions about anticoagulant therapy in patients with only asymptomatic AF and in those with very short atrial high-rate episodes.
- Anticoagulant therapy should be considered in patients who have a high risk of thromboembolism according to standard scoring systems.

Atrial fibrillation (AF) is found in up to 30% to 40% of patients with heart failure, depending on the underlying cause and severity of heart failure. Each complicates the course of the other. Paroxysmal AF is self-terminating, usually within 48 hours. Although AF paroxysms may continue for up to 7 days, the 48-hour time point is clinically important; after this period, the likelihood of spontaneous conversion is low and anticoagulation must be considered. Persistent AF is present when an AF episode either lasts longer than 7 days or requires termination by cardioversion, either with drugs or by direct current cardioversion. AF increases the risk of thromboembolic complications (particularly stroke) and may lead to worsening of symptoms. Heart failure can be both a consequence of AF (eg, tachycardiomyopathy or decompensation in acute-onset AF) and a cause of the arrhythmia as a result of increased atrial pressure, volume overload, or excessive neurohumoral stimulation. Patients with paroxysmal AF have a similar risk of thromboembolism to those with sustained AF. This risk can be significantly lowered by oral anticoagulation. Heart failure and AF share risk factors such as hypertension, valve disease, coronary artery disease, and diabetes mellitus. Both heart failure and AF independently increase the mortality risk, and, when both conditions occur together, the mortality risk is even higher.

Disclosures: Dr Herweg reports receiving fellowship support from Medtronic, and minor consulting fees from St. Jude Medical and Biosense-Webster. Dr Barold has no disclosures. Dr Steinberg reports receiving consulting fees from Medtronic, Boston-Scientific, Philips, St. Jude Medical, Janssen, Biosense-Webster and Sanofi. He is also receiving research grant support from Jansen, Medtronic and Biosense-Webster.

[a] Department of Cardiovascular Disease, University of South Florida Morsani College of Medicine, South Tampa Campus (5th Floor), Two Tampa General Circle, Tampa, FL 33606, USA; [b] 5806 Mariner's Watch Drive, Tampa, FL 33615, USA; [c] Arrhythmia Institute, Valley Health System, 223 North Van Dien Avenue, Ridgewood, NJ 07450, USA; [d] Department of Medicine, Columbia University College of Physicians & Surgeons, 630 W 168 Street, New York, NY 10032, USA

* Corresponding author. Department of Cardiovascular Disease, University of South Florida Morsani College of Medicine, South Tampa Campus (5th Floor), Two Tampa General Circle, Tampa, FL 33606.
E-mail address: bherweg@health.usf.edu

Heart Failure Clin 9 (2013) 385–395
http://dx.doi.org/10.1016/j.hfc.2013.06.002
1551-7136/13/$ – see front matter

heartfailure.theclinics.com

Detection of AF can be achieved by a 12-lead electrocardiogram (ECG), Holter (24 hour or 7 day), noninvasive and invasive event monitoring, and from data stored in a pacemaker, implantable cardioverter defibrillator (ICD), or a device for cardiac resynchronization therapy (CRT) by virtue of continuous monitoring via the atrial channel. Resting 12-lead ECGs and ambulatory monitoring (in the absence of an implanted device) provide only a snapshot of the ECG, with resulting limited information that underestimates the true prevalence of AF (**Fig. 1**). Asymptomatic AF may be as much as 6 to 8 times more common than symptomatic AF and seems to be a precursor of symptomatic AF.[1,2] In the last few years, research interest has grown in the clinical relevance of AF at an even earlier stage, before its clinical detection. Earlier detection of AF in the asymptomatic phase (as with cardiac rhythm devices) might allow the timely introduction of therapies to protect the patient, not only from the consequences of AF but also from progression from an easily treated condition into one that becomes refractory to therapy.

Contemporary pacemakers and CRT devices are equipped with reliable and extensive diagnostic and memory features yielding full disclosure of the number, duration, and overall burden of atrial tachyarrhythmias. These advanced diagnostic features have shown the high frequency of symptomatic and asymptomatic atrial arrhythmias in patients with heart failure and an implanted cardiac rhythm device. Device interrogation also provides estimates of the percentage of biventricular (BiV%) pacing in patients receiving CRT, a measurement of the utmost importance in achieving a satisfactory clinical response. Other important data from implanted devices include the ventricular rate (VR) during atrial tachyarrhythmias and stored electrograms that permit the precise diagnosis of the atrial tachyarrhythmia (eg, AF vs atrial flutter vs atrial tachycardia [AT]) and characterize the initiation/termination of arrhythmias. Many arrhythmias may not be true AF but rather ATs or atrial flutters with rates that exceed the programmable recording threshold. These arrhythmias are therefore referred to as atrial high-rate episodes (AHRE) and their therapy differs from that of AF. Manual overreading of all recorded episodes is good practice, because a device may not arrive at the correct diagnosis. Problematic situations include far-field R wave oversensing and other extraneous signals, such as external electromagnetic signals, which a device interprets and records as AF. Because of intermittent atrial undersensing, a single prolonged episode may be recorded as multiple shorter episodes, so that the overall arrhythmia burden may be more reliable than number of episodes. Many workers refer to all atrial tachyarrhythmias simply as AF, because AF constitutes most atrial arrhythmias in patients with cardiac rhythm devices.[2–6]

AF BURDEN

Over the last decade, the term burden has become frequently used when discussing AF. AF burden generally means the percentage of time that a patient is in AF calculated from the total time in AF divided by the total monitored time. AF burden using this definition can be adequately assessed only by some method of continuous monitoring for prolonged periods. Such assessments involve continuously applied monitors, implanted monitors, or interrogation of cardiac rhythm devices. The AF burden calculated from the ECG recordings in terms of total time in AF during a specific period is sometimes called the ECG AF burden. This burden can be further subdivided into total time in AF, the number of AF (re)occurrences in a specific period, or duration of the AF-free period until the recurrence of AF, or a combination of these. AF burden may provide a more clinically useful assessment of AF than the time to the first recurrence of AF. In addition, cardiac rhythm device–based AF recordings have become a useful guide to assess interventional procedures, the need for anticoagulation, and to understand the importance of asymptomatic AF. AF recurrence should not always be considered as treatment

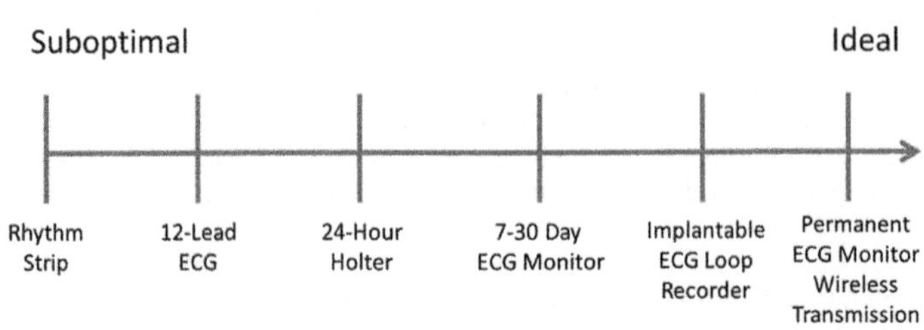

Fig. 1. The spectrum of ambulatory monitoring modalities. As one moves from left to right, the duration of monitoring increases, which in turn increases the diagnostic yield.

failure. A reduction of AF burden may constitute a therapeutic success because of less frequent, briefer, or less symptomatic episodes. However, in highly symptomatic patients, any AF recurrence may be unacceptable.

There is growing clinical interest in symptomatic and asymptomatic device-recorded AHRE as possible precursors of thromboembolic complications in patients with a pacemaker or ICD.[2–10] Timely diagnosis of both paroxysmal AF or atrial flutter has important implications for anticoagulant therapy for stroke prevention.[11–18]

INCIDENCE AND PROGNOSIS OF AF DURING CRT

Device-based continuous monitoring of AF in CRT patients has improved the diagnosis and therapy for AF in this group of patients. The bulk of our knowledge regarding the role of CRT in patients with permanent AF is based on nonrandomized, observational data. Marijon and colleagues[4] analyzed the incidence of AF in CRT patients in a prospective study and found that 34 of 173 (27.5%) patients developed paroxysmal AF during a follow-up of 9.9 ± 3.6 months. About half of the patients with AF had a past history of AF. Boriani and colleagues[19] evaluated 1404 CRT patients for a median follow-up of 18 months. All were in sinus rhythm at the time of entry into the study. AF was documented in 443 of 1404 patients (32%). The duration of AF ranged from more than 10 minutes to weeks. AF developed in 222 CRT patients without a previous history of AF (22%) and 221 CRT patients with a previous history of AF (16%). The observations of Leclercq and colleagues[5] involving 120 CRT patients followed for a mean of 183 ± 23 days showed an AF incidence of 21%. A previous history of AF was present in 29% of patients, and those with new-onset AF after CRT constituted 17% of all the patients. Thus, the incidence of AF in patients with heart failure treated with CRT ranges from 30% to 35% for paroxysmal AF and around 20% to 25% for permanent AF. This finding should not be surprising given the association of AF with the severity of heart failure. This association carries a worse prognosis than heart failure with sinus rhythm.

SIGNIFICANCE OF THE VR

A VR in AF controlled at rest may not be controlled during exercise. Furthermore, pronounced RR interval variability in AF may decrease the number of resynchronized beats. In the AF group (443 patients), Boriani and colleagues[19] calculated the average VR of each patient at 115 ± 15 bpm. An uncontrolled VR occurred in 150 of 443 (34%) of the patients. In the patients with new-onset AF, 93 of 222 (42%) were found to have uncontrolled VR, whereas in those with a known history of AF, 43 of 221 (26%) showed uncontrolled VR (P = .001). An uncontrolled VR, which occurred in one-third of CRT patients, was associated with a worse clinical outcome of combined heart failure hospitalization or death (P = .046).

The traditional recommendation in AF to control the resting VR at 80 bpm increasing to only 110 bpm with exertion is an effort that is difficult to achieve in heart failure. This arbitrary goal was recently challenged by the results of the Rate Control Efficacy in Permanent Atrial Fibrillation II (RACE II) trial, which showed that lenient rate control was not inferior to strict rate control in terms of cardiovascular morbidity and mortality. However, rate control between groups did not differ that much and the composite endpoint was very heterogenous. Furthermore, the trial did not evaluate the safety of a lenient strategy in patients with heart failure.[20] Consequently, it would be unwise to extrapolate the data from the RACE II trial to the management of patients with heart failure.

PROGNOSIS OF AF DURING CRT

Boriani and colleagues[19] found that age (P = .046) and uncontrolled VR (P = .028) in CRT patients with AF were the only independent predictors of clinical outcome assessed by the combined end point of heart failure hospitalizations or death. In a study involving 1193 CRT patients (initially all in sinus rhythm), Santini and colleagues[3] found AF in 361 patients (30%) over a mean follow-up of 13 months (the study overlapped that of Boriani and colleagues).[19] AF (especially persistent AF) correlated with the composite end point of death and heart failure hospitalization (P = .005). Prognostic data were also obtained in a recent subanalysis of MADIT-CRT (Multicenter Automatic Defibrillator Implantation Trial–Cardiac Resynchronization Therapy).[21] The cumulative probability of both the combined end point of heart failure or all-cause mortality was higher among patients who developed atrial tachyarrhythmia during the first year.

ABLATION OF THE ATRIOVENTRICULAR JUNCTION TO OPTIMIZE CRT

It seems reasonable to start with pharmacologic therapy to optimize rate control in AF patients requiring CRT. When after careful evaluation by device interrogation, Holter monitoring, and exercise testing, the amount of true BiV pacing is suboptimal, atrioventricular junctional (AVJ) ablation should be considered. The impressive results after AVJ ablation suggest that the procedure should be performed in most patients with permanent AF as well as in those with frequent and prolonged episodes of paroxysmal AF.[22–28] However, a few claim good results with rate control rather than ablation.[29] There are no reports of increased mortality associated with AVJ ablation. The procedure carries the theoretic risk of device failure and death in pacemaker-dependent patients and eliminates fusion with spontaneously conducted beats during sinus rhythm. A randomized clinical trial to test the value of routine AVJ ablation is desirable.

IMPORTANCE OF THE BIV%: MORE IS ALWAYS BETTER

In the study of Boriani and colleagues,[19] the BiV% in the AF group was 95% versus 98% in the entire patient population. When patients with AF were in sinus rhythm, the BiV% was 98% versus 71% during AF, *P*<.01). Suboptimal CRT was defined as BiV% less than 95%, which was predicted by the occurrence of persistent or permanent AF (*P*<.001), and uncontrolled VR (*P* = .002). BiV% was inversely correlated to the VR in AF, decreasing by 7% for each 10-bpm increase in VR.

Koplan and colleagues[30] conducted a retrospective analysis in 1800 of CRT patients to evaluate the significance of BiV% and its relationship to a combined clinical end point of death and heart failure hospitalization. Patients who showed a BiV% greater than 92% had a 44% reduction in clinical end points compared with patients with BiV% 0% to 92% (*P*<.00001). Patients with BiV % 98% to 99% had similar outcomes as the patients with BiV% 93% to 97% and also similar outcomes as patients paced 100% of the time. Patients with a history of atrial arrhythmias were more likely to pace 92% or lower (*P*<.001).

The importance of a high BiV% has recently been confirmed in a large cohort of 36,935 patients who participated in the US LATITUDE (LATITUDE, Patient Management System, Boston-Scientific, Natick, MA, USA) patient management system, in which the patients were followed in a remote monitoring network.[31] The mortality was inversely associated with BiV% in the presence of both normal sinus and atrial paced rhythm and with AF (**Fig. 2**). The greatest reduction in mortality was observed with BiV% greater than 98%. Patients with BiV% greater than 99.6% experienced a 24% reduction in mortality (*P*<.001), whereas those with BiV% less than 94.8% had a 19% increase in mortality. The optimal BiV% cut-point was 98.7%.

The delivery of a stimulus does not guarantee effective CRT. The BiV% based on device interrogation data overestimates the percentage of truly resynchronized beats, because it does not account for fusion and pseudofusion between intrinsic (not paced) and paced beats. Kamath and colleagues[32] used 12-lead Holter monitoring to assess the incidence of ineffective capture in 19 patients with AF undergoing CRT (**Fig. 3**). The study clearly showed that although device interrogation showed

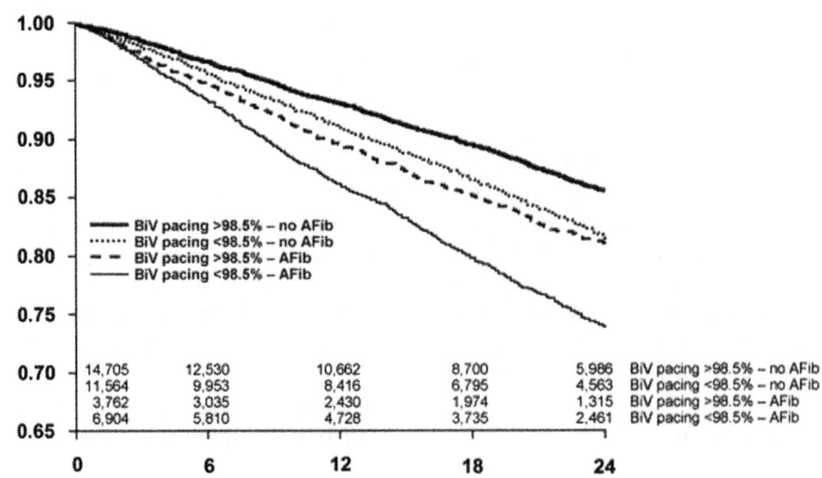

Fig. 2. In a large cohort of 36,935 patients followed up in a remote monitoring network (LATITUDE patient management system) a high BiV% achieved, specifically greater than 98.5%, was associated with a reduction in mortality. As expected, patients with AF had a worse outcome than those without AF. However, this was lessened if the high BiV% could be achieved in the AF population, usually after an AVJ ablation. (*From* Hayes DL, Boehmer JP, Day JD, et al. Cardiac resynchronization therapy and the relationship of percent biventricular pacing to symptoms and survival. Heart Rhythm 2011;8:1473; with permission.)

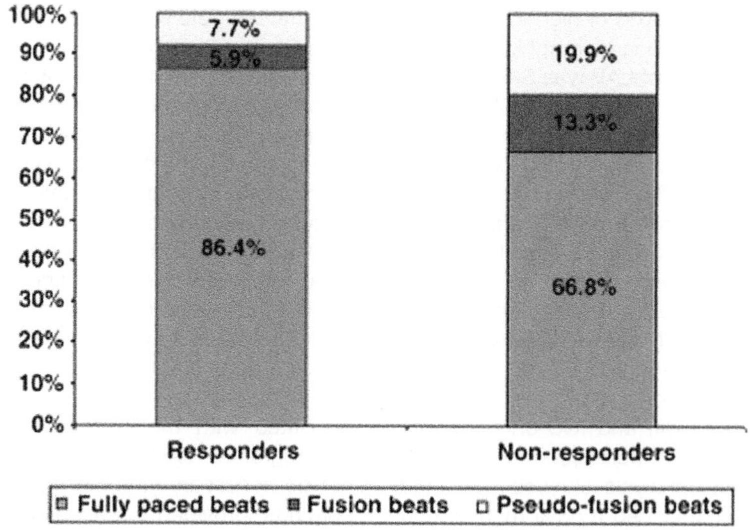

Fig. 3. 24-Hour Holter data for CRT responders and nonresponders with permanent AF. CRT responders had a higher percentage of fully paced beats than nonresponders. Nonresponders to CRT had a significantly higher percentage of ineffective pacing, because of a combination of fusion and pseudofusion beats. (*From* Kamath GS, Cotiga D, Koneru JN, et al. The utility of 12-lead Holter monitoring in patients with permanent atrial fibrillation for the identification of nonresponders after cardiac resynchronization therapy. J Am Coll Cardiol 2009;53:1050–5; with permission.)

more than 90% BiV pacing, only 9 patients (47%) received effective BiV pacing. It is imperative to examine rhythm strips and ECGs of nonresponders to verify that the beats are truly resynchronized. Certain device algorithms aimed at maximizing BiV pacing in patients with AF with a relatively fast VR may also lead to a false sense of reassurance about the BiV% pacing.

ANALYSIS OF THE RAFT STUDY IN PATIENTS WITH PERMANENT AF: SUBOPTIMAL DOSE OF CARDIAC RESYNCHRONIZATION?

The RAFT (Resynchronization for Ambulatory Heart Failure Trial) AF study constitutes the largest randomized report examining the role of CRT in patients with permanent AF.[33] Patients with permanent AF were randomized to CRT-ICD (n = 114) or ICD (n = 115). Cardiovascular death was similar between treatment arms (hazard ratio, 0.97; 95% confidence interval [CI], 0.55–1.71; *P* = .91); however, there was a trend for fewer heart failure hospitalizations with CRT-ICD (hazard ratio, 0.58; 95% CI, 0.38–1.01; *P* = .052). The findings were disappointing, contrary to prevailing belief that patients with AF improve with CRT, albeit less than in patients in sinus rhythm. To be eligible for the study, patients were required to have a resting heart rate of 60 beats per minute or lower and 90 beats per minute or lower after a 6-minute walk test. Only 1 patient underwent an AVJ ablation. There was no statistically significant difference of reaching a composite end point of all-cause mortality or heart failure hospitalization for those receiving BiV pacing less than 90% versus 90% or more or less than 95% versus 95% or more (only one-third of patients received BiV pacing ≥95%). Furthermore, the CRT-ICD arm had the conducted AF response algorithm (Medtronic, Minneapolis, MN, USA) enabled. This feature regularizes the pacing rate by adjusting the pacemaker escape interval after each ventricular beat. In this way, the delivery of BiV pacing was enhanced at a rate that closely matches the relatively fast spontaneous VR. Therefore, as a result of fusion and pseudofusion, the percentage of truly resynchronized beats was likely overestimated. The investigators of the RAFT study indicated that the standard medical rate control of permanent AF may have been insufficient to allow effective delivery of CRT therapy.

IMPACT OF STRUCTURAL CHANGES ON THE DEVELOPMENT OF ATRIAL TACHYARRHYTHMIAS DURING CARDIAC RESYNCHRONIZATION

The change in the left atrial volume (LAV) and incidence of atrial tachyarrhythmias was evaluated in a substudy of the MADIT-CRT trial.[21] In the total population of 1820 patients, there were 139 patients with atrial tachyarrhythmia (AF 47%). A low LAV reduction was defined as less than 20% and a high LAV reduction as 20% or higher. Based on the 1-year follow-up echocardiographic data, the mean percent reduction of LAV was 3-fold higher in patients treated with a CRT-D (D = ICD) device compared with the ICD-only group. The median reduction in LAV was 29% (20%–30%) in the CRT-D group versus 10% (5%–14%) in the ICD-only group (P<.001). As expected, reduction in LAV was highly correlated with reduction in the left ventricular end-systolic volume.

The cumulative probability of atrial tachyarrhythmias (at 2.5 years) in MADIT-CRT was lowest among high LAV responders to CRT-D (3%) and significantly higher among both low LAV responders to CRT-D (9%) and ICD-only patients (7%; P = .03 for the difference among the 3 groups). Multivariate analysis showed that high LAV responders experienced a 53% reduction in the risk of subsequent atrial tachyarrhythmia compared with low LAV responders in the CRT-D group and patients in the ICD-only group (P = .01).

REMOTE MONITORING

Implantable CRT devices are capable of automatic daily transmission of device data consisting of full interrogation and monitoring to a remote service center. Internet-based remote device interrogation systems provide clinicians with frequent (such as daily) and complete access to stored data. Easy access to these stored data permits clinicians to make diagnostic and therapeutic decisions sooner, thus avoiding potential long-term sequelae as a result of untreated clinical disorders. Such follow-up systems can automatically send reports and special alerts on a daily basis, thereby allowing physicians to respond more proactively to paroxysmal or asymptomatic AF. AF is more likely to be detected early with daily remote monitoring compared with traditional follow-up visits.[11–15,34]

MONITORING FOR AF BY CONVENTIONAL PACEMAKERS

Almost 10 years ago, in a landmark study of 110 patients with previous AF and a dual-chamber pacemaker, Israel and colleagues[35] reported recurrent AF in 88% of patients by review of stored electrograms and in 46% of patients by ECG recordings during follow-up (19 ± 11 months). AF lasted >48 hours in 50 patients, 19 of whom (38%) were completely asymptomatic and in sinus rhythm at subsequent follow-up. These observations clearly indicated clinical usefulness of pacemaker diagnostics. Continuous arrhythmia monitoring by cardiac rhythm devices has become the gold standard for AF diagnosis using continuous monitoring.

Devices vary in their capability to detect and record AHREs and are manufacturer specific. However, devices generally provide a reliable way to quantify AF burden. Devices do not simply average atrial cycles, and they vary in their rate detection and recordings. Therefore, evaluation of AHREs requires interpretation of the stored atrial rate data based on knowledge of how a particular device processes the data.

AHREs are not synonymous with AF, because they are dependent on the rate cut-off and duration of the high rate. As a rule, AHREs should be evaluated with the corresponding stored atrial electrograms. However, manual adjudication may not be necessary in some pacemaker-based recordings, provided the accuracy of AF detection without electrograms has been proven. Not all mode switches are necessarily caused by AF and should not be a surrogate for AF. Mode switches are less precise than full data disclosure with electrograms. Atrial oversensing can cause overestimation of AF episodes, whereas undersensing of AF may cause underestimation.

In 2003, Glotzer and colleagues[1] analyzed AHREs from MOST (Mode Selection Trial) and documented that AHREs greater than 5 minutes in duration and rate greater than 220 bpm were detected in 51% of patients during a mean of 27 months after implantation of a dual-chamber pacemaker for sinus node dysfunction. Patients with at least 1 episode of AHRE were 2.5 times more likely to die, 2.8 times more likely to die or have a nonfatal stroke, and nearly 6 times as likely to develop AF as patients without any AHRE. However, this was a retrospective analysis, including only 312 patients, and more than one-third of those with AHRE already had a clinical diagnosis of AF. In TRENDS (The Relationship Between Daily Atrial Tachyarrhythmia Burden From Implantable Device Diagnostics and Stroke Risks Study), it was shown that patients with a daily burden of AT of more than 5.5 hours had a 2.4-fold increase in the risk of thromboembolism, compared with patients with no AT.[2] In these trials, subclinical AF also increased the risk of clinical AF 5-fold to 6-fold, which suggests that subclinical AF could be regarded as a precursor to clinical AF. Whether the number of subclinical AF episodes, the AF burden (percentage of time spent in AF divided by total time), or the duration of the longest AF episode may be the best predictor for subsequent stroke, is still under debate.

Capucci and colleagues[36] reported the thromboembolic complications on a long-term follow-up (median 22 months) of 725 patients with permanent

Medtronic DDDR pacemakers for bradycardia and suffering from AF. Previous embolism, ischemic cardiomyopathy, hypertension, diabetes mellitus, and, in general, the presence of stroke risk factors resulted in the association of higher risk of embolism. Patients with device-detected AF recurrences longer than 1 day had a risk of embolism 3.1 times increased compared with patients without or with shorter AF recurrences, showing that AF recurrences longer than 1 day are independently associated with arterial embolism (*P*<.0001).

ASSERT (Asymptomatic Atrial Fibrillation and Stroke Evaluation in Pacemaker Patients and the AF Reduction Atrial Pacing Trial) enrolled 2580 patients, 65 years of age or older, with hypertension and no history of AF or related tachyarrhythmias in whom a pacemaker or defibrillator had recently been implanted (2451 pacemakers and 129 ICDs [St. Jude Medical, Saint Paul, MN, USA]), all capable of storing high-atrial-rate electrograms. The patients were monitored for 3 months to detect subclinical atrial tachyarrhythmias (episodes of atrial rate >190 bpm for >6 minutes) and then followed for a mean of 2.5 years for the primary outcome of ischemic stroke or systemic embolism (**Fig. 4**).[37–39] Kaufman and colleagues[38] reported the adjudicated AHREs derived from the programmed AT/AF algorithms. Of these AHREs, 82.7% were true AT/AF episodes, and 17.3%

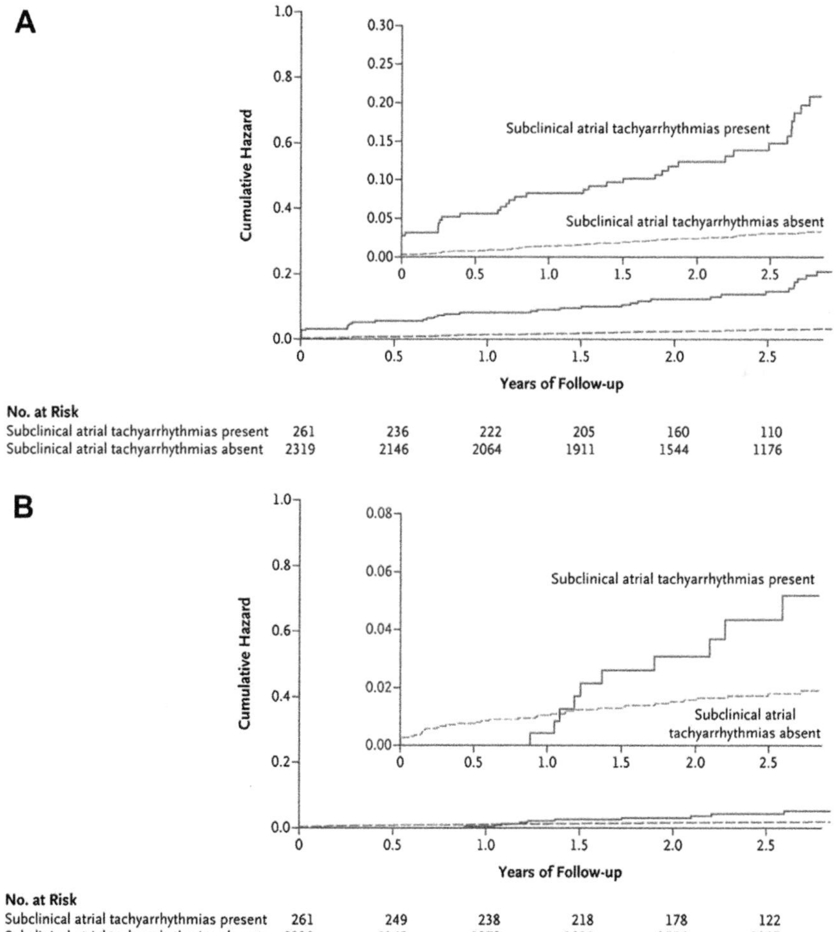

Fig. 4. The risk of clinical atrial tachyarrhythmias and of ischemic stroke or systemic embolism, according to the presence or absence of subclinical atrial tachyarrhythmia's (ASSERT trial). (*A*) The risk of electrocardiographically documented clinical atrial tachyarrhythmias after the 3-month visit, according to whether subclinical atrial tachyarrhythmias were or were not detected between enrollment and the 3-month visit. (*B*) The risk of ischemic stroke or systemic embolism after the 3-month visit, according to whether subclinical atrial tachyarrhythmias were or were not detected between enrollment and the 3-month visit. The insets show the same data on an enlarged y-axis. (*From* Healey JS, Connolly SJ, Gold MR, et al, ASSERT Investigators. Subclinical atrial fibrillation and the risk of stroke. N Engl J Med 2012;366:126; with permission.)

were inappropriate AT/AF episodes, highlighting the importance of individual electrogram review. The positive-predictive value for detecting true AT/AF improved with increased episode duration.

Subclinical (asymptomatic) atrial tachyarrhythmias were detected in 10% of the patients (n = 261) within 3 months after device implantation, and at least once in 34.7% of the patients during the follow-up of 2.5 years. Subclinical AF episodes were almost 8 times as common as clinical AF (*P*<.001). Subclinical atrial tachyarrhythmias often preceded the development of clinical AF. Clinical AF developed in only 15.7% of the patients with subclinical AF, suggesting that there is a time lag between subclinical events and clinical detection. Subclinical atrial tachyarrhythmias were associated with an increased risk of clinical AF (*P*<.001) and of ischemic stroke or systemic embolism (*P* = .007). The population attributable risk of stroke or systemic embolism associated with subclinical atrial tachyarrhythmias was 13%. The risk was virtually unchanged after adjustment for baseline risk factors for stroke (*P* = .008). During the follow-up period, 11 of the 261 patients (4.2%) in whom subclinical atrial tachyarrhythmias had been detected before 3 months had an ischemic stroke or systemic embolism (a rate of 1.69% per year), compared with 40 of the 2319 in whom subclinical atrial tachyarrhythmias had not been detected (1.7%, a rate of 0.69% per year, *P* = .007).

The ASSERT study did not show a strong temporal relationship between AHRE and thromboembolic events. The median interval between the most recent previous AHRE and the thromboembolic complication was 47 days, and only 27% of patients with AHRE who suffered a thromboembolic complication were in AF at the time of that event. This finding is in keeping with the published report from the TRENDS trial, which found that in patients with AHRE and a thromboembolic event, only 30% were in AF at the time of the event, and in the remaining patients, the most recent AHRE was an average of 168 $\pm$ 199 days earlier.[2]

MONITORING BY CARDIAC RESYNCHRONIZATION DEVICES

Shanmugam and colleagues[18] studied 560 patients with heart failure (median left ventricular ejection fraction 27%) with a CRT device (past history of paroxysmal AF in 178 patients). AHRE burden was defined as the duration of mode switch in a 24-hour period with atrial rates of more than 180 bpm. The investigators did not adjudicate the individual AHRE, but defined them as significant if they were documented for at least 1% of any day (14 minutes). Thromboembolic complications developed in 2% of patients overall and were 9 times more likely to develop among patients who had at least 3.8 hours of AHRE detected during any day. Sarkar and colleagues[40] retrospectively evaluated 519 CRT patients with paroxysmal AF (n = 519, 33% of all the CRT patients) and documented a greater risk of hospitalization for heart failure (*P*<.001) in patients with AF compared with patients with no AF. The risk increased further (*P*<.001) if there was 1 day of poor rate control during persistent AF or a high burden of paroxysmal AF in the last 30 days. Thus, a high burden of paroxysmal AF (>6 hours) with good or poor rate control is a risk factor for heart failure hospitalization in the next 30 days. The amount of AF, and the changes in rate control status during AF, may provide an opportunity to proactively reduce hospitalizations.

SUMMARY

In the last decade, our knowledge of AF in heart failure has increased dramatically, in large part because of the widespread use of continuous monitoring, mostly provided by implanted cardiac rhythm devices. Continuous monitoring has improved CRT management of patients with AF. New knowledge acquired from continuous monitoring has generated important questions, especially in patients with only asymptomatic AF and in those with very short AHREs. The answers to these questions require randomized trials.

- Several studies support a link between AHRE detected by implantable cardiac rhythm devices and the occurrence of stroke or systemic embolism. The minimum duration of subclinical or asymptomatic AF associated with a higher risk of thromboembolism remains debatable (ranging from 6 minutes in the ASSERT trial to 5.5 hours in the TRENDS study).
- Considering that there is frequently a long interval between AHRE and thromboembolic events, a causative relationship is questionable. It is more likely that AHRE are one of many features of the complex pathophysiologic mechanism that leads to cardioembolic events.
- The prevalence of subclinical atrial tachyarrhythmias may be higher in patients with pacemakers than in other high-risk patient groups. Sinus node dysfunction is associated with an increased risk of AF. Furthermore, patients with AV nodal disease may be more likely to be asymptomatic when atrial

tachyarrhythmias occur because of reduced AV conduction.

- Monitoring of the VR with ambulatory devices or implantable cardiac rhythm devices in patients with heart failure should be used to determine whether excessive VRs are present, targeting a resting VR of less than 80 bpm and peak activity rates of less than 110 to 120 bpm. The results of the RACE II trial that lenient rate control is not inferior to strict rate control should not be extrapolated to patients with heart failure.
- Although there is a strong association between AHRE and stroke, authorities believe that more data in the form of randomized studies are needed before routine oral anticoagulation can be recommended. Anticoagulant therapy should probably be considered in high-risk patients with asymptomatic AF from the CHADS2 score (or CHA2DS$_2$-VASc score) of 2 or greater (heart failure = 1) considering also the bleeding risk (HASBLED score, European Society of Cardiology).[41] In the ASSERT trial the absolute rate of stroke increased with increasing CHADS$_2$ score, reaching a rate of 3.78% per year in patients with subclinical atrial tachyarrhythmias and a CHADS2 score of greater than 2.
- The incidence of AF in patients with heart failure treated with CRT ranges from 30% to 35% for paroxysmal AF and around 20% to 25% for permanent AF. In CRT patients, AF is associated with an increase in heart failure hospitalizations and death. The greatest mortality reduction in CRT patients with AF was observed with BiV% greater than 98%. One should always aim for a BiV% of 100%. Small gains in BiV% are important. AVJ ablation will become more widely used, because it permits CRT delivery close to 100% of the time with regularization of the RR intervals, elimination of fusion and pseudofusion beats, and discontinuation of some AV nodal blocking drugs.

REFERENCES

1. Glotzer TV, Hellkamp AS, Zimmerman J, et al, MOST Investigators. Atrial high rate episodes detected by pacemaker diagnostics predict death and stroke: report of the Atrial Diagnostics Ancillary Study of the MOde Selection Trial (MOST). Circulation 2003; 107(12):1614–9.
2. Glotzer TV, Daoud EG, Wyse DG, et al. The relationship between daily atrial tachyarrhythmia burden from implantable device diagnostics and stroke risk: the TRENDS study. Circ Arrhythm Electrophysiol 2009;2:474–80.
3. Santini M, Gasparini M, Landolina M, et al, Cardiological centers participating in ClinicalService Project. Device-detected atrial tachyarrhythmias predict adverse outcome in real-world patients with implantable biventricular defibrillators. J Am Coll Cardiol 2011;57: 167–72.
4. Marijon E, Jacob S, Mouton E, et al, Mona Lisa Study Group. Frequency of atrial tachyarrhythmias in patients treated by cardiac resynchronization (from the Prospective, Multicenter Mona Lisa Study). Am J Cardiol 2010;106:688–93.
5. Leclercq C, Padeletti L, Cihák R, et al, CHAMP Study Investigators. Incidence of paroxysmal atrial tachycardias in patients treated with cardiac resynchronization therapy and continuously monitored by device diagnostics. Europace 2010;12:71–7.
6. Yannopoulos D, Lurie KG, Sakaguchi S, et al. Reduced atrial tachyarrhythmia susceptibility after upgrade of conventional pulse generator to cardiac resynchronization therapy in patients with heart failure. J Am Coll Cardiol 2007;50:1246–51.
7. Maisel WH, Stevenson LW. Atrial fibrillation in heart failure: epidemiology, pathophysiology, and rationale for therapy. Am J Cardiol 2003;91:2D–8D.
8. Tolosana JM, Hernandez Madrid A, Brugada J, et al, SPARE Investigators. Comparison of benefits and mortality in cardiac resynchronization therapy in patients with atrial fibrillation versus patients in sinus rhythm (Results of the Spanish Atrial Fibrillation and Resynchronization [SPARE] Study). Am J Cardiol 2008;102:444–9.
9. Molhoek SG, Bax JJ, Bleeker GB, et al. Comparison of response to cardiac resynchronization therapy in patients with sinus rhythm versus chronic atrial fibrillation. Am J Cardiol 2004;94:1506–9.
10. Linde C, Leclercq C, Rex S, et al. Long-term benefits of biventricular pacing in congestive heart failure: results from the MUltisite STimulation in cardiomyopathy (MUSTIC) study. J Am Coll Cardiol 2002;40: 111–8.
11. De Ruvo E, Gargaro A, Sciarra L, et al. Early detection of adverse events with daily remote monitoring versus quarterly standard follow-up program in patients with CRT-D. Pacing Clin Electrophysiol 2011; 34:208–16.
12. Burri H, Quesada A, Ricci RP, et al. The MOnitoring Resynchronization dEvices and CARdiac patiEnts (MORE-CARE) study: rationale and design. Am Heart J 2010;160:42–8.
13. Ricci RP, Morichelli L, Gargaro A, et al. Home monitoring in patients with implantable cardiac devices: is there a potential reduction of stroke risk? Results from a computer model tested through Monte Carlo simulations. J Cardiovasc Electrophysiol 2009;20: 1244–51.

14. Borleffs CJ, Ypenburg C, van Bommel RJ, et al. Clinical importance of new-onset atrial fibrillation after cardiac resynchronization therapy. Heart Rhythm 2009;6:305–10.
15. Crossley GH, Aonuma K, Haffajee C, et al, Concerto-AT Study Investigators. Atrial fibrillation therapy in patients with a CRT defibrillator with wireless telemetry. Pacing Clin Electrophysiol 2009;32:13–23.
16. Ip J, Waldo AL, Lip GY, et al, IMPACT Investigators. Multicenter randomized study of anticoagulation guided by remote rhythm monitoring in patients with implantable cardioverter-defibrillator and CRT-D devices: rationale, design, and clinical characteristics of the initially enrolled cohort. The IMPACT study. Am Heart J 2009;58:364–70.
17. Khoo CW, Krishnamoorthy S, Lim HS, et al. Atrial fibrillation, arrhythmia burden and thrombogenesis. Int J Cardiol 2012;157:318–23.
18. Shanmugam N, Boerdlein A, Proff J, et al. Detection of atrial high-rate events by continuous home monitoring: clinical significance in the heart failure-cardiac resynchronization therapy population. Europace 2012;14:230–7.
19. Boriani G, Gasparini M, Landolina M, et al, on behalf of the Clinical Service Cardiac Centres. Incidence and clinical relevance of uncontrolled ventricular rate during atrial fibrillation in heart failure patients treated with cardiac resynchronization therapy. Eur J Heart Fail 2011;13(8):868–76.
20. Van Gelder IC, Groenveld HF, Crijns HJ, RACE II Investigators. Lenient versus strict rate control in patients with atrial fibrillation. N Engl J Med 2010;362:1363–73.
21. Brenyo A, Link MS, Barsheshet A, et al. Cardiac resynchronization therapy reduces left atrial volume and the risk of atrial tachyarrhythmias in MADIT-CRT (Multicenter Automatic Defibrillator Implantation Trial with Cardiac Resynchronization Therapy). J Am Coll Cardiol 2011;58:1682–9.
22. Gasparini M, Auricchio A, Regoli F, et al. Four-year efficacy of cardiac resynchronization therapy on exercise tolerance and disease progression: the importance of performing atrioventricular junction ablation in patients with atrial fibrillation. J Am Coll Cardiol 2006;48:734–43.
23. Gasparini M, Auricchio A, Metra M, et al, Multicentre Longitudinal Observational Study (MILOS) Group. Long-term survival in patients undergoing cardiac resynchronization therapy: the importance of performing atrio-ventricular junction ablation in patients with permanent atrial fibrillation. Eur Heart J 2008;29:1644–52.
24. Ferreira AM, Adragão P, Cavaco DM, et al. Benefit of cardiac resynchronization therapy in atrial fibrillation patients vs. patients in sinus rhythm: the role of atrioventricular junction ablation. Europace 2008;10:809–15.
25. Dong K, Shen WK, Powell BD, et al. Atrioventricular nodal ablation predicts survival benefit in patients with atrial fibrillation receiving cardiac resynchronization therapy. Heart Rhythm 2010;7:1240–5.
26. Bradley DJ, Shen WK. Atrioventricular junction ablation combined with either right ventricular pacing or cardiac resynchronization therapy for atrial fibrillation: the need for large-scale randomized trials. Heart Rhythm 2007;4:224–32.
27. Foley PW, Leyva F. Long-term survival in patients undergoing cardiac resynchronization therapy: the importance of atrio-ventricular junction ablation in patients with permanent atrial fibrillation. Eur Heart J 2008;29:2182.
28. Kaszala K, Ellenbogen KA. Role of cardiac resynchronization therapy and atrioventricular junction ablation in patients with permanent atrial fibrillation. Eur Heart J 2011;32:2344–6.
29. Himmel F, Reppel M, Mortensen K, et al. A strategy to achieve CRT response in permanent atrial fibrillation without obligatory atrioventricular node ablation. Pacing Clin Electrophysiol 2012;35:943–7.
30. Koplan BA, Kaplan AJ, Weiner S, et al. Heart failure decompensation and all-cause mortality in relation to percent biventricular pacing in patients with heart failure: is a goal of 100% biventricular pacing necessary? J Am Coll Cardiol 2009;53:355–60.
31. Hayes DL, Boehmer JP, Day JD, et al. Cardiac resynchronization therapy and the relationship of percent biventricular pacing to symptoms and survival. Heart Rhythm 2011;8:1469–75.
32. Kamath GS, Cotiga D, Koneru JN, et al. The utility of 12-lead Holter monitoring in patients with permanent atrial fibrillation for the identification of nonresponders after cardiac resynchronization therapy. J Am Coll Cardiol 2009;53:1050–5.
33. Healey JS, Hohnloser SH, Exner DV, et al, RAFT Investigators. Cardiac resynchronization therapy in patients with permanent atrial fibrillation: results from the Resynchronization for Ambulatory Heart Failure Trial (RAFT). Circ Heart Fail 2012;5(5):566–70.
34. Caldwell JC, Contractor H, Petkar S, et al. Atrial fibrillation is under-recognized in chronic heart failure: insights from a heart failure cohort treated with cardiac resynchronization therapy. Europace 2009;11:1295–300.
35. Israel CW, Gronefeld G, Ehrlich JR, et al. Long-term risk of recurrent atrial fibrillation as documented by an implantable monitoring device: implications for optimal patient care. J Am Coll Cardiol 2004;43:47–52.
36. Capucci A, Santini M, Padeletti L, et al, Italian AT500 Registry Investigators. Monitored atrial fibrillation duration predicts arterial embolic events in patients suffering from bradycardia and atrial fibrillation

implanted with antitachycardia pacemakers. J Am Coll Cardiol 2005;46:1913–20.
37. Hohnloser SH, Capucci A, Fain E, et al. ASymptomatic atrial fibrillation and Stroke Evaluation in pacemaker patients and the atrial fibrillation reduction atrial pacing Trial (ASSERT). Am Heart J 2006;152: 442–7.
38. Kaufman ES, Israel CW, Nair GM, et al, ASSERT Steering Committee and Investigators. Positive predictive value of device-detected atrial high-rate episodes at different rates and durations: an analysis from ASSERT. Heart Rhythm 2012;9:1241–6.
39. Healey JS, Connolly SJ, Gold MR, et al, ASSERT Investigators. Subclinical atrial fibrillation and the risk of stroke. N Engl J Med 2012;366:120–9.
40. Sarkar S, Koehler J, Crossley GH, et al. Burden of atrial fibrillation and poor rate control detected by continuous monitoring and the risk for heart failure hospitalization. Am Heart J 2012;164:616–24.
41. Camm AJ, Kirchhof P, Lip GY, et al. Guidelines for the management of atrial fibrillation: the task force for the management of atrial fibrillation of the European Society of Cardiology (ESC). Eur Heart J 2010;31(19):2369–429.

Ventricular Rate Control of Atrial Fibrillation in Heart Failure

Michiel Rienstra, MD, PhD, Isabelle C. Van Gelder, MD, PhD*

KEYWORDS

• Atrial fibrillation • Heart failure • Ventricular rate • Treatment • Rate control

KEY POINTS

- Ventricular rate control in patients with atrial fibrillation (AF) and chronic heart failure (HF) is recommended as the first-line therapy in the acute phase.
- The decision for long-term ventricular rate control should be based on patient symptoms and the cause of HF.
- If the ventricular rate control is adopted, a target of less than 110 beats per minute is appropriate for most patients.
- Stricter rate control may be indicated in patients with persisting AF-related symptoms under lenient rate control or in the setting of HF with ongoing ischemia, severe diastolic dysfunction, hypertrophic cardiomyopathy, hypotension, or signs of pulmonary congestion, although the beneficial effects of stricter rate control have not yet been proven.
- Ventricular rate control is generally easy to achieve, although frequent dose adjustments, combinations of drugs, and medication changes may be needed.

INTRODUCTION

Atrial fibrillation (AF) and heart failure (HF) often coexist.[1,2] The prevalence of AF in patients with chronic HF in cardiology practices in Europe is 42%.[3] The incidence and the prevalence of AF increase with the severity of HF.[4] From several small studies, it is known that AF begets HF and HF begets AF in the first place because both have shared risk factors, like hypertension and ischemia.[5,6] The loss of atrioventricular synchrony (loss of atrial kick), the rapid ventricular rate, the irregular ventricular response (R-R irregularity), and the development of tachycardiomyopathy during AF may adversely affect ventricular function and overall hemodynamic status.[7–13] The onset of AF is associated with a worsening of the New York Heart Association (NYHA) functional class for HF and a decline in peak exercise capacity, a lower cardiac index, and increased mitral and tricuspid regurgitation in patients with mild to moderate chronic HF.[14] The increased atrial pressure and volume, the activation of the renin-angiotensin-aldosterone system, and the activation of the sympathetic nervous system that occurs in chronic HF may result in atrial stretch and interstitial fibrosis.[10,15–17]

In the last few years, there has been a major shift in the treatment of AF in the setting of HF, from rhythm to ventricular rate control in most patients with both conditions. In the present article, the authors focus on ventricular rate control and discuss

No conflicts of interest.

Department of Cardiology, University Medical Center Groningen, University of Groningen, Groningen, Hanzeplein 1, PO Box 30.001, Groningen 9700 RB, The Netherlands

* Corresponding author. Department of Cardiology, Thoraxcenter, University Medical Center Groningen, University of Groningen, Hanzeplein 1, PO Box 30.001, Groningen 9700 RB, The Netherlands.
E-mail address: I.C.van.Gelder@umcg.nl

Heart Failure Clin 9 (2013) 397–406
http://dx.doi.org/10.1016/j.hfc.2013.07.004
1551-7136/13/$ – see front matter

the indications; the optimal ventricular rate-control target, including detailed results of the Rate Control Efficacy in Permanent Atrial Fibrillation: a Comparison Between Lenient versus Strict Rate Control II (RACE II) study[18]; and the pharmacologic and nonpharmacologic options to control the ventricular rate during AF in the setting of HF.

INDICATIONS FOR VENTRICULAR RATE CONTROL OF AF IN HF

The treatment of patients with AF and chronic HF may differ from patient to patient. Initial acute therapy includes adequate ventricular rate control and anticoagulation based on the thromboembolic risk.[19] Before choosing ventricular rate control as a long-term strategy, symptoms and potential further deterioration of HF need to be considered.[19] Previously, 6 randomized controlled trials (the Atrial Fibrillation Follow-up Investigation of Rhythm Management [AFFIRM], the Rate Control versus Electrical Cardioversion for Persistent Atrial Fibrillation [RACE], the Pharmacologic Intervention in Atrial Fibrillation [PIAF], the Strategies of Treatment of Atrial Fibrillation [STAF], the How to Treat Chronic Atrial Fibrillation [HOT CAFE], and the Japanese Rhythm Management Trial for Atrial Fibrillation [J-RHYTHM]) showed that a ventricular rate-control strategy (see **Table 1** for the variety in ventricular rate-control criteria) is not inferior to rhythm control with regard to cardiovascular morbidity and mortality.[20–25] Although in most of these studies only a subset of patients had chronic HF, the large randomized Rhythm Control versus Rate Control for Atrial Fibrillation and Heart Failure trial confirmed that in 1376 patients with AF and chronic HF (AF-CHF), a routine strategy of rhythm control does not reduce the rate of death from cardiovascular causes, symptoms, functional status, quality of life, and left ventricular ejection fraction (LVEF), as compared with a ventricular rate-control strategy.[26–28]

Table 1
Heart rate criteria used in the rate versus rhythm control trials

Trial	Year	Primary Endpoint	Ventricular Rate Control Criteria
PIAF[22]	2000	Symptoms related to AF	Diltiazem 90 mg, 2–3 times per day, additional rate-control therapy at discretion of physician
AFFIRM[20]	2002	All-cause mortality	≤80 bpm and ≤110 bpm during moderate exercise; on Holter mean ventricular rate ≤100 bpm and not >110% of the maximum predicted heart rate
RACE[21]	2002	Composite of cardiovascular death, HF hospitalization, thromboembolic complications, bleeding, pacemaker implantation, and severe adverse effects or antiarrhythmic drugs	<100 bpm
STAF[23]	2003	Composite of all-cause mortality, stroke or transient ischemic attack, systemic embolism, and cardiopulmonary resuscitation	Not specified
HOT CAFE[24]	2004	All-cause mortality, thromboembolic complications and intracranial or other major hemorrhage	70–90 bpm, <140 bpm during moderate exercise
AF-CHF[26]	2008	Cardiovascular death	≤80 bpm and ≤110 bpm during 6-min walk test
J-RHYTHM[25]	2009	Composite of all-cause mortality, symptomatic cerebral infarction, systemic embolism, major bleeding, HF hospitalization, physical/ psychological disability requiring alteration of assigned strategy	60–80 bpm

Abbreviations: AF, atrial fibrillation; HF, heart failure; bpm, beat per minute.

Adapted from Groenveld HF, Crijns HJ, Tijssen JG, et al. Rate control in atrial fibrillation, insight into the RACE II study. Neth Heart J 2013;21(4):200; with permission.

However, since in the randomized controlled trials patients with severe symptoms were not included, rhythm control is still indicated in those patients who are severely symptomatic. But in the majority of patients with minor or absence of symptoms of AF long-term ventricular rate control is recommended. Previously, several small patient studies reported that AF adversely affects ventricular function and overall hemodynamic status.[7–13] Conversely, adequate ventricular rate control may improve left ventricular function.[13,29] In the aforementioned randomized controlled trials and their substudies, no evidence for the development of tachycardiomyopathy with ventricular rate control was found. In addition, in patients with chronic HF, no further deterioration of left ventricular function was observed.[26,28,30,31] Accordingly, no superior efficacy of rhythm control was observed. Furthermore, the safety of a rhythm-control strategy is a concern because patients with HF may be prone to proarrhythmic side effects of the antiarrhythmic drugs used to maintain sinus rhythm.[19] This inclination may further limit the applicability of a rhythm-control strategy in patients with HF. A rate-control strategy is, thus, established as one of the evidence-based strategies for managing patients with AF in the setting of chronic HF.

However, because the randomized controlled trials typically enrolled patients without severe symptoms, rhythm control should be strongly considered in the subset of patients who are severely symptomatic. In patients with HF with severe diastolic dysfunction or restrictive physiology (eg, hypertrophic cardiomyopathy), the loss of atrial kick during AF may be of great hemodynamic importance and lead to symptoms, and a rhythm-control strategy may still be indicated.

OPTIMAL VENTRICULAR RATE-CONTROL TARGET OF AF IN HF

The optimal target for ventricular rate control in patients with AF and chronic HF is the subject of an ongoing debate. So far, there has been 1 randomized controlled trial designed to address this specific question: the RACE II study.[18] In this pivotal trial, 614 patients with permanent AF and a resting ventricular rate of more than 80 beats per minute (bpm) were included. Of the total, 60 patients (10%) had a prior HF hospitalization, 93 patients (15%) had an LVEF of 40% or less, and 214 patients (35%) had dyspnea and were in the NYHA functional class II or III. The primary outcome was a composite of death from cardiovascular causes, hospitalization for HF and stroke, systemic embolism, bleeding, and life-threatening arrhythmic events and was assessed during 2 to 3 years of follow-up. The lenient ventricular rate-control target was a resting ventricular rate of less than 110 bpm, and the strict ventricular rate-control targets were a resting ventricular rate less than 80 bpm and a ventricular rate during moderate exercise of less than 110 bpm. During the dose-adjustment phase, patients were administered one or more negative dromotropic drugs (ie, beta-blockers, nondihydropyridine calcium channel blockers, and digoxin), used alone or in combination and at various doses, until the ventricular rate targets were achieved. The mean resting ventricular rate at the end of the dose-adjustment phase was 93 $\pm$ 9 bpm in the lenient-control group, as compared with 76 $\pm$ 12 bpm in the strict-control group ($P<.001$). There was no difference in the occurrence of the composite primary end point (38 in the lenient-control group and 43 in the strict-control group) or in its individual components. Furthermore, a predefined substudy of the RACE II trial was performed to assess the effect of the stringency of ventricular rate control on quality of life and symptoms.[32] General health-related quality of life was assessed using the Medical Outcomes Study 36-Item Short-Form Health Survey; the severity of AF-related symptoms was assessed with the University of Toronto AF Severity Scale (AF severity scale); and the severity of fatigue was measured using the Multidimensional Fatigue Inventory-20. At baseline, 58% of patients experienced symptoms of AF, predominantly dyspnea, fatigue, and palpitations. There were no differences in symptoms of AF at either baseline or at the end of the study between the lenient- and strict-control groups. Furthermore, the stringency of the rate control did not improve quality of life, measured on any of the used questionnaires. Instead, changes in quality of life were related to age, symptoms, severity of underlying disease, and female sex.[32] RACE II, thus, demonstrated that stringency of ventricular rate control had no influence on symptoms, quality of life, cardiovascular morbidity, and mortality. The main concern of high ventricular rates accompanying AF is the development of tachycardiomyopathy.[7–13] An echocardiographic substudy of RACE II investigated left ventricular and atrial remodeling in patients with permanent AF treated with lenient or strict rate control.[33] In general, no important adverse atrial or ventricular remodeling during the 3-year follow-up was observed. In addition, lenient rate control did not cause significant adverse atrial and ventricular remodeling compared with strict rate control.[33]

It is important to note that only a minority of patients with AF and HF were included in RACE II, although, as in the main trial, no effect of ventricular rate-control stringency on cardiovascular morbidity and mortality was consistently seen in those patients with AF and HF.[34] At this point, data from RACE II are some of the sparse data that are available on ventricular rate control in patients with AF and HF. Grogan and colleagues[13] reported in 1992 that adequate rate control, using mainly digoxin and amiodarone, improved left ventricular function in 10 patients with presumed idiopathic dilated cardiomyopathy with impaired left ventricular function. However, no specific rate-control target was defined. Khand and colleagues[35] performed the first randomized, double-blinded, placebo-controlled study. In total, 47 patients with persistent AF and systolic chronic HF were included. In the first 4 months, digoxin was compared with the combination of digoxin and carvedilol. In the 6 months thereafter, digoxin was withdrawn in a double-blinded manner in the carvedilol-treated arm, thus allowing a comparison between digoxin and carvedilol. Compared with digoxin alone, combination therapy lowered the ventricular rate on 24-hour Holter monitoring and during submaximal exercise, and LVEF and symptoms improved. There were no significant differences found between digoxin alone and carvedilol alone. Again, no prespecified ventricular rate-control targets were applied. More recently, Silvet and colleagues[36] performed an open-label, crossover, interventional study including patients with AF and chronic systolic HF. Quality of life and exercise tolerance were assessed before and after attempting strict ventricular rate control. Patients were treated with increasing doses of metoprolol succinate to achieve a target resting ventricular rate of less than 70 bpm. On monthly visits, the dose of the medication was increased in 25-mg to 50-mg steps until the ventricular rate target was reached or until side effects occurred. Quality of life and exercise tolerance were measured after at least 2 weeks of stable medication dose. After a mean follow-up of 98 days, the resting ventricular rate decreased from 94 $\pm$ 14 bpm to 85 $\pm$ 12 bpm (P = .005). Only 2 patients achieved the goal of a resting ventricular rate of less than 70 bpm. Side effects prevented further up-titration of metoprolol in the remaining patients. Both the primary outcome, meters walked during a 6-minute walk test, and quality of life as measured by the Minnesota Living With Heart Failure Questionnaire did not change.

Long-term prognostic information was provided by several subanalyses of randomized controlled trials and the aforementioned RACE II study.[18,37–40] A substudy of the Second Prospective Randomised Study of Ibopamine on Mortality and Efficacy (PRIME II) aimed to study heart rate in patients with AF and chronic systolic HF.[37] In total, 77 patients with AF at inclusion and advanced systolic HF were studied and dichotomized according to the median heart rate of 80 bpm at inclusion (39 patients with low heart rate and 38 patients with high heart rate). Both patient groups were remarkably comparable; after a mean follow-up of 3.3 $\pm$ 0.9 years, mortality was comparable (62% vs 55%). If anything, lower heart rates were related to impaired prognosis. The Candesartan in Heart Failure: Assessment of Reduction in Mortality and Morbidity (CHARM) Program enrolled 7599 patients with a clinical diagnosis of chronic HF that were enrolled in CHARM-Alternative (n = 2028, LVEF <40% and not receiving an angiotensin-converting enzyme inhibitor because of previous intolerance), CHARM-Added (n = 2548, LVEF <40% receiving angiotensin-converting enzyme inhibitor treatment), and the CHARM-Preserved study (n = 3023, LVEF >40%). Among all 3 CHARM studies, 1148 patients with AF at randomization were included. There was no association between ventricular rate and cardiovascular morbidity and mortality found in patients with AF; this is in great contrast to patients with sinus rhythm.[41] In the Permanent Atrial Fibrillation Outcome Study Using Dronedarone on Top of Standard Therapy (PALLAS), which was prematurely stopped for safety reasons, the high rate of cardiovascular events occurring directly after the institution of dronedarone may be related to excessive rate control. The ventricular rate at 1 month in survivors in the dronedarone arm had decreased by 7.6 $\pm$ 14.5 bpm.[42] Based on the studies described earlier, there is no evidence supporting the deleterious effects of a lenient ventricular rate-control approach in patients with AF.

At present, the European Society of Cardiology's 2010 AF guidelines[43] state that it is reasonable to initiate treatment with a lenient rate-control protocol aimed at a resting heart rate of less than 110 bpm and to adopt a stricter rate-control strategy (a resting heart rate of less than 80 bpm and heart rate during moderate exercise of less than 110 bpm) when symptoms persist or tachycardiomyopathy occurs, despite lenient rate control. After achieving the strict heart rate target, a 24-hour Holter monitor is recommended to assess safety (**Fig. 1**). No specific ventricular rate-control targets for patients with HF are described. The 2011 AF guidelines of the American College of Cardiology (ACC)/American Heart Association (AHA)/Heart Rhythm Society recommend strict ventricular rate control for patients with AF in the setting of chronic HF, with a ventricular rate target of 60 to 80 bpm at rest and 90 to 115 bpm during moderate exercise.[19] The 2009 chronic HF guidelines recommend a more lenient

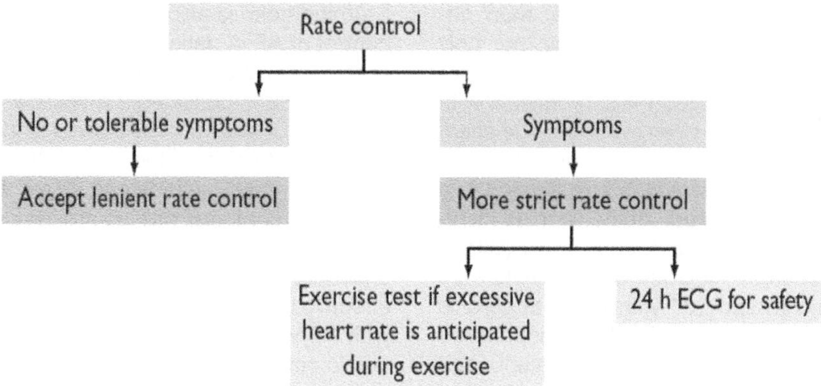

Fig. 1. Ventricular rate control approach according to the European Society of Cardiology's 2010 AF guidelines. (*Adapted from* Camm AJ, Kirchhof P, Lip GY, et al. Guidelines for the management of atrial fibrillation: the Task Force for the Management of Atrial Fibrillation of the European Society of Cardiology (ESC). Eur Heart J 2010;31:2369–429; with permission.)

approach, with a target ventricular rate of less than 80 to 90 bpm at rest and less than 110 to 130 during moderate exercise.[44]

Based on the available literature, there is no evidence supporting that different long-term ventricular rate-control targets should be recommended in patients with AF in the setting of chronic HF. In general, ventricular rates during AF of less than 110 bpm seem sufficient, although the persistence of symptoms or the presence of ongoing ischemia, signs of pulmonary congestion, severe diastolic dysfunction, and hypertrophic (obstructive) cardiomyopathy may warrant stricter targets; however, the beneficial effects of stricter rate control have not been proven.

PHARMACOLOGIC VENTRICULAR RATE CONTROL OF AF IN HF

Ventricular rate control is generally easy to achieve, although frequent dose adjustments, combinations of drugs, and medication changes may be needed.[18,36,45] In randomized controlled studies, pharmacologic ventricular rate control has been achieved in 70% to 80% of patients, dependent primarily on the rate-control target that was attempted.[18,45,46] As previously described, there is no evidence of any adverse influence on left ventricular function; serious adverse effects from rate-control drugs are uncommon. However, the rate-control strategy is not without adverse effects.[18,20,21] Negative dromotropic treatment that slows ventricular rates may lead to symptomatic bradycardia and eventually to otherwise unnecessary pacemaker implantation.

Ventricular rate control can be achieved by beta-blockers, nondihydropyridine calcium channel antagonists, digoxin, and amiodarone alone or in combination. Beta-blockers are the most effective rate-control agents[26] that reduce morbidity and mortality in HF patients and have a class IA recommendation[44] in the current chronic HF guidelines. This recommendation also holds for patients with AF and chronic HF, although the data are less convincing, as was shown in a recent meta-analysis including 8680 patients with chronic HF, of whom 1677 had AF from 4 selected randomized placebo-controlled beta-blocker trials.[47] In a systematic review by Segal and colleagues,[48] beta-blockers were proven safe and effective for control of heart rate in patients with AF and superior to placebo. Beta-blockers are effective for controlling ventricular rates in rest and during exercise[48] and provide better control of ventricular rates during exercise than digoxin.[49] Beta-blockers should be initiated cautiously in patients with AF and chronic systolic HF.[44] Patients taking beta-blockers may experience slow rates at rest or compromised exercise tolerance when the ventricular rate response is restrained excessively.[48]

Individual patient responses to a specific type of beta-blockers may depend on the presence of the beta-1-adrenoceptor Arg389Gly polymorphism; however, because data are sparse and sometimes conflicting, this has not yet found its way into clinical practice. The common single nucleotide polymorphism in the beta-1-adrenoceptor (Arg389Gly), a replacement of arginine with glycine at position 389, results in reduced cyclic adenosine monophosphate synthesis.[50,51] Around 40% of people of European ancestry are heterozygous and approximately 7% homozygous for the Gly389 genetic variant. Parvez and colleagues[52] reported that in the Vanderbilt AF registry, 543 patients with AF with the homozygous Arg389 genotype are more resistant to pharmacologic rate control (using different beta-blockers) than patients with AF with Gly389 genotypes; but only 11% of the patients in that study had HF. Two substudies of large randomized trials in patients with AF and chronic HF have been reported. The effect of this polymorphism on the ventricular rate response by beta-blockers was investigated in a pharmacogenetics substudy of the Cardiac Insufficiency Bisoprolol Study in Elderly study (CIBIS-ELD). This substudy included 528 patients (421 with sinus rhythm and 107 with AF) with chronic HF.[53] Patients were randomized to bisoprolol or carvedilol. Patients in sinus rhythm responded essentially identically to bisoprolol and carvedilol, independent of genotype. However, patients with AF who were homozygous for Arg389 had a 12-bpm lower response to carvedilol (but not bisoprolol) than carriers of at least one Gly389 allele. The immediate response to carvedilol did not differ between genotypes. Although intriguing, the absence of a ventricular rate response to carvedilol in Arg389-homozygous carriers contradicts a higher expected activity and prior reports of maintained responses to beta-blockers for this genotype. In a post hoc analysis of the Beta-Blocker Evaluation of Survival Trial (BEST), there was no difference observed in achieving the study-defined ventricular rate-control target in patients with AF and HF with the beta-1-adrenoceptor Arg389Gly polymorphism.[54]

Digoxin can be used for ventricular rate control in patients with AF and chronic systolic HF. A systematic review reported that digoxin slows the ventricular rate at rest, but not during exercise, in patients with AF.[48,49] The combination of a beta-blocker and digoxin improves ventricular rate control, reduces symptoms, and may improve ventricular function to a greater extent than either drug alone.[35] However, digoxin has a narrow therapeutic range; frequent drug interactions occur, so cautious use of low-dose digoxin is indicated in older patients, those with renal insufficiency, and those who are using other drugs that may raise digoxin concentrations. The most frequent adverse effects of digoxin are ventricular arrhythmias, atrioventricular block, and sinus pauses; all effects are dose dependent. Previously, concerns have been raised that digoxin use may be associated with mortality when used in patients with AF[55,56]; however, whether this is a true digoxin effect or is caused by bias by indication remains uncertain. It has been postulated that the excess mortality may result from high-dose digoxin because this was not observed in multiple other AF trials using lower-dose digoxin. At this point, recommendations for the use of low-dose digoxin have not been modified.

Amiodarone is also effective for ventricular rate control of AF in patients with chronic HF.[49] However, because of its potential noncardiac toxicity, amiodarone is considered a second-line drug for rate control after a beta-blocker and digoxin are proven ineffective. In the United States and some other countries, amiodarone is not approved for use as a ventricular rate-control drug, and its use is off label.[19] Acute ventricular rate control with amiodarone intravenously or at high oral doses is effective in lowering the ventricular rate in patients with AF with high ventricular rates and hemodynamic compromise, although strict hemodynamic monitoring is indicated.[57]

The nondihydropyridine calcium channel antagonists verapamil and diltiazem should be used cautiously or avoided in patients with HF caused by systolic dysfunction because of their negative inotropic effects, although these drugs seem to be useful in HF with preserved ejection fraction.[19]

NONPHARMACOLOGIC VENTRICULAR RATE CONTROL OF AF AND HF

Permanent complete atrioventricular node ablation provides highly effective ventricular rate control and improves symptoms in selected patients.[58–61] In general, patients most likely to benefit from this therapy are those who are severely symptomatic and with uncontrollable ventricular rates with antiarrhythmic or negative dromotropic drugs.[19,61] This approach has several limitations varying from the loss of atrioventricular synchrony if patients have intermittent sinus rhythm and an atrial lead is not present, lifelong pacemaker dependency, and the potential risk of development or deterioration of HF caused by right ventricular pacing-induced left ventricular dyssynchrony, affecting left ventricular structure and function.[62–68] The ACC/AHA/European Society of Cardiology's guidelines state that nonpharmacologic therapy should be considered when pharmacologic measures fails.[19] In patients with AF and chronic HF, lifelong right ventricular pacing is a great concern and biventricular pacing is an option. In several acute hemodynamic studies compared with right ventricular pacing, left ventricular pacing improves systolic function and diastolic filling and decreases mitral regurgitation.[69,70] Two randomized studies compared different pacing modes in patients undergoing atrioventricular node ablation for permanent AF. The Optimal Pacing Site study found that left ventricular and biventricular pacing provided modest or no additional favorable effect compared with right ventricular pacing.[71] The left ventricular–based cardiac stimulation study, Post

AtrioVentricular Nodal Ablation Evaluation, showed that biventricular pacing significantly improved the 6-minute walk test and LVEF compared with right ventricular pacing after 6 months of follow-up, with the greatest beneficial effects in those with impaired systolic function or with symptomatic HF.[72] Therefore, the guidelines[19] state that for those with impaired left ventricular function not caused by tachycardia, a biventricular pacemaker with or without defibrillator capability should be considered. Upgrading to a biventricular device should be considered for patients with chronic HF and a right ventricular pacing system who have undergone atrioventricular node ablation.[73]

NEW DEVELOPMENTS IN NONPHARMACOLOGIC VENTRICULAR RATE CONTROL OF AF IN HF

Diverse alternatives to permanent complete atrioventricular block have been studied to avoid lifelong pacemaker dependency and to allow native electrical conduction. However, these techniques have not yet found their way into daily clinical practice.

Selective atrioventricular node vagal stimulation is one technique under investigation. In animal models, the feasibility of selective vagal stimulation of the epicardial atrioventricular nodal fat pad that is located at the junction of the inferior vena cava and left atrium to achieve acute[74,75] and sustained (up to 6 weeks)[76] and reversible lowering of the ventricular response has been reported. It has been shown to be feasible in humans, using an endocardial neurostimulator.[77,78] Recently, research has been expanded to chronic HF whereby the vagal tone is reduced. Zhang and colleagues[79] demonstrated, in a canine model of pacing-induced HF and AF, that selective atrioventricular node vagal stimulation led to a decrease in ventricular rate and improvement in LVEF and remained present during 6 months of follow-up.

As an extension to selective atrioventricular node vagal stimulation, several other techniques of increasing vagal tone are under investigation, such as right cervical vagal nerve stimulation. Although right cervical vagal nerve stimulation seems to have beneficial effects in HF (eg, improvements in LVEF and left ventricular systolic volume, NYHA functional class, quality of life, and exercise tolerance), these effects were observed without a significant change the ventricular rate. Whether this approach is of use for ventricular rate control in patients with AF and HF is, therefore, uncertain.[80,81]

SUMMARY

Ventricular rate control in patients with AF and chronic HF is recommended as the first-line therapy in the acute phase. The decision for long-term ventricular rate control should be based on patient symptoms and the cause of heart failure. If ventricular rate control is adopted, a target of less than 110 bpm is appropriate for most patients. Stricter rate control may be indicated in patients with persisting AF-related symptoms under lenient rate control or in the setting of HF with ongoing ischemia, severe diastolic dysfunction, hypertrophic cardiomyopathy, hypotension, or signs of pulmonary congestion, although the beneficial effects of stricter rate control have not yet been proven. In general, rate control is easy to achieve with beta-blockers and digoxin alone or in combination. If unsuccessful, amiodarone or atrioventricular node ablation can be considered.

REFERENCES

1. Wang TJ, Larson MG, Levy D, et al. Temporal relations of atrial fibrillation and congestive heart failure and their joint influence on mortality: the Framingham Heart Study. Circulation 2003;107:2920–5.
2. Smit MD, Moes ML, Maass AH, et al. The importance of whether atrial fibrillation or heart failure develops first. Eur J Heart Fail 2012;14:1030–40.
3. Cleland JG, Swedberg K, Follath F, et al. The Euro-Heart Failure survey programme– a survey on the quality of care among patients with heart failure in Europe. Part 1: patient characteristics and diagnosis. Eur Heart J 2003;24:442–63.
4. Neuberger HR, Mewis C, van Veldhuisen DJ, et al. Management of atrial fibrillation in patients with heart failure. Eur Heart J 2007;28:2568–77.
5. Maisel WH, Stevenson LW. Atrial fibrillation in heart failure: epidemiology, pathophysiology, and rationale for therapy. Am J Cardiol 2003;91:2D–8D.
6. McManus DD, Shaikh AY, Abhishek F, et al. Atrial fibrillation and heart failure parallels: lessons for atrial fibrillation prevention. Crit Pathw Cardiol 2011;10:46–51.
7. Dries DL, Exner DV, Gersh BJ, et al. Atrial fibrillation is associated with an increased risk for mortality and heart failure progression in patients with asymptomatic and symptomatic left ventricular systolic dysfunction: a retrospective analysis of the solvd trials. Studies of left ventricular dysfunction. J Am Coll Cardiol 1998;32:695–703.
8. Shinbane JS, Wood MA, Jensen DN, et al. Tachycardia-induced cardiomyopathy: a review of animal models and clinical studies. J Am Coll Cardiol 1997;29:709–15.

9. Clark DM, Plumb VJ, Epstein AE, et al. Hemodynamic effects of an irregular sequence of ventricular cycle lengths during atrial fibrillation. J Am Coll Cardiol 1997;30:1039–45.
10. Van Den Berg MP, Tuinenburg AE, Crijns HJ, et al. Heart failure and atrial fibrillation: current concepts and controversies. Heart 1997;77:309–13.
11. Naito M, David D, Michelson EL, et al. The hemodynamic consequences of cardiac arrhythmias: evaluation of the relative roles of abnormal atrioventricular sequencing, irregularity of ventricular rhythm and atrial fibrillation in a canine model. Am Heart J 1983;106:284–91.
12. Daoud EG, Weiss R, Bahu M, et al. Effect of an irregular ventricular rhythm on cardiac output. Am J Cardiol 1996;78:1433–6.
13. Grogan M, Smith HC, Gersh BJ, et al. Left ventricular dysfunction due to atrial fibrillation in patients initially believed to have idiopathic dilated cardiomyopathy. Am J Cardiol 1992;69:1570–3.
14. Pozzoli M, Cioffi G, Traversi E, et al. Predictors of primary atrial fibrillation and concomitant clinical and hemodynamic changes in patients with chronic heart failure: a prospective study in 344 patients with baseline sinus rhythm. J Am Coll Cardiol 1998;32:197–204.
15. Li D, Fareh S, Leung TK, et al. Promotion of atrial fibrillation by heart failure in dogs: atrial remodeling of a different sort. Circulation 1999;100:87–95.
16. Li D, Shinagawa K, Pang L, et al. Effects of angiotensin-converting enzyme inhibition on the development of the atrial fibrillation substrate in dogs with ventricular tachypacing-induced congestive heart failure. Circulation 2001;104: 2608–14.
17. Shinagawa K, Shi YF, Tardif JC, et al. Dynamic nature of atrial fibrillation substrate during development and reversal of heart failure in dogs. Circulation 2002;105:2672–8.
18. Van Gelder IC, Groenveld HF, Crijns HJ, et al. Lenient versus strict rate control in patients with atrial fibrillation. N Engl J Med 2010;362:1363–73.
19. Fuster V, Ryden LE, Cannom DS, et al. 2011 ACCF/AHA/HRS focused updates incorporated into the ACC/AHA/ESC 2006 guidelines for the management of patients with atrial fibrillation: a report of the american college of cardiology foundation/american heart association task force on practice guidelines. Circulation 2011;123:e269–367.
20. Wyse DG, Waldo AL, DiMarco JP, et al. A comparison of rate control and rhythm control in patients with atrial fibrillation. N Engl J Med 2002;347:1825–33.
21. Van Gelder IC, Hagens VE, Bosker HA, et al. A comparison of rate control and rhythm control in patients with recurrent persistent atrial fibrillation. N Engl J Med 2002;347:1834–40.
22. Hohnloser SH, Kuck KH, Lilienthal J. Rhythm or rate control in atrial fibrillation–Pharmacological Intervention in Atrial Fibrillation (PIAF): a randomised trial. Lancet 2000;356:1789–94.
23. Carlsson J, Miketic S, Windeler J, et al. Randomized trail of rate-control versus rhythm-control in persistent atrial fibrillation: the Strategies of Treatment of Atrial Fibrillation (STAF) study. J Am Coll Cardiol 2003;41:1690–6.
24. Opolski G, Torbicki A, Kosior DA, et al. Rate control vs rhythm control in patients with nonvalvular persistent atrial fibrillation: the results of the Polish How to Treat Chronic Atrial Fibrillation (HOT CAFE) study. Chest 2004;126:476–86.
25. Ogawa S, Yamashita T, Yamazaki T, et al. Optimal treatment strategy for patients with paroxysmal atrial fibrillation: J-RHYTHM study. Circ J 2009;73:242–8.
26. Roy D, Talajic M, Nattel S, et al. Rhythm control versus rate control for atrial fibrillation and heart failure. N Engl J Med 2008;358:2667-77.
27. Suman-Horduna I, Roy D, Frasure-Smith N, et al. Quality of life and functional capacity in patients with atrial fibrillation and congestive heart failure. J Am Coll Cardiol 2013;61:455–60.
28. Henrard V, Ducharme A, Khairy P, et al. Cardiac remodeling with rhythm versus rate control strategies for atrial fibrillation in patients with heart failure: insights from the AF-CHF echocardiographic substudy. Int J Cardiol 2013;165(3):430–6.
29. Lazzari JO, Gonzalez J. Reversible high rate atrial fibrillation dilated cardiomyopathy. Heart 1997;77: 486.
30. Hagens VE, Crijns HJ, van Veldhuisen DJ, et al. Rate control versus rhythm control for patients with persistent atrial fibrillation with mild to moderate heart failure: results from the Rate Control versus Electrical Cardioversion (RACE) study. Am Heart J 2005;149:1106–11.
31. Hagens VE, van Veldhuisen DJ, Kamp O, et al. Effect of rate and rhythm control on left ventricular function and cardiac dimensions in patients with persistent atrial fibrillation: results from the Rate Control versus Electrical Cardioversion for Persistent Atrial Fibrillation (RACE) study. Heart Rhythm 2005;2:19–24.
32. Groenveld HF, Crijns HJ, Van den Berg MP, et al. The effect of rate control on quality of life in patients with permanent atrial fibrillation: data from the RACE II (Rate Control Efficacy in Permanent Atrial Fibrillation II) study. J Am Coll Cardiol 2011;58: 1795–803.
33. Smit MD, Crijns HJ, Tijssen JG, et al. Effect of lenient versus strict rate control on cardiac remodeling in patients with atrial fibrillation data of the RACE II (Rate Control Efficacy in Permanent Atrial Fibrillation II) study. J Am Coll Cardiol 2011;58: 942–9.

34. Mulder B, Tijssen J, Hillege H, et al. Stringency of rate control in patients with atrial fibrillation and heart failure: data of the Rate Control Efficacy in Permanent Atrial Fibrillation: a comparison between lenient versus strict rate control II (RACE II) study. Circulation 2010;122:A16829.
35. Khand AU, Rankin AC, Martin W, et al. Carvedilol alone or in combination with digoxin for the management of atrial fibrillation in patients with heart failure? J Am Coll Cardiol 2003;42:1944–51.
36. Silvet H, Hawkins LA, Jacobson AK. Heart rate control in patients with chronic atrial fibrillation and heart failure. Congest Heart Fail 2013;19:25–8.
37. Rienstra M, van Gelder IC, Van Den Berg MP, et al. A comparison of low versus high heart rate in patients with atrial fibrillation and advanced chronic heart failure: effects on clinical profile, neurohormones and survival. Int J Cardiol 2006;109:95–100.
38. Cooper HA, Bloomfield DA, Bush DE, et al. Relation between achieved heart rate and outcomes in patients with atrial fibrillation (from the Atrial Fibrillation Follow-up Investigation of Rhythm Management [AFFIRM] Study). Am J Cardiol 2004;93:1247–53.
39. Van Gelder IC, Wyse DG, Chandler ML, et al. Does intensity of rate-control influence outcome in atrial fibrillation? An analysis of pooled data from the race and affirm studies. Europace 2006;8:935–42.
40. Groenveld HF, Crijns HJ, Rienstra M, et al. Does intensity of rate control influence outcome in persistent atrial fibrillation? Data of the race study. Am Heart J 2009;158:785–91.
41. Castagno D, Skali H, Takeuchi M, et al. Association of heart rate and outcomes in a broad spectrum of patients with chronic heart failure: results from the CHARM (Candesartan in Heart Failure: Assessment of Reduction in Mortality and morbidity) program. J Am Coll Cardiol 2012;59:1785–95.
42. Connolly SJ, Camm AJ, Halperin JL, et al. Dronedarone in high-risk permanent atrial fibrillation. N Engl J Med 2011;365:2268–76.
43. Camm AJ, Kirchhof P, Lip GY, et al. Guidelines for the management of atrial fibrillation: the Task Force for the Management of Atrial Fibrillation of the European Society of Cardiology (ESC). Eur Heart J 2010;31:2369–429.
44. Hunt SA, Abraham WT, Chin MH, et al. 2009 focused update incorporated into the ACC/AHA 2005 guidelines for the diagnosis and management of heart failure in adults: a report of the American College of Cardiology Foundation/American Heart Association Task Force on Practice Guidelines: developed in collaboration with the International Society for Heart and Lung Transplantation. Circulation 2009;119:e391–479.
45. Olshansky B, Rosenfeld LE, Warner AL, et al. The Atrial Fibrillation Follow-up Investigation of Rhythm Management (AFFIRM) study: approaches to control rate in atrial fibrillation. J Am Coll Cardiol 2004;43:1201–8.
46. Weerasooriya R, Davis M, Powell A, et al. The Australian Intervention Randomized Control of Rate in Atrial Fibrillation Trial (AIRCRAFT). J Am Coll Cardiol 2003;41:1697–702.
47. Rienstra M, Damman K, Mulder B, et al. Beta-blockers and outcome in heart failure and atrial fibrillation: a meta-analysis. J Am Coll Cardiol HF 2013;1:21–8.
48. Segal JB, McNamara RL, Miller MR, et al. The evidence regarding the drugs used for ventricular rate control. J Fam Pract 2000;49:47–59.
49. Tamariz LJ, Bass EB. Pharmacological rate control of atrial fibrillation. Cardiol Clin 2004;22:35–45.
50. Mason DA, Moore JD, Green SA, et al. A gain-of-function polymorphism in a g-protein coupling domain of the human beta1-adrenergic receptor. J Biol Chem 1999;274:12670–4.
51. Joseph SS, Lynham JA, Grace AA, et al. Markedly reduced effects of (-)-isoprenaline but not of (-)-cgp12177 and unchanged affinity of beta-blockers at gly389-beta1-adrenoceptors compared to arg389-beta1-adrenoceptors. Br J Pharmacol 2004;142:51–6.
52. Parvez B, Chopra N, Rowan S, et al. A common beta1-adrenergic receptor polymorphism predicts favorable response to rate-control therapy in atrial fibrillation. J Am Coll Cardiol 2012;59:49–56.
53. Rau T, Dungen HD, Edelmann F, et al. Impact of the beta1-adrenoceptor Arg389Gly polymorphism on heart-rate responses to bisoprolol and carvedilol in heart-failure patients. Clin Pharmacol Ther 2012;92:21–8.
54. Kao DP, Davis G, Aleong R, et al. Effect of bucindolol on heart failure outcomes and heart rate response in patients with reduced ejection fraction heart failure and atrial fibrillation. Eur J Heart Fail 2013;15(3):324–33.
55. Corley SD, Epstein AE, DiMarco JP, et al. Relationships between sinus rhythm, treatment, and survival in the Atrial Fibrillation Follow-up Investigation of Rhythm Management (AFFIRM) study. Circulation 2004;109:1509–13.
56. Friberg L, Hammar N, Rosenqvist M. Digoxin in atrial fibrillation: report from the Stockholm cohort study of atrial fibrillation (SCAF). Heart 2010;96:275–80.
57. Hou ZY, Chang MS, Chen CY, et al. Acute treatment of recent-onset atrial fibrillation and flutter with a tailored dosing regimen of intravenous amiodarone. A randomized, digoxin-controlled study. Eur Heart J 1995;16:521–8.
58. Brignole M, Gianfranchi L, Menozzi C, et al. Assessment of atrioventricular junction ablation and DDDR mode- switching pacemaker versus pharmacological treatment in patients with

severely symptomatic paroxysmal atrial fibrillation: a randomized controlled study. Circulation 1997; 96:2617–24.

59. Brignole M, Menozzi C, Gianfranchi L, et al. Assessment of atrioventricular junction ablation and VVIR pacemaker versus pharmacological treatment in patients with heart failure and chronic atrial fibrillation: a randomized, controlled study. Circulation 1998;98:953–60.
60. Kay GN, Ellenbogen KA, Giudici M, et al. The Ablate and Pace trial: a prospective study of catheter ablation of the AV conduction system and permanent pacemaker implantation for treatment of atrial fibrillation. APT investigators. J Interv Card Electrophysiol 1998;2:121–35.
61. Wood MA, Brown-Mahoney C, Kay GN, et al. Clinical outcomes after ablation and pacing therapy for atrial fibrillation: a meta-analysis. Circulation 2000; 101:1138–44.
62. Moss AJ, Zareba W, Hall WJ, et al. Prophylactic implantation of a defibrillator in patients with myocardial infarction and reduced ejection fraction. N Engl J Med 2002;346:877–83.
63. Wilkoff BL, Cook JR, Epstein AE, et al. Dual-chamber pacing or ventricular backup pacing in patients with an implantable defibrillator: the Dual Chamber and VVI Implantable Defibrillator (DAVID) trial. JAMA 2002;288:3115–23.
64. Hohnloser SH, Kuck KH, Dorian P, et al. Prophylactic use of an implantable cardioverter-defibrillator after acute myocardial infarction. N Engl J Med 2004;351:2481–8.
65. Smit MD, Van Dessel PF, Nieuwland W, et al. Right ventricular pacing and the risk of heart failure in implantable cardioverter-defibrillator patients. Heart Rhythm 2006;3:1397–403.
66. Vernooy K, Dijkman B, Cheriex EC, et al. Ventricular remodeling during long-term right ventricular pacing following his bundle ablation. Am J Cardiol 2006;97:1223–7.
67. Tops LF, Schalij MJ, Holman ER, et al. Right ventricular pacing can induce ventricular dyssynchrony in patients with atrial fibrillation after atrioventricular node ablation. J Am Coll Cardiol 2006;48:1642–8.
68. Tan ES, Rienstra M, Wiesfeld AC, et al. Long-term outcome of the atrioventricular node ablation and pacemaker implantation for symptomatic refractory atrial fibrillation. Europace 2008;10:412–8.
69. Simantirakis EN, Vardakis KE, Kochiadakis GE, et al. Left ventricular mechanics during right ventricular apical or left ventricular-based pacing in patients with chronic atrial fibrillation after atrioventricular junction ablation. J Am Coll Cardiol 2004; 43:1013–8.
70. Puggioni E, Brignole M, Gammage M, et al. Acute comparative effect of right and left ventricular pacing in patients with permanent atrial fibrillation. J Am Coll Cardiol 2004;43:234–8.
71. Brignole M, Gammage M, Puggioni E, et al. Comparative assessment of right, left, and biventricular pacing in patients with permanent atrial fibrillation. Eur Heart J 2005;26:712–22.
72. Doshi RN, Daoud EG, Fellows C, et al. Left ventricular-based cardiac stimulation post AV nodal ablation evaluation (the PAVE study). J Cardiovasc Electrophysiol 2005;16:1160–5.
73. Leon AR, Greenberg JM, Kanuru N, et al. Cardiac resynchronization in patients with congestive heart failure and chronic atrial fibrillation: effect of upgrading to biventricular pacing after chronic right ventricular pacing. J Am Coll Cardiol 2002;39: 1258–63.
74. Wallick DW, Zhang Y, Tabata T, et al. Selective AV nodal vagal stimulation improves hemodynamics during acute atrial fibrillation in dogs. Am J Physiol Heart Circ Physiol 2001;281:H1490–7.
75. Zhuang S, Zhang Y, Mowrey KA, et al. Ventricular rate control by selective vagal stimulation is superior to rhythm regularization by atrioventricular nodal ablation and pacing during atrial fibrillation. Circulation 2002;106:1853–8.
76. Zhang Y, Yamada H, Bibevski S, et al. Chronic atrioventricular nodal vagal stimulation: first evidence for long-term ventricular rate control in canine atrial fibrillation model. Circulation 2005; 112:2904–11.
77. Mischke K, Zarse M, Schmid M, et al. Chronic augmentation of the parasympathetic tone to the atrioventricular node: a nonthoracotomy neurostimulation technique for ventricular rate control during atrial fibrillation. J Cardiovasc Electrophysiol 2010;21:193–9.
78. Schauerte P, Mischke K, Plisiene J, et al. Catheter stimulation of cardiac parasympathetic nerves in humans: a novel approach to the cardiac autonomic nervous system. Circulation 2001;104:2430–5.
79. Zhang Y, Popovic ZB, Kusunose K, et al. Therapeutic effects of selective atrioventricular node vagal stimulation in atrial fibrillation and heart failure. J Cardiovasc Electrophysiol 2013;24:86–91.
80. Zhang Y, Popovic ZB, Bibevski S, et al. Chronic vagus nerve stimulation improves autonomic control and attenuates systemic inflammation and heart failure progression in a canine high-rate pacing model. Circ Heart Fail 2009;2:692–9.
81. Field ME, Hamdan MH. AV nodal fat pad stimulation for rate control in atrial fibrillation and heart failure: a better solution? J Cardiovasc Electrophysiol 2013;24:92–3.

Rhythm Control of Atrial Fibrillation in Heart Failure

Jordi Heijman, PhD[a], Niels Voigt, MD[a,b],
Issam H. Abu-Taha, PhD[a], Dobromir Dobrev, MD[a,b,c,*]

KEYWORDS

• Antiarrhythmic drugs • Atrial fibrillation • Heart failure • Rhythm control

KEY POINTS

- Atrial fibrillation (AF) and heart failure (HF) are common cardiovascular pathologies with severe prognostic implications that show bidirectional interactions.
- Current rhythm-control strategies using antiarrhythmic drugs in patients with HF do not improve outcome, which may at least be partly due to the lack of safe and effective antiarrhythmic drugs for rhythm control of AF in HF.
- Amiodarone and dofetilide are the only antiarrhythmic drugs currently available for patients with HF but their success is limited by extracardiovascular toxicity and drug-induced proarrhythmia, respectively.
- Novel atrial-specific antiarrhythmic drugs or drugs targeting common arrhythmogenic pathways between AF and HF, and improved patient selection based on recent genetic data, may help to improve rhythm control of AF in HF.

INTRODUCTION

Atrial fibrillation (AF) and heart failure (HF) affect at least 2.7 and 5.1 million people in the United States alone,[1] figures which are expected to rise with the aging of the population, posing a significant burden on health care in the developed world. Both conditions are individually associated with increased morbidity and mortality.[1]

AF and HF frequently coexist and show bidirectional interactions. HF is a more powerful risk factor for AF than advanced age, hypertension, valvular heart disease, diabetes, or prior myocardial infarction, increasing the risk for AF by 4.5-fold to 5.9-fold.[2] The reported prevalence of AF in HF ranges from 13% to 27% and correlates with the severity of the left-ventricular (LV) dysfunction.[3] Initial studies failed to determine whether AF is an independent risk factor associated with worse outcome in HF or simply reflects increased overall risk. However, more recent studies and studies in larger populations, such

Funding Sources: The authors' work is supported by the European Network for Translational Research in Atrial Fibrillation (EUTRAF, No. 261057), the German Federal Ministry of Education and Research (AF Competence Network [01Gi0204] and DZHK [German Center for Cardiovascular Research]), the Deutsche Forschungsgemeinschaft (Do 769/1-3), and by a grant from Fondation Leducq (European-North American Atrial Fibrillation Research Alliance, ENAFRA, 07CVD03).
Conflicts of Interest: DD is an advisor and lecturer for Sanofi, Merck-Sharp-Dohme, Biotronik, Boehringer Ingelheim, and Boston Scientific. The other authors have no conflicts of interest to disclose.
[a] Institute of Pharmacology, Faculty of Medicine, University Duisburg-Essen, Hufelandstrasse 55, Essen 45122, Germany; [b] Division of Experimental Cardiology, Medical Faculty Mannheim, Heidelberg University, Theodor-Kutzer-Ufer 1-3, 68167 Mannheim, Germany; [c] DZHK (German Centre for Cardiovascular Research) Partner Site Mannheim/Heidelberg, Theodor-Kutzer-Ufer 1-3, 68167 Mannheim, Germany
* Corresponding author. Institute of Pharmacology, Faculty of Medicine, University Duisburg-Essen, Hufelandstrasse 55, Essen 45122, Germany.
E-mail address: dobromir.dobrev@uk-essen.de

Heart Failure Clin 9 (2013) 407–415
http://dx.doi.org/10.1016/j.hfc.2013.06.001
1551-7136/13/$ – see front matter

as the Studies of Left Ventricular Dysfunction (SOLVD)[4] and Valsartan in Acute Myocardial Infarction (VALIANT)[5] trials, have suggested that AF is independently associated with worse outcome in HF.[3] Moreover, even studies where baseline AF was not predictive of increased morbidity and mortality, such as the Carvedilol or Metroprolol European Trial (COMET), found that new-onset AF was associated with a particularly negative impact on HF prognosis.[6] In agreement, Smit and colleagues[7] have recently shown that despite the bidirectional interaction between AF and HF, the order in which both conditions develop matters. In particular, they showed that HF patients developing AF had a worse prognosis than AF patients who developed HF.

The severity and prevalence of both conditions make the treatment of AF in the setting of HF, including the associated risk of stroke, of critical importance. However, current therapeutic options for AF have important limitations including limited safety and efficacy,[8–10] a situation that is exacerbated in the presence of HF. A better understanding of the basic mechanisms underlying both pathologies and their interactions is required to facilitate the development of novel therapeutics.

RATE CONTROL VERSUS RHYTHM CONTROL

Rate control and rhythm control are the 2 predominant treatment strategies for AF. In the former (reviewed elsewhere in this edition), only the ventricular response is controlled, whereas in the latter the goal is to achieve normal sinus rhythm. Most clinical studies have failed to show a clear survival benefit in patients with pharmacologic rhythm control. In particular, the Atrial Fibrillation Follow-up Investigation of Rhythm Management (AFFIRM) and RAte Control versus Electrical cardioversion (RACE) trials found no benefit or even a trend toward harm with rhythm control of AF.[11,12] These findings were confirmed in the setting of HF by the Atrial Fibrillation and Congestive Heart Failure (AF-CHF) trial, where no differences in overall survival, cardiovascular death, worsened HF, or stroke were found between rate and rhythm control at 37 months' follow-up.[13] As such, rhythm control is currently only recommended in patients who remain symptomatic despite adequate rate control.[14,15] However, it is likely that the performance of rhythm control in these studies is negatively affected by the limited success to maintain sinus rhythm in patients, with success rates ranging from 26% to 64%.[16] Moreover, subsequent analysis of the data from the AFFIRM trial has shown that maintenance of sinus rhythm was associated with a survival benefit that was offset by the risk associated with antiarrhythmic drug therapy.[17] On the other hand, it cannot be ruled out that patients able to maintain sinus rhythm are simply healthier.[2] Safer and more effective antiarrhythmic drugs for the maintenance of sinus rhythm may help to determine whether rhythm control is indeed the preferred strategy for patients with AF and HF.

BASIC MECHANISMS UNDERLYING AF

Conceptually, AF is determined by factors controlling abnormal impulse formation and propagation (**Fig. 1**).[9,18] HF and AF share various risk factors, including age, hypertension, diabetes mellitus, valvular heart disease, and genetic factors, which create a vulnerable substrate for the initiation of atrial and ventricular arrhythmias. In the atria, impulse formation outside of the sinoatrial node (ectopic/triggered activity), particularly around the pulmonary veins (PV), can maintain AF when occurring repetitively ("driver") or can trigger reentry in a vulnerable substrate. Substantial experimental research has provided important insights into the molecular factors contributing to these arrhythmia mechanisms in AF and the contributing role of HF.

Ectopic Activity

In the atrial myocyte, the Na^+ current (I_{Na}) rapidly depolarizes the membrane potential, creating the upstroke of the atrial action potential (AP). Subsequent activation of voltage-gated L-type Ca^{2+} current ($I_{Ca,L}$) results in Ca^{2+} entry into the atrial myocyte, promoting a much larger Ca^{2+} release from the sarcoplasmic reticulum (SR) stores through the ryanodine receptor channel (RyR2), giving rise to the systolic Ca^{2+} transient, which controls myocyte contraction. The influx of Ca^{2+} is tightly controlled by inactivation of $I_{Ca,L}$, which, together with the activation of a complement of K^+ currents, is also responsible for the repolarization of the AP, determining AP duration.

Triggered activity is generally mediated by early or delayed afterdepolarizations. Early afterdepolarizations (EADs) are secondary depolarizations of the membrane potential that occur before final repolarization of the AP. They generally occur in the setting of AP prolongation, for example, due to loss-of-function mutations or pharmacologic inhibition of repolarizing K^+ currents. Prolongation of the AP allows $I_{Ca,L}$ to recover from nonconducting inactivated states, thereby depolarizing the membrane potential and causing the EAD upstroke.

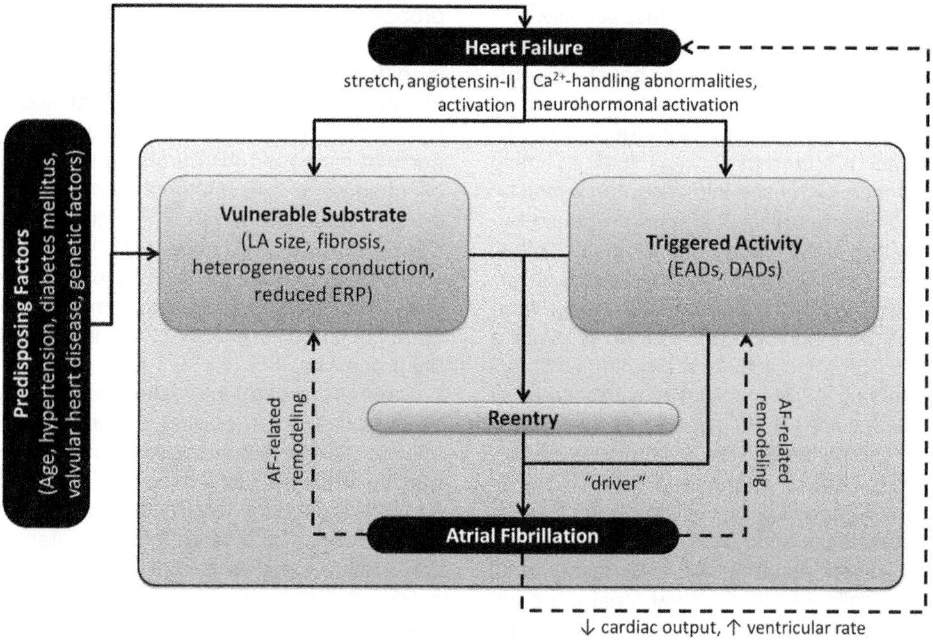

Fig. 1. Conceptual overview of the mechanisms underlying atrial fibrillation and the bidirectional interaction between atrial fibrillation and heart failure. LA, left atrium.

Delayed afterdepolarizations (DADs) occur after full repolarization of the AP and are caused by abnormalities in subcellular Ca^{2+} handling. Recent research has shown that dysfunction of RyR2 plays a critical role in AF, resulting in increased Ca^{2+} leak from the SR and spontaneous SR Ca^{2+}-release events.[19] Phosphorylation of RyR2 by Ca^{2+}/calmodulin-dependent protein kinase II (CaMKII) has been identified as an important contributor to this RyR2 dysfunction.[19] The Ca^{2+} released into the cytosol during spontaneous SR Ca^{2+}-release events is partly extruded via the Na^+/Ca^{2+} exchanger (NCX1), which brings in 3 Na^+ for every Ca^{2+} extruded, thereby causing a depolarizing transient-inward current (I_{NCX}), generating a DAD. The balance between I_{NCX} and the repolarizing inward-rectifier K^+ currents determines the DAD amplitude. If this amplitude is sufficiently large, Na^+ channels will be activated, giving rise to a triggered AP.

Reentry

Reentry is a central mechanism for maintaining AF, although the exact presentation remains a subject of debate and may vary from patient to patient.[20] Sustained reentry can occur in the presence or absence ("functional reentry") of fixed anatomic obstacles.[21] The leading circle and spiral wave concepts have been proposed as conceptual models of functional reentry. Although conceptually different, both models share several notions, including the predicted effects of K^+ channel alterations.[21] The spiral wave concept more accurately predicts the effect of I_{Na} blockade.[21] An advantage of the leading circle model is its definition by simple, clinically relevant electrophysiological concepts.[21] Leading circle reentry establishes itself in the smallest pathway that can support reentry such that all points in the reentrant path regain excitability before the arrival of the next impulse. As such, reentry is promoted by slow conduction velocity (CV) and a short effective refractory period (ERP), the product of which has been termed wavelength (wavelength $=$ CV $\times$ ERP).[20,21] CV is largely determined by the availability of I_{Na} to overcome the electrotonic load of the surrounding myocardium, the number of electrical connections (gap junctions) between myocytes, and the composition of the extracellular matrix, notably the amount of fibrosis.[9] ERP is determined by AP duration and the post-repolarization refractoriness, which is predominantly due to the recovery kinetics of I_{Na}.

AF-related Remodeling

When a rapid atrial rate is maintained, AF-related electrical and structural remodeling occur, further stabilizing the arrhythmia, contributing to the progression from paroxysmal to permanent AF, and making AF more difficult to treat.[22] Electrical remodeling is characterized by shortening of atrial ERP and abnormal Ca^{2+} handling, promoting reentry and ectopic activity, respectively.[23,24] Shortening of atrial ERP predominantly results from reduced $I_{Ca,L}$, increased basal inward-rectifier current (I_{K1}), and development of a "constitutively active" acetylcholine-dependent inward-rectifier K^+ current ($I_{K,AChc}$) that is active in the absence of muscarinic receptor agonists. Increased inward-rectifier K^+ currents cause hyperpolarization of the resting membrane potential, which has been shown to stabilize reentrant circuits ("rotors") by promoting recovery of I_{Na} from inactivation.[25] Abnormal Ca^{2+} handling plays a critical role in ectopic activity-promoting DAD formation. Chronic AF is associated with increased CaMKII expression, RyR2 hyperphosphorylation, and more spontaneous SR Ca^{2+}-release events, which lead to DADs and triggered APs.[19]

Structural remodeling of the atria can occur in various pathologic conditions, including HF, or can be a direct result of AF. Increased atrial fibrosis is a hallmark of structural atrial remodeling.[22] It contributes to conduction slowing and heterogeneous conduction, thereby promoting reentry. Proliferation of fibroblasts and differentiation into collagen-secreting myofibroblasts are main profibrotic mechanisms activated by a wide range of stimuli including myocardial injury, oxidative stress, inflammation, and stretch.[22] Angiotensin II and transforming growth factor-β1 are well-established profibrotic signaling molecules, and recent evidence also suggests roles for platelet-derived growth factor and connective tissue growth factor.[22] Interestingly, recent evidence suggests that AF may also promote ventricular remodeling. In particular, Ling and colleagues[26] found that AF was independently associated with increased LV interstitial fibrosis in patients.

The Role of HF in AF

HF and AF share numerous risk factors. In addition, various studies have highlighted pathways through which HF can directly promote AF. Congestive HF and the associated increased hemodynamic load cause abnormal atrial stretch, contributing to atrial dilatation and atrial myocyte hypertrophy.[27] Activation of stretch-sensitive ion channels may affect atrial electrophysiology, and Ca^{2+}-handling. Congestive HF is also associated with a pronounced increase in atrial fibrosis[3] and is accompanied by neurohormonal activation, which can promote atrial ectopic activity through abnormal Ca^{2+} handling and further amplify atrial fibrosis via increased angiotensin-II levels.[3] Together, these processes create a large vulnerable substrate with slow, heterogeneous conduction and spatially heterogeneous electrophysiological properties, strongly promoting atrial reentry. Congestive HF causes atrial ionic remodeling that is different from atrial tachycardia-related remodeling. Atrial AP duration is not substantially reduced by HF-related remodeling, with some reports of increased AP duration in animal models of congestive HF, although this may depend on the duration of HF.[28,29] Patients with HF-dependent AF will experience both HF- and AF-related remodeling. Due to cross-talk between both processes, the resulting remodeling is more complex and different from the sum of the individual processes.[22]

There are several interesting parallels between the ventricular remodeling observed in HF and chronic AF-related remodeling, notably with regard to abnormal Ca^{2+} handling.[29] The increased CaMKII-dependent RyR2 phosphorylation, increased SR Ca^{2+} leak, and spontaneous SR Ca^{2+}-release events had already been identified in HF before their discovery in AF.[19,29] In addition, both pathologies share an upregulation of NCX1, contributing to larger DAD amplitudes for a given Ca^{2+} release. Both conditions also result in reduced CV and increase conduction heterogeneity, promoting reentry.

ANTIARRHYTHMIC DRUGS FOR RHYTHM CONTROL IN AF IN THE PRESENCE OF HF

The class Ic drugs flecainide and propafenone predominantly inhibit voltage-gated Na^+ channels, thereby reducing atrial excitability, without affecting AP duration. They were shown to delay the first occurrence of AF and reduce the portion of time in AF in the structurally normal heart.[30,31] However, in patients with previous myocardial infarction or structural heart disease, class Ic antiarrhythmics have been associated with increased mortality[32] and are therefore contraindicated in patients with coronary artery disease or HF.[14,15] It is likely that under these conditions, the reentry-promoting effects of ventricular conduction slowing due to Na^+ channel inhibition outweigh antiarrhythmic effects due to reduced excitability.

Class III Drugs

Commonly used pure class III antiarrhythmic drugs include ibutilide, sotalol, and, in the United States, dofetilide.[30,31] These drugs predominantly block the rapidly activating delayed-rectifier K^+ current (I_{Kr}), thereby prolonging ERP and reducing the likelihood of reentry. The Danish Investigators of Arrhythmia and Mortality on Dofetilide trial (DIAMOND-CHF)[33] showed that dofetilide significantly reduced the risk of hospitalization for worsening HF, was more effective than placebo in maintaining sinus rhythm, and was not associated with increased mortality in patients with congestive HF. As such, dofetilide is an option for the maintenance of sinus rhythm in patients with HF in the United States.[15] However, in general all class III drugs can cause QT prolongation, carrying the risk of EADs and drug-induced torsades de pointes arrhythmias. Therefore, dofetilide dosage has to be personalized for each patient based on renal function, weight, and other clinical variables to prevent excessive QT prolongation.[15]

Multichannel Blockers

Although not officially approved for AF in the United States, amiodarone is the most-employed and most-successful antiarrhythmic drug for the maintenance of normal sinus rhythm in AF patients with and without HF.[30,31] Its reported efficacy for the maintenance of sinus rhythm lies between 50% and 78%.[31] Amiodarone is a class III antiarrhythmic drug, potently inhibiting I_{Kr}, but together with its active metabolite *N*-desethylamiodarone has a wide range of additional targets including I_{Na} and $I_{Ca,L}$ and also acts as a noncompetitive antagonist of α- and β-adrenoceptors, thereby showing actions of all 4 drug classes.[10,30] In addition, amiodarone and *N*-desethylamiodarone both cause venodilation,[34,35] potentially reducing preload, an effect that might contribute to its efficacy, especially in patients with HF. The Congestive Heart Failure Survival Trial of Antiarrhythmic Therapy (CHF-STAT) has shown that patients with congestive HF and AF treated with amiodarone were more likely to convert to sinus rhythm and had a reduced incidence of new-onset AF. However, the AF-CHF study has shown that this does not translate into improved survival compared with rate control.[13] Although amiodarone can cause QT-interval prolongation, it is not generally associated with development of torsades de pointes arrhythmias. Amiodarone has been associated with hepatotoxicity, photosensitivity, and pulmonary dysfunction (pneumonitis, fibrosis). Due to the iodine moieties, amiodarone frequently causes thyroid dysfunction, ranging from laboratory test abnormalities and thyreoiditis to hypothyreoidism and hyperthyreoidism. Treatment includes discontinuation of amiodarone, although due to its long half-time, thyroid dysfunction may persist for months after discontinuation. Overall, the substantial extracardiac side effects of amiodarone limit its use in a large proportion of patients.

Dronedarone was recently developed by altering the structure of amiodarone in an attempt to reduce its extracardiovascular toxicity. Like amiodarone, it blocks a wide range of ion channels and exhibits actions of all 4 drug classes.[36] Dronedarone was approved for the treatment of AF based on the results of the ATHENA (A Trial With Dronedarone to Prevent Hospitalization or Death in Patients With Atrial Fibrillation) trial, which showed that dronedarone reduced the rate of hospitalizations and cardiovascular death. In contrast, the ANDROMEDA (European Trial of Dronedarone in Moderate to Severe Congestive Heart Failure) trial found that dronedarone was associated with increased mortality in patients with severe HF.[37] Similarly, the Permanent Atrial Fibrillation Outcome Study Using Dronedarone on Top of Standard Therapy (PALLAS) trial, in which more than half of the patients had New York Heart Association class II or III congestive HF, was recently halted because of excess risk of stroke and cardiovascular death.[38] Overall, dronedarone is less effective compared with amiodarone and is not recommended for rhythm control of AF in patients with HF, except perhaps those with stable class I HF. Dronedarone is also not appropriate for patients with persistent/permanent AF.

Multichannel blockers have shown promise for the treatment of AF. Intravenous vernakalant was recently approved for the rapid conversion of recent-onset AF in Europe. Vernakalant targets multiple K^+-currents including the atrial-selective ultrarapid delayed-rectifier K^+ current (I_{Kur}) and $I_{K,ACh}$, which do not contribute to the ventricular AP, and uses differences between atrial and ventricular Na^+-channel properties to achieve an atrial-predominant action, thereby preventing ventricular proarrhythmia.[8] The safety and efficacy of vernakalant was evaluated in the AVRO and ACT trials, showing improved conversion to sinus rhythm compared with placebo and the slow-acting amiodarone, without ventricular arrhythmia.[31,39] However, the efficacy of vernakalant is substantially lower in patients with HF compared with hemodynamically stable patients.[39] Oral vernakalant has been evaluated for the long-term prevention of AF recurrence and has shown potential in several trials.[31] However, further development of oral vernakalant has recently been halted, likely because of low efficacy to maintain normal sinus rhythm.

Ranolazine is a multichannel blocker approved for the treatment of chronic angina. It is a potent inhibitor of I_{Na}, including its persistent (late) component ($I_{Na,late}$) and also inhibits I_{Kr} and RyR2 at clinically relevant concentrations.[10,40] Ranolazine has been shown to have antiarrhythmic properties at both the atrial and the ventricular level, including in dogs with HF, but is not yet approved for the treatment of AF.[40,41]

NONANTIARRHYTHMIC RHYTHM CONTROL OF AF IN HF

Several nonantiarrhythmic ("upstream") pharmacologic interventions including angiotensin-II converting enzyme inhibitors, angiotensin-II receptor blockers, β-adrenoceptor blockers, and statins are routinely used in the treatment of patients with AF (reviewed elsewhere in this edition) and have been suggested to be antiarrhythmic by limiting the deleterious effects of neurohormonal hyperactivity, oxidative stress, and inflammation.[3,42,43]

Catheter and surgical ablation of AF are the main nonpharmacologic approaches for rhythm control. Catheter ablation strategies aim to isolate the PV electrically, which is often sufficient to achieve sinus rhythm in patients with paroxysmal AF, whereas patients with persistent AF require additional lesions.[2,16] Surgical ablation techniques are advancing and might be used alone or in combination with endocardial catheter procedures. Adverse effects are more frequent with antiarrhythmic drugs than ablation. Hunter and colleagues[44] have recently shown that restoration of sinus rhythm by catheter ablation of AF is associated with a reduced incidence of stroke and death compared with predominantly pharmacologically treated patients from the Euro Heart Survey on AF. In patients with HF, Hsu and colleagues[45] have shown that AF ablation resulted in improved LV function, reduced LV dimensions, and increased exercise capacity. However, in a different cohort of patients with advanced HF, ablation restored long-term sinus rhythm in only 50% of patients and did not significantly improve LV ejection fraction assessed by cardiac magnetic resonance imaging.[46] Because of the paucity of available antiarrhythmic drugs for rhythm control of AF in patients with HF, ablation is recommended as a first-line treatment for patients with New York Heart Association class III and class IV HF in the European guidelines.[14] However, more data about the long-term efficacy of ablation from prospective studies are required.[16] Moreover, the complexity of the procedure, the frequent requirement of additional ablations, and the costs involved prohibit the use of ablation for the large number of AF patients. As such, careful patient selection, better antiarrhythmic drugs, and advances in ablation technology remain a requirement for optimal rhythm control.

Antiarrhythmic drugs may be used in conjunction with ablation procedures to prevent AF recurrence (**Fig. 2**). The PABA-CHF (Pulmonary Vein Antrum Isolation vs AV Node Ablation With Biventricular Pacing for Treatment of Atrial Fibrillation in Patients With Congestive Heart Failure) trial reported maintenance of sinus rhythm in 71% of HF patients following PV isolation alone and in 88% of HF patients with PV isolation and antiarrhythmic drug therapy at 6 months' follow-up.[47] Moreover, because catheter ablation and surgical ablation modify the arrhythmogenic substrate, previously ineffective antiarrhythmic drugs may be reevaluated following ablation procedures.[48] Finally, the performance of antiarrhythmic, ablative, and combined rhythm-control strategies

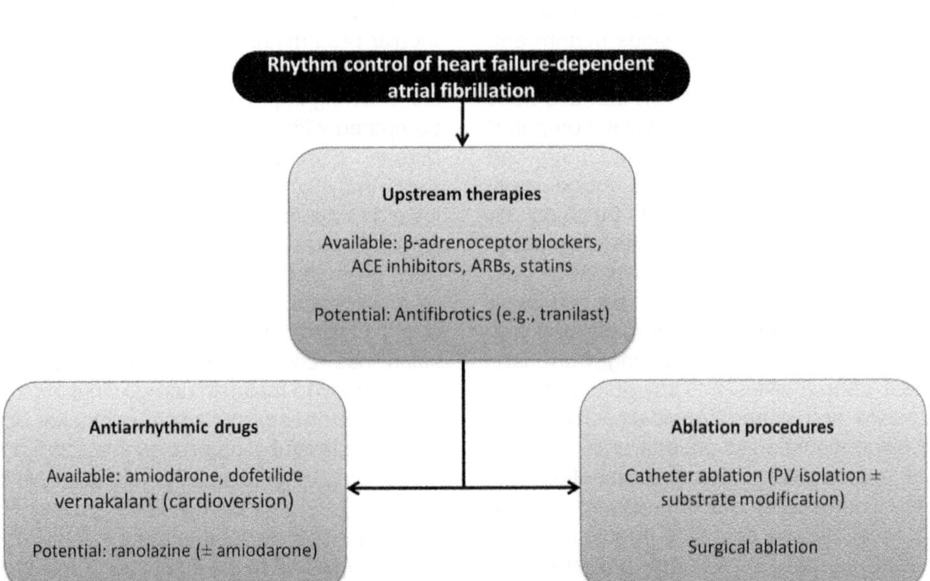

Fig. 2. Therapeutic options for rhythm control of HF -dependent AF. ACE, angiotensin-II converting enzyme; ARB, angiotensin-II type-1 receptor blockers; PV, pulmonary veins.

may be supported by upstream therapy to limit AF-related and HF-related remodeling.

FUTURE PERSPECTIVES

Novel Antiarrhythmic Strategies and Agents

Patients with HF often take multiple medications, making unwanted drug interactions likely and further necessitating the development of safe atrial-specific and pathology-specific antiarrhythmics for rhythm control of AF. Novel atrial-specific antiarrhythmic drugs targeting I_{Kur} and $I_{K,ACh}$ and/or showing atrial-predominant I_{Na} inhibition may facilitate rhythm control of AF without ventricular proarrhythmia.[9,10] A recent study found that bolus injection of the novel I_{Kur} inhibitor MK-0448 could abolish AF in a canine HF model, but had no effect on atrial or ventricular refractoriness in human subjects,[49] suggesting that I_{Kur} inhibition alone may not be sufficient to prevent AF in patients.

An alternative strategy for rhythm control of AF in patients with HF is to target pathologic processes or arrhythmogenic mechanisms common to AF and HF. Recent research strongly suggests that abnormal Ca^{2+} handling is a prime candidate for such dual antiarrhythmic therapy.[9,19] For example, the dual antiarrhythmic actions of ranolazine[40] may at least partly be due to its effects on Ca^{2+} handling, by both direct RyR2 inhibition and lowering intracellular Ca^{2+} through $I_{Na,late}$ inhibition, thereby reducing Na^+ load and promoting Ca^{2+} extrusion via NCX. In addition, several lead compounds that stabilize RyR2 and reduce SR Ca^{2+} leak have been identified and shown to have antiarrhythmic properties in several preclinical models.[9,10] Of particular interest in this group is the β-adrenoceptor blocker carvedilol, which was shown to be more effective than β_1-adrenoceptor selective blockers in reducing all-cause mortality in patients with HF in a recent meta-analysis.[50] Carvedilol and its newer analogues also inhibit RyR2 and this may importantly contribute to their antiarrhythmic action.[9]

Recent research has shown that gene transfer of connexin gap-junction proteins responsible for cell-to-cell communication improves atrial conduction and reduces AF occurrence in a large-animal model of rapid atrial pacing.[51] HF-dependent AF is also associated with changes in connexins,[51] suggesting that pharmacologic or gene therapy for connexins may have potential in the treatment of HF-dependent AF.[9] Finally, the transforming growth factor-β1 blocker tranilast prevents profibrotic atrial remodeling and suppresses AF development in a canine model of tachycardiomyopathy, highlighting the clinical potential of antifibrotic drugs for the treatment of AF in the context of HF.[52]

Patient Selection and Personalized Treatment

Genome-wide association studies have identified several genetic polymorphisms that influence the risk of AF in the general population. Interestingly, Smith and colleagues[53] have recently shown that at least one of these polymorphisms in the *ZFHX3* gene on chromosome 16q22 also associated with an increased risk for AF in patients with HF. Moreover, Parvez and colleagues[54] recently discovered that successful rhythm control of AF partly depends on a common variant on chromosome 4q25 near the *PITX2* gene. In the future, such genetic information may help to identify patients that are likely to benefit from rhythm control and may suggest which approach to use.

SUMMARY

AF and HF are prevalent conditions with serious prognostic implications that frequently coexist. Although it remains unclear whether AF is an independent risk factor for worse outcomes in patients with HF and whether rhythm control is superior to rate control, it is clear that there is a dire need for safer and more effective antiarrhythmic drugs for AF in patients with and without HF. Amiodarone and dofetilide are currently the only antiarrhythmic drugs available for rhythm control in HF patients but their success is limited by extracardiovascular toxicity and substantial risk of proarrhythmia, respectively. Recent antiarrhythmic drugs such as ranolazine show promising results and an improved understanding of AF and HF pathophysiology has facilitated the development of several interesting lead compounds for atrial antiarrhythmic drugs. However, more extensive experimental testing and long-term follow-up in patients with HF of different causes is required to assess their safety and efficacy.

REFERENCES

1. Go AS, Mozaffarian D, Roger VL, et al. Heart disease and stroke statistics–2013 update a report from the American Heart Association. Circulation 2012;127(1):e6–245.
2. Darby AE, Dimarco JP. Management of atrial fibrillation in patients with structural heart disease. Circulation 2012;125(7):945–57.
3. Anter E, Jessup M, Callans DJ. Atrial fibrillation and heart failure: treatment considerations for a dual epidemic. Circulation 2009;119(18):2516–25.
4. Dries DL, Exner DV, Gersh BJ, et al. Atrial fibrillation is associated with an increased risk for mortality and

heart failure progression in patients with asymptomatic and symptomatic left ventricular systolic dysfunction: a retrospective analysis of the SOLVD trials. Studies of Left Ventricular Dysfunction. J Am Coll Cardiol 1998;32(3):695–703.
5. Køber L, Swedberg K, McMurray JJ, et al. Previously known and newly diagnosed atrial fibrillation: a major risk indicator after a myocardial infarction complicated by heart failure or left ventricular dysfunction. Eur J Heart Fail 2006;8(6):591–8.
6. Swedberg K, Olsson LG, Charlesworth A, et al. Prognostic relevance of atrial fibrillation in patients with chronic heart failure on long-term treatment with beta-blockers: results from COMET. Eur Heart J 2005;26(13):1303–8.
7. Smit MD, Moes ML, Maass AH, et al. The importance of whether atrial fibrillation or heart failure develops first. Eur J Heart Fail 2012;14(9):1030–40.
8. Dobrev D, Nattel S. New antiarrhythmic drugs for treatment of atrial fibrillation. Lancet 2010; 375(9721):1212–23.
9. Dobrev D, Carlsson L, Nattel S. Novel molecular targets for atrial fibrillation therapy. Nat Rev Drug Discov 2012;11(4):275–91.
10. Heijman J, Voigt N, Dobrev D. New directions in antiarrhythmic drug therapy for atrial fibrillation. Future Cardiol 2013;9(1):71–88.
11. Van Gelder IC, Hagens VE, Bosker HA, et al. A comparison of rate control and rhythm control in patients with recurrent persistent atrial fibrillation. N Engl J Med 2002;347(23):1834–40.
12. Wyse DG, Waldo AL, DiMarco JP, et al. A comparison of rate control and rhythm control in patients with atrial fibrillation. N Engl J Med 2002;347(23):1825–33.
13. Roy D, Talajic M, Nattel S, et al. Rhythm control versus rate control for atrial fibrillation and heart failure. N Engl J Med 2008;358(25):2667–77.
14. Camm AJ, Kirchhof P, Lip GY, et al. Guidelines for the management of atrial fibrillation: the Task Force for the Management of Atrial Fibrillation of the European Society of Cardiology (ESC). Europace 2010;12(10):1360–420.
15. Fuster V, Ryden LE, Cannom DS, et al. ACC/AHA/ESC 2006 guidelines for the management of patients with atrial fibrillation: a report of the American College of Cardiology/American Heart Association Task Force on Practice Guidelines and the European Society of Cardiology Committee for Practice Guidelines (Writing Committee to Revise the 2001 Guidelines for the Management of Patients With Atrial Fibrillation): developed in collaboration with the European Heart Rhythm Association and the Heart Rhythm Society. Circulation 2006;114(7):e257–354.
16. Chinitz JS, Halperin JL, Reddy VY, et al. Rate or rhythm control for atrial fibrillation: update and controversies. Am J Med 2012;125(11):1049–56.
17. Corley SD, Epstein AE, DiMarco JP, et al. Relationships between sinus rhythm, treatment, and survival in the Atrial Fibrillation Follow-Up Investigation of Rhythm Management (AFFIRM) Study. Circulation 2004;109(12):1509–13.
18. Wakili R, Voigt N, Kaab S, et al. Recent advances in the molecular pathophysiology of atrial fibrillation. J Clin Invest 2011;121(8):2955–68.
19. Voigt N, Li N, Wang Q, et al. Enhanced sarcoplasmic reticulum Ca^{2+} leak and increased Na^{+}-Ca^{2+} exchanger function underlie delayed afterdepolarizations in patients with chronic atrial fibrillation. Circulation 2012;125(17):2059–70.
20. Atienza F, Martins RP, Jalife J. Translational research in atrial fibrillation: a quest for mechanistically based diagnosis and therapy. Circ Arrhythm Electrophysiol 2012;5(6):1207–15.
21. Comtois P, Kneller J, Nattel S. Of circles and spirals: bridging the gap between the leading circle and spiral wave concepts of cardiac reentry. Europace 2005;7(Suppl 2):10–20.
22. Nattel S, Burstein B, Dobrev D. Atrial remodeling and atrial fibrillation: mechanisms and implications. Circ Arrhythm Electrophysiol 2008;1(1):62–73.
23. Dobrev D. Electrical remodeling in atrial fibrillation. Herz 2006;31(2):108–12 [quiz: 142–143].
24. Nattel S, Dobrev D. The multidimensional role of calcium in atrial fibrillation pathophysiology: mechanistic insights and therapeutic opportunities. Eur Heart J 2012;33(15):1870–7.
25. Pandit SV, Berenfeld O, Anumonwo JM, et al. Ionic determinants of functional reentry in a 2-D model of human atrial cells during simulated chronic atrial fibrillation. Biophys J 2005;88(6):3806–21.
26. Ling LH, Kistler PM, Ellims AH, et al. Diffuse ventricular fibrosis in atrial fibrillation: noninvasive evaluation and relationships with aging and systolic dysfunction. J Am Coll Cardiol 2012;60(23): 2402–8.
27. De Jong AM, Maass AH, Oberdorf-Maass SU, et al. Mechanisms of atrial structural changes caused by stretch occurring before and during early atrial fibrillation. Cardiovasc Res 2011;89(4): 754–65.
28. Rankin AC, Workman AJ. Duration of heart failure and the risk of atrial fibrillation: different mechanisms at different times? Cardiovasc Res 2009; 84(2):180–1.
29. Nattel S, Maguy A, Le Bouter S, et al. Arrhythmogenic ion-channel remodeling in the heart: heart failure, myocardial infarction, and atrial fibrillation. Physiol Rev 2007;87(2):425–56.
30. Zimetbaum P. Antiarrhythmic drug therapy for atrial fibrillation. Circulation 2012;125(2):381–9.
31. Camm J. Antiarrhythmic drugs for the maintenance of sinus rhythm: risks and benefits. Int J Cardiol 2012;155(3):362–71.

32. Akiyama T, Pawitan Y, Greenberg H, et al. Increased risk of death and cardiac arrest from encainide and flecainide in patients after non-Q-wave acute myocardial infarction in the Cardiac Arrhythmia Suppression Trial. CAST Investigators. Am J Cardiol 1991;68(17):1551–5.
33. Torp-Pedersen C, Moller M, Bloch-Thomsen PE, et al. Dofetilide in patients with congestive heart failure and left ventricular dysfunction. Danish Investigations of Arrhythmia and Mortality on Dofetilide Study Group. N Engl J Med 1999;341(12): 857–65.
34. Grossmann M, Dobrev D, Kirch W. Amiodarone causes endothelium-dependent vasodilation in human hand veins in vivo. Clin Pharmacol Ther 1998;64:302–11.
35. Grossmann M, Dobrev D, Himmel HM, et al. Local venous response to N-desethylamiodarone in humans. Clin Pharmacol Ther 2000;67(1):22–31.
36. Patel C, Yan GX, Kowey PR. Dronedarone. Circulation 2009;120(7):636–44.
37. Køber L, Torp-Pedersen C, McMurray JJ, et al. Increased mortality after dronedarone therapy for severe heart failure. N Engl J Med 2008;358(25): 2678–87.
38. Connolly SJ, Camm AJ, Halperin JL, et al. Dronedarone in high-risk permanent atrial fibrillation. N Engl J Med 2011;365(24):2268–76.
39. Dobrev D, Hamad B, Kirkpatrick P. Vernakalant. Nat Rev Drug Discov 2010;9(12):915–6.
40. Verrier RL, Kumar K, Nieminen T, et al. Mechanisms of ranolazine's dual protection against atrial and ventricular fibrillation. Europace 2013;15(3):317–24. http://dx.doi.org/10.1093/europace/eus380.
41. Frommeyer G, Schmidt M, Clauss C, et al. Further insights into the underlying electrophysiological mechanisms for reduction of atrial fibrillation by ranolazine in an experimental model of chronic heart failure. Eur J Heart Fail 2012; 14(12):1322–31.
42. Savelieva I, Kakouros N, Kourliouros A, et al. Upstream therapies for management of atrial fibrillation: review of clinical evidence and implications for European Society of Cardiology guidelines. Part I: primary prevention. Europace 2011;13(3): 308–28.
43. Goette A, Bukowska A, Dobrev D, et al. Acute atrial tachyarrhythmia induces angiotensin II type 1 receptor-mediated oxidative stress and microvascular flow abnormalities in the ventricles. Eur Heart J 2009;30(11):1411–20.
44. Hunter RJ, McCready J, Diab I, et al. Maintenance of sinus rhythm with an ablation strategy in patients with atrial fibrillation is associated with a lower risk of stroke and death. Heart 2012;98(1):48–53.
45. Hsu LF, Jais P, Sanders P, et al. Catheter ablation for atrial fibrillation in congestive heart failure. N Engl J Med 2004;351(23):2373–83.
46. MacDonald MR, Connelly DT, Hawkins NM, et al. Radiofrequency ablation for persistent atrial fibrillation in patients with advanced heart failure and severe left ventricular systolic dysfunction: a randomised controlled trial. Heart 2011;97(9):740–7.
47. Khan MN, Jais P, Cummings J, et al. Pulmonary-vein isolation for atrial fibrillation in patients with heart failure. N Engl J Med 2008;359(17):1778–85.
48. Naccarelli GV, Gonzalez MD. Atrial fibrillation and the expanding role of catheter ablation: do antiarrhythmic drugs have a future? J Cardiovasc Pharmacol 2008;52(3):203–9.
49. Pavri BB, Greenberg HE, Kraft WK, et al. MK-0448, a specific Kv1.5 inhibitor: safety, pharmacokinetics, and pharmacodynamic electrophysiology in experimental animal models and humans. Circ Arrhythm Electrophysiol 2012;5(6):1193–201.
50. Dinicolantonio JJ, Lavie CJ, Fares H, et al. Meta-analysis of carvedilol versus beta 1 selective beta-blockers (atenolol, bisoprolol, metoprolol, and nebivolol). Am J Cardiol 2013;111(5):765–9.
51. Kato T, Iwasaki YK, Nattel S. Connexins and atrial fibrillation: filling in the gaps. Circulation 2012; 125(2):203–6.
52. Nakatani Y, Nishida K, Sakabe M, et al. Tranilast prevents atrial remodeling and development of atrial fibrillation in a canine model of atrial tachycardia and left ventricular dysfunction. J Am Coll Cardiol 2013;61(5):582–8.
53. Smith JG, Melander O, Sjogren M, et al. Genetic polymorphisms confer risk of atrial fibrillation in patients with heart failure: a population-based study. Eur J Heart Fail 2012;15(3):250–7.
54. Parvez B, Vaglio J, Rowan S, et al. Symptomatic response to antiarrhythmic drug therapy is modulated by a common single nucleotide polymorphism in atrial fibrillation. J Am Coll Cardiol 2012; 60(6):539–45.

Upstream Therapy for Atrial Fibrillation in Heart Failure

Andreas Goette, MD

KEYWORDS

• Atrial fibrillation • Heart failure • Upstream therapy • Statins • Prevention

KEY POINTS

- Heart failure is a major factor that increases the likelihood for atrial fibrillation (AF).
- Several aspects of the morphologic and electrophysiologic alterations promoting AF in heart failure (congestive heart failure [CHF]) have been studied in animal models and in patients with CHF; under these conditions, ectopic activity originating from the pulmonary veins or other sites is more likely to occur and to trigger longer episodes of AF.
- Angiotensin-converting enzyme inhibitors, angiotensin receptor blockers, and spironolactone may help to reduce the occurrence of AF.
- Statins are indicated if patients have an indication for their use, such as increased low-density lipoprotein levels or established coronary artery disease.
- Results for secondary prevention are very heterogeneous, and the effect of upstream therapy is less well established in this clinical setting.

PATHOPHYSIOLOGY OF ATRIAL FIBRILLATION IN HEART FAILURE

Atrial fibrillation (AF) is the most common sustained arrhythmia in humans, causing an increasing number of complications and deaths.[1–3] Reports suggest that approximately 1% of the total population is affected.[4] The number of patients with AF is likely to double or triple within the next 2 to 3 decades.[5] The prevalence of AF is clearly age dependent. Patients with AF usually seek medical attention because of AF-related symptoms, and the treatment of these symptoms has been the main motivation for AF therapy in the past. However, even the presence of asymptomatic AF markedly decreases quality of life.[2,6] AF also doubles mortality independently of other known disease-causing factors and is one of the most common causes for stroke. Left ventricular function, the best-validated clinical parameter for cardiac prognosis, can be markedly impaired in patients with AF and improves when sinus rhythm is maintained for a longer period of time.[2,7] Heart failure with dyspnea on exertion (New York Heart Association [NYHA] classes II–IV) is found in 30% of patients with AF,[8] and AF is found in 30% to 40% of patients with heart failure.[2,9] Heart failure and AF seem to promote each other, with AF compromising left ventricular function and left ventricular dysfunction causing atrial dilation and pressure overload. Treatment of heart failure is able to prevent AF,[2,10] adding to the evidence that AF is promoted by these conditions.

In order to investigate how congestive heart failure (CHF) promotes AF, experimental models of CHF have been described.[11] When CHF was induced by pacing with a ventricular pacemaker at a high rate (>200 beats per minute) for 5 weeks, atrial fibrosis was dramatically increased in dogs with CHF,[11] with large areas of connective tissue. These structural abnormalities were accompanied

Disclosures: The author has nothing to disclose.
Department of Cardiology and Intensive Care Medicine, St. Vincenz Hospital Paderborn GmbH, EUTRAF Working Group, University Hospital Magdeburg, Am Busdorf 2, Paderborn 33098, Germany
E-mail address: andreas.goette@med.ovgu.de

Heart Failure Clin 9 (2013) 417–425
http://dx.doi.org/10.1016/j.hfc.2013.07.010
1551-7136/13/$ – see front matter

heartfailure.theclinics.com

by regional conduction heterogeneity. Studies have supported the role of atrial fibrosis in the promotion of AF in CHF.[2,12,13] Atrial damage in the CHF model occurs rapidly, with a peak in inflammation, apoptosis, and necrosis within 24 hours after activation of the ventricular pacemaker.[2,14] The renin-angiotensin system is an important mediator in the development of an AF substrate in CHF. Inhibition of angiotensin II (AT II) production by the angiotensin-converting enzyme (ACE) blocker enalapril not only attenuated CHF-induced atrial fibrosis but also reduced conduction heterogeneity and AF stability.[2,15,16] Atrial fibrosis and increased AF stability in the canine CHF model can also be inhibited by simvastatin,[17] pirfenidone,[18] polyunsaturated ω-3 fatty acids,[19] and sprionolactone.[20] The peroxisome proliferator-activated receptor α (PPARα) activator fenofibrate was not effective in this model[17]; but in rabbits with tachycardiomyopathy-induced CHF, the PPARγ activator pioglitazone did reduce atrial structural remodeling and AF stability.[2,21]

MOLECULAR DRUG TARGETS FOR UPSTREAM THERAPY

Chronic atrial stretch seems to be one of the most prominent trigger mechanisms for signaling changes involved in the pathogenesis of AF. Atria seem to react much faster and more strongly to increased wall stress caused by atrial dilatation than ventricular myocardium.[14] The induction of heart failure by rapid ventricular pacing induces the development of apoptosis and increased collagen synthesis in the atria within a couple of days, whereas the degree of such changes is substantially smaller and the time course much slower in the ventricles.[2,11] At the molecular level, the development of atrial fibrosis caused by pressure and/or volume overload is mediated by both angiotensin II-dependent and independent mechanisms.[2,15,17] Left ventricular failure increases atrial synthesis of angiotensin II, and thereby atrial fibrosis is induced via activation of mitogen-activated protein (MAP) kinases.[2,22] Signaling pathways mediated by angiotensin II type 1 receptors (AT-1 receptors) are linked to G proteins. Studies have shown a linear correlation between angiotensin II, MAP kinase activation, and the degree of atrial fibrosis.[15] Another tyrosine kinase that is activated by angiotensin II is Janus kinase 2 (JAK2).[22] JAK2 initiates the activation of transcription factors signal transducer and activator of transcription (STAT)-1 and STAT-3. A recent study demonstrated that the angiotensin II/Rac1/STAT3 pathway is an important signaling pathway involved in atrial structural remodeling.[23]

In addition to angiotensin II, pacing-induced ventricular failure also increases atrial transforming growth factor (TGF)-β and platelet-derived growth factor (PDGF) levels. TGF-β operates predominantly by autocrine and paracrine mechanisms. Binding of a TGF-β homodimer to 2 TGF-β type II receptors causes phosphorylation of signaling molecules belonging to the family known as SMADs. When phosphorylated, SMADs aggregate and enter the nucleus to induce myocardial fibrosis.[24] In addition, TGF-β1 can redirect protein synthesis to favor expression of fetal genes as described in fibrillating atria.[25] Atrial fibroblasts are activated significantly faster than ventricular fibroblasts in the CHF models, explaining the rapid and more severe degree of interstitial fibrosis in the atria.[26]

Another important contributor to atrial remodeling in CHF is oxidative stress.[27] The PPARγ activator pioglitazone antagonizes angiotensin II actions and possesses antiinflammatory and antioxidant properties. Pioglitazone attenuated CHF-induced atrial structural remodeling and AF vulnerability.[2] In the same study, both pioglitazone and candesartan reduced TGF-β, tumor necrosis factor α, and MAP kinase, but neither affected p38 kinase or c-Jun N-terminal kinase activation. In contrast, ω-3 polyunsaturated fatty acids attenuate CHF-related phosphorylation of the MAP kinases ERK and p38.[2,19] In failing human myocardium, NADPH oxidase-related reactive oxygen species (ROS) production increases, with enhanced expression and activity of Rac1. The application of 3-hydroxy-3-methylglutaryl coenzyme A reductase inhibitors (statins) like simvastatin inhibits myocardial Rac1-GTPase activity.[17] The small GTPase Rac1 regulates NADPH oxidase activity. Statins downregulate Rac1-GTPase activity by reducing isoprenylation and translocation of Rac1 to the cell membrane.[28] The inhibition of Rac1 by statins decreases NADPH oxidase-related reactive oxygen species production in cardiac myocytes and reduces myocardial hypertrophy. Furthermore, simvastatin reduces human atrial myofibroblast proliferation via a RhoA pathway.[29] In addition, simvastatin, but not fenofibrate (PPARα agonist), inhibits canine atrial fibroblast proliferation, which paralleled collagen-synthetic fibroblast function.[2] Thus, statins and PPARα agonists have very different efficacy in preventing CHF-related atrial structural remodeling.

In addition to cellular effects, atrial stretch is also associated with an altered expression of matrix metalloproteinases (MMP). In patients with AF with congestive heart failure, an increased collagen I fraction seems to be associated with upregulation of MMP-2 and downregulation of tissue inhibitor of metalloprotease-1.[2,30,31] In addition to MMPs,

ADAMs (a disintegrin and metalloproteinase) also influence interstitial matrix composition and cell-cell and cell-matrix interactions. ADAMs form a large family of membrane-bound glycoproteins that function in proteolysis, signaling, cell adhesion, and cleavage-secretion of membrane-bound proteins.[2] Arndt and colleagues[32] described the effect of AF in patients with concomitant heart diseases on the regulation of ADAMs. Atrial tissue of patients with permanent AF shows increased levels of ADAM10 and ADAM15. Membrane expression of ADAM15 is significantly upregulated during AF, whereas most ADAM15 is retarded in the cytoplasm during sinus rhythm. The ADAM15/integrin β1 ratio is significantly increased in fibrillating tissue and correlates with the left atrial diameter and the duration of fibrillation. Thus, the regulation of MMPs and ADAMs influences the composition of interstitial matrix and contributes to geometric changes and dilatation of the atria and ventricles.[2,33]

Although atrial fibrosis is proarrhythmic in some animal models,[2,34,35] the quantitative association between atrial fibrosis and AF is not very strong. Some but not all human studies have found that atrial fibrosis is more pronounced in patients with chronic AF than in patients in sinus rhythm.[2,36] The degree of atrial fibrosis and fibrogenic activity correlates with the persistence of AF.[2,37] However, from these studies, it is unclear whether increased fibrosis is caused by underlying structural disease or by AF itself.[2]

UPSTREAM THERAPY FOR AF

As described, the treatment of CHF has been shown to reduce the incidence of AF in experimental models and clinical studies. Animal studies showed that the antiarrhythmic effects of ACE inhibitors and angiotensin receptor blockers (ARB) are related to their effect on atrial morphology.[38,39] The results are supported by analyses of several clinical trials: Valsartan Heart Failure Trial (Val-HeFT), Studies of Left Ventricular Dysfunction (SOLVD), and Candesartan in Heart Failure: Assessment of Reduction in Mortality and Morbidity (CHARM).[40] Furthermore, the Randomized Aldactone Evaluation Study (RALES) trial showed that spironolactone (an aldosterone antagonist) reduces circulating procollagen I and III levels in patients with CHF, which was associated with an improved survival.[41] Other targets and drugs for upstream therapy like statins, polyunsaturated fatty acids are less well studied in clinical trials so far. Of note, the results for primary prevention are significantly better than data for secondary prevention of AF in patients with CHF.

RENIN-ANGIOTENSIN-ALDOSTERONE SYSTEM INHIBITION IN CHF

In patients, several post hoc analyses of clinical trials suggest that therapy with ACE inhibitors, AT-1-receptor blocker, statins, and polyunsaturated fatty acids (PUFAs) are useful to prevent AF (**Table 1**). CHF is one of the most important risk factors for AF and, as evidenced by multivariate analysis from the Framingham Study, increases the risk of AF by 4.5-fold in men and 5.9-fold in women.[42,43] Diastolic left ventricular dysfunction is associated with a 5.26-fold increased risk of AF.[43,44] The occurrence of CHF in middle age confers an 8% risk of developing AF over a 10-year period if the patient's age at the time of CHF diagnosis was 55 to 64 years, which increases to 30% if CHF was diagnosed at 45 to 54 years of age.[43,45] Furthermore, the presence of CHF not only increases the likelihood of developing AF but is also the leading independent predictor of progression to permanent AF, with an odds ratio of 2.2.[46] New-onset AF in CHF is associated with clinical deterioration and poor prognosis.[43,47] There are reports that the absence of AF is associated with fewer symptoms and better functional status and left ventricular function in patients with CHF.[43,48,49] The true benefit of preserving sinus rhythm in patients with CHF in the AF-CHF and other secondary prevention studies might have been offset by the relatively low efficacy and adverse effects of antiarrhythmic drugs. Thus, upstream therapies (eg, renin-angiotensin-aldosterone system [RAAS] inhibitors) that target both the underlying condition and the substrate formation for AF may offer a greater benefit than specific antiarrhythmic drugs.[43,50]

The first large study to report the beneficial effect of RAAS inhibition on the occurrence of new-onset AF was the Trandolapril Cardiac Evaluation (TRACE) study in patients with recent myocardial infarction and an ejection fraction of 35% or less.[10] Patients who received trandolapril were less likely to develop new-onset AF during 2 to 4 years of follow-up compared with the placebo group (2.8% vs 5.3%). The report from the TRACE study was followed by similar retrospective analysis of the single-center results from the SOLVD trial, which also demonstrated less AF occurrence in patients with CHF and an ejection fraction of 35% or less with enalapril as opposed to placebo after 2.9 years of follow-up (5.4% vs 24.0%).[43] Later studies with ARBs yielded similar results.

In the Val-HeFT study, in 4395 patients with symptomatic CHF, therapy with valsartan was associated with a 37% reduction in relative risk of newly detected AF compared with placebo

Table 1
Clinical trials of renin-angiotensin systems inhibition to prevent new-onset AF in patients with CHF or AMI (primary prevention)

References	Study Design	Patients	Intervention	Primary Outcome
Pedersen et al,[10] 1999	TRACE study (post hoc analysis)	1577 with AMI and reduced LVEF	Trandolapril vs placebo Follow-up: 2–4 y	Reduced incidence of new-onset AF
Pizetti et al	GISSI-3 study (post hoc analysis)	17,749 with AMI	Lisinopril vs no lisinopril Follow-up: 4 y	No difference in new-onset AF
Vermes et al	SOLVD study (post hoc analysis)	347 with LV dysfunction	Enalapril vs placebo Follow-up: 2.9 y	Reduced incidence of new-onset AF
Alsheikh-Ali et al	SOLVD study (post hoc analysis)	6797 with LV dysfunction	Enalapril vs placebo Follow-up: 34 mo	Reduced incidence of hospitalization with AF
Maggioni et al	Val-HeFT study (post hoc analysis)	4395 with chronic symptomatic HF	Valsartan vs placebo Follow-up: 23 mo	Reduced incidence of new-onset AF
Ducharme et al,[52] 2006	CHARM study (prespecified secondary end point)	6379 with symptomatic CHF	Candesartan vs placebo Follow-up: 37.7 mo	Reduced incidence of new-onset AF
Hansson et al	CAPPP study (randomized, open label [analysis on adverse event reports])	10,985 with hypertension	Captopril vs diuretics ± beta-blocker Follow-up: 6.1 y	No difference in new-onset AF
Hansson et al	STOP-2 study (randomized, open label)	6628 with hypertension	Enalapril/lisinopril vs CCB vs diuretics ± beta-blocker Study duration: 4 y	No difference in new-onset AF
Lh'Allier et al	Retrospective longitudinal cohort study	10,926 with hypertension	ACEI vs CCB Average follow-up: 4.5 y	Reduced incidence of new-onset AF
Wachtell et al,[64] 2005	LIFE study (randomized, double blind)	8851 with hypertension + ECG LVH	Losartan vs atenolol Follow-up: 4.8 y	Reduced incidence of new-onset AF

Abbreviations: ACEI, ACE inhibitor; AMI, acute myocardial infarction; CCB, calcium channel blockers; ECG, electrocardiogram; GISSI, Gruppo Italiano per lo Studio della Sopravvivenza nell'Insufficienza cardiaca; HF, heart failure; LIFE, Losartan Intervention For End Point Reduction in Hypertension; LV, left ventricular; LVEF, left ventricular ejection fraction; LVH, left ventricular hypertrophy.

Adapted from Savelieva I, Kakouros N, Kourliouros A, et al. Upstream therapies for management of atrial fibrillation. Part I: primary prevention. Europace 2011;13:308–28; with permission.

(5.12% vs 7.95%) during 1.9 years.[43,51] This benefit from an ARB was present despite a high (93%) rate of concomitant use of ACE inhibitors (ACEIs). This study has also demonstrated that the occurrence of AF was independently associated with adverse major outcomes, such as all-cause death and combined mortality and morbidity, which increased by 40% and 38%, respectively, in the presence of AF. However, whether valsartan therapy improved the outcome within the new-onset AF group compared with placebo has not been reported.[43]

One of the limitations of these retrospective analyses was that AF was not a prespecified end point, and a significant proportion of asymptomatic or mildly symptomatic episodes might not have been reported. The CHARM program designated AF as one of the secondary end points.[43] The AF substudy from the CHARM trials has shown that adding candesartan to conventional CHF therapy in 6379 patients with symptomatic CHF and without a history of AF at enrollment led to a lower incidence of new-onset AF compared with placebo, albeit this reduction was not as significant as in the previous reports (5.55% vs 6.74%).[43,52] Of note, the magnitude of the preventative effect of RAAS inhibition varies in patients according to the degree of impairment of left ventricular function. Thus, although statistically there was no heterogeneity of the effect of candesartan on AF between the 3 component trials in the CHARM program, the greatest benefit was seen in patients with impaired systolic function and without the concurrent use of ACEIs enrolled in the CHARM-alternative study and the least in patients with CHF and preserved systolic function.[51]

Similarly, irbesartan did not influence the incidence of AF reported as an adverse event in the Irbesartan in Patients with Heart Failure and Preserved Ejection Fraction trial.[53] Four meta-analyses have shown that the risk of new-onset AF in patients with CHF was reduced by 30% to 48%, suggesting that ACEIs and ARBs may be effective in the primary prevention of AF in this clinical setting.[38,54–56] This finding is consistent with experimental evidence of atrial fibrosis as the leading mechanism of AF in CHF models and evidence of antifibrotic effects of RAAS inhibition. It is unclear whether therapy with ACEIs and ARBs can prevent or delay the occurrence of AF in patients with CHF and preserved systolic function. There is no direct evidence that upstream therapies with RAAS inhibitors can reduce morbidity and mortality in patients with CHF by deterring AF.[43]

STATINS IN CHF

Retrospective analyses from randomized controlled trials (RCTs) and registries in patients with CHF have suggested a modest reduction in the incidence of AF, mainly newly detected AF, although the differentiation between truly new-onset AF and recurrent AF has not always been possible.[43,57–59] In the AdvancentSM registry of 25,268 patients with an ejection fraction of 40% or less and left ventricular dysfunction of an ischemic cause in 72%, lipid-lowering therapy (mostly statins or combination therapy) was associated with a 31% reduction in relative risk of developing AF compared with no therapy.[57] This effect was greater than that of beta-blockers and RAAS inhibitors. The Sudden Cardiac Death in Heart Failure Trial investigators reported a similar 28% reduction in relative risk of AF, which was comparable with that of amiodarone.[43,58]

The GISSI-HF (Gruppo Italiano per lo Studio della Sopravvivenza nell'Insufficienza cardiaca Heart Failure) study enrolled 3690 patients with sinus rhythm. Therapy with rosuvastatin reduced the risk of any AF during the study by only 13%. The difference with the placebo arm became statistically significant only after adjustment for clinical variables, laboratory findings, and concomitant therapy.[59] In the prespecified subgroup of patients with no history of paroxysmal AF, the incidence of new-onset AF was 9.8% in the rosuvastatin arm and 11.6% in the placebo arm. Patients in whom AF was present on the baseline electrocardiogram (19.3%) were excluded, but it could not be ascertained whether all patients who developed AF in the course of the study had new-onset AF.[43] There was a nonsignificant difference between the rosuvastatin and placebo arms in the proportion of patients with AF at study entry who were excluded from analysis (18.8% vs 19.8%). During the study, AF occurred in 15% patients: 13.9% in the rosuvastatin group and 16.0% in the placebo group (absolute difference 2.1%). It is possible that more patients in the rosuvastatin arm may have had unrecognized AF at baseline and, hence, a greater likelihood of recurrent AF.[43] Because of the retrospective nature of these reports, much important information is not available. One brief report from a large cohort of patients with CHF who were prescribed statins has suggested that the intensity of treatment might play a role; thus, in this study, AF was less common in those who received high doses (atorvastatin 80 mg, simvastatin 80 mg, and lovastatin 40 mg) as opposed to lower doses of the same agent.[43,60]

Table 2
Clinical trials of statins to prevent new-onset and progression of AF (primary and secondary prevention)

References	Study Design	Patients	Intervention	Primary Outcome
Hanna et al	Retrospective	25,268 with CHF	Lipid-lowering drug use vs no use	Reduced incidence of new-onset AF
Adabag et al	Retrospective	13,783 with CHD	Statins vs no statins Average follow-up: 4.8 y	No difference in new-onset AF

Abbreviation: CHD, coronary heart diseases.

Adapted from Savelieva I, Kakouros N, Kourliouros A, et al. Upstream therapies for management of atrial fibrillation. Part I: primary prevention. Europace 2011;13:308–28; with permission.

Table 3
Clinical trials of ω-3 (omega-3) polyunsaturated fatty acids to prevent AF in patients without CHF

References	Study Design	Patients	Intervention	Primary Outcome
Mozaffarian et al	Cardiovascular Health Study (population-based, prospective cohort)	4815	Dietary intake assessment Follow-up: 12 y	Reduced incidence of AF
Frost et al	Danish Diet, Cancer and Health study (population-based, prospective cohort)	47,949	Dietary intake assessment Mean follow-up: 5.4 y	No difference in incidence of AF
Brouwer et al	Rotterdam study: (population-based, prospective cohort)	5184	Dietary intake assessment Follow-up: 6.4 y	No difference in incidence of AF

Adapted from Savelieva I, Kakouros N, Kourliouros A, et al. Upstream therapies for management of atrial fibrillation. Part I: primary prevention. Europace 2011;13:308–28; with permission.

META-ANALYSES OF STATIN TRIALS

Other meta-analyses of the efficacy of statins for primary prevention of AF in different clinical settings have yielded controversial results (**Table 2**).[43,60,61] The first meta-analysis by Fauchier and colleagues,[60] which included 3 RCTs of primary prevention (one in ACS and 2 in postoperative AF) in 3101 patients, has shown a nonsignificant trend toward fewer AF events. In a meta-analysis by Liu and colleagues,[61] statin treatment was associated with a reduction in new-onset AF both after cardiac surgery and in the nonsurgical setting but only in the observational studies. No effect on AF was seen when the results of RCTs were analyzed. The most recent meta-analysis, which has not yet been published in full, has confirmed the previous findings by showing a 30% reduction in relative risk of new-onset or recurrent AF with statins compared with control in 7 hypothesis-generating relatively small and short-term studies in mixed populations, including patients with acute coronary syndrome (ACS), cardiac surgery, and after electrical cardioversion (411 events in 3609 patients).[62] However, in 15 (1514 events in 68,504 patients) hypothesis-testing long-term prospective RCTs in large patient populations with and without cardiovascular pathologic conditions, the use of statins had no effect on the occurrence of (mainly) new-onset AF compared with control or placebo.[43] Further analysis revealed no difference in the effects of statins in patients with coronary artery disease (CAD) versus other underlying cardiovascular pathology. Thus, the value of statins for the primary prevention of AF has not been sufficiently demonstrated, except perhaps for patients undergoing cardiac surgery. Nevertheless, several positive reports suggest some benefit of statins in patients with underlying heart disease, particularly CHF.[43,63]

SUMMARY

CHF induces substantial molecular alteration in atrial tissue. These changes are proarrhythmic and increase the likelihood for AF. Thus, aggressive therapy for CHF has been shown to be useful for the primary prevention of AF in these patients; in particular, ACE inhibitors, ARBs, and spironolactone may help to reduce the occurrence of AF. Statins are indicated if patients have an indication for their use, such as increased low-density lipoprotein levels or established CAD. Results for secondary prevention are very heterogeneous, and the effect of upstream therapy is less well established in this clinical setting. This point may be explained by the fact that an established proarrhythmic atrial fibrosis is not reversible; therefore, the burden of AF cannot be decreased by such therapies. The impact of PUFA therapy is not established in patients with CHF (**Table 3**). Although there are experimental data showing antiarrhythmic effects, the true clinical benefit of long-term PUFA application is very vague in patients with CHF.[2,43,47,64–70]

There is a good deal of supporting evidence for the use of upstream therapies, mostly in favor of modification of the RAAS axis. It is, therefore, entirely appropriate that drugs acting beneficially on the RAAS are prescribed in the heart failure population using the additional benefit on the predisposition to AF to provide supporting arguments.

REFERENCES

1. Fuster V, Ryden LE, Cannom DS, et al. ACC/AHA/ESC 2006 guidelines for the management of patients with atrial fibrillation-executive summary: A report of the American College of Cardiology/American Heart Association Task Force on practice

guidelines and the European Society of Cardiology Committee for Practice Guidelines (Writing Committee to Revise the 2001 Guidelines for the Management of Patients with Atrial Fibrillation) developed in collaboration with the European Heart Rhythm Association and the Heart Rhythm Society. Eur Heart J 2006;27:1979–2030.
2. Schotten U, Verheule S, Kirchhof P, et al. Pathophysiological mechanisms of atrial fibrillation: a translational appraisal. Physiol Rev 2011;91(1): 265–325.
3. Kirchhof P, Auricchio A, Bax J, et al. Outcome parameters for trials in atrial fibrillation: executive summary: recommendations from a consensus conference organized by the German Atrial Fibrillation Competence NETwork (AFNET) and the European Heart Rhythm Association (EHRA). Eur Heart J 2007;28:2803–17.
4. Kannel WB, Wolf PA, Benjamin EJ, et al. Prevalence, incidence, prognosis, and predisposing conditions for atrial fibrillation: population-based estimates. Am J Cardiol 1998;82:2N–9N.
5. Hobbs FD, Fitzmaurice DA, Mant J, et al. A randomised controlled trial and cost-effectiveness study of systematic screening (targeted and total population screening) versus routine practice for the detection of atrial fibrillation in people aged 65 and over. The SAFE study. Health Technol Assess 2005;9:1–74, iii–iv, ix–x.
6. Wilhelmsen L, Rosengren A, Lappas G. Hospitalizations for atrial fibrillation in the general male population: morbidity and risk factors. J Intern Med 2001;250:382–9.
7. Khan MN, Jais P, Cummings J, et al. Pulmonary-vein isolation for atrial fibrillation in patients with heart failure. N Engl J Med 2008;359:1778–85.
8. Nieuwlaat R, Capucci A, Camm AJ, et al. Atrial fibrillation management: a prospective survey in ESC member countries: the Euro Heart Survey on Atrial Fibrillation. Eur Heart J 2005;26:2422–34.
9. Cleland JG, Swedberg K, Follath F, et al. The Euro-Heart Failure survey programme: a survey on the quality of care among patients with heart failure in Europe. Part 1: patient characteristics and diagnosis. Eur Heart J 2003;24:442–63.
10. Pedersen OD, Bagger H, Kober L, et al. Trandolapril reduces the incidence of atrial fibrillation after acute myocardial infarction in patients with left ventricular dysfunction. Circulation 1999;100:376–80.
11. Li D, Fareh S, Leung TK, et al. Promotion of atrial fibrillation by heart failure in dogs: atrial remodeling of a different sort. Circulation 1999;100:87–95.
12. Cha TJ, Ehrlich JR, Zhang L, et al. Dissociation between ionic remodeling and ability to sustain atrial fibrillation during recovery from experimental congestive heart failure. Circulation 2004;109: 412–8.
13. Shinagawa K, Shi Y, Tardif JC, et al. Dynamic nature of atrial fibrillation substrate during development and reversal of heart failure in dogs. Circulation 2002;105:2672–8.
14. Hanna N, Cardin S, Leung TK, et al. Differences in atrial versus ventricular remodeling in dogs with ventricular tachypacing-induced congestive heart failure. Cardiovasc Res 2004;63(2):236–44.
15. Li D, Shinagawa K, Pang L, et al. Effects of angiotensin-converting enzyme inhibition on the development of the atrial fibrillation substrate in dogs with ventricular tachypacing-induced congestive heart failure. Circulation 2001;104:2608–14.
16. Shi Y, Li D, Tardif JC, et al. Enalapril effects on atrial remodeling and atrial fibrillation in experimental congestive heart failure. Cardiovasc Res 2002;54: 456–61.
17. Shiroshita-Takeshita A, Brundel BJ, Burstein B, et al. Effects of simvastatin on the development of the atrial fibrillation substrate in dogs with congestive heart failure. Cardiovasc Res 2007; 74:75–84.
18. Lee KW, Everett TH, Rahmutula D, et al. Pirfenidone prevents the development of a vulnerable substrate for atrial fibrillation in a canine model of heart failure. Circulation 2006;114:1703–12.
19. Sakabe M, Shiroshita-Takeshita A, Maguy A, et al. Omega-3 polyunsaturated fatty acids prevent atrial fibrillation associated with heart failure but not atrial tachycardia remodeling. Circulation 2007;116: 2101–9.
20. Yang SS, Han W, Zhou HY, et al. Effects of spironolactone on electrical and structural remodeling of atrium in congestive heart failure dogs. Chin Med J 2008;121:38–42.
21. Shimano M, Tsuji Y, Inden Y, et al. Pioglitazone, a peroxisome proliferator-activated receptor-gamma activator, attenuates atrial fibrosis and atrial fibrillation promotion in rabbits with congestive heart failure. Heart Rhythm 2008;5(3):451–9.
22. Goette A, Staack T, Röcken C, et al. Increased expression of extracellular-signal regulated kinase and angiotensin-converting enzyme in human atria during atrial fibrillation. J Am Coll Cardiol 2000;35: 1669–77.
23. Tsai CT, Lai LP, Kuo KT, et al. Angiotensin II activates signal transducer and activators of transcription 3 via Rac1 in atrial myocytes and fibroblasts: implication for the therapeutic effect of statin in atrial structural remodeling. Circulation 2008; 117(3):344–55.
24. Brand T, Schneider MD. Transforming growth factor-β signal transduction. Circ Res 1996;78:173–9.
25. Parker TG, Packer SE, Schneider MD. Peptide growth factors can provoke fetal contractile proteins gene expression in rat cardiac myocytes. J Clin Invest 1990;85:507–14.

26. Burstein B, Libby E, Calderone A, et al. Differential behaviors of atrial versus ventricular fibroblasts: a potential role for platelet-derived growth factor in atrial-ventricular remodeling differences. Circulation 2008;117(13):1630–41.
27. Cha YM, Shen WK, Jahangir A, et al. Failing atrial myocardium: energetic deficits accompany structural remodeling and electrical instability. Am J Physiol Heart Circ Physiol 2003;284(4):H1313–20.
28. Adam O, Neuberger HR, Böhm M, et al. Prevention of atrial fibrillation with 3-hydroxy-3-methylglutaryl coenzyme A reductase inhibitors. Circulation 2008;118:1285–93.
29. Porter KE, O'Regan DJ, Balmforth AJ, et al. Simvastatin reduces human atrial myofibroblast proliferation independently of cholesterol lowering via inhibition of RhoA. Cardiovasc Res 2004;61:745–55.
30. Cooradi D, Callegari S, Benussi S, et al. Regional left atrial interstitial remodeling in patients with chronic atrial fibrillation undergoing mitral-valve surgery. Virchows Arch 2004;445(5):498–505.
31. Xu J, Cui G, Esmailian F, et al. Atrial extracellular matrix remodeling and the maintenance of atrial fibrillation. Circulation 2004;109:363–8.
32. Arndt M, Röcken C, Nepple K, et al. Altered expression of ADAMs (a disintegrin and metalloproteinase) in fibrillating human atria. Circulation 2002;105:720–5.
33. Hunt MJ, Aru GM, Hayden MR, et al. Induction of oxidative stress and disintegrin metalloproteinase in human heart end-stage failure. Am J Physiol Lung Cell Mol Physiol 2002;283:L239–45.
34. Burstein B, Nattel S. Atrial fibrosis: mechanisms and clinical relevance in atrial fibrillation. J Am Coll Cardiol 2008;51:802–9.
35. Everett TH, Olgin JE. Atrial fibrosis and the mechanisms of atrial fibrillation. Heart Rhythm 2007;4: S24–7.
36. Boldt A, Wetzel U, Lauschke J, et al. Fibrosis in left atrial tissue of patients with atrial fibrillation with and without underlying mitral valve disease. Heart 2004;90:400–5.
37. Gramley F, Lorenzen J, Plisiene J, et al. Decreased plasminogen activator inhibitor and tissue metalloproteinase inhibitor expression may promote increased metalloproteinase activity with increasing duration of human atrial fibrillation. J Cardiovasc Electrophysiol 2007;18:1076–82.
38. Healey JS, Baranchuk A, Crystal E, et al. Prevention of atrial fibrillation with angiotensin-converting enzyme inhibitors and angiotensin receptor blockers: a meta-analysis. J Am Coll Cardiol 2005;45(11):1832–9.
39. Hammwöhner M, D'Alessandro A, Dobrev D, et al. New antiarrhythmic drugs for therapy of atrial fibrillation: II. Non-ion channel blockers. Herzschrittmacherther Elektrophysiol 2006;17(2):73–80.
40. Ehrlich JR, Hohnloser SH, Nattel S. Role of angiotensin system and effects of its inhibition in atrial fibrillation: clinical and experimental evidence. Eur Heart J 2006;27(5):512–8.
41. Zannad F, Alla F, Dousset B, et al. Limitation of excessive extracellular matrix turnover may contribute to survival benefit of spironolactone therapy in patients with congestive heart failure: insights from the randomized Aldactone evaluation study (RALES). Rales Investigators. Circulation 2000;102(22):2700–6.
42. Benjamin EJ, Levy D, Vaziri SM, et al. Independent risk factors for atrial fibrillation in a population-based cohort: the Framingham Heart Study. JAMA 1994;271:840–4.
43. Savelieva I, Kakouros N, Kourliouros A, et al. Upstream therapies for management of atrial fibrillation. Part I: primary prevention. Europace 2011; 13:308–28.
44. Tsang TS, Gersh BJ, Appleton CP, et al. Left ventricular diastolic dysfunction as a predictor of the first diagnosed nonvalvular atrial fibrillation in 840 elderly men and women. J Am Coll Cardiol 2002; 40:1636–44.
45. Schnabel RB, Sullivan LM, Levy D, et al. Development of a risk score for atrial fibrillation (Framingham Heart Study): a community-based cohort study. Lancet 2009;373:739–45.
46. De Vos CB, Pisters R, Nieuwlaat R, et al. Progression from paroxysmal to persistent atrial fibrillation clinical correlates and prognosis. J Am Coll Cardiol 2010;55:725–31.
47. Wang TJ, Larson MG, Levy D, et al. Temporal relations of atrial fibrillation and congestive heart failure and their joint influence on mortality: the Framingham Heart Study. Circulation 2003;107(23):2920–5.
48. Shelton RJ, Clark AL, Goode K, et al. A randomised, controlled study of rate versus rhythm control in patients with chronic atrial fibrillation and heart failure: (CAFE-II Study). Heart 2009; 95:924–30.
49. Guglin M, Chen R, Curtis AB. Sinus rhythm is associated with fewer heart failure symptoms: insights from the AFFIRM trial. Heart Rhythm 2010; 7:596–601.
50. Savelieva I, Camm AJ. Atrial fibrillation and heart failure: natural history and pharmacological treatment. Europace 2004;5:S5–19.
51. Maggioni AP, Latini R, Carson PE, et al. Valsartan reduces the incidence of atrial fibrillation in patients with heart failure: results from the Valsartan Heart Failure Trial (Val-HeFT). Am Heart J 2005;149: 548–57.
52. Ducharme A, Swedberg K, Pfeffer MA, et al. Prevention of atrial fibrillation in patients with symptomatic chronic heart failure by candesartan in the Candesartan in Heart failure: Assessment of

Reduction in Mortality and Morbidity (CHARM) program. Am Heart J 2006;152:86–92.
53. Massie BM, Carson PE, McMurray JJ, et al. Irbesartan in patients with heart failure and preserved ejection fraction. N Engl J Med 2008;359:2456–67.
54. Anand K, Mooss AN, Hee TT, et al. Meta-analysis: inhibition of renin–angiotensin system prevents new-onset atrial fibrillation. Am Heart J 2006;152:217–22.
55. Jibrini MB, Molnar J, Arora RR. Prevention of atrial fibrillation by way of abrogation of the renin–angiotensin system: a systematic review and meta-analysis. Am J Ther 2008;15:36–43.
56. Schneider MP, Hua TA, Boehm M, et al. Prevention of atrial fibrillation by renin–angiotensin system inhibition a meta-analysis. J Am Coll Cardiol 2010; 55:2299–307.
57. Hanna IR, Heeke B, Bush H, et al. Lipid-lowering drug use is associated with reduced prevalence of atrial fibrillation in patients with left ventricular systolic dysfunction. Heart Rhythm 2006;3:881–6.
58. Dickinson MG, Hellkamp AS, Ip JH, et al. Statin therapy was associated with reduced atrial fibrillation and flutter in heart failure patients in SCD-HEFT [abstract]. Heart Rhythm 2006;3:S49.
59. Maggioni AP, Fabbri G, Lucci D, et al. Effects of rosuvastatin on atrial fibrillation occurrence: ancillary results of the GISSI-HF trial. Eur Heart J 2009;19: 2327–36.
60. Fauchier L, Pierre B, de Labriolle A, et al. Antiarrhythmic effect of statin therapy and atrial fibrillation a meta-analysis of randomized controlled trials. J Am Coll Cardiol 2008;51:828–35.
61. Liu T, Li G, Korantzopoulos P, et al. Statin use and development of atrial fibrillation: a systematic review and meta-analysis of randomized clinical trials and observational studies. Int J Cardiol 2008;126: 160–70.
62. Rahimi K, Emberson J, Mcgale P, et al. Effect of statins on atrial fibrillation: a collaborative meta-analysis of randomised controlled trials. Eur Heart J 2009 [abstract 2782].
63. Savelieva I, Camm J. Statins and polyunsaturated fatty acids for treatment of atrial fibrillation. Nat Clin Pract Cardiovasc Med 2008;5:30–41.
64. Wachtell K, Lehto M, Gerdts E, et al. Angiotensin II receptor blockade reduces new-onset atrial fibrillation and subsequent stroke compared to atenolol: the Losartan Intervention For End Point Reduction in Hypertension (LIFE) study. J Am Coll Cardiol 2005;45(5):712–9.
65. Ueng KC, Tsai TP, Yu WC, et al. Use of enalapril to facilitate sinus rhythm maintenance after external cardioversion of long-standing persistent atrial fibrillation. Results of a prospective and controlled study. Eur Heart J 2003;24(23):2090–8.
66. Heckbert SR, Wiggins KL, Glazer NL, et al. Antihypertensive treatment with ACE inhibitors or beta-blockers and risk of incident atrial fibrillation in a general hypertensive population. Am J Hypertens 2009;22(5):538–44.
67. Dagres N, Karatasakis G, Panou F, et al. Pre-treatment with Irbesartan attenuates left atrial stunning after electrical cardioversion of atrial fibrillation. Eur Heart J 2006;27(17):2062–8.
68. Verdecchia P, Reboldi G, Gattobigio R, et al. Atrial fibrillation in hypertension: predictors and outcome. Hypertension 2003;41(2):218–23.
69. Hammwöhner M, Smid J, Lendeckel U, et al. New drugs for atrial fibrillation. J Interv Card Electrophysiol 2008;35:55–62.
70. Goette A, Schön N, Kirchhof P, et al. Angiotensin II-antagonist in paroxysmal atrial fibrillation (ANTIPAF) trial. Circ Arrhythm Electrophysiol 2012;5(1): 43–51.

Stroke Prevention in Atrial Fibrillation in Heart Failure

Eduard Shantsila, PhD, Gregory Y.H. Lip, MD*

KEYWORDS

• Heart failure • Atrial fibrillation • Anticoagulation • Stroke • Prevention

KEY POINTS

- Patients with atrial fibrillation associated with heart failure have a high risk of stroke.
- Oral anticoagulation with vitamin K antagonists or novel licensed medicines should be considered in all such patients unless contraindicated.
- A risk of anticoagulation-related bleeding should be assessed and regularly reviewed.
- Possible benefits of sinus rhythm maintenance for stroke prevention in heart failure are not entirely clear and may need to be explored further as new treatment options emerge.
- Relatively scarce data are available on stroke prevention in atrial fibrillation in heart failure with preserved ejection fraction, which requires further research.

INTRODUCTION

Heart failure (HF) and atrial fibrillation (AF) represent two major problems of modern cardiology with important clinical, prognostic, and socioeconomic implications. Each of these clinical entities poses high morbidity, impaired quality of life, and poor outcome, including increased risk of stroke. Of importance, these two conditions share several common pathophysiological mechanisms and risk factors (ie, hypertension, cardiac ischemia), which potentiate the associated health risks.

AF and HF often coexist. The prevalence of AF in patients with HF ranges from 13% to 40%, showing comparable rates in systolic HF and HF with preserved ejection fraction (HFpEF).[1–3] The recent EuroHeart Failure Survey II (EHFS II) confirmed the role of AF as one of the most common underlying conditions among patients admitted with acute HF.[4] Among patients with HF, those with AF have worse functional class, quality of life, and lower exercise tolerance.[5]

These conditions contribute to the pathogenesis of each other. AF promotes HF development and progression, primarily via triggering tachycardia-induced cardiomyopathy, loss of effective atrial systole, irregularity of ventricular contractions, and impairment of cardiac filling. In a large population of 360,000 subjects, AF was independently associated with a doubled risk of HF development.[6] Atrial systole can contribute up to 25% of the cardiac output, and as much as 50% in patients with preexisting valvular disease or ventricular dysfunction.[7,8]

In addition, a drastic shift in cardiac hemodynamics in HF provides a background for AF development. HF can increase the risk for the development of AF in several ways, including elevation of cardiac filling pressures with mechanical stretching of the atria, dysregulation of intracellular calcium, and neurohormonal changes, linked to atrial remodeling and fibrosis.[9,10] In the Framingham Study, HF was the strongest predictor for AF onset, with an increased risk of almost

Disclosures: The authors have nothing to disclose.
University of Birmingham Centre for Cardiovascular Sciences, City Hospital, Birmingham B18 7QH, UK
* Corresponding author.
E-mail address: g.y.h.lip@bham.ac.uk

Heart Failure Clin 9 (2013) 427–435
http://dx.doi.org/10.1016/j.hfc.2013.07.008

fivefold in men and sixfold in women.[11] A third of HF patients free of AF developed the arrhythmia within the following 4 years.[12] Of note, the prevalence of AF in patients with HF increased in parallel with the severity of the disease, ranging from 4% in patients with mild HF to 50% in the most severe forms of HF.[13] In those with AF, the presence of HF predicts progression to more persistent patterns of AF.[14]

In the Candesartan in Heart Failure-Assessment of Reduction in Mortality and morbidity (CHARM) program, which covered 7599 patients with symptomatic HF with a 3-year follow-up, AF predicted a high risk of cardiovascular morbidity and mortality and all-cause mortality regardless of baseline cardiac contractility.[2] In an even larger population of almost 100,000 patients admitted with HF and enrolled in Get With The Guidelines-Heart Failure program, AF was independently associated with adverse outcomes.[15] Indeed, a meta-analysis of clinical trials of patients with AF confirmed a significantly higher risk of death with AF compared with subjects in sinus rhythm.[16]

Importantly, HF is a major risk factor of stroke in patients with AF. Its presence almost doubles the risk of ischemic stroke and systemic embolism.[17] Independent risk factors for stroke in AF include recent cardiac failure or moderately-to-severely impaired left ventricular ejection fraction (LVEF).[17] As an example, Pozzoli and colleagues[18] prospectively followed patients with mild HF in sinus rhythm and confirmed that the onset of AF was linked with a significant predisposition to systemic thromboembolism, as well as an increased incidence of clinical and hemodynamic complications and a poorer outlook. Of note, accumulating data point toward prognostic relevance of both systolic HF and HFpEF as risk factors for future strokes. In a recent, relatively small study, rates of ischemic stroke over 3-year follow-up were about threefold higher in patients with AF with HFpEF than in those with AF without HF (hazard ratio 3.29; 95% CI 1.58–6.86; $P = .001$).[19]

THE PROTHROMBOTIC STATE IN AF AND HF

Both AF and HF predispose to thrombogenesis. The association between AF and the risk of stroke has been recognized for decades and recently similar links have been established for HF. Both conditions present components of Virchow's triad for thrombus formation (ie, abnormal blood stasis, endothelial or endocardial damage, or dysfunction), and abnormal hemostasis.

The left atrial appendage is a small but long sack located on the lateral aspect of the left atrium. Having a relatively narrow inlet, this structure clearly predisposes to blood stasis and represents the usual site of intra-atrial thrombus generation, particularly in patients with AF.[20,21] Additionally, AF is often associated with an increased left atrial size, further predisposing to stasis and cardiac thrombus formation.[22] The implication of left atrial enlargement in thrombogenesis is supported by evidence of a significant and independent association between the left atrial size, adjusted for body surface area and risk of stroke.[23,24]

It is important to emphasize that the pathogenesis of thrombogenesis in AF is multifactorial and is not solely related to blood stasis in a poorly contractile left atrium and left atrial appendage.[25] Endothelial and endocardial damage and/or dysfunction are also well documented in both AF and HF.[26,27] Small areas of endothelial denudation and thrombotic aggregation have been noted in patients with AF and cerebral embolism. The diverse and complex pattern of endothelial dysfunction in HF has been extensively documented and discussed in detail elsewhere.[28] Also, AF and HF can be considered as conditions characterized by systemic and local cardiac inflammation.[25,29] The final component of Virchow's triad in AF and HF is the presence of abnormal hemostasis and coagulation (eg, elevated levels of fibrin turnover products).[25,27,30,31]

ANTICOAGULATION IN AF WITH HF

Given the high prevalence of AF in patients with HF and its implications for the management of HF, patients' peripheral pulses should be checked during each visit. If AF is suspected, the diagnosis of AF needs to be documented by an ECG. Pharmacologic thromboembolism prophylaxis is of paramount importance for stroke prevention in AF with HF.

According to current guidelines, risk assessment for stroke in such patients should be based on the CHA_2DS_2-VASc score (**Table 1**).[32,33] It is crucial to appreciate that chronic oral anticoagulation is preferable in most AF patients with systolic HF (score $\geq$1) because most have a firm indication for the treatment (ie, score $\geq$2). In parallel to HF as an important risk factor of stroke in AF, such patients often have other comorbidities, such as coronary artery disease, hypertension, valvular heart disease, renal dysfunction, and diabetes, which further increase the risk of AF-related stroke.[34,35] In fact, both European and American guidelines on the management of HF advocate routine use of oral anticoagulation in all patients with HF and a history of AF.[32,36]

In addition to universal contraindications to oral anticoagulants, such therapy in subjects with HF

Table 1
The CHA_2DS_2-VASc stroke risk score

Letter	Risk Factor	Points
C	Congestive HF or left ventricular dysfunction	1
H	Hypertension	1
A	Age >75 y	2
D	Diabetes mellitus	1
S	Stroke, transient ischemic attack, or thromboembolism	2
V	Vascular disease	1
A	Age 65–74 y	1
S	Sex category (ie, female sex)	1

Maximum 9 points.

Adapted from Lip GY, Frison L, Halperin JL, et al. Identifying patients at high risk for stroke despite anticoagulation: a comparison of contemporary stroke risk stratification schemes in an anticoagulated atrial fibrillation cohort. Stroke 2010;41:2731–8; with permission.

may be restricted by a high bleeding risk. Consequently, every patient with AF and HF considered for anticoagulation should have a formal bleeding risk estimation based on the validated HAS-BLED score (**Table 2**).[32,37,38] Careful considerations of the initiation and regular review of anticoagulant therapy should be ensured in patients with HF with a HAS-BLED score greater than or equal to 3 and modifiable risk factors of bleeding have to be addressed.

All patients receiving oral anticoagulation with vitamin K antagonists (VKAs) should have regular monitoring of the degree of anticoagulation based on international normalized ratio (INR), which is the ratio of the actual prothrombin time and of a standardized control serum. The suggested optimal range of INR in nonvalvular AF is 2.0 to 3.0 to allow optimal balance of effective stroke prevention and small risk of bleeding.[39,40]

The early period following initiation of anticoagulation with VKA bears considerable risk for both over- and under-coagulation despite following established protocols of initiation of VKA.[41] Given the complicated pharmacologic features of warfarin and other VKAs, all patients should be given advice on the importance of INR monitoring due to high interindividual and intraindividual variations in response to medications. The patients must also be advised on lifestyle, food, alcohol consumption, and relevant drug interactions. The need to seek immediate medical help in cases of bleeding should be emphasized.

Of note, at present there is little role for aspirin in stroke prevention in patients with AF and HF. In the minority of patients not suitable for oral

Table 2
The HAS-BLED bleeding risk score

Letter	Clinical Characteristic	Points	Definition
H	Hypertension	1	Systolic blood pressure >160 mm Hg
A	Abnormal renal	1	Presence of chronic dialysis or renal transplantation or serum creatinine ≥200 mmol/L
	Abnormal liver function	1	Chronic hepatic disease (eg, cirrhosis) or biochemical evidence of significant hepatic derangement (eg, bilirubin .2 × upper limit of normal, in association with aspartate aminotransferase-alanine aminotransferase-alkaline phosphatase .3 × upper limit normal)
S	Stroke	1	History of stroke
B	Bleeding	1	Previous bleeding history and/or predisposition to bleeding (eg, bleeding diathesis, anemia)
L	Labile INRs	1	Unstable or high INRs or poor time in therapeutic range (eg, 60%).
E	Elderly	1	Age >65 y, frail condition
D	Drugs or alcohol (1 point each)	1 or 2	Concomitant use of drugs (eg, antiplatelet agents, nonsteroidal antiinflammatory drugs, or alcohol abuse)

Maximum 9 points.

Abbreviation: INRs, international normalized ratios.

Adapted from Pisters R, Lane DA, Nieuwlaat R, et al. A novel user-friendly score (HAS-BLED) to assess 1-year risk of major bleeding in patients with atrial fibrillation: the euro heart survey. Chest 2010;138:1093–1100; with permission.

anticoagulation due to contraindications or high risk of bleeding, aspirin is unlikely to provide adequate stroke prevention and bears a risk of bleeding comparable to warfarin. The efficacy and clinical place of interventional percutaneous left atrial appendage closure is insufficiently established in AF patients with HF.

Of note, although discontinuation of oral anticoagulation may be required in patients undergoing surgery it can usually be continued at modified doses in most patients undergoing cardiac catheterization, especially if the radial approach is used. Catheter ablation for AF and the implantation of cardiac electronic devices are now widely performed on uninterrupted warfarin with an INR within the therapeutic range.

ORAL ANTICOAGULANTS FOR USE IN AF WITH HF

Oral anticoagulation is effective through inhibition of different coagulation factors. VKAs such as warfarin have been used for more than 50 years, providing effective stroke prevention in AF. The pharmacologic effects of VKAs are based on their ability to downregulate the levels of factors II (prothrombin), VII, IX, and X by interrupting carboxylation of these vitamin K-dependent factors.[42] Vitamin K availability depends on normal activity of the enzyme vitamin K epoxide reductase. Its inhibition by warfarin results in vitamin K depletion and production of functionally inactive factors, thus disrupting coagulation cascades mediated by these factors. However, the usefulness of VKAs is complicated by the need for cumbersome monitoring and numerous food and drug interactions leading to substantial variability in their oral absorption and bioavailability. Warfarin is mainly bound to albumin in the plasma and is metabolized by the liver. It has a relatively long half-life of around 40 hours, which means it often takes several days to reach the therapeutic level. Foods that contain a high level of vitamin K, such as broccoli, reduce the effect of warfarin. Excessive use of alcohol interferes with function of liver enzymes and affects the metabolism of VKAs.[43]

Novel oral anticoagulants have recently focused on selective inhibitors of coagulation factor. Inhibition of the two key factors of the coagulation cascade, factor Xa and factor IIa (thrombin), blocks both extrinsic and intrinsic coagulation cascades (**Table 3**). These two factors are considered the most promising targets for novel anticoagulants.

To ensure effective anticoagulation, it is desirable to block activity of both free and fibrin-bound thrombin. This can be achieved using direct thrombin inhibitors that provide potent inhibition of both forms of thrombin and prevent generation of fibrin from fibrinogen. Dabigatran etexilate, a second-generation, reversible, direct thrombin inhibitor, has been recently licensed for thromboembolism prevention in AF.[44] Dabigatran etexilate possesses the desirable qualities of effective anticoagulant with predictable pharmacokinetics and pharmacodynamics. The drug is rapidly absorbed with therapeutic concentrations achieved within 2 hours, with estimated half-lives of 14 to 17 hours when administered regularly. The drug shows an average bioavailability of 6.5%, thus it requires high doses to maintain therapeutic plasma levels. Simultaneous administration of proton pump inhibitors reduced the absorption of the drug by 20% to 25%.[44] About 80% of dabigatran etexilate is eliminated by the kidneys without biotransformation; therefore, its use is restricted in patients with severe renal dysfunction. These novel oral anticoagulants are usually well tolerated by patients AF with bleeding complications being the most serious reported side-effect.

Direct factor Xa inhibitors, rivaroxaban, and apixaban reversibly inhibit free plasma factor Xa and block factor Xa bound to platelets as part of

Table 3
Mode of action and characteristics of new oral anticoagulants

	Dabigatran	Rivaroxaban	Apixaban
Mode of action	Direct thrombin inhibitor	Direct factor Xa inhibitor	Direct factor Xa inhibitor
Prodrug	Yes	No	No
Dosing	Twice daily	Once daily	Twice daily
Time to peak drug level	2 h	3 h	3 h
Bioavailability	6.5%	60%–80%	>50%
Half-life	14–17 h	9 h	9–14 h
Elimination	80% renal	65% renal, 35% liver	25% renal, 75% fecal
Interaction	Proton pump inhibitors	Potent CYP3A4 inhibitors	Potent CYP3A4 inhibitors

the prothrombinase complex.[45] Both rivaroxaban and apixaban are selective oral direct factor Xa inhibitors with favorable pharmacokinetic profile. Rivaroxaban has a bioavailability of 60% to 80% and its peak plasma levels are reached within 3 hours after administration. The medication has a half-life of 9 hours in young subjects, but it can be longer (about 12 hours) in the older age typical of patients with AF and HF; therefore, it has a potential for one-daily administration. Rivaroxaban is metabolized by the liver via CYP3A4 with about 65% of the metabolite cleared out by the kidneys and the rest eliminated by the liver.[46] Apixaban is a potent and highly selective inhibitor of factor Xa with bioavailability of more than 50% and a half-life of 9 to 14 hours. The drug is metabolized in the liver via CYP3A4 and predominantly excreted by the intestines with about 25% eliminated by the kidneys.[45]

All three novel anticoagulants do not need monitoring of parameters of coagulation but require monitoring of renal function, especially given that there are no established protocols to reverse their anticoagulant action.

The use of dabigatran, rivaroxban, or apixaban for thromboembolism prevention in AF has been tested in large, multicenter, randomized clinical trials. Three key clinical trials, RE-LY (the Randomized Evaluation of Long-Term Anticoagulation Therapy), ROCKET-AF (the Rivaroxaban Once Daily Oral Direct Factor Xa Inhibition Compared with Vitamin K Antagonism for Prevention of Stroke and Embolism Trial in Atrial Fibrillation), and ARISTOTLE (Apixaban for reduction in stroke and other ThromboemboLic events in atrial fibrillation), confirmed the efficacy and good safety profiles of the new drugs, which were at least noninferior to VKAs in thromboprophylaxis and had lower risk of intracranial hemorrhage than warfarin (**Table 4**).[47–49] Moreover, compared with VKAs, twice-daily apixaban and dabigatran 150 mg significantly reduced risk of stroke.[47,49] In addition, treatment with apixaban was associated with lower mortality compared with warfarin.[49] Finally, lower rates of major bleedings were seen in patients receiving dabigatran 110 mg twice daily or apixaban.[47,49] Although these trial were not specifically devoted to patients with HF, such subjects represented a sizable proportion of the participants and subgroup analyses of these three trials have not found any significant detrimental effect of coexisting HF on the treatment effects.[47–49]

The 2012 focused update of the European Society of Cardiology guidelines on the management of AF highlights dabigatran, apixaban, and rivaroxaban as first-line choices of oral anticoagulation.[38] However, their cost is high and this needs to be weighed against the benefits, such as clinical safety, efficacy, and convenience of use. One special consideration relates to patients with renal dysfunction, which is common in HF. The currently approved new oral anticoagulant drugs are contraindicated in severe renal impairment (ie, creatinine clearance <30 mL/min) and lowering of the dose was required in RE-LY, ROCKET-AF, and ARISTOTLE trials in subjects

Table 4
Major clinical trial on new oral anticoagulants in AF

	RE-LY	ROCKET-AF	ARISTOTLE
Active medication	Dabigatran	Rivaroxaban	Apixaban
Participant number	18,113	14,264	18,201
Age	72 ± 9 y	73 (65–78) y	70 (63–76) y
Follow-up duration	2.1 y	3.5 y	2.1 y
Mean $CHADS_2$ score	2.1 ± 1.1	3.5 ± 0.9	2.1 ± 1.1
Paroxysmal AF	32.8%	17.6%	15.3%
Subjects with HF	5793 (32%)	8908 (63%)	6451 (35%)
HF criteria	LVEF <40%, NYHA class ≥II HF symptoms within 6 mo before screening	Symptomatic HF or LVEF ≤35%	Symptomatic HF within the previous 3 mo or LVEF ≤40%
Stroke or systemic thromboembolism	1.5% for 110 mg dose 1.1% for 150 mg dose	2.1%	1.3%
Major bleeding	2.7% for 110 mg dose 3.1% for 150 mg dose	3.6%	1.8%
Interaction with HF	No ($P = .42$ or $P = .33$)	No	No ($P = .50$)

Data from Refs.[47–49]

with moderate kidney dysfunction (creatinine clearance 30–50 mL/min).[47–49]

RATE CONTROL VERSUS RHYTHM CONTROL: DOES IT MATTER FOR STROKE PREVENTION IN HF?

The main clinical trials, which directly compared rate control versus rhythm control strategy for stroke prevention in AF generally failed to prove superiority of one strategy over another. However, these trials provide limited specific evidence in relation to patients with HF. In the Atrial Fibrillation Follow-up Investigation of Rhythm Management (AFFIRM) study,[50,51] only 26% of subjects had evidence of reduced LVEF, and 23% of participants had a history of congestive HF, but only 9% of the subjects had symptoms compatible with New York Heart Association (NYHA) functional class of II or greater. Overall LVEF in the AFFIRM study was relatively good (ie, 55 ± 14%). Of interest, the rhythm control approach was associated with a higher risk of death than the rate control approach only in subjects without congestive HF, with no difference seen in those having HF.

Subjects with HF were better represented in the RAte Control versus Electrical cardioversion for Persistent Atrial Fibrillation (RACE)[52,53] trial with about half of the 512 participants having a history of symptomatic HF and with average left ventricular fractional shortening of 30%. After a mean 2.3-year follow-up, the composite primary end point of death from cardiovascular causes, HF, thromboembolic complications, bleeding, implantation of a pacemaker, and severe adverse effects of drugs developed in 17.2% of those randomized for the rate control strategy and 22.6% of those aiming to maintain sinus rhythm. Although there was a numerical trend toward lower HF rates in the rate control group (3.5% vs 4.5% in the rhythm control group), the difference was not statistically significant, perhaps due to the relatively small study population. Unfortunately, the published data do not provide specific information on how the observed trends could affect risk of stroke in subjects with HF.

According to the results of the How to Treat Chronic Atrial Fibrillation (HOT CAFE) trial,[54] all participants had a certain degree of congestive HF at baseline, although almost half of the subjects had only mild HF symptoms equivalent to NYHA class I. NYHA class 2 to 3 was present in 53% of those randomized to the rate control approach versus 71% of those subjected to the rhythm control strategy, with overall average left ventricular fractional shortening of 31%. In the rhythm control arm only, a significant improvement in exercise tolerance was noticed with a rise in maximal workload ($P<.001$). In addition, rhythm control was linked favorably with left and right atrial remodeling and improvement in left ventricular contractility. However, this did not translate into any significant benefits for stroke or death prevention.

A comparison of the two strategies of AF management in HF was performed in the randomized Atrial Fibrillation and Congestive Heart Failure (AF-CHF) trial[55] of 1376 patients with LVEF <35% (mean LVEF 27 ± 6%) followed for an average for 3 years. Amiodarone was the predominant pharmacologic agent used to achieve rhythm control. There was no difference in mortality or HF-related hospitalizations between the groups. In addition, there was no difference in stroke rates ($P = .68$), but the number of such events was low: 9 (1%) in rhythm control group and 11 (2%) in the rate control group.

It is important to acknowledge that all of these studies have certain limitations requiring cautious interpretation of their results. For example, potential benefits of maintenance of sinus rhythm could have been masked by side effects of currently available treatments. In addition, a sizable proportion of subjects assigned for rhythm control failed to preserve sinus rhythm during the study period.[56] Finally, conditions of strict rate control under the clinical trial environment may not be entirely applicable in real-life settings. Indeed, according to a large population-based observational study of over 40,000 subjects with AF (30% of whom had HF, stroke, or TIA), incidence rate was lower in patients treated with rhythm control than in those on rate control therapy.[57] This was particularly true in patients with moderate-to-high-risk of stroke and the association remained significant in multivariate analysis. In addition, in a substudy from the Danish Investigations of Arrhythmia and Mortality on Dofetilide (DIAMOND) trials, in subjects with AF or atrial flutter and severe systolic left ventricular dysfunction, restoration of sinus rhythm was associated with a significant reduction in mortality.[58] Accordingly, available data on clinical potential of sinus rhythm preservation in patients with AF and HF for stroke prevention are inconclusive and merit further investigation.

SUMMARY

Patients with AF associated with HF have a high risk of stroke. Oral anticoagulation with VKAs or novel licensed medicines should be considered in all such patients unless contraindicated. A risk of anticoagulation-related bleeding should be assessed and regularly reviewed. Possible benefits of sinus rhythm maintenance for stroke prevention in HF are not entirely clear and may need to be explored further as new treatment options emerge. Relatively scarce data are available in relation to HFpEF with further research needed on this clinically and socially important problem.

REFERENCES

1. Linssen GC, Rienstra M, Jaarsma T, et al. Clinical and prognostic effects of atrial fibrillation in heart failure patients with reduced and preserved left ventricular ejection fraction. Eur J Heart Fail 2011; 13:1111–20.
2. Olsson LG, Swedberg K, Ducharme A, et al. Atrial fibrillation and risk of clinical events in chronic heart failure with and without left ventricular systolic dysfunction: results from the Candesartan in Heart Failure-Assessment of Reduction in Mortality and morbidity (CHARM) program. J Am Coll Cardiol 2006;47:1997–2004.
3. Carson PE, Johnson GR, Dunkman WB, et al. The influence of atrial fibrillation on prognosis in mild to moderate heart failure. The V-HeFT Studies. The V-HeFT VA Cooperative Studies Group. Circulation 1993;87:VI102–10.
4. Nieminen MS, Brutsaert D, Dickstein K, et al. EuroHeart Failure Survey II (EHFS II): a survey on hospitalized acute heart failure patients: description of population. Eur Heart J 2006;27:2725–36.
5. Fung JW, Sanderson JE, Yip GW, et al. Impact of atrial fibrillation in heart failure with normal ejection fraction: a clinical and echocardiographic study. J Card Fail 2007;13:649–55.
6. Goyal A, Norton CR, Thomas TN, et al. Predictors of incident heart failure in a large insured population: a one million person-year follow-up study. Circ Heart Fail 2010;3:698–705.
7. Leonard JJ, Shaver J, Thompson M. Left atrial transport function. Trans Am Clin Climatol Assoc 1981;92:133–41.
8. Rahimtoola SH, Ehsani A, Sinno MZ, et al. Left atrial transport function in myocardial infarction. Importance of its booster pump function. Am J Med 1975;59:686–94.
9. Cha YM, Dzeja PP, Shen WK, et al. Failing atrial myocardium: energetic deficits accompany structural remodeling and electrical instability. Am J Physiol Heart Circ Physiol 2003;284:H1313–20.
10. Li D, Shinagawa K, Pang L, et al. Effects of angiotensin-converting enzyme inhibition on the development of the atrial fibrillation substrate in dogs with ventricular tachypacing-induced congestive heart failure. Circulation 2001;104:2608–14.
11. Benjamin EJ, Levy D, Vaziri SM, et al. Independent risk factors for atrial fibrillation in a population-based cohort. The Framingham Heart Study. JAMA 1994;271:840–4.
12. Chamberlain AM, Redfield MM, Alonso A, et al. Atrial fibrillation and mortality in heart failure: a community study. Circ Heart Fail 2011;4:740–6.
13. Maisel WH, Stevenson LW. Atrial fibrillation in heart failure: epidemiology, pathophysiology, and rationale for therapy. Am J Cardiol 2003;91:2D–8D.
14. Camm AJ, Breithardt G, Crijns H, et al. Real-life observations of clinical outcomes with rhythm- and rate-control therapies for atrial fibrillation RECORDAF (Registry on Cardiac Rhythm Disorders Assessing the Control of Atrial Fibrillation). J Am Coll Cardiol 2011;58:493–501.
15. Mountantonakis SE, Grau-Sepulveda MV, Bhatt DL, et al. Presence of atrial fibrillation is independently associated with adverse outcomes in patients hospitalized with heart failure: an analysis of get with the guidelines-heart failure. Circ Heart Fail 2012; 5:191–201.
16. Wasywich CA, Pope AJ, Somaratne J, et al. Atrial fibrillation and the risk of death in patients with heart failure: a literature-based meta-analysis. Intern Med J 2010;40:347–56.
17. Risk factors for stroke and efficacy of antithrombotic therapy in atrial fibrillation. Analysis of pooled data from five randomized controlled trials. Arch Intern Med 1994;154:1449–57.
18. Pozzoli M, Cioffi G, Traversi E, et al. Predictors of primary atrial fibrillation and concomitant clinical and hemodynamic changes in patients with chronic heart failure: a prospective study in 344 patients with baseline sinus rhythm. J Am Coll Cardiol 1998;32:197–204.
19. Jang SJ, Kim MS, Park HJ, et al. Impact of heart failure with normal ejection fraction on the occurrence of ischaemic stroke in patients with atrial fibrillation. Heart 2013;99(1):17–21.
20. Blackshear JL, Odell JA. Appendage obliteration to reduce stroke in cardiac surgical patients with atrial fibrillation. Ann Thorac Surg 1996;61:755–9.
21. Pollick C, Taylor D. Assessment of left atrial appendage function by transesophageal echocardiography. Implications for the development of thrombus. Circulation 1991;84:223–31.
22. Sanfilippo AJ, Abascal VM, Sheehan M, et al. Atrial enlargement as a consequence of atrial fibrillation. A prospective echocardiographic study. Circulation 1990;82:792–7.
23. Predictors of thromboembolism in atrial fibrillation: II. Echocardiographic features of patients at risk. The Stroke Prevention in Atrial Fibrillation Investigators. Ann Intern Med 1992;116:6–12.
24. Di Tullio MR, Sacco RL, Sciacca RR, et al. Left atrial size and the risk of ischemic stroke in an ethnically mixed population. Stroke 1999;30:2019–24.
25. Watson T, Shantsila E, Lip GY. Mechanisms of thrombogenesis in atrial fibrillation: Virchow's triad revisited. Lancet 2009;373:155–66.

26. Masawa N, Yoshida Y, Yamada T, et al. Diagnosis of cardiac thrombosis in patients with atrial fibrillation in the absence of macroscopically visible thrombi. Virchows Arch A Pathol Anat Histopathol 1993;422:67–71.
27. Marin F, Roldan V, Climent VE, et al. Plasma von Willebrand factor, soluble thrombomodulin, and fibrin D-dimer concentrations in acute onset nonrheumatic atrial fibrillation. Heart 2004;90:1162–6.
28. Shantsila E, Wrigley BJ, Blann AD, et al. A contemporary view on endothelial function in heart failure. Eur J Heart Fail 2012;14:873–81.
29. Vaduganathan M, Greene SJ, Butler J, et al. The immunological axis in heart failure: importance of the leukocyte differential. Heart Fail Rev 2013; 99(1):17–21.
30. Watson T, Shantsila E, Lip GY. Fibrin d-dimer levels and thromboembolic events in patients with atrial fibrillation. Int J Cardiol 2007;120:123–4 [author reply 125–6].
31. Lip GY, Lowe GD, Rumley A, et al. Increased markers of thrombogenesis in chronic atrial fibrillation: effects of warfarin treatment. Br Heart J 1995; 73:527–33.
32. McMurray JJ, Adamopoulos S, Anker SD, et al. ESC guidelines for the diagnosis and treatment of acute and chronic heart failure 2012: the Task Force for the Diagnosis and Treatment of Acute and Chronic Heart Failure 2012 of the European Society of Cardiology. Developed in collaboration with the Heart Failure Association (HFA) of the ESC. Eur Heart J 2012;33:1787–847.
33. Lip GY, Nieuwlaat R, Pisters R, et al. Refining clinical risk stratification for predicting stroke and thromboembolism in atrial fibrillation using a novel risk factor-based approach: the euro heart survey on atrial fibrillation. Chest 2010;137:263–72.
34. Gheorghiade M, Pang PS. Acute heart failure syndromes. J Am Coll Cardiol 2009;53:557–73.
35. Gheorghiade M, Abraham WT, Albert NM, et al. Systolic blood pressure at admission, clinical characteristics, and outcomes in patients hospitalized with acute heart failure. JAMA 2006;296:2217–26.
36. Jessup M, Abraham WT, Casey DE, et al. 2009 focused update: ACCF/AHA Guidelines for the Diagnosis and Management of Heart Failure in Adults: a report of the American College of Cardiology Foundation/American Heart Association Task Force on Practice Guidelines: developed in collaboration with the International Society for Heart and Lung Transplantation. Circulation 2009;119: 1977–2016.
37. Pisters R, Lane DA, Nieuwlaat R, et al. A novel user-friendly score (HAS-BLED) to assess 1-year risk of major bleeding in patients with atrial fibrillation: the Euro Heart survey. Chest 2010;138:1093–100.
38. Camm AJ, Lip GY, De Caterina R, et al. 2012 focused update of the ESC Guidelines for the management of atrial fibrillation: an update of the 2010 ESC Guidelines for the management of atrial fibrillation. Developed with the special contribution of the European Heart Rhythm Association. Eur Heart J 2012;33:2719–47.
39. Camm AJ, Kirchhof P, Lip GY, et al. Guidelines for the management of atrial fibrillation: the Task Force for the Management of Atrial Fibrillation of the European Society of Cardiology (ESC). Eur Heart J 2010;31:2369–429.
40. You JJ, Singer DE, Howard PA, et al. Antithrombotic therapy for atrial fibrillation: antithrombotic therapy and prevention of thrombosis, 9th ed: American college of chest physicians evidence-based clinical practice guidelines. Chest 2012; 141:e531S–75S.
41. Roberts GW, Helboe T, Nielsen CB, et al. Assessment of an age-adjusted warfarin initiation protocol. Ann Pharmacother 2003;37:799–803.
42. Ansell J, Hirsh J, Poller L, et al. The pharmacology and management of the vitamin k antagonists: the Seventh ACCP Conference on Antithrombotic and Thrombolytic Therapy. Chest 2004;126:204S–33S.
43. Holbrook AM, Pereira JA, Labiris R, et al. Systematic overview of warfarin and its drug and food interactions. Arch Intern Med 2005;165: 1095–106.
44. Stangier J, Rathgen K, Stahle H, et al. The pharmacokinetics, pharmacodynamics and tolerability of dabigatran etexilate, a new oral direct thrombin inhibitor, in healthy male subjects. Br J Clin Pharmacol 2007;64:292–303.
45. Khoo CW, Tay KH, Shantsila E, et al. Novel oral anticoagulants. Int J Clin Pract 2009;63:630–41.
46. Kubitza D, Becka M, Voith B, et al. Safety, pharmacodynamics, and pharmacokinetics of single doses of bay 59-7939, an oral, direct factor xa inhibitor. Clin Pharmacol Ther 2005;78:412–21.
47. Connolly SJ, Ezekowitz MD, Yusuf S, et al. Dabigatran versus warfarin in patients with atrial fibrillation. N Engl J Med 2009;361:1139–51.
48. Granger CB, Alexander JH, McMurray JJ, et al. Apixaban versus warfarin in patients with atrial fibrillation. N Engl J Med 2011;365:981–92.
49. Patel MR, Mahaffey KW, Garg J, et al. Rivaroxaban versus warfarin in nonvalvular atrial fibrillation. N Engl J Med 2011;365:883–91.
50. Wyse DG, Waldo AL, DiMarco JP, et al. A comparison of rate control and rhythm control in patients with atrial fibrillation. N Engl J Med 2002;347:1825–33.
51. Corley SD, Epstein AE, DiMarco JP, et al. Relationships between sinus rhythm, treatment, and survival in the Atrial Fibrillation Follow-Up Investigation of

Rhythm Management (AFFIRM) Study. Circulation 2004;109:1509–13.
52. Van Gelder IC, Hagens VE, Bosker HA, et al. A comparison of rate control and rhythm control in patients with recurrent persistent atrial fibrillation. N Engl J Med 2002;347:1834–40.
53. Hagens VE, Crijns HJ, Van Veldhuisen DJ, et al. Rate control versus rhythm control for patients with persistent atrial fibrillation with mild to moderate heart failure: results from the RAte Control versus Electrical cardioversion (RACE) study. Am Heart J 2005;149:1106–11.
54. Opolski G, Torbicki A, Kosior DA, et al. Rate control vs rhythm control in patients with nonvalvular persistent atrial fibrillation: the results of the Polish How to Treat Chronic Atrial Fibrillation (HOT CAFE) Study. Chest 2004;126:476–86.
55. Roy D, Talajic M, Nattel S, et al. Rhythm control versus rate control for atrial fibrillation and heart failure. N Engl J Med 2008;358:2667–77.
56. Humphries KH, Kerr CR, Steinbuch M, et al. Limitations to antiarrhythmic drug use in patients with atrial fibrillation. CMAJ 2004;171:741–5.
57. Tsadok MA, Jackevicius CA, Essebag V, et al. Rhythm versus rate control therapy and subsequent stroke or transient ischemic attack in patients with atrial fibrillation. Circulation 2012;126:2680–7.
58. Pedersen OD, Bagger H, Keller N, et al. Efficacy of dofetilide in the treatment of atrial fibrillation-flutter in patients with reduced left ventricular function: a Danish investigations of arrhythmia and mortality on dofetilide (diamond) substudy. Circulation 2001;104:292–6.

Impact of Atrial Fibrillation on Outcomes in Heart Failure

Eugene C. DePasquale, MD, Gregg C. Fonarow, MD*

KEYWORDS

• Atrial fibrillation • Heart failure treatment • Prognosis • Antiarrhythmic therapy
• Antithrombotic therapy • Catheter ablation

KEY POINTS

- The presence of atrial fibrillation (AF) is a marker of worse prognosis in patients with heart failure (HF), associated with increased morbidity and mortality.
- Management strategies are aimed at limiting symptoms through rate or rhythm control as well as anticoagulation to prevent systemic embolization and stroke, avoiding therapies that increase mortality in the population with HF.
- Current data suggest that pharmacologic rhythm control has no advantage over rate control.
- It remains unknown whether prompt restoration of sinus rhythm or aggressive rate control in patients hospitalized with new-onset AF is beneficial; further study is required.
- Improvements in invasive strategies to restore sinus rhythm have resulted in increased efficacy and safety; however, further data are warranted to determine their role in the treatment of AF in HF.
- New anticoagulants have emerged and present their unique advantages and challenges.
- Advances in pharmacotherapy, nonpharmacologic therapies, and treatment strategies have benefited patients with AF and heart failure.

Atrial fibrillation (AF) affects many patients with heart failure (HF). The prevalence of both AF and HF increases with advancing age, and the 2 conditions can precipitate one another. It is estimated that the annual incidence of AF in the general HF population is approximately 5%, whereas as many as 40% of patients with advanced HF have AF. Like the general population of patients with AF, the main goals of therapy in patients with HF and AF are symptom control and prevention of arterial thromboembolism. The adverse hemodynamic events of AF may quickly lead to symptom deterioration and reduced exercise capacity, providing significant management challenges.[1–3] This review addresses the impact of AF on HF outcomes as they pertain to prognosis and management.

EPIDEMIOLOGY

AF and HF are both major causes of cardiovascular morbidity and mortality. Decompensated HF may be precipitated by loss of atrial contraction and rapid irregular heart rates, whereas HF progression may lead to AF through increased left atrial stretch. The incidence of AF was examined in a Framingham Heart Study (n = 1470) in which 22% of 708 patients who developed HF without previous AF subsequently developed AF (incidence rate 5.4% per year).[4,5] A subsequent study

Disclosures: None (E.C. DePasquale). NHLBI, research, significant; AHRQ, research, significant; Novartis, consultant, significant; Medtronic, consultant, modest (G.C. Fonarow).
Ahmanson-UCLA Cardiomyopathy Center, Division of Cardiology, David Geffen School of Medicine, 100 UCLA Medical Plaza, Suite 630 East, Los Angeles, CA 90095, USA
* Corresponding author. Ahmanson-UCLA Cardiomyopathy Center, Ronald Reagan UCLA Medical Center, 10833 LeConte Avenue, Room 47-123 CHS, Los Angeles, CA 90095-1679.
E-mail address: gfonarow@mednet.ucla.edu

Heart Failure Clin 9 (2013) 437–449
http://dx.doi.org/10.1016/j.hfc.2013.07.009

from Framingham reported that the odds ratio (OR) for developing AF among patients with HF was 4.5 for men and 4.9 for women over a 2-year period[6,7] compared with patients without HF.

The prevalence of AF in the HF population increases with advancing age and has been reported from less than 10% up to 50%, with variations depending on New York Heart Association (NYHA) class and severity of HF.[8–13] A direct relationship between NYHA class and the occurrence of AF has been shown, with prevalence increasing from 4% to 40% with progression from NYHA I to NYHA IV.[14–22]

DOES AF INDEPENDENTLY PREDICT MORTALITY?

Data conflict as to whether AF is an independent predictor of mortality in patients with HF. Three-year follow-up of the SOLVD (Studies of Left Ventricular Dysfunction) trial (n = 6517), which consisted of patients with asymptomatic left ventricular dysfunction or NYHA class II to III HF, showed that AF (present in 6.4%) was a significant predictor of all-cause mortality (34 vs 23%) and was maintained after multivariate analysis.[14,23] In CHARM (Candesartan in Heart Failure Assessment of Reduction in Mortality and Morbidity), 7599 patients with symptomatic HF with either reduced or preserved ejection fraction were enrolled, of which baseline AF was present in approximately 18%. AF was shown to be an independent predictor of all-cause mortality in this population in both HF with reduced ejection fraction (37 vs 28% in patients without AF) or preserved ejection fraction (24 vs 14%).[24,25]

However, the V-HeFT (Vasodilator Heart Failure Trial) trials of 1427 patients with NYHA class II to III, of whom 14% had AF, did not show a significant difference in 2-year mortality or hospitalization for HF.[9,26] Similarly, a study examining the prognostic effect of AF on HF in both a national population in New Zealand (n = 55,106) and a cohort of 197 patients recruited after HF admission into the Auckland Heart Failure Management Study reported that the presence of AF in these 2 populations was not associated with an adverse prognosis.[27,28]

However, more recent data from the Get With The Guidelines Heart Failure Registry suggest otherwise. In 99,810 patients with HF enrolled in the registry between 2005 and 2010, patients with AF on admission (31.4%) were compared with those in sinus rhythm. In this cohort, AF was found to be independently associated with adverse hospital outcomes (hospital mortality 4.0% vs 2.6%, *P*<.001) and increased length of stay (>4 days: 48.8% vs 41.5%, *P*<.001). Analysis also showed that hospital outcomes were worse in those with newly diagnosed AF (adjusted OR for mortality [95% confidence internal (CI)] 1.29 [1.10–1.52] vs 1.17 [1.05–1.29]) (**Fig. 1**).[26,29] It remains unknown whether the association between new-onset AF and mortality is causative or whether the development of AF is a marker of more advanced disease. Despite conflicting reports in the literature, more recent data show that AF is at minimum a marker of adverse

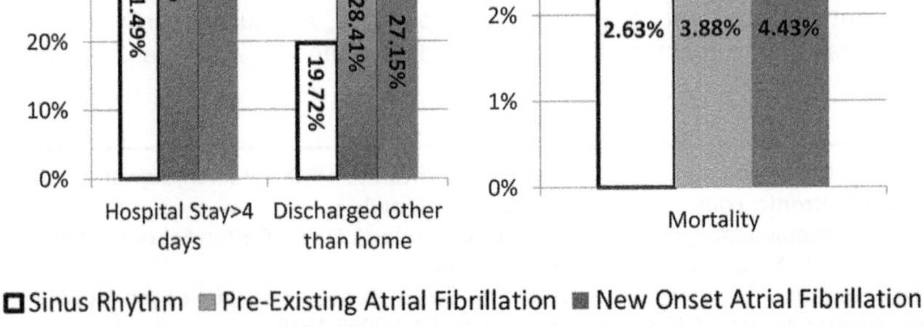

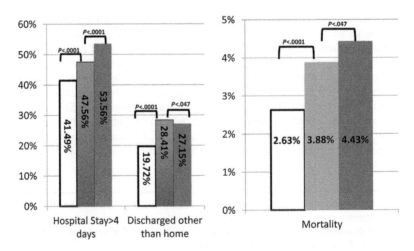

Fig. 1. Hospital outcomes stratified by AF groups. (*From* Mountantonakis SE, Grau-Sepulveda MV, Bhatt DL, et al. Presence of atrial fibrillation is independently associated with adverse outcomes in patients hospitalized with heart failure. Circ Heart Fail 2012;5(2):198; with permission.)

outcomes in this population, if not a mediator of adverse outcomes.

AF MANAGEMENT IN THE SETTING OF HF

AF can lead to worsening symptoms in patients with HF, and uncontrolled HF may precipitate or accelerate the ventricular response of AF or result in AF in those in sinus rhythm. It is critical that all reversible causes of both AF and HF be identified and corrected. Symptomatic patients with AF with rapid ventricular rates may require therapy to slow the ventricular response before any considerations of rate versus rhythm control strategies.

Rhythm Versus Rate Control

Rate and rhythm control strategies have been tested in various studies with the hypothesis that restoration and maintenance of sinus rhythm allow HF symptoms to be more easily controlled. The AF and Congestive Heart Failure (AF-CHF) trial was designed to determine whether long-term rhythm control is superior to rate control in patients with HF with reduced ejection fraction and AF. In this trial, 1376 patients with left ventricular dysfunction were randomized to a strategy of rhythm control (amiodarone, sotalol, or dofetilide) or rate control. No significant difference was observed between groups in the primary outcome of cardiovascular death or outcome of event-free survival (mean follow-up 37 months) (**Fig. 2**).[30–32] There was also no difference in quality of life with similar 6-minute walk distance assessments and NYHA class.[33–36] However, evidence from subsets of patients with HF in the AFFIRM (Atrial Fibrillation Follow-Up Investigation of Rhythm Management), RACE (Rate Control vs Electrical Cardioversion for Persistent Atrial Fibrillation Study) and DIAMOND (Danish Investigations of Arrhythmia and Mortality ON Dofetilide) trials have presented conflicting data on mortality, thromboembolic complications, and hospitalization in patients receiving rhythm control therapy.[24,25,36–41]

Rate Control

Rate control to prevent AF with rapid ventricular response may lead to improvement in symptoms in those with HF. Post hoc analysis of the US Carvedilol Heart Failure Trials (n = 1094) showed the potential benefit of rate control in 136 patients with HF with reduced left ventricular ejection fraction and AF, with resulting improved ejection fraction and a trend toward reduction in the combined end point of death and HF hospitalization.[11,42] It remains unknown if the improved outcomes observed are caused by rate control or the beneficial effect of the β-blocker in HF.

Initiation or increase of β-blockers in patients with decompensated HF is contraindicated.[33,43] In this setting, the use of digoxin for rate control may be beneficial. However, digoxin may be ineffective when used alone, particularly in patients with increased sympathetic tone.[44–46] Nondihydropyridine calcium channel blockers (ie, diltiazem, verapamil) should be used sparingly and

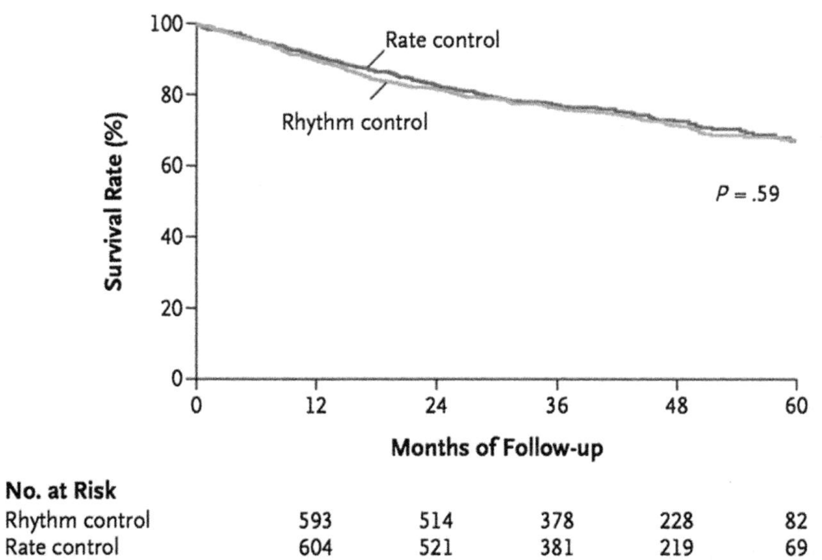

Fig. 2. Kaplan-Meier estimates of death from cardiovascular causes in patients with AF and HF treated with rhythm or rate control strategies in the AF-CHF trial. (*From* Roy D, Talajic M, Nattel S, et al. Rhythm control versus rate control for atrial fibrillation and heart failure. N Engl J Med 2008;358(25):2667–77; with permission.)

with caution, because there is significant risk of worsening HF in those with reduced ejection fraction. However, nondihydropyridine calcium channel blockers may be a reasonable choice for rate control of AF in HF with preserved ejection fraction.[4,33,47] Amiodarone may be useful as an adjunct when the use of β-blocker or combination therapy with digoxin does not achieve rate control. Amiodarone is not recommended as a chronic rate control therapy, and therapeutic anticoagulation should be maintained, because there is a possibility of pharmacologically restoring sinus rhythm.[8,33]

The strictness of rate control was examined in RACE II (The Rate Control Efficacy in Permanent Atrial Fibrillation: a Comparison Between Lenient vs Strict Rate Control II trial). In this trial, 614 patients with permanent AF (of whom approximately 10% had history of hospitalization because of HF) were randomized to either a strict (resting heart rate <80 beats per minute [bpm] and heart rate during moderate exercise <110 bpm) or lenient (resting heart rate <110 bpm) rate control strategy. There was no difference in the composite primary outcome of death from cardiovascular causes, hospitalization for HF, and stroke, systemic embolism, bleeding, and life-threatening arrhythmic events (**Fig. 3**).[10,48–50] It is unclear how well this trial applies to the HF population, because there were few patients with HF or reduced ejection fraction in the study. Nevertheless, it may be reasonable to start with a lenient approach and convert to a strict approach in patients who remain symptomatic.

Other strategies for rate control may include a more invasive approach in those in whom pharmacologic rate control has been ineffective or contraindicated. Rate control may be accomplished with radiofrequency ablation of the atrioventricular node and permanent pacemaker placement.[4,51,52] In patients with HF with reduced ejection fraction in whom ventricular pacing may occur greater than 40% of the time, cardiac resynchronization therapy should be strongly considered, because isolated right ventricular pacing may worsen HF and increase frequency of AF, as shown in the DAVID (Dual Chamber and VVI Implantable Defibrillator) and MOST (Mode Selection Trial) trials.[51–54]

The SHIFT trial (Systolic Heart Failure Treatment with the I_f Inhibitor Ivabradine Trial) was a randomized double-blind placebo-controlled parallel group study for patients who were symptomatic with HF with reduced ejection fraction who were in sinus rhythm with heart rate 70 bpm or higher admitted within the previous year for HF on baseline β-blockade in which patients were randomized to ivabradine (n = 3241) or placebo (n = 3264). Although AF was an exclusion criterion for this trial, approximately 8% of patients in each group had history of AF or atrial flutter. The primary end point (composite of cardiovascular death or admission

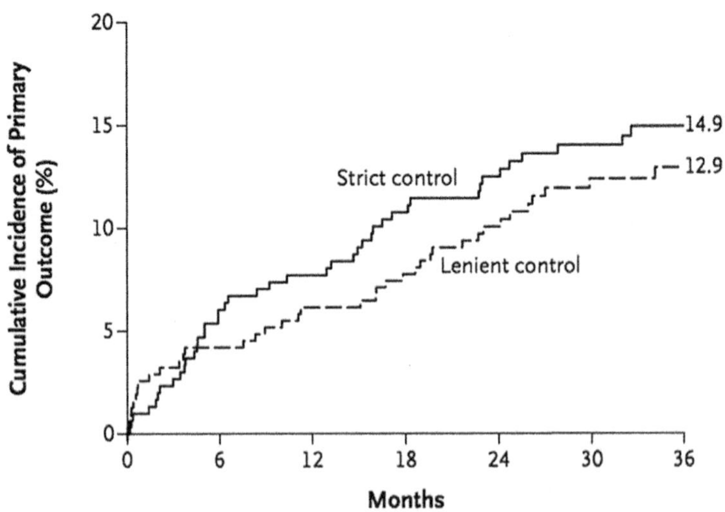

No. at Risk							
Strict control	303	282	273	262	246	212	131
Lenient control	311	298	290	285	255	218	138

Fig. 3. Kaplan-Meier estimates of the cumulative incidence of major adverse cardiac events in patients with AF treated with either strict or lenient rate control strategies in the RACE II trial. (*From* Van Gelder IC, Groenveld HF, Crijns HJ, et al. Lenient versus strict rate control in patients with atrial fibrillation. N Engl J Med 2010;362(15):1371; with permission.)

for worsening HF) was lower in the ivabradine group (24% compared with 29% in the placebo group). This finding was driven by reduction in HF admissions (16% vs 21%, hazard ratio 0.74, 95% CI 0.66–0.83, $P<.001$) and deaths caused by HF (3% vs 5%, hazard ratio 0.74, 95% CI 0.58–0.94, $P = .014$).[55–57] This trial showed that heart rate reduction led to improvement in HF outcomes. These findings are interesting and raise new questions in light of studies showing no significant difference between strict and lenient rate control in RACE II.

Rhythm Control

Rhythm control may be reasonable in patients with HF with AF who are hemodynamically unstable or symptomatic despite rate control.[45] Rhythm control typically commences with direct current cardioversion, particularly in those with sudden-onset HF. Attempts at stabilization and rate control should be pursued before anticipated acute cardioversion. Some practitioners advocate cardioversion without adjunctive antiarrhythmic therapies for an initial episode of AF, and antiarrhythmic therapy in those with recurrent AF episodes. However, in patients with HF, antiarrhythmic agents are typically required to maintain sinus rhythm after cardioversion, especially if there is significant left atrial dilatation.

Rhythm control is usually undertaken with the premise that maintenance of sinus rhythm leads to improved outcomes (eg, reduced symptoms or HF admissions). However, as previously discussed, current evidence suggests no significant difference in mortality or event-free survival between rate or rhythm control approaches. Antiarrhythmic therapies to maintain sinus rhythm are not without risk or side effects and in some cases have raised concerns about increased mortality.[33,58] Current guidelines from the American College of Cardiology (ACC)/American Heart Association (AHA)/Heart Rhythm Society recommend amiodarone and dofetilide as first-line therapy to maintain sinus rhythm in patients with HF and AF.[33,59] However, the European Society of Cardiology (ESC) does not recommend dofetilide (which has limited availability in Europe, anyway) in AF.[60] In addition, dronedarone is not recommended for patients with NYHA class II HF with recent exacerbation and is contraindicated in patients with NYHA class III or IV HF.[60]

Pharmacotherapy

β-blockers

Most patients with HF and AF require a β-blocker to reduce the ventricular rate as well as part of guideline-directed medical therapy for HF with reduced ejection fraction. A meta-analysis of 8680 patients, representing 4 randomized trials, of β-blockade therapy in patients with HF evaluated outcomes in those with AF (n = 1677) and those without AF. No mortality benefit of β-blockers was observed in patients with HF and AF (OR 0.86, 95% CI 0.66–1.13), which may reflect the low event rate in the meta-analysis.[1] However, in general, β-blockade is recommended as guideline-directed medical therapy in HF with reduced ejection fraction.[4]

Amiodarone

Amiodarone at lower doses does not have a negative inotropic effect. In addition, there is a low incidence of QT prolongation and little proarrhythmia, as shown in a meta-analysis (n = 1465) in which 738 patients received low doses of amiodarone. Amiodarone also tends to slow ventricular rates in AF because of its β-blocking and calcium channel–blocking activity.[6] CHF-STAT (Congestive Heart Failure Trial of Antiarrhythmic Therapy) randomized 667 patients with HF with reduced ejection fraction, of whom 15% had AF at baseline, to amiodarone or placebo. This trial reported that amiodarone was able to prevent the development of new-onset AF (4.1% vs 8.3%) and significantly reduce ventricular rate in patients with persistent AF. In addition, amiodarone showed the ability to spontaneously convert AF to sinus rhythm (31% vs 8% in control individuals).[8] However, there are potential adverse events that may occur during the loading phase. In a series of 37 consecutive patients with HF with reduced ejection fraction initiated on amiodarone therapy for AF or atrial flutter,[14] 32% developed bradycardia and 19% required a permanent pacemaker. Amiodarone has many well-documented side effects, including but not limited to pulmonary toxicity, thyroid abnormalities (hypothyroidism and hyperthyroidism), dermatologic manifestations, and gastrointestinal side effects. Amiodarone may be initiated as an outpatient and has low risk of torsades de pointe.[14]

Dofetilide

Dofetilide is a class III antiarrhythmic drug that has been shown to be effective in preventing recurrent AF in patients with HF. In the DIAMOND studies, 506 patients with HF with reduced ejection fraction and baseline AF or atrial flutter were randomized to placebo or dofetilide (n = 234). During the study, those treated with dofetilide were more likely to convert to sinus rhythm (59 vs 34%), with 79% (vs 42%) maintaining sinus rhythm at 1 year.[24] In the larger DIAMOND-CHF trial, in which 1518 patients with HF with reduced ejection fraction (391 with baseline AF) were enrolled and randomized to either dofetilide or placebo, dofetilide showed a significant association with conversion to sinus rhythm at 1 year with no mortality difference at a mean follow-up of 18 months (41 vs 42%). In those with restoration and maintenance of sinus rhythm, mortality was lower independent of therapy. The risk of HF hospitalization was also significantly reduced in the dofetilide treatment group (risk ratio 0.75, 95% CI 0.63–0.89).[26] In addition, a mortality difference was observed when analyzed by baseline corrected QT (QTc) interval. In those with a normal QTc, dofetilide was associated with mortality reduction (risk ratio 0.4, 95% CI 0.3–0.8). However, mortality increased when the QTc was greater than 479 milliseconds (risk ratio 1.3, 95% CI 0.8–1.9). The most clinically important side effect observed was torsades de pointes occurring in 3.3% (n = 25).[27] Patients must be hospitalized to initiate dofetilide to allow for assessment of creatinine clearance and cardiac monitoring, because most episodes of torsades occurred during the initial 3-day period of initiation of therapy.[26]

Dronedarone

Dronedarone has been shown to be effective in maintaining sinus rhythm, reducing ventricular rate during arrhythmia recurrence, and reducing hospitalization caused by cardiovascular events or death in a broad population.[30,32] However, current guidelines do not support the use of dronedarone in patients with NYHA class III to IV HF or HF with reduced ejection fraction.[33,35,36] The US Food and Drug Administration and European Medicines Agency offered similar recommendations in 2011. In ANDROMEDA (Antiarrhythmic Trial with Dronedarone in Moderate to Severe CHF Evaluating Morbidity Decrease),[36] the safety and efficacy of dronedarone (n = 310) was compared with placebo (n = 317) in symptomatic patients with HF with reduced ejection fraction. This trial was discontinued early because of a significant increase in mortality in those assigned to the dronedarone group (8.1% vs 3.8%) at 2 months follow-up related to HF worsening. The safety and efficacy of dronedarone in NYHA class I/II patients with HF are unclear. In addition, there are concerns regarding use of dronedarone in permanent AF. In the PALLAS trial (n = 3236), of which the majority were NYHA class I/II, patients were randomized to dronedarone or placebo. The study was terminated early because of increased rates of HF, stroke, and death from cardiovascular causes.[42]

Sotalol

Sotalol should be used with great caution if at all in patients with HF. Sotalol may increase the risk of torsades de pointes, which is enhanced in the setting of electrolyte abnormalities, reduced ejection fraction, acute-onset or decompensated HF, or renal dysfunction. In 1 large study (n = 3135),[43] 5.0% of patients with HF history experienced torsades with sotalol (compared with 1.7% with no previous history). A meta-analysis examining the safety of sotalol showed that proarrhythmia was associated with HF history, sustained ventricular tachycardia, and myocardial infarction.[44] The SWORD (Survival With Oral D-sotalol) trial reported that sotalol was associated with higher relative risk of mortality than placebo in those with an ejection fraction of 40% or less.[47] ACC/AHA guidelines do not support the use of sotalol in this population.[33]

Class IC antiarrhythmic drugs

Class IC drugs such as flecainide and propafenone are associated with increased risk for proarrhythmias and sudden cardiac death. These medications are not recommended for use in patients with HF. A meta-analysis reported that with increasing HF severity, there was increased risk of spontaneous complex ventricular arrhythmias.[10,48,50]

Angiotensin-converting enzyme inhibitors and angiotensin receptor blockers

Initial studies have suggested that angiotensin-converting enzyme inhibitors (ACEIs) and angiotensin receptor blockers (ARBs) may reduce major adverse cardiovascular events in AF and prevent new-onset and recurrent AF. However, although there are no data to suggest these therapies for this primary purpose, ACEIs and ARBs have been shown to be efficacious in HF, particularly HF with reduced ejection fraction.[4] In the TRACE (Trandolapril Cardiac Evaluation) study of patients with left ventricular dysfunction and sinus rhythm after an acute myocardial infarction,[53] trandolapril was associated with a significant reduction in subsequent development of AF in follow-up at 2 to 4 years compared with placebo. Similar findings were noted in the SOLVD and Val-HeFT (Valsartan Heart Failure Trial) trials.[55,57] However, the ACTIVE I (Atrial Fibrillation Clopidogrel Trial with Irbesartan for Prevention of Vascular Events) trial presented contrary data in 9016 patients with AF history, stroke risk factors, and systolic blood pressure of at least 110 mm Hg randomized to either irbesartan or placebo. Those receiving irbesartan were not more likely to remain in sinus rhythm at baseline, regardless of baseline rhythm (risk ratio

0.97, $P = .61$).[61] Given limited evidence, the guidelines do not support ACEI or ARB therapy for prevention of new-onset AF or secondary prevention of AF, although these agents are recommended for HF and reduced ejection fraction.

Nonpharmacologic Approaches

AF is often triggered by ectopic atrial beats originating from the pulmonary vein ostia. Ablation of these foci or the complete electrical isolation of the pulmonary veins may be accomplished by radiofrequency catheter ablation or surgically.[62,63] This strategy may be beneficial when rate and rhythm control strategies have been unsuccessful. In a matched study of 58 consecutive patients (NYHA class II-IV) with ejection fraction less than 45% who underwent pulmonary vein isolation,[62] successful ablation was achieved without antiarrhythmic therapy in 69% of those with HF (vs 71% without HF) noted at 1 year after the last procedure. NYHA class, quality of life, exercise capacity, and exercise time had significant improvements in both groups. Long-term efficacy in this population remains uncertain.

The Pulmonary Vein Antrum Isolation versus AV Node Ablation with Bi-Ventricular Pacing for Treatment of Atrial Fibrillation in Patients with Congestive Heart Failure Trial (PABA-CHF)[64] examined the efficacy of pulmonary vein isolation ablation compared with atrioventricular node ablation with biventricular pacing for rate control in a randomized trial of 81 patients with NYHA class II/III HF with symptomatic AF refractory to medical therapy. At 6 months, pulmonary vein isolation was associated with significant improvements in quality of life, left ventricular ejection fraction, and 6-minute walk distance. However, longer follow-up periods and larger studies are warranted to confirm these findings.

ANTICOAGULATION

Most patients with AF with HF meet criteria for long-term anticoagulation because of increased risk of embolization, whether or not a rate control or rhythm control strategy is used. There are various risk models that can guide choice of therapy for anticoagulation. A detailed discussion of these models is beyond the scope of this review. However, one of the best validated models is the CHADS2 risk score, which incorporates the presence of HF, hypertension, age greater than 75 years, diabetes, and previous transient ischemic attack or stroke as variables in the model, all of which are weighted with 1 point, except for stroke or transient ischemic attack, which is weighted as 2 points. The more sensitive CHA2DS2-VASc score adds weight to those older than 74 years and incorporates female sex and vascular disease as additional risk factors.[65]

The risks and benefits of anticoagulation must be evaluated before selecting an agent. The HF population have CHADS2 or CHA2DS2-VASc scores of at least 1 by definition. Aspirin therapy (81–325 mg daily) or warfarin (international normalized ratio [INR] 2.0–3.0) is recommended for patients with a CHADS2 score of 1 alone, although this choice may be mitigated by other clinical characteristics (ie, prosthetic valve) as well as physician and patient preference. Patients with CHADS2/CHA2DS2-VASc scores of 2 or greater are at relatively high risk of stroke (annual risk of at least 4%), and anticoagulant therapy is strongly recommended.[33] Warfarin and newer anticoagulants are available to reduce stroke risk in these patients. Warfarin significantly lowers risk of embolism and stroke compared with placebo. Multiple studies have concluded that newer agents (dabigatran, apixaban, rivaroxaban) have similar or lower rates of both ischemic stroke and bleeding, which may support the use of these therapies as alternatives to warfarin.

Warfarin

Several trials with more than 4000 patients randomizing those with nonvalvular/nonrheumatic AF to aspirin, warfarin, or placebo have shown significantly reduced stroke risk with warfarin compared with aspirin or placebo. Mortality was also significantly reduced compared with no antithrombotic therapy with warfarin.[66–69] More recent studies continue to support warfarin efficacy; however, lower absolute levels of stroke risk have been recently observed, which result in a smaller absolute benefit of therapy.[70] In the RE-LY (Randomized Evaluation of Long-Term Anticoagulation Therapy), ROCKET AF (Rivaroxaban Once Daily Oral Direct Factor Xa Inhibition Compared with Vitamin K Antagonism for Prevention of Stroke and Embolism Trial in Atrial Fibrillation), and ARISTOTLE (Apixaban for Reduction in Stroke and Other Thromboembolic Events in Atrial Fibrillation) trials, the risk of stroke or systemic embolism in more than 20,000 patients was 1.7%, 2.2%, and 1.6% per year, respectively. A meta-analysis of 8 randomized trials with more than 55,000 patients treated with warfarin found an annual incidence of stroke or embolism of 1.66%.[71] A major safety concern of warfarin and all anticoagulants is bleeding risk. The absolute rate of major bleeding (bleeding requiring hospitalization, transfusion, surgery, or certain anatomic locations) with warfarin was significantly higher compared with aspirin in a meta-analysis of 6 randomized controlled trials (2.2 vs 1.3 events per 100 patient-years).[72] There is also underutilization of anticoagulation.[65,73] In the ORBIT-AF (Outcomes Registry for Better Informed Treatment of AF) registry of 10,098 patients, more than 70% had CHADS2 scores greater than or equal to 2; however, more than 25% were not treated with systemic anticoagulation (warfarin or dabigatran), despite relative or absolute contraindications in only 14%.[65]

Direct Thrombin and Factor Xa Inhibitors

Dabigatran (direct thrombin inhibitor), apixaban, and rivaroxaban (factor Xa inhibitors) have been compared with warfarin in large randomized trials of intermediate-risk to high-risk patients. These therapies have shown similar or better efficacy and safety compared with warfarin, but do not have the advantage of long-term data. These newer agents do not require INR monitoring. These agents are less affected by dietary and drug interactions. However, these therapies may require twice-daily dosing and may be higher in cost. These agents lack a reversal agent and may require dose adjustment in chronic kidney disease.[74] The ACC/AHA guidelines recommend dabigatran as an alternative to warfarin; however, although approved by the Food and Drug Administration, there are currently no ACC/AHA recommendations regarding the use of apixaban and rivaroxaban.[59] However, the ESC does recommend these 3 agents as alternatives to warfarin in nonvalvular AF.[75] These agents are not recommended in patients with prosthetic valves.

The RE-LY noninferiority trial assessed the safety and efficacy of dabigatran compared with warfarin in 18,113 patients with nonvalvular AF and intermediate risk (mean CHADS2 score of 2.1). The rate of the primary outcome of stroke or systemic embolization was 1.52%, 1.11%, and 1.69% per year in the dabigatran 110 mg, dabigatran 150 mg and warfarin groups, respectively.[76] The risk of major bleeding was significantly lower in the dabigatran 110 mg group compared with warfarin, whereas the dabigatran 150 mg group was equivalent in safety to warfarin.[77–79] Post hoc evaluation of the RE-LY trial reported a nonsignificantly increased rate of myocardial infarction for both doses of dabigatran compared with warfarin.[80] These findings were confirmed in a meta-analysis of 7 trials comparing dabigatran with warfarin, enoxaparin or placebo for either stroke prophylaxis in AF, treatment of deep venous thrombosis, short-term prophylaxis of deep venous thrombosis, or treatment of acute coronary syndrome. Dabigatran was associated with a significantly increased risk of myocardial infarction, cardiac death, or unstable angina compared with the control group (OR 1.27, 95% CI 1.00–1.61).[81] These findings warrant further investigation.

Rivaroxaban was studied in the ROCKET AF trial, in which 14,264 patients with AF at intermediate to high risk of stroke (mean CHADS2 score of 3.5) were randomized to rivaroxaban or warfarin. Similar proportions of patients with HF were in both groups (approximately 62%). Rivaroxaban was shown to be noninferior to warfarin (1.7 vs 2.2% per year, hazard ratio 0.79, 95% CI 0.66–0.96). There was no significant difference in bleeding (major or nonmajor) as well.[82]

Apixaban was studied in the ARISTOTLE trial of 18,201 patients with intermediate risk (mean CHADS2 score 2.1) who were randomized to apixaban or warfarin. There were similar proportions of patients with HF in each group (approximately 36%). Apixaban was shown to be noninferior, because the composite primary end point of stroke and systemic embolism was significantly reduced in the apixaban group (1.3 vs 1.6% per year, hazard ratio 0.79, 95% CI 0.66–0.95). In addition, the rate of major bleeding was significantly lower in the apixaban group, with a significant reduction in the hemorrhagic stroke rate. This trial also showed a significant reduction in the secondary efficacy outcome of all-cause mortality compared with warfarin (3.52 vs 3.94% per year, $P = .047$).[83]

HF WITH PRESERVED EJECTION FRACTION

AF can impair left ventricular filling in late diastole in HF with preserved ejection fraction, because HF with preserved ejection fraction (HFpEF) may be more dependent on atrial contraction. Rapid ventricular response caused by AF may also impair filling by shortening diastole. Restoration and maintenance of sinus rhythm may be beneficial in this population; however, observational data ($n = 382$) suggest that there was no survival advantage with this approach.[84] Further study is warranted to assess morbidity and mortality with rate versus rhythm control approaches in a larger randomized cohort. β-blockers and calcium channel blockers are first-line therapies. Digoxin may be beneficial as well.[33] HF with preserved ejection fraction has also been reported to have a higher risk of death, hospitalization from HF, and hospitalization from any cause, although similar to that of patients with reduced ejection fraction in a study of 23,644 patients with HF (HFpEF $n = 14,295$).[85] However, these findings have not been consistent across all studies.[86–88]

FUTURE DIRECTIONS

Although there is evidence that rate and rhythm control approaches to AF may produce similar outcomes in patients with HF, there are conflicting data with respect to degree of rate control. Lenient and strict rate control were shown to be similar; however, the SHIFT study, although representing differing populations, seemingly indicates that rate control of patients with HF without AF is efficacious. A subset of patients in SHIFT had a history of AF (approximately 8%), and it is unknown if a difference was seen in this population. Data from the Get With The Guidelines Heart Failure Registry have shown that higher admission heart rates are independently associated with worse outcomes in those admitted for HF, irrespective of rhythm. It may be beneficial to further study rate reduction in HF and AF.[89] Long-term follow-up and refinement of patient selection for AF ablation as well as improved algorithms for anticoagulant therapies are needed.[90,91] Cost-effectiveness studies to assess these strategies are also crucial. In addition, further study is warranted in the population with HFpEF, because current therapies may not apply to this cohort of patients, particularly because most standard therapies for HF with reduced ejection fraction have not been efficacious in HFpEF.

SUMMARY

AF affects many patients with HF, and both disorders impose a significant burden on the health care system. The presence of AF is a marker of worse prognosis in this population, associated with increased morbidity and mortality. Management strategies are aimed at limiting symptoms through rate or rhythm control as well as anticoagulation to prevent systemic embolization and stroke, avoiding therapies that increase mortality in the HF population. Current data suggest that pharmacologic rhythm control has no advantage over rate control. It remains unknown whether prompt restoration of sinus rhythm or aggressive rate control in patients hospitalized with new-onset AF is beneficial, and this aspect requires further study. Improvements in invasive strategies to restore sinus rhythm have resulted in increased efficacy and safety; however, further data are warranted to determine their role in the treatment of AF in HF. New anticoagulants have emerged and present their unique advantages and challenges. Advances in pharmacotherapy, nonpharmacologic therapies, and treatment strategies have benefited patients with AF and HF.

REFERENCES

1. Rienstra M, Damman K, Mulder BA, et al. Beta-blockers and outcome in heart failure and atrial fibrillation. JACC Heart Fail 2013;1(1):21–8. http://dx.doi.org/10.1016/j.jchf.2012.09.002.
2. Parthenakis FI, Patrianakos AP, Skalidis EI, et al. Atrial fibrillation is associated with increased neurohumoral activation and reduced exercise tolerance in patients with non-ischemic dilated cardiomyopathy. Int J Cardiol 2007;118(2):206–14. http://dx.doi.org/10.1016/j.ijcard.2006.03.090.
3. Pardaens K, Van Cleemput J, Vanhaecke J, et al. Atrial fibrillation is associated with a lower exercise capacity in male chronic heart failure patients. Heart 1997;78(6):564–8.
4. Yancy CW, Jessup M, Bozkurt B, et al. 2013 ACCF/AHA guideline for the management of heart failure. J Am Coll Cardiol 2013. http://dx.doi.org/10.1016/j.jacc.2013.05.019.
5. Wang TJ, Larson MG, Levy D, et al. Temporal relations of atrial fibrillation and congestive heart failure and their joint influence on mortality. Circulation 2003;107:2920–5.
6. Vorperian VR, Havighurst TC, Miller S, et al. Adverse effects of low dose amiodarone: a meta-analysis. J Am Coll Cardiol 1997;30(3):791–8. http://dx.doi.org/10.1016/S0735-1097(97)00220-9.
7. Benjamin EJ, Levy D, Vaziri SM, et al. Independent risk factors for atrial fibrillation in a population-based cohort. The Framingham Heart Study. JAMA 1994;271(11):840–4. http://dx.doi.org/10.1001/jama.1994.03510350050036.
8. Deedwania PC, Singh BN, Ellenbogen K, et al. Spontaneous conversion and maintenance of sinus rhythm by amiodarone in patients with heart failure and atrial fibrillation: observations from the veterans affairs congestive heart failure survival trial of antiarrhythmic therapy (CHF-STAT). The Department of Veterans Affairs CHF-STAT Investigators. Circulation 1998;98(23):2574–9.
9. Carson PE, Johnson GR, Dunkman WB, et al. The influence of atrial fibrillation on prognosis in mild to moderate heart failure. The V-HeFT Studies. The V-HeFT VA Cooperative Studies Group. Circulation 1993;87(Suppl 6):VI102–10.
10. Stevenson WG, Stevenson LW, Middlekauff HR, et al. Improving survival for patients with atrial fibrillation and advanced heart failure. J Am Coll Cardiol 1996;28(6):1458–63. http://dx.doi.org/10.1016/S0735-1097(96)00358-0.
11. Joglar JA, Acusta AP, Shusterman NH, et al. Effect of carvedilol on survival and hemodynamics in patients with atrial fibrillation and left ventricular dysfunction: retrospective analysis of the US Carvedilol Heart Failure Trials Program. Am Heart J 2001;142(3):498–501. http://dx.doi.org/10.1067/mhj.2001.117318.

12. Mahoney P, Kimmel S, DeNofrio D, et al. Prognostic significance of atrial fibrillation in patients at a tertiary medical center referred for heart transplantation because of severe heart failure. Am J Cardiol 1999;83(11):1544–7. http://dx.doi.org/10.1016/S0002-9149(99)00144-7.
13. Maisel WH, Stevenson LW. Atrial fibrillation in heart failure: epidemiology, pathophysiology, and rationale for therapy. Am J Cardiol 2003;91(Suppl): 2D–8D. http://dx.doi.org/10.1016/S0002-9149(02)03373-8.
14. Weinfeld MS, Drazner MH, Stevenson WG, et al. Early outcome of initiating amiodarone for atrial fibrillation in advanced heart failure. J Heart Lung Transplant 2000;19(7):638–43.
15. Cohn JN, Johnson G, Ziesche S, et al. A comparison of enalapril with hydralazine-isosorbide dinitrate in the treatment of chronic congestive heart failure. N Engl J Med 1991;325(5):303–10. http://dx.doi.org/10.1056/NEJM199108013250502.
16. Cohn JN, Archibald DG, Ziesche S, et al. Effect of vasodilator therapy on mortality in chronic congestive heart failure. Results of a Veterans Administration Cooperative Study. N Engl J Med 1986;314(24):1547–52. http://dx.doi.org/10.1056/NEJM198606123142404.
17. Doval HC, Nul DR, Grancelli HO, et al. Randomised trial of low-dose amiodarone in severe congestive heart failure. Lancet 1994;344(8921): 493–8. http://dx.doi.org/10.1016/S0140-6736(94)91895-3.
18. Packer M, Poole-Wilson PA, Armstrong PW, et al. Comparative effects of low and high doses of the angiotensin-converting enzyme inhibitor, lisinopril, on morbidity and mortality in chronic heart failure. ATLAS Study Group. Circulation 1999;100(23): 2312–8.
19. Johnstone D, Limacher M, Rousseau M, et al. Clinical characteristics of patients in studies of left ventricular dysfunction (SOLVD). Am J Cardiol 1992; 70(9):894–900. http://dx.doi.org/10.1016/0002-9149(92)90734-G.
20. Singh SN, Fletcher RD, Fisher SG, et al. Amiodarone in patients with congestive heart failure and asymptomatic ventricular arrhythmia. N Engl J Med 1995;333(2):77–82. http://dx.doi.org/10.1056/NEJM199507133330201.
21. Group TCTS. Effects of enalapril on mortality in severe congestive heart failure. Results of the Cooperative North Scandinavian Enalapril Survival Study (CONSENSUS). N Engl J Med 1987; 316(23):1429–35. http://dx.doi.org/10.1056/NEJM198706043162301.
22. Yusuf S, Pepine CJ, Garces C, et al. Effect of enalapril on myocardial infarction and unstable angina in patients with low ejection fractions. Lancet 1992; 340(8829):1173–8.
23. Dries DL, Exner DV, Gersh BJ, et al. Atrial fibrillation is associated with an increased risk for mortality and heart failure progression in patients with asymptomatic and symptomatic left ventricular systolic dysfunction: a retrospective analysis of the SOLVD trials. Studies of Left Ventricular Dysfunction. J Am Coll Cardiol 1998;32(3):695–703.
24. Pedersen OD, Bagger H, Keller N, et al. Efficacy of dofetilide in the treatment of atrial fibrillation-flutter in patients with reduced left ventricular function: a Danish investigations of arrhythmia and mortality on dofetilide (DIAMOND) substudy. Circulation 2001;104(3):292–6.
25. Olsson LG, Swedberg KK, Ducharme AA, et al. Atrial fibrillation and risk of clinical events in chronic heart failure with and without left ventricular systolic dysfunction. J Am Coll Cardiol 2006; 47(10):1997–2004. http://dx.doi.org/10.1016/j.jacc.2006.01.060.
26. Torp-Pedersen C, Møller M, Bloch-Thomsen PE, et al. Dofetilide in patients with congestive heart failure and left ventricular dysfunction. N Engl J Med 1999;341(12):857–65. http://dx.doi.org/10.1056/NEJM199909163411201.
27. Brendorp B, Elming H, Jun L, et al. Qtc interval as a guide to select those patients with congestive heart failure and reduced left ventricular systolic function who will benefit from antiarrhythmic treatment with dofetilide. Circulation 2001;103(10):1422–7.
28. Wasywich CA, Whalley GA, Gamble GD, et al. Does rhythm matter? The prognostic importance of atrial fibrillation in heart failure. Heart Lung Circ 2006;15(6):353–7. http://dx.doi.org/10.1016/j.hlc.2006.07.011.
29. Mountantonakis SE, Grau-Sepulveda MV, Bhatt DL, et al. Presence of atrial fibrillation is independently associated with adverse outcomes in patients hospitalized with heart failure. Circ Heart Fail 2012;5(2):191–201. http://dx.doi.org/10.1161/CIRCHEARTFAILURE.111.965681.
30. Singh BN, Connolly SJ, Crijns HJ, et al. Dronedarone for maintenance of sinus rhythm in atrial fibrillation or flutter. N Engl J Med 2007;357(10):987–99. http://dx.doi.org/10.1056/NEJMoa054686.
31. Roy D, Talajic M, Nattel S, et al. Rhythm control versus rate control for atrial fibrillation and heart failure. N Engl J Med 2008;358(25):2667–77. http://dx.doi.org/10.1056/NEJMoa0708789.
32. Hohnloser SH, Crijns HJ, van Eickels M, et al. Effect of dronedarone on cardiovascular events in atrial fibrillation. N Engl J Med 2009;360(7):668–78. http://dx.doi.org/10.1056/NEJMoa0803778.
33. Fuster V, Ryden LE, Cannom DS, et al. ACC/AHA/ESC 2006 guidelines for the management of patients with atrial fibrillation–executive summary. Circulation 2006;114(7):700–52. http://dx.doi.org/10.1161/CIRCULATIONAHA.106.177031.

34. Suman-Horduna I, Roy D, Frasure-Smith N, et al. Quality of life and functional capacity in patients with atrial fibrillation and congestive heart failure. J Am Coll Cardiol 2013;61:455–60. http://dx.doi.org/10.1016/j.jacc.2012.10.031.
35. Hohnloser SH, Crijns HJ, van Eickels M, et al. Dronedarone in patients with congestive heart failure: insights from ATHENA. Eur Heart J 2010;31(14):1717–21. http://dx.doi.org/10.1093/eurheartj/ehq113.
36. Kober L, Torp-Pedersen C, McMurray JJ, et al. Increased mortality after dronedarone therapy for severe heart failure. N Engl J Med 2008;358(25):2678–87. http://dx.doi.org/10.1056/NEJMoa0800456.
37. Pozzoli M, Cioffi G, Traversi E, et al. Predictors of primary atrial fibrillation and concomitant clinical and hemodynamic changes in patients with chronic heart failure: a prospective study in 344 patients with baseline sinus rhythm. J Am Coll Cardiol 1998;32(1):197–204. http://dx.doi.org/10.1016/S0735-1097(98)00221-6.
38. Crijns HJ, Tjeerdsma G, de Kam PJ, et al. Prognostic value of the presence and development of atrial fibrillation in patients with advanced chronic heart failure. Eur Heart J 2000;21(15):1238–45. http://dx.doi.org/10.1053/euhj.1999.2107.
39. Khand AU, Rankin AC, Kaye GC, et al. Systematic review of the management of atrial fibrillation in patients with heart failure. Eur Heart J 2000;21(8):614–32. http://dx.doi.org/10.1053/euhj.1999.1767.
40. Wyse DG, Waldo AL, DiMarco JP, et al. A comparison of rate control and rhythm control in patients with atrial fibrillation. N Engl J Med 2002;347(23):1825–33. http://dx.doi.org/10.1056/NEJMoa021328.
41. Van Gelder IC, Hagens VE, Bosker HA, et al. A comparison of rate control and rhythm control in patients with recurrent persistent atrial fibrillation. N Engl J Med 2002;347(23):1834–40. http://dx.doi.org/10.1056/NEJMoa021375.
42. Connolly SJ, Camm AJ, Halperin JL, et al. Dronedarone in high-risk permanent atrial fibrillation. N Engl J Med 2011;365(24):2268–76. http://dx.doi.org/10.1056/NEJMoa1109867.
43. Lehmann MH, Hardy S, Archibald D, et al. Sex difference in risk of torsade de pointes with d, l-sotalol. Circulation 1996;94(10):2535–41.
44. Soyka LF, Wirtz C, Spangenberg RB. Clinical safety profile of sotalol in patients with arrhythmias. Am J Cardiol 1990;65(2):74A–83A.
45. Cha YM, Redfield MM, Shen WK, et al. Atrial fibrillation and ventricular dysfunction: a vicious electromechanical cycle. Circulation 2004;109(23):2839–43. http://dx.doi.org/10.1161/01.CIR.0000132470.78896.A8.
46. Gheorghiade M, Fonarow GC, van Veldhuisen DJ, et al. Lack of evidence of increased mortality among patients with atrial fibrillation taking digoxin: findings from post hoc propensity-matched analysis of the AFFIRM trial. Eur Heart J 2013;34(20):1489–97. http://dx.doi.org/10.1093/eurheartj/eht120.
47. Waldo AL, Camm AJ, deRuyter H, et al. Effect of d-sotalol on mortality in patients with left ventricular dysfunction after recent and remote myocardial infarction. The SWORD Investigators. Survival With Oral d-Sotalol. Lancet 1996;348(9019):7–12.
48. Kjekshus J. Arrhythmias and mortality in congestive heart failure. Am J Cardiol 1990;65(19):42I–8I.
49. Van Gelder IC, Groenveld HF, Crijns HJ, et al. Lenient versus strict rate control in patients with atrial fibrillation. N Engl J Med 2010;362(15):1363–73. http://dx.doi.org/10.1056/NEJMoa1001337.
50. Amabile CM, Spencer AP. Keeping your patient with heart failure safe–a review of potentially dangerous medications. Arch Intern Med 2004;164(7):709–20. http://dx.doi.org/10.1001/archinte.164.7.709.
51. Wilkoff BL, Cook JR, Epstein AE, et al. Dual-chamber pacing or ventricular backup pacing in patients with an implantable defibrillator: the Dual Chamber and VVI Implantable Defibrillator (DAVID) Trial. JAMA 2002;288(24):3115–23. http://dx.doi.org/10.1001/jama.288.24.3115.
52. Sweeney MO, Hellkamp AS, Ellenbogen KA, et al. Adverse effect of ventricular pacing on heart failure and atrial fibrillation among patients with normal baseline QRS duration in a clinical trial of pacemaker therapy for sinus node dysfunction. Circulation 2003;107(23):2932–7. http://dx.doi.org/10.1161/01.CIR.0000072769.17295.B1.
53. Pedersen OD, Bagger H, Kober L, et al. Trandolapril reduces the incidence of atrial fibrillation after acute myocardial infarction in patients with left ventricular dysfunction. Circulation 1999;100(4):376–80.
54. Gasparini M, Regoli F, Galimberti P, et al. Cardiac resynchronization therapy in heart failure patients with atrial fibrillation. Europace 2009;11(Suppl 5):v82–6. http://dx.doi.org/10.1093/europace/eup273.
55. Vermes E, Tardif JC, Bourassa MG, et al. Enalapril decreases the incidence of atrial fibrillation in patients with left ventricular dysfunction: insight from the Studies Of Left Ventricular Dysfunction (SOLVD) trials. Circulation 2003;107(23):2926–31. http://dx.doi.org/10.1161/01.CIR.0000072793.81076.D4.
56. Swedberg K, Komajda M, Böhm M, et al. Ivabradine and outcomes in chronic heart failure (SHIFT): a randomised placebo-controlled study. Lancet 2010;376(9744):875–85. http://dx.doi.org/10.1016/S0140-6736(10)61198-1.
57. Maggioni AP, Latini R, Carson PE, et al. Valsartan reduces the incidence of atrial fibrillation in patients with heart failure: results from the Valsartan Heart Failure Trial (Val-HeFT). Am Heart J 2005;149(3):548–57. http://dx.doi.org/10.1016/j.ahj.2004.09.033.

58. Flaker GC, Blackshear JL, McBride R, et al. Antiarrhythmic drug therapy and cardiac mortality in atrial fibrillation. The Stroke Prevention in Atrial Fibrillation Investigators. J Am Coll Cardiol 1992;20(3):527–32. http://dx.doi.org/10.1016/0735-1097(92)90003-6.
59. Fuster V, Ryden LE, Cannom DS, et al. 2011 ACCF/AHA/HRS focused updates incorporated into the ACC/AHA/ESC 2006 Guidelines for the management of patients with atrial fibrillation. J Am Coll Cardiol 2011;57(11):e101–98. http://dx.doi.org/10.1016/j.jacc.2010.09.013.
60. European Heart Rhythm Association, European Association for Cardio-Thoracic Surgery, Camm AJ, et al. Guidelines for the management of atrial fibrillation: the Task Force for the Management of Atrial Fibrillation of the European Society of Cardiology (ESC). Eur Heart J 2010;31(19):2369–429. http://dx.doi.org/10.1093/eurheartj/ehq278.
61. Investigators TAI. Irbesartan in patients with atrial fibrillation. N Engl J Med 2011;364(10):928–38. http://dx.doi.org/10.1056/NEJMoa1008816.
62. Hsu LF, Jaïs P, Sanders P, et al. Catheter ablation for atrial fibrillation in congestive heart failure. N Engl J Med 2004;351(23):2373–83. http://dx.doi.org/10.1056/NEJMoa041018.
63. Chen MS, Marrouche NF, Khaykin Y, et al. Pulmonary vein isolation for the treatment of atrial fibrillation in patients with impaired systolic function. J Am Coll Cardiol 2004;43(6):1004–9. http://dx.doi.org/10.1016/j.jacc.2003.09.056.
64. Khan MN, Jaïs P, Cummings J, et al. Pulmonary-vein isolation for atrial fibrillation in patients with heart failure. N Engl J Med 2008;359(17):1778–85. http://dx.doi.org/10.1056/NEJMoa0708234.
65. Cullen MW, Kim S, Piccini JP, et al. Risks and benefits of anticoagulation in atrial fibrillation: insights from the outcomes registry for better informed treatment of atrial fibrillation (ORBIT-AF) registry. Circ Cardiovasc Qual Outcomes 2013;6(4):461–9. http://dx.doi.org/10.1161/CIRCOUTCOMES.113.000127.
66. The Effect of Low-Dose Warfarin on the Risk of Stroke in Patients with Nonrheumatic Atrial Fibrillation. N Engl J Med 1990;323(22):1505–11. http://dx.doi.org/10.1056/NEJM199011293232201.
67. Warfarin versus aspirin for prevention of thromboembolism in atrial fibrillation: stroke prevention in atrial fibrillation II study. Lancet 1994;343:687–91.
68. Petersen P, Boysen G, Godtfredsen J. Placebo-controlled, randomised trial of warfarin and aspirin for prevention of thromboembolic complications in chronic atrial fibrillation. The Copenhagen AFASAK study. Lancet 1989;1:175–9. Available at: http://www.uptodate.com/contents/antithrombotic-therapy-to-prevent-embolization-in-atrial-fibrillation/abstract-text/2563096/pubmed. Accessed July 4, 2013.
69. Ezekowitz MD, Bridgers SL, James KE, et al. Warfarin in the prevention of stroke associated with nonrheumatic atrial fibrillation. N Engl J Med 1992;327:1406–12. http://dx.doi.org/10.1056/NEJM199301143280227.
70. Singer DE, Chang Y, Fang MC, et al. The net clinical benefit of warfarin anticoagulation in atrial fibrillation. Ann Intern Med 2009;151(5):297–305. http://dx.doi.org/10.7326/0003-4819-151-5-200909010-00003.
71. Agarwal S, Hachamovitch R, Menon V. Current trial-associated outcomes with warfarin in prevention of stroke in patients with nonvalvular atrial fibrillation–a meta-analysis. Arch Intern Med 2012;172(8):623–31. http://dx.doi.org/10.1001/archinternmed.2012.121.
72. van Walraven C, Hart RG, Singer DE, et al. Oral anticoagulants vs aspirin in nonvalvular atrial fibrillation–an individual patient meta-analysis. JAMA 2002;288(19):2441–8. http://dx.doi.org/10.1001/jama.288.19.2441.
73. Piccini JP, Hernandez AF, Zhao X, et al. Quality of care for atrial fibrillation among patients hospitalized for heart failure. J Am Coll Cardiol 2009;54(14):1280–9. http://dx.doi.org/10.1016/j.jacc.2009.04.091.
74. Gong IY, Kim RB. Importance of pharmacokinetic profile and variability as determinants of dose and response to dabigatran, rivaroxaban, and apixaban. Can J Cardiol 2013;29(7):S24–33. http://dx.doi.org/10.1016/j.cjca.2013.04.002.
75. Camm AJ, Lip GY, De Caterina R, et al. 2012 focused update of the ESC guidelines for the management of atrial fibrillation: an update of the 2010 ESC guidelines for the management of atrial fibrillation. Developed with the special contribution of the European Heart Rhythm Association. Eur Heart J 2012;33(21):2719–47. http://dx.doi.org/10.1093/eurheartj/ehs253.
76. Connolly SJ, Ezekowitz MD, Yusuf S, et al. Dabigatran versus warfarin in patients with atrial fibrillation. N Engl J Med 2009;361(12):1139–51. http://dx.doi.org/10.1056/NEJMoa0905561.
77. Connolly SJ, Ezekowitz MD, Yusuf S, et al. Newly identified events in the RE-LY trial. N Engl J Med 2010;363(19):1875–6. http://dx.doi.org/10.1056/NEJMc1007378.
78. Ezekowitz MD, Wallentin L, Connolly SJ, et al. Dabigatran and warfarin in vitamin K antagonist-naive and -experienced cohorts with atrial fibrillation. Circulation 2010;122(22):2246–53. http://dx.doi.org/10.1161/CIRCULATIONAHA.110.973735.
79. Eikelboom JW, Wallentin L, Connolly SJ, et al. Risk of bleeding with 2 doses of dabigatran compared with warfarin in older and younger patients with atrial fibrillation: an analysis of the randomized evaluation of long-term anticoagulant therapy (RE-LY) trial. Circulation 2011;123(21):2363–72. http://dx.doi.org/10.1161/CIRCULATIONAHA.110.004747.
80. Hohnloser SH, Oldgren JJ, Yang SS, et al. Myocardial ischemic events in patients with atrial

fibrillation treated with dabigatran or warfarin in the RE-LY (Randomized Evaluation of Long-Term Anticoagulation Therapy) trial. Circulation 2012; 125(5):669–76. http://dx.doi.org/10.1161/CIRCULATIONAHA.111.055970.

81. Uchino K, Hernandez AV. Dabigatran association with higher risk of acute coronary events–meta-analysis of noninferiority randomized controlled trials. Arch Intern Med 2012;172(5):397–402. http://dx.doi.org/10.1001/archinternmed.2011.1666.
82. Patel MR, Mahaffey KW, Garg J, et al. Rivaroxaban versus warfarin in nonvalvular atrial fibrillation. N Engl J Med 2011;365(10):883–91. http://dx.doi.org/10.1056/NEJMoa1009638.
83. Granger CB, Alexander JH, McMurray JJ, et al. Apixaban versus warfarin in patients with atrial fibrillation. N Engl J Med 2011;365(11):981–92. http://dx.doi.org/10.1056/NEJMoa1107039.
84. Kong MH, Shaw LK, O'Connor C, et al. Is rhythm-control superior to rate-control in patients with atrial fibrillation and diastolic heart failure? Ann Noninvasive Electrocardiol 2010;15(3):209–17. http://dx.doi.org/10.1111/j.1542-474X.2010.00365.x.
85. McManus DD, Hsu G, Sung SH, et al. Atrial fibrillation and outcomes in heart failure with preserved versus reduced left ventricular ejection fraction. J Am Heart Assoc 2012;2(1):e005694. http://dx.doi.org/10.1161/JAHA.112.005694.
86. Badheka AO, Rathod A, Kizilbash MA, et al. Comparison of mortality and morbidity in patients with atrial fibrillation and heart failure with preserved versus decreased left ventricular ejection fraction. Am J Cardiol 2011;108(9):1283–8. http://dx.doi.org/10.1016/j.amjcard.2011.06.045.
87. Linssen GC, Rienstra M, Jaarsma T, et al. Clinical and prognostic effects of atrial fibrillation in heart failure patients with reduced and preserved left ventricular ejection fraction. Eur J Heart Fail 2011;13(10): 1111–20. http://dx.doi.org/10.1093/eurjhf/hfr066.
88. Rusinaru D, Leborgne L, Peltier M, et al. Effect of atrial fibrillation on long-term survival in patients hospitalised for heart failure with preserved ejection fraction. Eur J Heart Fail 2008;10(6):566–72. http://dx.doi.org/10.1016/j.ejheart.2008.04.002.
89. Alings M, Smit MD, Moes ML, et al. Routine versus aggressive upstream rhythm control for prevention of early atrial fibrillation in heart failure: background, aims and design of the RACE 3 study. Neth Heart J 2013. http://dx.doi.org/10.1007/s12471-013-0428-5.
90. Jones DG, Haldar SK, Hussain W, et al. A randomized trial to assess catheter ablation versus rate control in the management of persistent atrial fibrillation in heart failure. J Am Coll Cardiol 2013;61(18):1894–903. http://dx.doi.org/10.1016/j.jacc.2013.01.069.
91. Gheorghiade M, Vaduganathan M, Fonarow GC, et al. Anticoagulation in heart failure: current status and future direction. Heart Fail Rev 2012. http://dx.doi.org/10.1007/s10741-012-9343-x.

Atrial Fibrillation in Heart Failure in the Older Population

Patrick M. Heck, BM BCh[a,*], Justin M.S. Lee, BM BCh[a], Peter M. Kistler, MBBS, PhD[b,c]

KEYWORDS

• Atrial fibrillation • Heart failure • Elderly • Ablation • Anticoagulation

KEY POINTS

- Atrial fibrillation (AF) and heart failure (HF) both have a higher incidence in the older patient and this is increasing.
- Older patients are more likely to have additional comorbidities that can make the management of AF and HF more complex.
- The risk of stroke secondary to AF in this population is high, making consideration of anticoagulation crucially important.
- Although data specifically targeting this patient group is scarce, it would appear that AF ablation can be undertaken safely, is as effective and superior to medical therapy.

INTRODUCTION

Atrial fibrillation (AF) is an important and often-underrecognized cause of cardiovascular morbidity and mortality. It is an arrhythmia that is commonly seen in the older patient, indeed the median age of patients with AF in early studies was 75 years.[1] Heart failure (HF) is also more frequently seen in the older patient with an approximate doubling of HF prevalence with each decade of life.[2] There is clear interaction between AF and HF, with evidence that HF can lead to AF and AF exacerbates HF. The prevalence of AF in individuals with HF is considerably greater than the general population and has been reported to be as high as 25%.[3] This increased prevalence appears related to the severity of the HF and ranges from 5% to 50% as the New York Heart Association (NYHA) classification of the patient increases from I to IV.[4] Taken together, these data make it apparent that AF and HF are frequently going to be encountered in the elderly patient. Elderly patients are more likely to have multiple comorbidities and polypharmacy, which complicate their management compared with their younger counterparts. This review focuses on the specific aspect of AF management in elderly (aged 70 years or more) patients with HF.

PHARMACOLOGIC MANAGEMENT

Older patients are often underrepresented in clinical trials. Pharmacokinetics are significantly altered in the elderly.[5] There is relatively lower muscle mass and higher body fat content, which alters the volume of distribution of drugs such as amiodarone. Hepatic drug metabolism is diminished, affecting drugs including propranolol,

None of the authors have any conflicts of interests to report.
Professor Peter M. Kistler is supported by a practitioner fellowship from the NHMRC. This research is supported in part by the Victorian Government's Operational Infrastructure Funding.
[a] Department of Cardiology, Papworth Hospital, Papworth Everard, Cambridge CB23 3RE, UK; [b] Department of Cardiology, Baker IDI, Melbourne, Australia; [c] Department of Cardiovascular Medicine, Alfred Heart Centre, Alfred Hospital, Baker IDI Heart and Diabetes Institute, University of Melbourne, Victoria 3004, Australia
* Corresponding author.
E-mail address: Patrick.heck@nhs.net

Heart Failure Clin 9 (2013) 451–459
http://dx.doi.org/10.1016/j.hfc.2013.07.007
1551-7136/13/$ – see front matter

verapamil, and diltiazem. Renal dysfunction is also more common, reducing the elimination of drugs, including digoxin and sotalol. The older population has comorbidities, and polypharmacy can result in significant drug interactions.

Rate Versus Rhythm Control

The major decision in treatment of AF is whether to pursue a strategy to maintain sinus rhythm (SR) with potentially toxic antiarrhythmic drugs or to accept AF and target rate control; this is explored in detail in other articles in this issue. Current evidence indicates that in the absence of significant symptoms due to AF, clinical outcomes from rate control are equivalent to rhythm control.[6,7] Rhythm control should be favored in symptomatic patients. SR can be achieved with Class Ic or Class III antiarrhythmic drugs and/or electrical cardioversion. In the presence of structural heart disease Class Ic agents, such as flecainide, are generally avoided.[8,9] Rate control can be achieved with beta-blockers, calcium channel blockers or digoxin. Previously, guidelines have advocated the use of "strict" rate control[10] with resting heart rate less than 80 beats per minute, but recent evidence suggests that a more lenient target of less than 110 beats per minute could be adopted.[11]

The Atrial Fibrillation Follow-up Investigation of Rhythm Management (AFFIRM) study recruited more than 4000 patients with a mean age of 70 years, including 23% with a history of HF.[6] In the rhythm control arm, SR was maintained in 73% of patients at 3 years and 63% at 5 years and did not confer a survival advantage over rate control. Subgroup analysis did not identify a survival advantage according to left ventricular (LV) function.[12] However, in a post hoc "on-treatment" analysis, warfarin use and presence of SR were associated with a significant reduction in mortality, but the use of antiarrhythmic drugs was not.[13] This emphasizes the importance of anticoagulation and suggests that adverse effects of antiarrhythmic drugs may counteract the benefits of SR.

Similarly, the RAte Control versus Electrical cardioversion for atrial fibrillation (RACE) study randomized 522 patients (mean age 68 years) with persistent AF (median AF duration>300 days) to rate or rhythm control.[7] After a mean of 2.3 years, 39% of the rhythm-control group were in SR, compared with 10% of the rate-control group. Rate control was noninferior to rhythm control for the prevention of death and cardiovascular morbidity.

The Atrial Fibrillation and Congestive Heart Failure (AF-CHF) study randomized 1376 patients (mean age 67 years) to rate versus rhythm control in an HF population with NYHA class II to IV symptoms and LV ejection fraction (EF) less than 35%.[14] Once again, there was no significant difference between strategies in cardiovascular death, death from any cause, stroke, or worsening HF. Rhythm control was associated with an increase in hospitalization.

To date, clinical trials have used medical therapy in the rhythm control arm with few patients undergoing catheter ablation and this is explored in detail later. The benefits of rhythm control may be offset by the relative inefficacy and toxicity of current drugs. In the Carvedilol in Atrial Fibrillation Evaluation (CAFÉ) II trial of 61 patients comparing pharmacological rate versus rhythm control, NYHA class and 6-minute walk time (6MWT) distance were similar between patients assigned to rate or rhythm control, but those assigned to rhythm control had improved LV function, N-terminal pro-brain natriuretic peptide (NT-proBNP) concentration, and quality of life compared with those assigned to rate control.[15]

Pharmacologic Management

In the setting of significant structural heart disease, in particular HF, pharmacologic options for rhythm control of AF are almost exclusively limited to amiodarone according to European guidelines,[16] although US guidelines support the use of dofetilide as well.[17] A detailed review of pharmacological treatments in AF and HF is published elsewhere in this issue. This section will focus on the specific additional considerations in the elderly although there are limited data available specifically targeting this patient group.

Dofetilide is used infrequently because of the need for in-hospital initiation and the risks of proarrhythmia due to QT prolongation. In the Danish Investigations of Arrhythmia and Mortality ON Dofetilide (DIAMOND) study of dofetilide versus placebo in LV dysfunction post myocardial infarction, there was no effect on all-cause mortality.[20] Dofetilide was effective in converting AF and SR was maintained at 1 year in 79%.[21] Maintenance of SR was associated with significant reduction in mortality, whereas dofetilide therapy was associated with a significantly lower risk of congestive HF rehospitalization.

Dronedarone was developed as a modification of amiodarone in an attempt to maintain efficacy without toxicity and has shown some promise in studies.[22,23] In the ANDROMEDA study, dronedarone was trialed in patients with HF, with the study stopped early because of excess mortality in the dronedarone arm.[24] The current role of dronedarone is limited and is probably reserved for maintenance of SR in paroxysmal patients with AF with preserved systolic function.

Sotalol has a combined beta-blocker and class III effect. In the Sotalol Amiodarone Atrial Fibrillation Efficacy Trial (SAFE-T) study of patients with persistent AF, amiodarone and sotalol were equally efficacious in converting AF to SR, although amiodarone was superior for maintaining SR following electrical cardioversion.[18] Sotalol is renally excreted and at higher doses can lead to significant QT prolongation with risk of proarrhythmia in the elderly with HF. In addition, unlike other beta-blockers, such as bisoprolol and carvedilol, sotalol has no proven benefit in HF and so its use is not recommended in patients with AF and HF.[16,17]

Beta-blockers, in particular carvedilol, bisoprolol, and metoprolol, are recommended in current guidelines for treatment of HF because of their proven prognostic and symptomatic benefits.[19] In the Study of Effects of Nebivolol Intervention on Outcomes and Rehospitalization in Seniors (SENIORS) study, nebivolol, a beta-blocker with vasodilator properties, resulted in a reduction in the combined end point of death and hospital admissions in patients older than 70 years.[20] However, more recent data from the SENIORS study showed that nebivolol did not appear to confer clinical benefit in the AF subgroup, irrespective of ejection fraction.[21] In the Carvedilol Or Metoprolol European Trial (COMET)[22] study, although presence of AF was a poor prognostic factor, there was a relative benefit of carvedilol versus metoprolol in patients with AF and HF.

Digoxin is a second-line therapy for AF rate control and is also used in HF as a weak inotrope. Advanced age may predispose patients to an increased risk for digoxin toxicity because of decreased renal function, low body mass, and electrical conduction abnormalities. However, this was not observed in the Digitalis Investigation Group (DIG) trial, in which advanced age was not associated with an increased risk of digoxin toxicity.[23] These findings demonstrate that digoxin remains a useful agent in elderly patients with HF, although patients in this study were in SR. The combination of carvedilol and digoxin was better than either used alone in AF and HF, in terms of symptom control and ejection fraction in a small study by Khand and colleagues.[24]

Calcium channel blockers (eg, diltiazem and verapamil) are another option for rate control of AF when beta-blockers are contraindicated. A recent study compared the use of four different single dose drug regimens for rate control of AF in patients with a mean age of 71 years. This showed diltiazem 360 mg/d to be superior both in heart rate control and symptom improvement, although HF was an exclusion crtieria for this study.[25]

THROMBOPROPHYLAXIS FOR AF IN THE OLDER PATIENT

Perhaps the most feared complication associated with AF is that of embolic stroke. Cardioembolic strokes tend to be more severe and are more likely to be fatal.[26] The risk of stroke attributable to AF increases markedly with age, such that in patients aged 80 to 89 years, AF accounts for more than 20% of their stroke risk, compared with only 1.5% in patients aged 50 to 59 years.[27] Using the recently validated risk-scoring tool for estimating stroke risk in AF, CHA_2DS_2-VASc (Congestive heart failure, Hypertension, Age >75, Diabetes, Stroke, Vascular disease, Age 65–75, Sex category), patients aged 75 years or more with HF (CHA_2DS_2-VASc of 3) have an annual risk of stroke or thromboembolism in excess of 5%.[28] Addressing thromboprophylaxis is fundamental to the management of any patient with AF.

Anticoagulation remains the cornerstone of treatment for the prevention of stroke in AF and this has been looked at in some detail earlier in this series. Oral anticoagulation (OAC) is recommended for anyone with a CHA_2DS_2-VASc score of 2 or higher and the improved safety profile afforded by the novel oral anticoagulants (NOACs) has led to the European Society of Cardiology extending this recommendation to those with a CHA_2DS_2-VASc score of 1 or higher. Generally, older patients with AF and HF require anticoagulation unless the bleeding risk is considered prohibitive.

Bleeding Risk in the Older Patient

OAC therapy in the elderly patient with AF and HF is not without potential risk of significant bleeding. Just as advancing age increases an individual's risk of stroke in AF and hence their potential gain from treatment with OAC, older patients are at higher risk of bleeding when taking OAC therapy.[29]

There are many potential barriers that can lead to the underprescription of OACs, but bleeding risk is the most frequently cited reason among elderly patients, with aspirin typically being used as an alternative. This is now a growing body of evidence to show that aspirin use in the elderly is not as benign as previously thought, with several studies reporting bleeding rates in the elderly taking aspirin equivalent to those receiving warfarin.[30–32] Concerns regarding bleeding risk, susceptibility to falls, patient avoidance of anticoagulation, and the requirement for international normalized ratio (INR) monitoring have resulted in a significant number of elderly patents not being anticoagulated and thus being inadequately protected against stroke.[33,34]

Several bleeding risk scores have been introduced (Anticoagulation and Risk Factors in Atrial Fibrillation [ATRIA][35] and HAS-BLED[36] [hypertension, abnormal renal/liver function, stroke, bleeding history or predisposition, labile INR, elderly, drugs/alcohol concomitantly]) to provide physicians with the tools to objectively assess an individual's bleeding risk, enabling more informed discussions with the patient and family. In addition, 3 of the risk factors in the HAS-BLED scoring system are potentially reversible (*uncontrolled* hypertension, labile INRs, and drugs, such as aspirin or nonsteroidal anti-inflammatory drugs), thereby prompting the physician to minimize an individual's bleeding risk where possible.

The NOACs

The underuse of warfarin in the elderly with AF is multifactorial. In addition to the overestimation of bleeding risk in the older patient, another major deterrent is its fairly unappealing characteristics: narrow therapeutic range, variable dose response necessitating monitoring, and slow onset and offset of action. The NOACs have several distinct advantages in the older patient with AF. First, they have significantly fewer drug interactions than warfarin and older patients with HF are more likely to have comorbidities requiring the use of drugs that interfere with stable warfarin therapy.[37] The pharmacodynamics of the NOACs are more predictable and do not require monitoring.[38] In addition, the reduced need for frequent monitoring will be especially advantageous in the elderly where mobility and access to anticoagulation services might be problematic.

At the time of writing this article, 3 new agents had received Food and Drug Administration approval for the use of stroke prevention in nonvalvular AF: dabigatran etexilate, rivaroxaban, and apixaban. The data from trials leading to the approval of these drugs has been looked at in some detail elsewhere in this issue. In essence, the pivotal studies for each agent, in which they were compared with warfarin in nonvalvular AF, concluded *at least* noninferiority to warfarin in stroke prevention with a bleeding profile that was comparable or better.[39–41] There was a nonsignificant trend to increased extracranial hemorrhage in the elderly patients on higher dose (150 mg twice a day) dabigatran in the Randomized Evaluation of Long Term Anticoagulant Therapy (REL-Y) study, perhaps favoring the 110 mg twice a day in this population.

The place of the NOACs in the management of AF in older patients remains to be firmly established. It is likely that a greater proportion of eligible patients with AF will now receive oral anticoagulation therapy. Caution should be exercised when considering these agents in the very elderly, as these patients have been underrepresented in the NOAC trials, with the mean ages between 70 and 73 years. As with any new medication, ongoing surveillance on the safety and efficacy of NOACs in real-world medicine is critically important.

CATHETER ABLATION IN THE OLDER PATIENT

When discussing ablation for AF, it is important to make the distinction between ablation undertaken with the expectation of achieving SR and ablation of the atrioventricular node (AVN) combined with a pacemaker for optimizing rate control in AF. Ablation strategies in the nonelderly patient have been discussed elsewhere in this issue.

Catheter Ablation to Achieve SR

In appropriately selected patients with atrial fibrillation catheter ablation of AF, with or without the use of antiarrhythmic drugs, is widely acknowledged as being superior to pharmacologic therapy alone in maintaining SR.[42,43] At present there are limited data that specifically address the issue of catheter ablation for the older patient with symptomatic AF and HF. A recent meta-analysis on the role of AF ablation in patients with HF concluded an overall improvement in symptoms and EF with catheter ablation,[44] however the mean age of patients in the studies analyzed ranged from 49 to 62 years. CABANA (catheter ablation vs antiarrhythmic drug therapy for AF) is a multicenter international randomized trial on catheter ablation for AF compared with medical therapy (without HF) targeting older patients or those with elevated stroke risk, with the primary end point of mortality. Unfortunately, the results are not yet available and we can only consider retrospective analyses and nonrandomized studies to provide guidance (**Table 1**).[45–47,49–54]

There are 2 fundamental questions that need to be answered. First, is the ablation of AF in the older patient with HF effective? Second, is it safe? Neither question can be answered directly from the literature at present, but CASTLE-AF (Catheter Ablation vs Standard conventional Treatment in patients with LEft ventricular dysfunction and Atrial Fibrillation)[55] is an ongoing study aiming to

Table 1
Reported success rates for atrial fibrillation ablation in older patients

Study	No. of Patients	Age (y)	PAF (%)	Success Rate (%)	Follow-up (mo)
Bhargava et al,[45] 2004	103	>60	52	82	14.7
Bunch et al,[46] 2010	35	≥80	46	78	12
Corrado et al,[47] 2008	174	>75	55	95	20
Haegeli et al,[48] 2010	45	≥65	87	74	6
Hsieh et al,[49] 2005	37	>65	100	81	52
Kusumoto et al,[50] 2009	61	>75	34	82	12
Nademanee et al,[51] 2008	635	>65	40	81	27
Tan et al,[52] 2010	200	≥70	54	71	18
Traub et al,[53] 2009	15	≥70	100	60	12
Zado et al,[54] 2008	32	≥75	53	86	27

Abbreviation: PAF, paroxysmal atrial fibrillation.
Data from Refs.[45–54]

address this question in patients with AF and HF without an age cutoff.

Although the number of patients in most studies is small and there is some heterogeneity in the reported success rates, catheter ablation of AF is associated with equivalent success rates to younger patients when undertaken in *highly selected* elderly patients.[56] In the series by Zado and colleagues,[54] the success rate was more than 85% in the group of patients older than 75; however, older patients were less likely to undergo a repeat ablation and more likely to remain on antiarrhythmic drugs, but only represented a small proportion of the study group overall. Similar findings on antiarrhythmic drug use after ablation were demonstrated in the series by Traub and colleagues[53] and Kusumoto and colleagues.[50]

Taken together, there are data to support the efficacy of AF ablation in nonelderly patients with HF and data to support the efficacy of AF ablation in the older patient without HF. However, we await the outcomes of large randomized studies, such as CABANA and CASTLE-AF[55] enrolling older patients with AF and structural heart disease before defining the role of catheter ablation in the older patient with AF and HF.

Safety is important in assessing the role of catheter ablation of AF in older patients with HF. In general terms, older patients are widely acknowledged to have higher complication rates for most medical or surgical interventions. Early data support this, with age older than 70 years shown to be associated with a fourfold increase in risk of major complications from AF ablation in a retrospective, single-center series reported by Spragg and colleagues.[57] This result was consistent with an earlier report by Oral and Morady[58] showing a fourfold increase in risk of tamponade or stroke in patients older than 70 years.

However, with increasing experience and better tools to guide and deliver ablation, the procedure has become safer. More recent studies demonstrate equivalent safety in elderly compared with younger patients, although it must be acknowledged that these are *carefully selected* elderly patients.[46,47,50,53] Changes in ablation techniques combined with irrigated ablation, and refinement of periprocedural anticoagulation protocols are possibly responsible for the reduction in increased risk observed in earlier reports of ablation in the elderly.

Although there are no prospective, randomized trials to guide decision making in the elderly with AF and HF, catheter ablation appears to be effective and can be undertaken safely by experienced operators. This is reflected in the change in patient demographics reported in the most recent worldwide survey on AF reported by Cappato and colleagues.[59] Catheter ablation for AF is being undertaken in older patients and patients with worse LV function.[9,42]

Pacemaker Combined with AVN Ablation

The role of AVN ablation combined with permanent pacing is discussed in detail elsewhere.[60] AVN ablation provides effective rate control in drug-refractory AF, but must be preceded by pacemaker implantation.[61] Catheter "modification" of the AVN has also been described in an attempt to avoid pacemaker implantation, but the effects are not predictable, with potential complications, including polymorphic ventricular tachycardia or late atrioventricular block, and this is not recommended.[62,63] Brignole and colleagues[64] showed that a "pace and ablate" approach was superior to pharmacologic therapy in symptom control for AF. Significant improvement of LV function is seen in most patients following this procedure.[65] However, randomized trials support pulmonary vein isolation over AVN ablation in younger patients with AF and HF.[49,66]

AVN ablation and permanent pacing is often viewed as a more attractive therapy for the elderly.[67] However, there remains a paucity of randomized data comparing it to optimal medical therapy or catheter ablation of AF in elderly patients with AF and HF. Ablation of the AVN combined with permanent pacing does not prevent AF, and physicians must ensure appropriate anticoagulation is continued.

The choice of pacing system is important, especially in patients with HF. The clinician treating the patient with HF and uncontrolled AF with "pace and ablate" must consider whether it is appropriate to place a single-chamber pacemaker on the assumption that a tachycardia-mediated cardiomyopathy is present and will improve.[68] However, if there is a primary cardiomyopathy, chronic pacing of the right ventricle (RV) can be deleterious.[69–71] The Post AV Nodal Ablation Evaluation (PAVE) trial randomized patients (mean age 69 years and mean EF 46%) undergoing AVN ablation to receive either RV-only or biventricular pacing.[72] Biventricular pacing was shown to be superior to RV-only pacing, particularly in more severe LV function. Accordingly, major cardiology guidelines[42,73] advocate the implantation of a biventricular pacemaker to prevent deterioration in LV function when performing AVN ablation in a patient with AF and HF.[59,73]

AVN ablation is also recommended in guidelines to ensure complete biventricular capture in patients with HF and AF who already have a biventricular pacemaker implanted.[74,75] A recent meta-analysis by Ganesan and colleagues[76] reported that AVN ablation in patients with HF and biventricular pacemakers was associated with significant reductions in all-cause mortality and an improvement in NYHA functional class. The mean age of patients in this analysis ranged from 63 to 72 years.

SUMMARY

There are few randomized control trials that specifically assess the optimal management of AF in the older patient with HF. Studies are ongoing that will hopefully provide more evidence in this area.

Older patients with AF and HF are at significant risk for thromboembolic complications and should be anticoagulated unless the bleeding risk is considered prohibitive.

Rate control is equivalent to rhythm control in minimally symptomatic patients with AF. Rate control can be achieved medically, but often drugs are less well tolerated in the older patient and in these cases AVN ablation combined with biventricular pacing can be very effective.

Rhythm control for symptomatic benefit can be achieved pharmacologically or by catheter ablation, and there is growing evidence that catheter ablation of AF in older patients with HF is effective, superior to medical therapy alone, and can be delivered safely.

REFERENCES

1. Feinberg WM, Blackshear JL, Laupacis A, et al. Prevalence, age distribution, and gender of patients with atrial fibrillation. Analysis and implications. Arch Intern Med 1995;155(5):469–73.
2. Kannel WB, Belanger AJ. Epidemiology of heart failure. Am Heart J 1991;121(3 Pt 1):951–7.
3. Cleland JG, Swedberg K, Follath F, et al. The EuroHeart Failure survey programme—a survey on the quality of care among patients with heart failure in Europe. Part 1: patient characteristics and diagnosis. Eur Heart J 2003;24(5):442–63.
4. Maisel WH, Stevenson LW. Atrial fibrillation in heart failure: epidemiology, pathophysiology, and rationale for therapy. Am J Cardiol 2003;91(6A):2D–8D.
5. Shi S, Klotz U. Age-related changes in pharmacokinetics. Curr Drug Metab 2011;12(7):601–10.
6. Wyse DG, Waldo AL, DiMarco JP, et al. A comparison of rate control and rhythm control in patients with atrial fibrillation. N Engl J Med 2002;347(23):1825–33.
7. Van Gelder IC, Hagens VE, Bosker HA, et al. A comparison of rate control and rhythm control in patients with recurrent persistent atrial fibrillation. N Engl J Med 2002;347(23):1834–40.
8. Echt DS, Liebson PR, Mitchell LB, et al. Mortality and morbidity in patients receiving encainide, flecainide, or placebo. The Cardiac Arrhythmia Suppression Trial. N Engl J Med 1991;324(12):781–8.
9. Akiyama T, Pawitan Y, Campbell WB, et al. Effects of advancing age on the efficacy and side effects of antiarrhythmic drugs in post-myocardial infarction patients with ventricular arrhythmias. The CAST Investigators. J Am Geriatr Soc 1992;40(7):666–72.
10. Fuster V, Ryden LE, Cannom DS, et al. ACC/AHA/ESC 2006 Guidelines for the Management of Patients with Atrial Fibrillation: a report of the American College of Cardiology/American Heart Association Task Force on Practice Guidelines and the European Society of Cardiology Committee

for Practice Guidelines (Writing Committee to Revise the 2001 Guidelines for the Management of Patients With Atrial Fibrillation): developed in collaboration with the European Heart Rhythm Association and the Heart Rhythm Society. Circulation 2006;114(7):e257–354.

11. Van Gelder IC, Groenveld HF, Crijns HJ, et al. Lenient versus strict rate control in patients with atrial fibrillation. N Engl J Med 2010;362(15): 1363–73.
12. Freudenberger RS, Wilson AC, Kostis JB. Comparison of rate versus rhythm control for atrial fibrillation in patients with left ventricular dysfunction (from the AFFIRM Study). Am J Cardiol 2007; 100(2):247–52.
13. Corley SD, Epstein AE, DiMarco JP, et al. Relationships between sinus rhythm, treatment, and survival in the Atrial Fibrillation Follow-Up Investigation of Rhythm Management (AFFIRM) Study. Circulation 2004;109(12):1509–13.
14. Roy D, Talajic M, Nattel S, et al. Rhythm control versus rate control for atrial fibrillation and heart failure. N Engl J Med 2008;358(25):2667–77.
15. Shelton RJ, Clark AL, Goode K, et al. A randomised, controlled study of rate versus rhythm control in patients with chronic atrial fibrillation and heart failure: (CAFE-II Study). Heart 2009; 95(11):924–30.
16. Camm AJ, Lip GY, De Caterina R, et al. 2012 focused update of the ESC Guidelines for the management of atrial fibrillation: an update of the 2010 ESC Guidelines for the management of atrial fibrillation. Developed with the special contribution of the European Heart Rhythm Association. Eur Heart J 2012;33(21):2719–47.
17. Wann LS, Curtis AB, Ellenbogen KA, et al. 2011 ACCF/AHA/HRS focused update on the management of patients with atrial fibrillation (update on dabigatran). A report of the American College of Cardiology Foundation/American Heart Association Task Force on Practice Guidelines. Heart Rhythm 2011;8(3):e1–8.
18. Singh BN, Singh SN, Reda DJ, et al. Amiodarone versus sotalol for atrial fibrillation. N Engl J Med 2005;352(18):1861–72.
19. Hunt SA, Abraham WT, Chin MH, et al. 2009 Focused update incorporated into the ACC/AHA 2005 Guidelines for the Diagnosis and Management of Heart Failure in Adults. A report of the American College of Cardiology Foundation/American Heart Association Task Force on Practice Guidelines developed in collaboration with the International Society for Heart and Lung Transplantation. J Am Coll Cardiol 2009;53(15):e1–90.
20. Flather MD, Shibata MC, Coats AJ, et al. Randomized trial to determine the effect of nebivolol on mortality and cardiovascular hospital admission in elderly patients with heart failure (SENIORS). Eur Heart J 2005;26(3):215–25.
21. Mulder BA, van Veldhuisen DJ, Crijns HJ, et al. Effect of nebivolol on outcome in elderly patients with heart failure and atrial fibrillation: insights from SENIORS. Eur J Heart Fail 2012;14(10): 1171–8.
22. Poole-Wilson PA, Swedberg K, Cleland JG, et al. Comparison of carvedilol and metoprolol on clinical outcomes in patients with chronic heart failure in the Carvedilol Or Metoprolol European Trial (COMET): randomised controlled trial. Lancet 2003;362(9377):7–13.
23. Ahmed A, Rich MW, Love TE, et al. Digoxin and reduction in mortality and hospitalization in heart failure: a comprehensive post hoc analysis of the DIG trial. Eur Heart J 2006;27(2):178–86.
24. Khand AU, Rankin AC, Martin W, et al. Carvedilol alone or in combination with digoxin for the management of atrial fibrillation in patients with heart failure? J Am Coll Cardiol 2003;42(11):1944–51.
25. Ulimoen SR, Enger S, Carlson J, et al. Comparison of four single-drug regimens on ventricular rate and arrhythmia-related symptoms in patients with permanent atrial fibrillation. Am J Cardiol 2013; 111(2):225–30.
26. Lin HJ, Wolf PA, Kelly-Hayes M, et al. Stroke severity in atrial fibrillation. The Framingham Study. Stroke 1996;27(10):1760–4.
27. Wolf PA, Abbott RD, Kannel WB. Atrial fibrillation as an independent risk factor for stroke: the Framingham Study. Stroke 1991;22(8):983–8.
28. Olesen JB, Lip GY, Hansen ML, et al. Validation of risk stratification schemes for predicting stroke and thromboembolism in patients with atrial fibrillation: nationwide cohort study. BMJ 2011;342:d124.
29. Fang MC, Go AS, Hylek EM, et al. Age and the risk of warfarin-associated hemorrhage: the anticoagulation and risk factors in atrial fibrillation study. J Am Geriatr Soc 2006;54(8):1231–6.
30. Rash A, Downes T, Portner R, et al. A randomised controlled trial of warfarin versus aspirin for stroke prevention in octogenarians with atrial fibrillation (WASPO). Age Ageing 2007;36(2):151–6.
31. Mant J, Hobbs FD, Fletcher K, et al. Warfarin versus aspirin for stroke prevention in an elderly community population with atrial fibrillation (the Birmingham Atrial Fibrillation Treatment of the Aged Study, BAFTA): a randomised controlled trial. Lancet 2007;370(9586):493–503.
32. Friberg L, Rosenqvist M, Lip GY. Evaluation of risk stratification schemes for ischaemic stroke and bleeding in 182 678 patients with atrial fibrillation: the Swedish Atrial Fibrillation cohort study. Eur Heart J 2012;33(12):1500–10.
33. Nieuwlaat R, Capucci A, Camm AJ, et al. Atrial fibrillation management: a prospective survey in

ESC member countries: the Euro Heart Survey on Atrial Fibrillation. Eur Heart J 2005;26(22):2422–34.
34. Man-Son-Hing M, Laupacis A. Anticoagulant-related bleeding in older persons with atrial fibrillation: physicians' fears often unfounded. Arch Intern Med 2003;163(13):1580–6.
35. Fang MC, Go AS, Chang Y, et al. A new risk scheme to predict warfarin-associated hemorrhage: the ATRIA (Anticoagulation and Risk Factors in Atrial Fibrillation) Study. J Am Coll Cardiol 2011; 58(4):395–401.
36. Pisters R, Lane DA, Nieuwlaat R, et al. A novel user-friendly score (HAS-BLED) to assess 1-year risk of major bleeding in patients with atrial fibrillation: the Euro Heart Survey. Chest 2010;138(5):1093–100.
37. Holbrook AM, Pereira JA, Labiris R, et al. Systematic overview of warfarin and its drug and food interactions. Arch Intern Med 2005;165(10): 1095–106.
38. De Caterina R, Husted S, Wallentin L, et al. New oral anticoagulants in atrial fibrillation and acute coronary syndromes: ESC Working Group on Thrombosis-Task Force on Anticoagulants in Heart Disease position paper. J Am Coll Cardiol 2012; 59(16):1413–25.
39. Connolly SJ, Ezekowitz MD, Yusuf S, et al. Dabigatran versus warfarin in patients with atrial fibrillation. N Engl J Med 2009;361(12):1139–51.
40. Granger CB, Alexander JH, McMurray JJ, et al. Apixaban versus warfarin in patients with atrial fibrillation. N Engl J Med 2011;365(11):981–92.
41. Patel MR, Mahaffey KW, Garg J, et al. Rivaroxaban versus warfarin in nonvalvular atrial fibrillation. N Engl J Med 2011;365(10):883–91.
42. Camm AJ, Lip GY, De Caterina R, et al. 2012 focused update of the ESC Guidelines for the management of atrial fibrillation: an update of the 2010 ESC Guidelines for the management of atrial fibrillation—developed with the special contribution of the European Heart Rhythm Association. Europace 2012;14(10):1385–413.
43. Wilber DJ, Pappone C, Neuzil P, et al. Comparison of antiarrhythmic drug therapy and radiofrequency catheter ablation in patients with paroxysmal atrial fibrillation: a randomized controlled trial. JAMA 2010;303(4):333–40.
44. Dagres N, Varounis C, Gaspar T, et al. Catheter ablation for atrial fibrillation in patients with left ventricular systolic dysfunction. A systematic review and meta-analysis. J Card Fail 2011;17(11):964–70.
45. Bhargava M, Marrouche NF, Martin DO, et al. Impact of age on the outcome of pulmonary vein isolation for atrial fibrillation using circular mapping technique and cooled-tip ablation catheter. J Cardiovasc Electrophysiol 2004;15(1):8–13.
46. Bunch TJ, Weiss JP, Crandall BG, et al. Long-term clinical efficacy and risk of catheter ablation for atrial fibrillation in octogenarians. Pacing Clin Electrophysiol 2010;33(2):146–52.
47. Corrado A, Patel D, Riedlbauchova L, et al. Efficacy, safety, and outcome of atrial fibrillation ablation in septuagenarians. J Cardiovasc Electrophysiol 2008;19(8):807–11.
48. Haegeli LM, Duru F, Lockwood EE, et al. Ablation of atrial fibrillation after the retirement age: considerations on safety and outcome. J Interv Card Electrophysiol 2010;28(3):193–7.
49. Hsieh MH, Tai CT, Lee SH, et al. Catheter ablation of atrial fibrillation versus atrioventricular junction ablation plus pacing therapy for elderly patients with medically refractory paroxysmal atrial fibrillation. J Cardiovasc Electrophysiol 2005;16(5):457–61.
50. Kusumoto F, Prussak K, Wiesinger M, et al. Radiofrequency catheter ablation of atrial fibrillation in older patients: outcomes and complications. J Interv Card Electrophysiol 2009;25(1):31–5.
51. Nademanee K, Schwab MC, Kosar EM, et al. Clinical outcomes of catheter substrate ablation for high-risk patients with atrial fibrillation. J Am Coll Cardiol 2008;51(8):843–9.
52. Tan HW, Wang XH, Shi HF, et al. Efficacy, safety and outcome of catheter ablation for atrial fibrillation in octogenarians. Int J Cardiol 2010;145(1): 147–8.
53. Traub D, Daubert JP, McNitt S, et al. Catheter ablation of atrial fibrillation in the elderly: where do we stand? Cardiol J 2009;16(2):113–20.
54. Zado E, Callans DJ, Riley M, et al. Long-term clinical efficacy and risk of catheter ablation for atrial fibrillation in the elderly. J Cardiovasc Electrophysiol 2008;19(6):621–6.
55. Marrouche NF, Brachmann J. Catheter ablation versus standard conventional treatment in patients with left ventricular dysfunction and atrial fibrillation (CASTLE-AF)—study design. Pacing Clin Electrophysiol 2009;32(8):987–94.
56. Yamada T, Kay GN. Catheter ablation of atrial fibrillation in the elderly. Pacing Clin Electrophysiol 2009;32(8):1085–91.
57. Spragg DD, Dalal D, Cheema A, et al. Complications of catheter ablation for atrial fibrillation: incidence and predictors. J Cardiovasc Electrophysiol 2008;19(6):627–31.
58. Oral H, Morady F. How to select patients for atrial fibrillation ablation. Heart Rhythm 2006;3(5):615–8.
59. Cappato R, Calkins H, Chen SA, et al. Updated worldwide survey on the methods, efficacy, and safety of catheter ablation for human atrial fibrillation. Circ Arrhythm Electrophysiol 2010;3(1):32–8.
60. Hoffmayer KS, Scheinman M. Current role of atrioventricular junction (AVJ) ablation. Pacing Clin Electrophysiol 2013;36(2):257–65.
61. Langberg JJ, Chin M, Schamp DJ, et al. Ablation of the atrioventricular junction with radiofrequency

energy using a new electrode catheter. Am J Cardiol 1991;67(2):142–7.

62. Menozzi C, Brignole M, Gianfranchi L, et al. Radiofrequency catheter ablation and modulation of atrioventricular conduction in patients with atrial fibrillation. Pacing Clin Electrophysiol 1994;17(11 Pt 2):2143–9.
63. Morady F, Hasse C, Strickberger SA, et al. Long-term follow-up after radiofrequency modification of the atrioventricular node in patients with atrial fibrillation. J Am Coll Cardiol 1997;29(1):113–21.
64. Brignole M, Menozzi C, Gianfranchi L, et al. Assessment of atrioventricular junction ablation and VVIR pacemaker versus pharmacological treatment in patients with heart failure and chronic atrial fibrillation: a randomized, controlled study. Circulation 1998;98(10):953–60.
65. Wood MA, Brown-Mahoney C, Kay GN, et al. Clinical outcomes after ablation and pacing therapy for atrial fibrillation: a meta-analysis. Circulation 2000; 101(10):1138–44.
66. Khan MN, Jais P, Cummings J, et al. Pulmonary-vein isolation for atrial fibrillation in patients with heart failure. N Engl J Med 2008;359(17):1778–85.
67. Hindricks G. The Multicentre European Radiofrequency Survey (MERFS): complications of radiofrequency catheter ablation of arrhythmias. The Multicentre European Radiofrequency Survey (MERFS) investigators of the Working Group on Arrhythmias of the European Society of Cardiology. Eur Heart J 1993;14(12):1644–53.
68. Lemery R, Brugada P, Cheriex E, et al. Reversibility of tachycardia-induced left ventricular dysfunction after closed-chest catheter ablation of the atrioventricular junction for intractable atrial fibrillation. Am J Cardiol 1987;60(16):1406–8.
69. Leong DP, Mitchell AM, Salna I, et al. Long-term mechanical consequences of permanent right ventricular pacing: effect of pacing site. J Cardiovasc Electrophysiol 2010;21(10):1120–6.
70. Sharma AD, Rizo-Patron C, Hallstrom AP, et al. Percent right ventricular pacing predicts outcomes in the DAVID trial. Heart Rhythm 2005;2(8):830–4.
71. Wilkoff BL, Cook JR, Epstein AE, et al. Dual-chamber pacing or ventricular backup pacing in patients with an implantable defibrillator: the Dual Chamber and VVI Implantable Defibrillator (DAVID) Trial. JAMA 2002;288(24):3115–23.
72. Doshi RN, Daoud EG, Fellows C, et al. Left ventricular-based cardiac stimulation post AV nodal ablation evaluation (the PAVE study). J Cardiovasc Electrophysiol 2005;16(11):1160–5.
73. Fuster V, Ryden LE, Cannom DS, et al. 2011 ACCF/AHA/HRS focused updates incorporated into the ACC/AHA/ESC 2006 Guidelines for the management of patients with atrial fibrillation: a report of the American College of Cardiology Foundation/American Heart Association Task Force on Practice Guidelines developed in partnership with the European Society of Cardiology and in collaboration with the European Heart Rhythm Association and the Heart Rhythm Society. J Am Coll Cardiol 2011;57(11):e101–98.
74. Dickstein K, Vardas PE, Auricchio A, et al. 2010 Focused Update of ESC Guidelines on device therapy in heart failure: an update of the 2008 ESC Guidelines for the diagnosis and treatment of acute and chronic heart failure and the 2007 ESC Guidelines for cardiac and resynchronization therapy. Developed with the special contribution of the Heart Failure Association and the European Heart Rhythm Association. Europace 2010;12(11):1526–36.
75. Epstein AE, Dimarco JP, Ellenbogen KA, et al. ACC/AHA/HRS 2008 guidelines for Device-Based Therapy of Cardiac Rhythm Abnormalities: executive summary. Heart Rhythm 2008;5(6):934–55.
76. Ganesan AN, Brooks AG, Roberts-Thomson KC, et al. Role of AV nodal ablation in cardiac resynchronization in patients with coexistent atrial fibrillation and heart failure. J Am Coll Cardiol 2012;59(8):719–26.

Case Selection for Cardiac Resynchronization in Atrial Fibrillation

John G.F. Cleland, MD, FRCP, FESC*,
Freidoon Keshavarzi, MD, MRCP, Pierpaolo Pellicori, MD,
Benjamin Dicken, MBBS, MRCP

KEYWORDS

- Cardiac resynchronization therapy • Atrial fibrillation • Atrioventricular resynchronization
- Biventricular capture • Heart failure

KEY POINTS

- Several guidelines make strong recommendations in favor of cardiac resynchronization therapy (CRT) for patients with atrial fibrillation (AF); however, avoiding implantation of CRT in patients with AF is more consistent with current evidence and reasonable clinical practice.
- Circumstances in which implantation of CRT into patients with AF should at least be considered include (1) those in whom a return to sinus rhythm is anticipated; (2) as a last resort in patients who lack better alternatives; and, perhaps, (3) patients with AF who otherwise are indicated for CRT and are about to receive either a standard pacemaker or an implantable defibrillator.
- Biventricular pacing cannot be effective unless AV conduction is suppressed.
- Failure of biventricular capture might explain the lack of benefit of CRT in AF; however, providing a possible explanation for failure does not constitute proof of efficacy. Further trials are required.

BACKGROUND

The prevalence of atrial fibrillation (AF) ranges from about 5% in patients with asymptomatic cardiac dysfunction to more than 50% of those with severe symptomatic heart failure.[1,2] In many patients, the onset of heart failure and AF coincide. Hypertension and coronary disease will often cause chronic cardiac dysfunction that progresses silently until symptoms are precipitated by an event such as the onset of AF or acute myocardial infarction.[3–5] In this sense, AF is the cause of heart failure, although rarely in isolation. Aggressive restoration of sinus rhythm may improve symptoms and quality of life in selected patients, although this has not yet been translated into an improvement in outcome.[6,7] The benefits of restoring sinus rhythm in the one large trial that addressed this issue may have been offset by the adverse effects of amiodarone.[6]

The onset of AF in patients with preexisting heart failure indicates a poor prognosis.[8] Patients who develop heart failure as a consequence of AF (about 75% of those admitted when these two conditions coexist) have a better outcome than those who develop AF after the onset of heart failure.[9] Patients with chronic heart failure receiving contemporary therapy for heart failure, including beta-blockers, have a similar outcome, after adjusting for age and symptom severity, whether they are in persistent AF or in sinus rhythm, although patients with left bundle branch block might have a worse prognosis if in AF.[8,10,11]

Disclosures: Professor Cleland has received honoraria from Medtronic, Sorin and St Jude within the last 5 years for speaking at symposia and on advisory committees. Prof Cleland and Dr Dicken are investigators for the RESPOND study, funded by Sorin.
Department of Cardiology, Castle Hill Hospital, Hull York Medical School, University of Hull, Kingston-upon-Hull HU6 5JQ, UK
* Corresponding author.
E-mail address: j.g.cleland@hull.ac.uk

Heart Failure Clin 9 (2013) 461–474
http://dx.doi.org/10.1016/j.hfc.2013.07.001

Among patients with an implanted device that can record atrial arrhythmias, otherwise undetected paroxysmal AF may be present in more than 40% of patients[12–21]; when the burden is high (>3.8 hours per day), the risk of thromboembolic events, hospitalization for heart failure, and death increases substantially.[18] Studies in patients with less severe disease have also noted that only prolonged episodes of AF (>18 hours) seem to predict adverse outcomes.[22,23] Preimplant history is important both for predicting recurrent AF and the subsequent risk of embolic events.[18] About one-third of patients with a prior history of AF will develop a clinical overt recurrence in the following 1 to 2 years compared with about 10% without such a history (**Table 1**).[12–21] Device-detected episodes lasting more than 24 hours probably occur in only 5% to 10% of those without a history of AF but perhaps more than 20% of those with such a history (see **Table 1**). Clearly, AF is an important issue for many patients both before and after the implantation of a CRT device.

Pharmacologic treatment of heart failure can alter the risk of developing AF. Angiotensin-converting enzyme inhibitors, beta-blockers, and aldosterone antagonists have all been shown to reduce the incidence of AF in patients with heart failure and left ventricular systolic dysfunction (LVSD), whereas ivabradine, an agent that slows the rate of sinus node discharge, has been shown to increase the risk of AF.[1,2,24,25] The presence of AF may also alter the impact of treatment on the outcome. Patients with AF and LVSD do not seem to benefit from beta-1-selective blockers and may have a reduced response to carvedilol.[26] Drug therapy aimed at rhythm control for AF does not seem to improve the outcome of patients with heart failure and LVSD.[6] For patients in sinus rhythm, the optimal heart rate seems to be between 50 to 60 beats per minute (bpm); but for patients in AF, the optimal resting ventricular rate as observed in the clinic seems to be closer to 80 bpm.[27–29] The reason for this difference in optimal heart rate is unknown but could be related to excessive slowing of nocturnal ventricular rate with increased exposure to pause-dependent ventricular tachycardia.[29–31]

POTENTIAL MECHANISMS OF BENEFIT OF CARDIAC RESYNCHRONIZATION THERAPY

There is no doubt that cardiac resynchronization therapy (CRT) works, but exactly how it works remains elusive. It is likely that there are at least 4 major mechanisms in play, with the relative importance of each varying from one patient to the next and, perhaps, over time.

Studies attempting to predict the benefit from CRT have come up with remarkably little evidence to support any particular patient characteristic before implantation other than the QRS duration.[32] There are lots of observational studies purporting to show differences according to sex, cause of ventricular dysfunction, or QRS morphology; but these fail to disentangle factors reflecting the natural history of the disease from the effects of CRT. Identifying markers that predict the response to intervention rather than merely predictors of outcome in patients who have had the intervention requires randomized trials.[33] Further confusion has been caused by using improvements in LV function as a surrogate for response. It is true that patients with dilated cardiomyopathy have a greater improvement in LV function in response to CRT and a better prognosis compared with patients with ischemic heart disease (IHD). However, the change in prognosis wrought by CRT is similar or greater in patients with IHD.[32,34–36] So in population terms, if we want to improve the echocardiogram, we should implant CRT devices into patients with dilated cardiomyopathy; but if we want to prolong life, then we should choose to implant them into patients with LVSD caused by IHD.

Studies conducted at the time of CRT implantation provide some further insights into the likely mechanisms of benefit from CRT. The LV pacing site seems to be important. Pacing scarred regions should be avoided. Pacing regions exhibiting dyssynchrony that are far from the right ventricular (RV) pacing site seem successful.[37,38] The choice of LV pacing site can make a large difference to the effects of CRT on raising blood pressure, a candidate predictor of the longer-term benefits of CRT.[37,39]

Randomized controlled trials of device programming after implantation have been marred by the inclusion of all-comers, whether they have responded to the initial implantation or not and, therefore, provide little help in determining the importance of individualized programming among patients with a poor response to CRT.[40–44] Many patients respond to the standard factory CRT settings and may not benefit from reprogramming. Acute studies of programming suggest little effect of altering the inter-ventricular (VV) pacing interval on blood pressure or cardiac function in most patients but substantial differences with atrioventricular (AV) programming.[45,46] This finding implies that AV resynchronization might be more clinically important than VV resynchronization, as also suggested by a recent analysis of the MADIT-CRT (Multicenter Automatic Defibrillator Implantation with Cardiac Resynchronization Therapy) study.[47] If this is true, then CRT may deliver little or even no

Table 1
Studies investigating the incidence of AF in patients receiving CRT (where n >100)

Author, Pub Year	PAF if Reported	N =	Age (y)	IHD (%)	FU	Min Dur AF	AF: Device Diagnostics (%)	AF: Clinical n = (%)	Effect of AF on Clinical Outcome
Puglisi et al,[12] 2008	No	249	69	—	13 mo	>5 min (24 h)	42 (6)	—	Reduced activity
	Yes	161	—	—			47 (22)	—	
Borleffs et al,[13] 2009	No	223	—	—	32 mo	—	25	unknown	Less improvement
Caldwell et al,[14] 2009	No	101	66	60	—	30 s	27	—	Higher mortality if AF
	Yes	18			—		*High*	—	
Leclerq et al, 2010	No	82	70	28	6 mo	—	17	—	Less improvement
	Yes	38	—	—		—	29	—	
Marijon et al,[16] 2010	No	173	70	—	10 mo	—	28	—	Predicted clinical AF
Boriani et al,[17] 2011	—	1404		—	—	—	32	—	—
Shanmugam et al,[18] 2012	—	560	66	54	—	—	—	—	—
CARE-HF Control,[66] 2005	No	314	67	—	29 mo	—	Not applicable	30 (10)	Outcome worse in patients who developed AF who were assigned to either strategy; some attenuation of effect of CRT on M/M
	Yes	90						28 (31)	
CARE-HF CRT	No	330				>10 min (48 h)	93 (28)[a]	40 (12)	
	Yes	79					20 (25)[a]	26 (33)	
Padeletti et al,[20] 2008	No	323	68	49	12 mo	—	unknown	26 (8)	—
	Yes	71		—		—	unknown	25 (35)	—
MADIT-CRT 2011	—	1820	—	—	—	—	8	—	—
Santini et al,[21] 2011	—	—	—	—	13 mo	—	30	—	—

Abbreviations: Dur, duration; FU, follow-up; IHD, ischemic heart disease; MADIT-CRT, multicenter automatic defibrillator implantation with cardiac resynchronization therapy trial; Min, minimum; M/M, morbidity and mortality; PAF, paroxysmal atrial fibrillation; Pub, publication.

[a] This value does not include patients who were detected during clinical follow-up.

Data from Refs.[12–21,75]

benefit in the absence of atrial systole. However, the most striking marker of super response is the correction of mitral regurgitation.[34,48] The effects of CRT on mitral regurgitation are almost immediate,[34] and it is possible that it is the ventricular stimulation site that exerts the greater reduction in mitral regurgitation that is the optimal pacing site. Clearly, only patients who have mitral regurgitation can benefit from CRT by this mechanism.

To summarize, of the 4 likely main mechanisms of CRT benefit, 3 can be observed at the initial clinical assessment and are (1) correction of ventricular dyssynchrony; (2) correction of AV dyssynchrony including diastolic mitral regurgitation; and (3) reduction, when present, of mitral systolic regurgitation by resynchronizing papillary muscle contraction. These effects are then likely to lead to favorable LV remodeling, especially if the left ventricle is not heavily scarred. The fourth mechanism, the effects of CRT on arrhythmias, still requires longer-term verification and may be secondary to ventricular remodeling or caused by the prevention of pauses.

Patients with AF cannot benefit from AV resynchronization and can only benefit from VV resynchronization if ventricular capture occurs. This requires AV conduction to be slow or absent, which may be achieved by AV conduction system disease, by drugs, or (most reliably) by AV ablation. It is also possible that a more regular ventricular rhythm may improve cardiac performance as varying ventricular filling periods may lead to wide variations in filling pressures and autonomic feedback from one cardiac cycle to the next and long diastolic periods will lead to diastolic mitral regurgitation. The alternative to controlling ventricular rate is to try and restore sinus rhythm, either by pharmacologic or electrical cardioversion or by catheter ablation.[49,50]

CRT could affect the incidence of several arrhythmias. Reductions in atrial pressure should lead to a reduction in recurrent AF. Although some observational trials have suggested that CRT may reduce the AF burden according to the device diagnostics, randomized trials have been unable to show an effect on clinically relevant AF,[19,51] although longer-term follow-up suggests there may be delayed benefits perhaps consequent on late ventricular remodeling.[52] Possibly, the presence of a wire and the associated fibrotic reaction in the atrial wall is a stimulus to developing AF that negates the early hemodynamic benefits of CRT. However, it is likely, as with most treatments, that some patients benefit and some are harmed. With respect to the incidence of AF, harm and benefit seem to be in equilibrium.

CRT could also reduce the risk of ventricular arrhythmias. In the MADIT-CRT trial, implantation of CRT-defibrillator (D) rather than an implantable cardioverter defibrillator (ICD) was associated with a lower rate of ventricular arrhythmias requiring therapy, although there was no difference in mortality.[53] In CARE-HF (Cardiac Resynchronization-Heart Failure) trial, the implantation of a CRT pacemaker was associated with a reduction in sudden death compared with medical treatment alone.[36,53] The reduction in sudden death may have occurred only after the first year of follow-up, suggesting that ventricular remodeling may have played a role. However, it is possible that the greatest effect of CRT is in preventing pauses that represent a potentially significant direct cause of sudden death in advanced heart failure or a trigger for ventricular tachycardia.[31] This effect will only be observed in studies if the comparator group has no device. An important effect of CRT on prognosis may be its ability to prevent pauses without exacerbating dyssynchrony.

MANAGING AF IN PATIENTS WITH HEART FAILURE

Although there is no substantial study specifically investigating anticoagulants in patients with heart failure and AF, subgroup analyses and consensus generally support the use of anticoagulants.[54] Some observational trials have not supported this view.[55]

As noted earlier, the optimal ventricular rate in patients with heart failure and AF is uncertain and may be substantially higher than for patients in sinus rhythm.[29] Beta-blockers reduce the sympathetically driven component of heart rate, predominantly during the daytime and exercise; digoxin enhances the parasympathetic component, predominantly at rest and at night.[56] Beta-1-selective blockers seem less effective in improving the outcome of patients with heart failure if they are in AF rather than sinus rhythm.[9] The effects of digoxin on the outcome in patients with heart failure and AF remain unclear.[57]

Restoring sinus rhythm is intuitively appealing providing that treatment is not more toxic than the disease. The potential prognostic benefits of restoring the sinus rhythm with amiodarone or dronedarone seem to be neutralized by adverse effects of these drugs, although they might still improve the quality of life for some patients.[58–61] The benefits and risks of AV node or catheter ablation have not yet been adequately studied.[50] One small study suggested that pulmonary vein isolation was superior to biventricular pacing with AV node ablation in patients with heart failure and AF, again suggesting the importance of restoring atrial function and AV synchrony.[50] Another recent study in which 52 patients, most of whom did not have CRT devices, were randomly assigned to pharmacological ventricular rate control or pulmonary vein ablation, suggested that the latter strategy was associated with a greater improvement in quality of life and exercise capacity.[62] The rate and consequences of silent cerebral infarction after catheter ablation for AF are incompletely understood.[63] Unfortunately, a randomized trial of atrial overdrive pacing in patients with CRT failed to alter the incidence of AF.[20]

A further problem associated with AF in patients who receive a defibrillator in addition to CRT is an increased risk of inappropriate shocks, although contemporary conservative programming schemes with longer diagnostic delays (typically 20–30 beats) and widespread use of beta-blockers that reduce the risk of rapid ventricular response rates may have reduced this problem.[64,65]

CLINICAL EVIDENCE FOR CRT

Observational data are an unreliable guide to the benefits of therapy, especially when putative benefits, such as symptoms or ventricular function, have such a large subjective component.

When interpreting a clinical trial, it is important to consider what is being compared. Whether or not to implant a CRT device in patients on a background of pharmacologic therapy is one question (CARE-HF,[66] COMPANION [Comparison of Medical Therapy, Pacing, and Defibrillation in Heart Failure][67]); but whether or not to implant CRT or a backup pacemaker (MUSTIC [Multisite Stimulation in Cardiomyopathies],[68,69] MIRACLE [Multicenter InSync ICD Randomized Clinical Evaluation],[70] REVERSE [Resynchronization Reverses Remodeling in Systolic Left Ventricular Dysfunction trial][71]) or an ICD (MIRACLE-ICD,[72] MADIT-CRT,[73] REVERSE,[71] and RAFT [Resynchronization for Ambulatory Heart Failure Trial][74]) is quite another. The full potential range of CRT's benefit and harm can only be properly addressed in studies that have a device-free control group. Most studies comparing CRT with a control device programmed backup pacing at relatively low rates; this will have prevented profound bradycardia and its consequences. Studies comparing biventricular pacing and RV pacing after AV node ablation should be interpreted with caution. It is likely that AV node ablation with RV pacing is deleterious in patients with LVSD, although it may be innocuous in those without heart failure. This topic is discussed later. Better outcomes with biventricular pacing after AV node ablation may indicate that it is less harmful than RV pacing but do not prove that it is better or safer than avoiding AV node ablation in the first place.

RANDOMIZED TRIALS OF CRT OR CRT-D COMPARED WITH NO DEVICE

The COMPANION study has not reported information on AF. In CARE-HF, patients assigned to CRT were slightly more likely to develop clinically overt AF.[19] This finding could reflect an increased rate of clinical detection of AF caused by the presence of the device, in addition to the obvious increase in detection of asymptomatic AF. Patients with new-onset AF did have a worse outcome, but this was largely explained by their intrinsically worse prognostic profile before the onset of AF. Prior history of AF, left atrial systolic volume, and plasma concentration of NT-proBNP predicted the development of AF.[19] The development of AF did not seem to detract from the benefits of CRT. Several explanations of these findings should be considered: CRT may have delivered benefits before AF developed; AF may have reverted spontaneously or with treatment; ventricular rate control may have been sufficient to ensure a high rate of ventricular capture; or it could be that simply preventing excessive bradycardia in these patients may be beneficial. In other words, CARE-HF does not provide robust evidence that CRT is effective in patients with AF.

RANDOMIZED TRIALS OF CRT COMPARED WITH BACKUP PACING WITHOUT AV NODE ABLATION

The MIRACLE studies have not reported information on AF. MADIT-CRT showed no overall difference between CRT-D and ICD on device-related occurrence of atrial arrhythmias, although the analysis suggested that patients who developed a marked reduction in left atrial volume had a lower incidence of atrial arrhythmias and a markedly better prognosis.[75] In this sense, the left atrium seems to be a good barometer of LV and overall cardiac performance. The RAFT study failed to show a difference between treatments in patients with AF despite a powerful reduction in morbidity and mortality in patients in sinus rhythm (**Fig. 1**).[76] However, only one patient received AV node ablation, and insufficient ventricular rate control probably prevented a high rate of biventricular capture. RAFT did suggest trends to improved quality of life and reductions in heart failure hospitalization among patients with AF.[76]

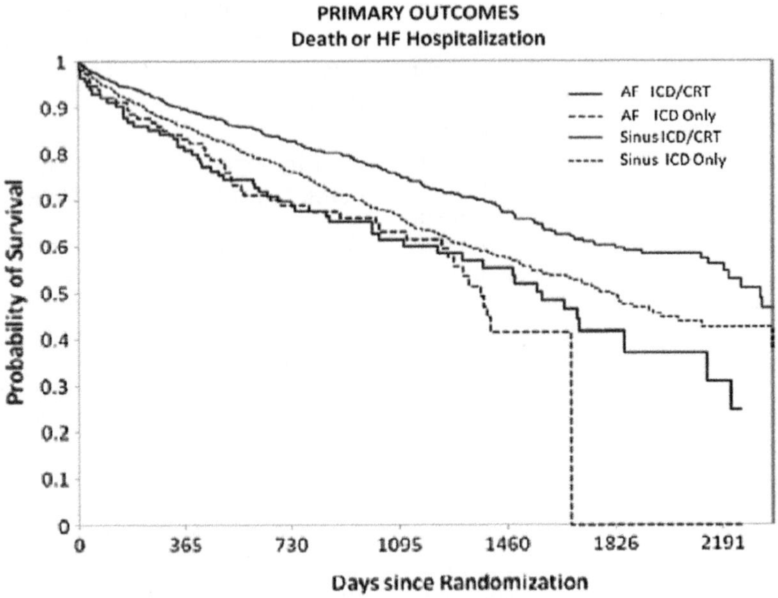

Fig. 1. Effects of cardiac resynchronization on the primary outcome of death or heart failure (HF) hospitalization. (*From* Healey JS, Hohnloser SH, Exner DV, et al, RAFT Investigators. Cardiac resynchronization therapy in patients with permanent atrial fibrillation: results from the Resynchronization for Ambulatory Heart Failure Trial (RAFT). Circ Heart Fail 2012;5(5):568; with permission.)

RANDOMIZED TRIALS COMPARING AV NODE ABLATION AND PACING WITH MEDICAL THERAPY

Although some advocate routine AV node ablation to ensure high rates of ventricular capture, others suggest that AV node ablation is only required in a minority of patients.[77–79]

There are no relevant randomized trials among patients with heart failure and a low LV ejection fraction (LVEF). A meta-analysis of trials including 314 patients mostly with a normal ejection fraction has been conducted.[80] Symptoms generally improved with AV node ablation, but there was insufficient information to identify whether the procedure increased or reduced risks. In a subgroup with a mean ejection fraction of 44%, a 4% improvement in ejection fraction was observed. Many experts advise an increased ventricular pacing rate after AV node ablation to reduce the risk of sudden death.[80,81]

RANDOMIZED TRIALS OF CRT COMPARED WITH BACKUP PACING WITH ROUTINE AV NODE ABLATION

Five trials (**Table 2**), including 637 patients, have compared RV backup pacing with CRT, although only one, MUSTIC-AF, was conducted exclusively in patients with heart failure and a LVEF of 35% or less.[82] Overall, these trials suggested a favorable trend on mortality (risk ratio 0.75, 95% confidence interval [CI] 0.43–1.30; P = .30), a substantial reduction in hospitalization for heart failure (risk ratio 0.38, 95% CI 0.17–0.85; P = .02), and improvement in LVEF by about 2% but no benefit on quality of life or walking distance.[82,83] The results of MUSTIC-AF are consistent with the pooled data.[69] The largest of these studies was the PAVE (Post AV Nodal Ablation Evaluation) study, which enrolled 252 patients with a mean LVEF of 46%.[84] By 6 months, patients assigned to CRT improved their 6-minute walk test more than those assigned to RV pacing. LVEF was unchanged with CRT but decreased with RV pacing. The deterioration in LV function with RV pacing may have accounted for the significantly worse survival of those assigned to RV pacing.

Two small, randomized, crossover trials have compared LV pacing with CRT in patients with AF. One trial of 13 patients suggested that cardiac function and symptom improvement might be superior with CRT compared with LV pacing.[85] The other trial of 56 patients suggested little incremental benefit of either LV pacing or CRT compared with RV pacing on symptoms or walking distance; but both LV pacing and CRT improved LVEF, LV volumes, and mitral regurgitation by similar amounts.[86]

Other studies, such as RD-HF,[87] Homburg Biventricular Pacing Evaluation,[88] and BLOCK-HF (Biventricular Pacing for Atrio-ventricular Block

Table 2
Randomized trials of CRT compared with backup pacing with routine AV node ablation

Comparison	Reference	N with AF	Comparison	Outcome
CRT vs no device			No relevant trials	
CRT vs backup pacing without AVNA	RAFT	229	ICD vs CRT-D	No benefit
RCTs of AVNA	AVERT-AF[90]	180	ICD vs CRT-D + AVNA	Ongoing
	CAAN-HF	550	CRT-D vs CRT-D + AVNA	Ongoing (ClinicalTrials.gov: NCT01522898)
	RAFT-AF	1000	Rhythm control (drugs ± CA) vs rate control (drugs ± AVNA and pacing)	ClinicalTrials.gov: NCT01420393
RCTs of device after routine AVNA	Meta-analysis[82]		RVP (± ICD) vs CRT-D	Favorable trend on mortality. Significant reduction in hospitalizations for heart failure.

Abbreviations: AVNA, atrioventricular node ablation; CA, catheter ablation; CAAN-HF, cardiac resynchronization therapy and AV nodal ablation trial in atrial fibrillation; RCTs, randomized controlled trials; RVP, right ventricular pacing.

and Systolic Dysfunction in Heart Failure),[89] have compared RV pacing with CRT in patients with high-grade AV block who may or may not have been in AF. These studies have also suggested a benefit, but it remains unclear whether the presence of AF influenced the response to CRT or whether, in the absence of atrial systole, differences merely reflect the avoidance of RV-only pacing rather than an intrinsic benefit from CRT.

In summary, these trials strongly suggest that CRT is superior to RV pacing; but this may be because CRT prevents the adverse effects of RV pacing rather than an intrinsic benefit of CRT in patients with AF.

RANDOMIZED TRIALS OF AV NODE ABLATION

No randomized study has specifically compared medical management without AV node ablation with CRT and AV node ablation as necessary to ensure high rates of biventricular capture, and yet this is what guidelines generally advocate. For patients with AF who have received a CRT device, no randomized study has compared medical management with AV node ablation; but such a study is now underway (see **Table 2** CAAN-HF [Cardiac Resynchronization Therapy and AV Nodal Ablation Trial in Atrial Fibrillation]) (ClinicalTrials.gov: NCT01522898). A randomized study, the AVERT-AF trial (Atrio-VEntricular Junction Ablation Followed by Resynchronization Therapy in patients with CHF and AF) is testing the hypothesis that AV node ablation followed by CRT improves symptoms and exercise capacity compared with pharmacologic rate control and an ICD in patients with chronic AF and depressed ejection fraction, regardless of ventricular rate or QRS duration.[90] This study, which should now be complete, will not address the issue of whether patients with a prolonged QRS duration who are in AF should receive CRT or, indeed, any device at all.

OBSERVATIONAL STUDIES

Observational studies provide important information on prognosis and outcome with therapy and to that extent provide insights into met and unmet needs.[33] Cohort studies are a poor substitute for randomized trials but can help create hypotheses.

One of the earliest reports of CRT for AF was a study in which patients who had severe heart failure consequent on AV node ablation and RV pacing. Patients improved with an upgrade to CRT.[91] The extent to which this was caused by better care or correcting problems caused by RV pacing is not clear.

In a meta-analysis of 5 observational studies including 1164 patients, of whom 367 had AF (207 of whom had AV node ablation), mortality and improvement in symptoms after CRT were similar regardless of cardiac rhythm, although patients with AF may have fared less well in terms of exercise capacity and quality of life.[92] In a meta-analysis of 6 observational studies including 768 with AF, the 339 patients who had an AV node ablation to ensure ventricular capture with CRT had a substantially better prognosis than those who did not (risk ratio 0.42, 95% CI 0.26–0.68) and a greater improvement in New York Heart Association functional class (risk ratio −0.52, 95% CI −0.87 to −0.17).[93] This is illustrated by the largest of these reports from Gasparini and colleagues (**Figs. 2** and **3**).[94,95] However, higher-risk patients may have been less likely to receive AV node ablation and more likely to receive medications with adverse effects on outcome; therefore, these results may be biased. Reducing a ventricular rate to less than about 80 bpm is associated with a worse outcome in patients with heart failure and AF, perhaps because of exacerbation of nocturnal pauses that provoke lethal arrhythmias.[29]

If biventricular pacing is an important mechanism for the effect of CRT, then ensuring ventricular capture will be important. Two substantial observational studies[94–96] have suggested that for patients with AF, very high rates of capture (in excess of 95%) according to the device diagnostic algorithms, which might only be achieved by AV node ablation, are associated with dramatically better outcomes (**Fig. 4**). It is not immediately clear why such high rates of capture are required for CRT to be effective. One explanation is that the device diagnostics are only the tip of the iceberg reflecting a much more serious loss of ventricular capture rate. In some patients, a 5% to 10% loss of capture according to device diagnostics may be associated with more than 40% loss of capture when analyzed by Holter monitoring.[97]

SPECIFIC CASE SELECTION

Scenario 1: Patients are Expected to Return to Sinus Rhythm

A substantial proportion of younger patients who have a short history both of heart failure and of AF should return to sinus rhythm after implantation of CRT, especially if echocardiography shows that the left atrium is not grossly dilated. Such patients should be selected for CRT as though they were in sinus rhythm. Cardioversion may be considered at the time of implantation provided that patients are anticoagulated. Patients who fail initial attempts at cardioversion should have a further attempt after a few months once the LV lead has been shown to be in a stable position. Short-term use of amiodarone may increase the chance of a return of sinus rhythm.

Scenario 2: Patients are Indicated for an ICD and, Apart From AF, are Indicated for CRT

Devices are expensive, and all procedures carry a risk. Implanting the right device at the first attempt reduces patient morbidity and costs. Although the RAFT trial provides the largest body of evidence that upgrading an ICD to CRT-D has no effect on prognosis, there are several arguments against

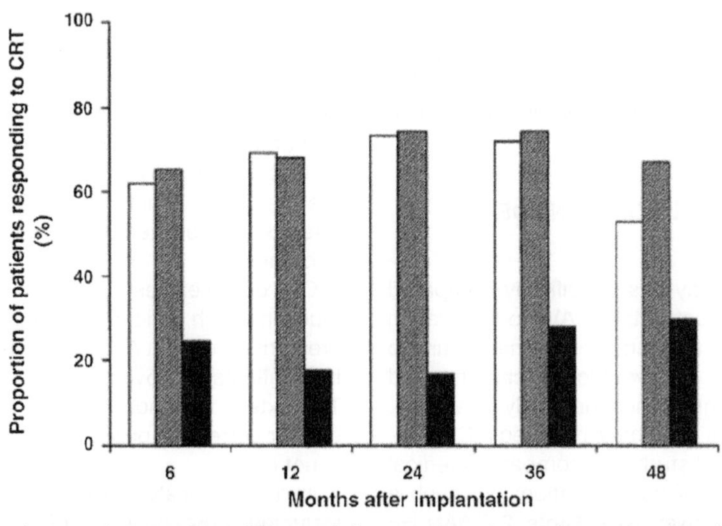

Fig. 2. Percentage of responders to CRT at different follow-up times in an observational study is presented. The open bars refer to sinus rhythm patients; the ruled bars relate to AF with AV junction ablation; and, finally, the solid bars refer to AF without AV junction ablation. There was a significantly higher proportion of responders in patients with sinus rhythm or AF with AF junction ablation compared with patients with AF without AF junction ablation. (*From* Gasparini M, Auricchio A, Regoli F, et al. Four-year efficacy of cardiac resynchronization therapy on exercise tolerance and disease progression: the importance of performing atrioventricular junction ablation in patients with atrial fibrillation. J Am Coll Cardiol 2006;48(4):741; with permission.)

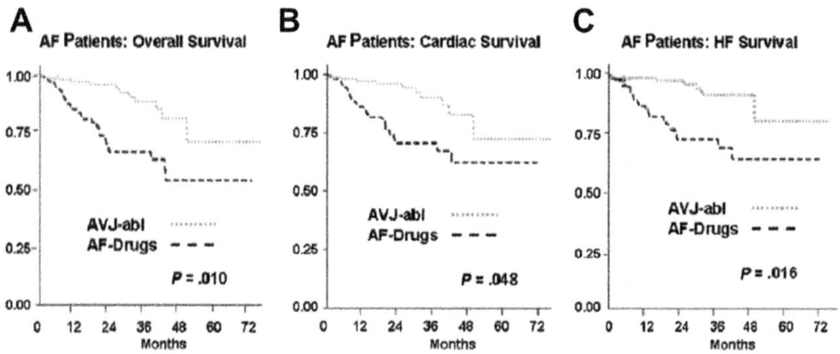

Fig. 3. Pharmacologic therapy for rate control in 125 patients and AV node ablation done in 118. Comparison of Kaplan-Meier estimates of overall (*A*), cardiac (*B*), and heart failure (*C*) survival between patients with AF who underwent AV junction ablation (AVJ-abl) and patients with AF treated only with negative chronotropic drugs. *P* values shown derived from the adjusted hazards ratio analysis stratified according to the corresponding cause of death. (*From* Gasparini M, Auricchio A, Metra M, et al. Long-term survival in patients undergoing cardiac resynchronization therapy: the importance of performing atrio-ventricular junction ablation in patients with permanent atrial fibrillation. Eur Heart J 2008;29(13):1648; with permission.)

ICD as the preferred option in patients otherwise indicated for CRT. RAFT did suggest some improvement in symptoms and reduction in heart failure hospitalization among patients with AF.[76] Only one patient had AV node ablation in RAFT. It is possible that the benefits would have been greater had a more aggressive strategy to ensure biventricular capture been adopted, although clearly this is speculation. If an ICD is implanted but subsequently an upgrade to CRT-D is considered appropriate, this creates a dilemma. Should the potential benefits of an early upgrade be foregone to incur the risk and costs of a potential second procedure? Ultimately, implanting a CRT-D device with selective AV node ablation depending on the progression of symptoms may be the best strategy. On current evidence, any patient with substantial LVSD who is in AF and who is going to receive a device and who is otherwise indicated for CRT should have a CRT device rather than RV pacing or an ICD.

Scenario 3: Patients have AF, Severe Heart Failure Recalcitrant to Best Drug Therapy, and are Otherwise Indicated for CRT

These patients have a limited number of options: LV assist device or a heart transplant. Under these circumstances, in the absence of the possibility of participating in a randomized controlled trial, it seems reasonable to consider CRT if the other alternatives are considered unattractive.

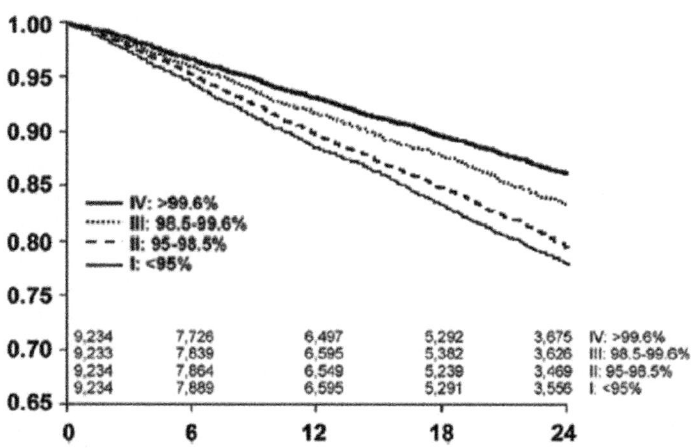

Fig. 4. Probability of survival in biventricular pacing patients with or without AF as a function of percentage of biventricular pacing capture. Patients with biventricular pacing greater than 99.6% experienced a 24% reduction in mortality compared with the other groups (hazard ration 0.76, *P*<.001). (*Adapted from* Hayes DL, Boehmer JP, Day JD, et al. Cardiac resynchronization therapy and the relationship of percent biventricular pacing to symptoms and survival. Heart Rhythm 2011;8:1469–75; with permission.)

Scenario 4: Patients have AF and Mild to Moderate Heart Failure on Pharmacologic Therapy but are Otherwise Indicated for CRT but have no Mandate for or are Unwilling to Have an ICD

These patients should not have CRT based on current evidence. CRT might be superior to AV node ablation and RV pacing, but then what is the evidence in support of the latter strategy? Ideally, they should be enrolled in a randomized controlled trial comparing CRT (or CRT-D) with no device in patients who would be indicated for a CRT if they were in sinus rhythm (LVEF <40%, QRS duration >140 ms).[32] Unfortunately, no trial fits these criteria that the authors are aware of.

REFERENCES

1. Khand A, Rankin AC, Kaye GC, et al. Systematic review of the management of atrial fibrillation in patients with heart failure. Eur Heart J 2000;21:614–32.
2. Khand A, Cleland JG, Deedwania P. Prevention of and medical therapy for atrial arrhythmias in heart failure. Heart Fail Rev 2002;7:267–83.
3. Shelton RJ, Clark AL, Kaye GC, et al. The atrial fibrillation paradox of heart failure. Congest Heart Fail 2010;16(1):3–9.
4. Khand AU, Shaw M, Gemmel I, et al. Do discharge codes underestimate hospitalisation due to heart failure? Validation study of hospital discharge coding for heart failure. Eur J Heart Fail 2005;7(5):792–7.
5. Khand AU, Gemmell I, Rankin AC, et al. Clinical events leading to the progression of heart failure: insights from a national database of hospital discharges. Eur Heart J 2001;22:153–64.
6. Roy D, Talajic M, Nattel S, et al. Rhythm control versus rate control for atrial fibrillation and heart failure. N Engl J Med 2008;358(25):2667–77.
7. Shelton RJ, Clark AL, Goode KM, et al. A randomized controlled study of rate versus rhythm control in patients with chronic atrial fibrillation and heart failure: (CAFE-II Study). Heart 2009;95(11):924–30.
8. Swedberg K, Olsson LG, Charlesworth A, et al. Prognostic relevance of atrial fibrillation in patients with chronic heart failure on long-term treatment with beta-blockers: results from COMET. Eur Heart J 2005;26:1303–8.
9. Smit MD, Moes ML, Maass AH, et al. The importance of whether atrial fibrillation or heart failure develops first. Eur J Heart Fail 2012;14(9):1030–40.
10. Baldasseroni S, De BL, Fresco C, et al. Cumulative effect of complete left bundle-branch block and chronic atrial fibrillation on 1-year mortality and hospitalization in patients with congestive heart failure. A report from the Italian network on congestive heart failure (in-CHF database). Eur Heart J 2002;23(21):1692–8.
11. Mamas MA, Caldwell JC, Chacko S, et al. A meta-analysis of the prognostic significance of atrial fibrillation in chronic heart failure. Eur J Heart Fail 2009;11(7):676–83.
12. Puglisi A, Gasparini M, Lunati M, et al. Persistent atrial fibrillation worsens heart rate variability, activity and heart rate, as shown by a continuous monitoring by implantable biventricular pacemakers in heart failure patients. J Cardiovasc Electrophysiol 2008;19(7):693–701.
13. Borleffs CJ, Ypenburg C, van Bommel RJ, et al. Clinical importance of new-onset atrial fibrillation after cardiac resynchronization therapy. Heart Rhythm 2009;6(3):305–10.
14. Caldwell JC, Contractor H, Petkar S, et al. Atrial fibrillation is under-recognized in chronic heart failure: insights from a heart failure cohort treated with cardiac resynchronization therapy. Europace 2009;11(10):1295–300.
15. Leclercq C, Padeletti L, Cihak R, et al. Incidence of paroxysmal atrial tachycardias in patients treated with cardiac resynchronization therapy and continuously monitored by device diagnostics. Europace 2010;12(1):71–7.
16. Marijon E, Jacob S, Mouton E, et al. Frequency of atrial tachyarrhythmias in patients treated by cardiac resynchronization (from the Prospective, Multicenter Mona Lisa Study). Am J Cardiol 2010;106(5):688–93.
17. Boriani G, Gasparini M, Landolina M, et al. Incidence and clinical relevance of uncontrolled ventricular rate during atrial fibrillation in heart failure patients treated with cardiac resynchronization therapy. Eur J Heart Fail 2011;13(8):868–76.
18. Shanmugam N, Boerdlein A, Proff J, et al. Detection of atrial high-rate events by continuous home monitoring: clinical significance in the heart failure-cardiac resynchronization therapy population. Europace 2012;14(2):230–7.
19. Hoppe UC, Casares JM, Eiskjaer H, et al. Effect of cardiac resynchronization on the incidence of atrial fibrillation in patients with severe heart failure. Circulation 2006;114(1):18–25.
20. Padeletti L, Muto C, Maounis T, et al. Atrial fibrillation in recipients of cardiac resynchronization therapy device: 1-year results of the randomized MASCOT trial. Am Heart J 2008;156(3):520–6.
21. Santini M, Gasparini M, Landolina M, et al. Device-detected atrial tachyarrhythmias predict adverse outcome in real-world patients with implantable biventricular defibrillators. J Am Coll Cardiol 2011;57(2):167–72.

22. Healey JS, Connolly SJ, Gold MR, et al. Subclinical atrial fibrillation and the risk of stroke. N Engl J Med 2012;366(2):120–9.
23. Capucci A, Santini M, Padeletti L, et al. Monitored atrial fibrillation duration predicts arterial embolic events in patients suffering from bradycardia and atrial fibrillation implanted with antitachycardia pacemakers. J Am Coll Cardiol 2005;46(10):1913–20.
24. Swedberg K, Komajda M, Bohm M, et al, on behalf of the SHIFT Investigators. Ivabradine and outcomes in chronic heart failure (SHIFT): a randomised controlled study. Lancet 2010;376:875–85.
25. Swedberg K, Zannad F, McMurray JJ, et al. Eplerenone and atrial fibrillation in mild systolic heart failure: results from the EMPHASIS-HF (Eplerenone in Mild Patients Hospitalization And Survival Study in Heart Failure) study. J Am Coll Cardiol 2012;59(18):1598–603.
26. Rienstra M, Damman K, Mulder BA, et al. Beta-blockers and outcome in heart failure and atrial fibrillation; a meta-analysis. J Am Coll Cardiol HF 2013;1(1):21–8.
27. Bohm M, Borer J, Ford I, et al. Heart rate at baseline influences the effect of ivabradine on cardiovascular outcomes in chronic heart failure: analysis from the SHIFT study. Clin Res Cardiol 2013;102(1):11–22.
28. Cullington D, Goode KM, Clark AL, et al. Heart rate achieved or beta-blocker dose in patients with chronic heart failure: which is the better target? Eur J Heart Fail 2012;14(7):737–47.
29. Cullington D, Goode KM, Cleland JG, et al. Is heart rate important for patients with heart failure in atrial fibrillation? 2013.
30. Gronefeld GC, Israel CW, Padmanabhan V, et al. Ventricular rate stabilization for the prevention of pause dependent ventricular tachyarrhythmias: results from a prospective study in 309 ICD recipients. Pacing Clin Electrophysiol 2002;25(12):1708–14.
31. Aizawa Y, Sato A, Watanabe H, et al. Dynamicity of the J-wave in idiopathic ventricular fibrillation with a special reference to pause-dependent augmentation of the J-wave. J Am Coll Cardiol 2012;59(22):1948–53.
32. Cleland JG, Abraham WT, Linde C, et al. An individual patient meta-analysis of five randomized trials assessing the effects of cardiac resynchronization therapy on morbidity and mortality in patients with symptomatic heart failure. Eur Heart J 2013. [E-pub ahead of print].
33. Cleland JG, Tavazzi L, Daubert JC, et al. Cardiac resynchronization therapy. Are modern myths preventing appropriate use? J Am Coll Cardiol 2009;53(7):608–11.
34. Ghio S, Freemantle N, Scelsi L, et al. Long term left ventricular reverse remodelling with cardiac resynchronization therapy. Results from the CARE-HF trial. Eur J Heart Fail 2009;11(5):480–8.
35. Cleland JG, Freemantle N, Erdmann E, et al. Long-term mortality with cardiac resynchronization therapy in the Cardiac Resynchronization-Heart Failure (CARE-HF) trial. Eur J Heart Fail 2012;14(6):628–34.
36. Cleland JG, Daubert JC, Erdmann E, et al, on behalf of the CARE-HF Study Investigators. Longer-term effects of cardiac resynchronization therapy on mortality in heart failure {the Cardiac Resynchronization - Heart Failure (CARE-HF) trial extension phase}. Eur Heart J 2006;27(16):1928–32.
37. Cowburn PJ, Leclercq C. How to improve outcomes with cardiac resynchronisation therapy: importance of lead positioning. Heart Fail Rev 2012;17(6):781–9.
38. Khan FZ, Virdee MS, Palmer CR, et al. Targeted left ventricular lead placement to guide cardiac resynchronization therapy: the TARGET study: a randomized, controlled trial. J Am Coll Cardiol 2012;59(17):1509–18.
39. Richardson M, Freemantle N, Calvert MJ, et al. Predictors and treatment response with cardiac resynchronisation therapy in patients with heart failure characterised by dyssynchrony: a predefined analysis from the CARE-HF Trial. Eur Heart J 2007;28(15):1827–34.
40. Ellenbogen KA, Gold MR, Meyer TE, et al. Primary results from the SmartDelay determined AV optimization: a comparison to other delay methods used in cardiac resynchronization therapy (SMART-AV) trial: a randomized trial comparing empirical, echocardiography-guided and algorithmic atrioventricular delay programming in cardiac resynchronization therapy. Circulation 2010;122:2660–8.
41. Boriani G, Biffi M, Muller CP, et al. A prospective randomized evaluation of VV delay optimization in CRT-D recipients: echocardiographic observations from the RHYTHM II ICD study. Pacing Clin Electrophysiol 2009;32(Suppl 1):S120–5.
42. Rao RK, Kumar UN, Schafer J, et al. Reduced ventricular volumes and improved systolic function with cardiac resynchronization therapy: a randomized trial comparing simultaneous biventricular pacing, sequential biventricular pacing, and left ventricular pacing. Circulation 2007;115:2136–44.
43. Abraham WT, Leon AR, St John Sutton MG, et al. Randomized controlled trial comparing simultaneous versus optimized sequential interventricular stimulation during cardiac resynchronization therapy. Am Heart J 2012;164(5):735–41.
44. Ritter P, Delnoy PP, Padeletti L, et al. A randomized pilot study of optimization of cardiac

resynchronization therapy in sinus rhythm patients using a peak endocardial acceleration sensor vs. standard methods. Europace 2012;14(9):1324–33.
45. Whinnett ZI, Davies JE, Willson K, et al. Haemodynamic effects of changes in atrioventricular and interventricular delay in cardiac resynchronisation therapy show a consistent pattern: analysis of shape, magnitude and relative importance of atrioventricular and interventricular delay. Heart 2006; 92(11):1628–34.
46. Whinnett ZI, Francis DP, Denis A, et al. Comparison of different invasive hemodynamic methods for AV delay optimization in patients with cardiac resynchronization therapy: implications for clinical trial design and clinical practice. Int J Cardiol 2013. [Epub ahead of print].
47. Brenyo A, Kutyifa V, Moss AJ, et al. Atrioventricular delay programming and the benefit of cardiac resynchronization therapy in MADIT-CRT. Heart Rhythm 2013;10(8):1136–43.
48. Cleland JG, Freemantle N, Ghio S, et al. Predicting the long-term effects of cardiac resynchronisation therapy on mortality from baseline variables and the early response: a report from CARE-HF (Cardiac Resynchronisation in Heart Failure). J Am Coll Cardiol 2008;52:438–45.
49. Hsu LF, Jais P, Sanders P, et al. Catheter ablation for atrial fibrillation in congestive heart failure. N Engl J Med 2004;351(23):2373–83.
50. Khan MN, Jais P, Cummings J, et al. Pulmonary-vein isolation for atrial fibrillation in patients with heart failure. N Engl J Med 2008;359(17):1778–85.
51. Kies P, Leclercq C, Bleeker GB, et al. Cardiac resynchronisation therapy in chronic atrial fibrillation: impact on left atrial size and reversal to sinus rhythm. Heart 2006;92(4):490–4.
52. Hugl B, Bruns HJ, Unterberg-Buchwald C, et al. Atrial fibrillation burden during the post-implant period after CRT using device-based diagnostics. J Cardiovasc Electrophysiol 2006;17(8):813–7.
53. Ouellet G, Huang DT, Moss AJ, et al. Effect of cardiac resynchronization therapy on the risk of first and recurrent ventricular tachyarrhythmic events in MADIT-CRT. J Am Coll Cardiol 2012;60(18): 1809–16.
54. McMurray JJ, Adamopoulos S, Anker SD, et al. ESC guidelines for the diagnosis and treatment of acute and chronic heart failure 2012: the task force for the diagnosis and treatment of acute and chronic heart failure 2012 of the European Society of Cardiology. Developed in collaboration with the Heart Failure Association (HFA) of the ESC. Eur J Heart Fail 2012;14(8):803–69.
55. Carson PE, Johnson GR, Dunkman WB, et al. The influence of atrial fibrillation on prognosis in mild to moderate heart failure: the V-HeFT studies. Circulation 1993;87:VI102–10.
56. Khand AU, Rankin AC, Martin W, et al. Carvedilol alone or in combination with digoxin for the management of atrial fibrillation in patients with heart failure. J Am Coll Cardiol 2003;42:1944–51.
57. Gheorghiade M, Fonarow GC, Van Veldhuisen DJ, et al. Lack of evidence of increased mortality among patients with atrial fibrillation taking digoxin: findings from post hoc propensity-matched analysis of the AFFIRM trial. Eur Heart J 2013;34(20): 1489–97.
58. Chatterjee S, Ghosh J, Lichstein E, et al. Meta-analysis of cardiovascular outcomes with dronedarone in patients with atrial fibrillation or heart failure. Am J Cardiol 2012;110(4):607–13.
59. Connolly SJ, Camm AJ, Halperin JL, et al. Dronedarone in high-risk permanent atrial fibrillation. N Engl J Med 2011;365(24):2268–76.
60. Torp-Pedersen C, Metra M, Spark P, et al, for the COMET Investigators. The safety of amiodarone in patients with heart failure. J Card Fail 2007; 13(5):340–5.
61. Kober L, Torp-Pedersen C, McMurray JJ, et al. Increased mortality after dronedarone therapy for severe heart failure. N Engl J Med 2008;358(25): 2678–87.
62. Jones DG, Haldar SK, Hussain W, et al. A randomized trial to assess catheter ablation versus rate control in the management of persistent atrial fibrillation in heart failure. J Am Coll Cardiol 2013; 61(18):1894–903.
63. Gaita F, Caponi D, Pianelli M, et al. Radiofrequency catheter ablation of atrial fibrillation: a cause of silent thromboembolism? Magnetic resonance imaging assessment of cerebral thromboembolism in patients undergoing ablation of atrial fibrillation. Circulation 2010;122(17):1667–73.
64. Daubert JP, Zareba W, Cannom DS, et al. Inappropriate implantable cardioverter-defibrillator shocks in MADIT II: frequency, mechanisms, predictors, and survival impact. J Am Coll Cardiol 2008; 51(14):1357–65.
65. Cleland JG, Buga L. Defibrillators - a shocking therapy for cardiomyopathy? Nat Rev Cardiol 2010; 7(2):69–70.
66. Cleland JG, Daubert JC, Erdmann E, et al, for the Cardiac Resynchronisation - Heart Failure (CARE-HF) Study Investigators. The effect of cardiac resynchronization on morbidity and mortality in heart failure. N Engl J Med 2005;352(15): 1539–49.
67. Bristow MR, Saxon LA, Boehmer J, et al, for the Comparison of Medical Therapy, Pacing, and Defibrillation in Heart Failure (COMPANION) Investigators. Cardiac-resynchronization therapy with or without an implantable defibrillator in advanced chronic heart failure. N Engl J Med 2004;350: 2140–50.

68. Cazeau S, Leclerc C, Lavergne T, et al, Multisite Stimulation in Cardiomyopathies (MUSTIC) Study Investigators. Effects of multisite biventricular pacing in patients with heart failure and intraventricular conduction delay. N Engl J Med 2001; 344:873–80.
69. Leclercq C, Walker S, Linde C, et al. Comparative effects of permanent biventricular and right-univentricular pacing in heart failure patients with chronic atrial fibrillation. Eur Heart J 2002;23: 1780–7.
70. Abraham WT, Fisher WG, Smith AL, et al, for the MIRACLE Study Group. Cardiac resynchronisation in chronic heart failure. N Engl J Med 2002;346(24): 1845–53.
71. Daubert JC, Gold MR, Abraham WT, et al, on behalf of the REVERSE Study Group. Prevention of disease progression by cardiac resynchronization therapy in patients with asymptomatic or mildly symptomatic left ventricular dysfunction. J Am Coll Cardiol 2009;54:1837–46.
72. Young J, Abraham WT, Smith AL, et al, Multicenter InSync ICD Randomized Clinical Evaluation (MIRACLE ICD) Trial Investigators. Combined cardiac resynchronisation and implantable cardioversion defibrillation in advanced chronic heart failure. The MIRACLE ICD trial. JAMA 2003;289: 2685–94.
73. Moss AJ, Hall WJ, Cannom DS, et al. Cardiac-resynchronization therapy for the prevention of heart-failure events. N Engl J Med 2009;361(14): 1329–38.
74. Tang AS, Wells GA, Talajic M, et al. Cardiac-resynchronization therapy for mild-to-moderate heart failure. N Engl J Med 2010;363(25):2385–95.
75. Brenyo A, Link MS, Barsheshet A, et al. Cardiac resynchronization therapy reduces left atrial volume and the risk of atrial tachyarrhythmias in MADIT-CRT (Multicenter Automatic Defibrillator Implantation Trial with Cardiac Resynchronization Therapy). J Am Coll Cardiol 2011;58(16):1682–9.
76. Healey JS, Hohnloser SH, Exner DV, et al. Cardiac resynchronization therapy in patients with permanent atrial fibrillation: results from the Resynchronization for Ambulatory Heart Failure Trial (RAFT). Circ Heart Fail 2012;5(5):566–70.
77. Tolosana JM, Arnau AM, Madrid AH, et al. Cardiac resynchronization therapy in patients with permanent atrial fibrillation. Is it mandatory to ablate the atrioventricular junction to obtain a good response? Eur J Heart Fail 2012;14(6):635–41.
78. Khadjooi K, Foley PW, Chalil S, et al. Long-term effects of cardiac resynchronisation therapy in patients with atrial fibrillation. Heart 2008;94(7): 879–83.
79. Schutte F, Ludorff G, Grove R, et al. Atrioventricular node ablation is not a prerequisite for cardiac resynchronization therapy in patients with chronic atrial fibrillation. Cardiol J 2009;16(3):246–9.
80. Chatterjee NA, Upadhyay GA, Ellenbogen KA, et al. Atrioventricular nodal ablation in atrial fibrillation: a meta-analysis and systematic review. Circ Arrhythm Electrophysiol 2012;5(1):68–76.
81. Geelen P, Brugada J, Andries E, et al. Ventricular fibrillation and sudden death after radiofrequency catheter ablation of the atrioventricular junction. Pacing Clin Electrophysiol 1997; 20(2 Pt 1):343–8.
82. Stavrakis S, Garabelli P, Reynolds DW. Cardiac resynchronization therapy after atrioventricular junction ablation for symptomatic atrial fibrillation: a meta-analysis. Europace 2012;14:1490–7.
83. Chatterjee NA, Upadhyay GA, Ellenbogen KA, et al. Atrioventricular nodal ablation in atrial fibrillation: a meta-analysis of biventricular vs. right ventricular pacing mode. Eur J Heart Fail 2012;14(6): 661–7.
84. Doshi RN, Daoud EG, Fellows C, et al, for the PAVE Study Group. Left ventricular-based cardiac stimulation Post AV Nodal Ablation Evaluation (The PAVE Study). J Cardiovasc Electrophysiol 2005; 16:1160–5.
85. Garrigue S, Bordachar P, Reuter S, et al. Comparison of permanent left ventricular and biventricular pacing in patients with heart failure and chronic atrial fibrillation: prospective haemodynamic study. Heart 2002;87(6):529–34.
86. Brignole M, Gammage M, Puggioni E, et al. Comparative assessment of right, left, and biventricular pacing in patients with permanent atrial fibrillation. Eur Heart J 2005;26(7):712–22.
87. Leclercq C, Cazeau S, Lellouche D, et al. Upgrading from single chamber right ventricular to biventricular pacing in permanently paced patients with worsening heart failure: The RD-CHF Study. Pacing Clin Electrophysiol 2007;30(Suppl 1):S23–30.
88. Kindermann M, Hennen B, Jung J, et al. Biventricular versus conventional right ventricular stimulation for patients with standard pacing indication and left ventricular dysfunction: the Homburg Biventricular Pacing Evaluation (HOBIPACE). J Am Coll Cardiol 2006;47(10):1927–37.
89. Curtis AB, Worley SJ, Adamson PB, et al. Biventricular pacing for atrioventricular block and systolic dysfunction. N Engl J Med 2013;368(17):1585–93.
90. Hamdan MH, Freedman RA, Gilbert EM, et al. Atrioventricular junction ablation followed by resynchronization therapy in patients with congestive heart failure and atrial fibrillation (AVERT-AF) study design. Pacing Clin Electrophysiol 2006;29(10): 1081–8.
91. Leon AR, Greenberg JM, Kanuru N, et al. Cardiac resynchronization in patients with congestive heart failure and chronic atrial fibrillation: effect of

upgrading to biventricular pacing after chronic right ventricular pacing. J Am Coll Cardiol 2002; 39:1258–63.
92. Upadhyay GA, Choudhry NK, Auricchio A, et al. Cardiac resynchronization in patients with atrial fibrillation: a meta-analysis of prospective cohort studies. J Am Coll Cardiol 2008;52(15): 1239–46.
93. Ganesan AN, Brooks AG, Roberts-Thomson KC, et al. Role of AV nodal ablation in cardiac resynchronization in patients with coexistent atrial fibrillation and heart failure: a systematic review. J Am Coll Cardiol 2012;59(8):719–26.
94. Gasparini M, Auricchio A, Metra M, et al. Long-term survival in patients undergoing cardiac resynchronization therapy: the importance of performing atrio-ventricular junction ablation in patients with permanent atrial fibrillation. Eur Heart J 2008; 29(13):1644–52.
95. Gasparini M, Auricchio A, Regoli F, et al. Four-year efficacy of cardiac resynchronization therapy on exercise tolerance and disease progression: the importance of performing atrioventricular junction ablation in patients with atrial fibrillation. J Am Coll Cardiol 2006;48(4):734–43.
96. Hayes DL, Boehmer JP, Day JD, et al. Cardiac resynchronization therapy and the relationship of percent biventricular pacing to symptoms and survival. Heart Rhythm 2011;8(9):1469–75.
97. Kamath GS, Cotiga D, Koneru JN, et al. The utility of 12-lead Holter monitoring in patients with permanent atrial fibrillation for the identification of nonresponders after cardiac resynchronization therapy. J Am Coll Cardiol 2009;53(12):1050–5.

Cardiac Resynchronization Therapy Mechanisms in Atrial Fibrillation

Zachary I. Whinnett, BMedSci, BMBS, MRCP, PhD*,
Darrel P. Francis, FRCP, MD

KEYWORDS

• Biventricular pacing • Cardiac resynchronization therapy • Atrial fibrillation

KEY POINTS

- The process of comparing multiple settings is the acid test of the resynchronization hypothesis, largely unacknowledged by the clinical and scientific community.
- Lack of a visible prominent effect of interventricular (VV) adjustment on hemodynamics is proof that either the resynchronization concept is plain wrong or the measurement protocol was designed to be so vulnerable to error that it cannot detect this important effect.
- The hazard of VV delay optimization lies in the widespread failure to perceive natural biologic variability, which is often mistaken for failure of the operator to make measurements correctly. Measurement variability causes false optima to appear with VV delay adjustment and makes the size of the optimization benefit become exaggerated.
- Using sensitive (narrow-error-bar) methods, VV delay optimization produces relatively small increments in hemodynamic effects over and above programming a nominal setting of VV 0 ms.

INTRODUCTION

It has been commonly assumed that the mechanism through which biventricular pacemakers (BVPs) improve cardiac function is by resynchronization of ventricular activation, which is why it is commonly referred to as cardiac resynchronization therapy (CRT). Resynchronization means restoration of simultaneity, which can only mean of the ventricles (because the atria are never supposed to contract simultaneously with the ventricles). The mental picture conjured by that term and conveyed when speaking to nonspecialists is almost always that of ventricular walls contracting incoordinately under native conduction and then brought back into correct mutual timing by the pacemaker. The visual impact and cognitive catchiness of the concept is overwhelming.

Under this hypothesis, patients with atrial fibrillation (AF) should be in as strong a position to benefit from BVP as those in sinus rhythm, because both groups are equally liable to ventricular dyssynchrony.

In routine clinical practice, BVPs are frequently implanted into patients who are in permanent AF (23% in a large European survey[1]).

After implantation of a BVP in a patient with AF, there are 2 main targets for optimizing therapy. First, measures can be taken to ensure high percentages of ventricular pacing that allow adequate

Funding Sources: The authors would like to acknowledge support from the British Heart Foundation DF (FS/10/38/28268).

International Centre for Circulatory Health, National Heart and Lung Institute, Imperial College London, 59-61 North Wharf Road, London W2 1LA, UK
* Corresponding author.
E-mail address: z.whinnett@imperial.ac.uk

Heart Failure Clin 9 (2013) 475–488
http://dx.doi.org/10.1016/j.hfc.2013.07.005
1551-7136/13/$ – see front matter

delivery of therapy. Second, the relative timing of stimulation of the 2 pacing leads can be adjusted (VV delay). If the mechanism through which BVP delivers its beneficial effect is predominantly ventricular resynchronization, then adjusting VV delay would be expected to produce large changes in cardiac function.

This article examines how to assess the reliability of potential techniques for performing optimization and explores whether the effort required for optimization is likely worthwhile.

CRT IN PATIENTS WITH ATRIAL FIBRILLATION

Would a patient with AF and left bundle branch block (LBBB) stand to benefit from BVP? Even a devotee of the resynchronization concept accepts that the presence of AF might impair the ability of BVP to give benefit. The variable intrinsic atrioventricular (AV) conduction might cause some beats to not have BV capture by the pacemaker and, therefore, incomplete delivery of biventricular pacing.

Therefore, it is not possible to simply assume that the benefit observed in patients with sinus rhythm also applies to patients in AF.

The evidence base for BVP in patients with AF has been predominantly derived from observational case series.[2–10] These data suggest that the benefits seem attenuated compared with patients in sinus rhythm.[11,12]

Only small numbers of patients with permanent AF have been included in the landmark randomized studies to assess the impact of CRT on clinical outcome measures. It is difficult to understand why these randomized trials—outwardly designated trials of cardiac resynchronization—were not designed to cover a full spread of patients with heart failure and LBBB. Until new studies are carried out, guidance is based on interpretation of the data that did arise.[13,14]

In a predefined substudy of the RAFT (Resynchronization–Defibrillation for Ambulatory Heart Failure Trial), patients with permanent AF, New York Heart Association class II or III heart failure, left ventricular (LV) ejection fraction less than or equal to 30%, and QRS duration greater than or equal to 120 ms were randomized to receive BVP or no BVP, with all patients receiving a defibrillator; 229 patients were randomized. The principal result of the study is that the event rate was low in both arms and, therefore, the CI for the primary outcome of death or heart failure hospitalization between those assigned to CRT–implantable cardioverter defibrillator (ICD) and those assigned ICD was wide,[15] ranging from 0.65 to 1.41. The point estimate was 0.96 (P = .82), but the CI includes an effect as strong as seen in CARE-HF (Cardiac Resynchronization-Heart failure) trial, for instance.

The MUSTIC-AF (Multisite Stimulation in Cardiomyopathy Atrial Fibrillation) trial, which deliberately focused on AF and addressed symptoms, did find evidence of symptomatic advantage of BVP over pure right ventricular (RV) pacing[13] but it should be borne in mind that RV pacing on its own was found harmful in the DAVID (Dual Chamber and VVI Implantable Defibrillator) trial,[16] so the favorable outcome in the BVP arm should not be assumed due to a salutary effect of BVP: it may simply be a neutral alternative to harmful RV pacing.

The absence of conclusive evidence of benefit from randomized studies to support the use of CRT in patients with AF may be explained by the following:

1. Insufficient numbers of patients entered into randomized studies

Many more sinus rhythm patients than AF patients have been entered into randomized studies. Therefore, even if BVP is equally effective in both groups, the AF studies are likely to be underpowered.

2. Lack of consistent biventricular capture through lack of AV node ablation

In AF, native RR interval varies because of variable arrival of atrial wavefronts and possibly also variable AV node conduction. This means that a regular programmed ventricular pacing rate may fail to capture every beat consistently, because of intermittent breakthrough of native conduction.[17] If there is reduced delivery of therapy, perhaps in the 60% to 75% range, then a study approximately 2.5 times as large as those performed in sinus rhythm is required. In reality, AF studies have been smaller than their sinus rhythm counterparts.

3. The effect may be smaller in AF

Even if ventricular resynchronization is the primary driver of the benefit of CRT in sinus rhythm, there may be a contribution from coordination of atrial versus ventricular contraction (this is not resynchronization but might be called euchronization).[18] The beneficial effect of BVP in AF might, therefore, be smaller than in sinus rhythm.

OPTIMIZING DELIVERY OF BIVENTRICULAR PACING

In order to ensure high percentages of ventricular pacing, hence, the opportunity for adequate delivery of therapy, it is important to ensure that native conduction does not unfavorably compete with BVP, so that ventricular resynchronization is successfully delivered.

High percentages of ventricular pacing may be achieved pharmacologically by adequate uptitration of medication to control ventricular rate. Relying on the percent biventricular pacing data stored in the pacemaker to determine this may be misleading, because these rates may include fusion and pseudofusion between pacing from the device and intrinsic atrioventricular conduction.[19]

AV node ablation can deliver a more powerful guarantee of the effectiveness of adequate rate control. Some operators are anxious about the potential adverse consequences of converting a patient with stable status, who is nonpacemaker dependent, into a patient who is totally dependent on the pacemaker for survival.

Although observational studies report strong symptomatic responses to ablation plus BVP[3,6–9,20] there are 2 limitations. First, these procedures are by their nature only likely to be carried out by groups with a strong belief in the rationale and, therefore, any outcome markers that require human judgment should not be assumed free of innocent bias. Second, they have all covered only the short term. Adverse consequences that take longer to materialize, such as the undesirable sequelae of total pacing dependency, may not have manifested at the time the studies were evaluated.

The net clinical effect of biventricular pacing in AF is difficult to guess from the clinical outcome data that exist to date. The randomized experience is small, and the nonrandomized experience (like all observational data) is open to an unquantifiable degree of natural observer bias.

What is needed are reliable experimental data, which may take the form of physiologic measurements with and without BVP, with careful attention to bias-resistance and reliability of the data within individual patients. Alternatively, they may take the form of outcome trials with event endpoints, although, for the reasons described previously, these have to be much larger than their sinus rhythm predecessors to achieve the same degree of statistical power.

OPTIMIZATION OF INTERVENTRICULAR DELAY

The typical nominal VV delay is close to 0 ms (ie, virtually simultaneous onset of stimulation). Adjusting the VV delay is expected to change the degree of ventricular resynchronization. There are theoretic reasons why it may be necessary to adjust the VV delay in order to obtain maximal improvements in ventricular resynchronization. For example, if the LV lead is positioned in an area of slow conduction, there may be a significant time delay before the pacing stimulus spreads to activate the left ventricle. In this case, it may be rational to program the LV lead to pace before the RV lead in order to allow a greater bulk of the ventricular myocardium to be activated approximately synchronously.

Several different methods have been proposed to guide the process of assessing the impact of adjusting the VV delay. Because supporting evidence on the long-term benefit of BVP optimization from large clinical trials is lacking, guidelines provide little scientifically supported guidance on how to program VV delay in AF.[21]

The lack of supporting evidence for optimization may be because there is no or little incremental benefit to be obtained from optimizing VV delay over and above the nominal delay. Alternatively, it may be that there are advantageous VV delays, but the methods used for optimization were unreliable and did not identify them correctly.

In order to establish which of these explanations is most likely, there must be a mechanism for assessing the reliability of an optimization method. Before proceeding to clinical outcome studies, simple steps can be taken to determine whether an optimization method has a high likelihood of delivering reliable results. A rigorously conducted large-scale clinical outcome study assessing an optimization method that does not reliably identify the true optimal VV delay will not find a beneficial effect for VV optimization. It will not be possible to determine whether the lack of benefit is because VV optimization is not important or whether it is simply due to the failure of the optimization method tested.

IS A PROPOSED OPTIMIZATION METHOD SUFFICIENTLY RELIABLE TO DELIVER CLINICALLY USEFUL RESULTS?

It is unwise to proceed directly to a clinical trial with an optimization scheme before establishing its reliability; this can be done cheaply. This article sets out a series of steps that can be used to assess any optimization method, beginning with simple tests that can be done in a few minutes in 1 or 2 patients.

Step 1: Does the Proposed Optimization Scheme Identify a Singular Optimal Value?

An optimization scheme must select a single VV delay (or a narrow range of VV delays) if it is to make any meaningful claim of being an optimization scheme at all.

For example, a scheme that selects a broad range, such as "anywhere from LV first by 80 ms to RV first by 80 ms," is so vague as to be little better than completely uninformative. Taken to its extreme, a scheme could declare all possible VV delays to be optimal: there is no reason to consider this an optimization scheme.

Ideally, a scheme should provide the optimum to the level of precision to which a device can be programmed. For devices that can only be programmed to the nearest 10-ms step, there is no need to know the optimum to any greater degree of precision than this. Despite being easy to determine, the majority of optimization schemes do not report a degree of precision for the value determined as the optimum.

Aside from a too-wide range of proposed optimality, the second undesirable pattern is the dual-peaked optimum. How can LV first by 20 ms and RV first by 40 ms be equally optimal, with intervening settings worse? Uncritical acceptance of dual-peaked optima allows virtually any pattern to be taken as a valid set of optimization measurements. There is little physiologic justification for dual peaks. At the least, a dual-peaked pattern should be the subject of blinded verification from separate data by an independent observer, and, if confirmed, patients should undergo detailed assessment of the physiologic process underlying the phenomenon, which might turn out to be a landmark finding in fundamental mechanisms.

The ability to identify a singular region on the VV delay spectrum as optimal is the most basic requirement for an optimization scheme. It takes only a handful of patients to test singularity of most of the proposed methods. For example, to assess whether optimization performed using left ventricular outflow tract (LVOT) velocity-time integral (VTI) measurements identify a singular region would only require about 7 minutes per patient (3 beats per VV delay, across 7 VV delays, allowing 20 seconds per VTI measurement). Readers are encouraged to test this.

Step 2: Is It Reproducible?

Once a scheme has demonstrated adequate singularity, it can then go forward for the slightly more time-consuming test of reproducibility. If a test is not singular, there is no point assessing it for reproducibility. The reason for this is as follows. A scheme that is not singular either provides too broad a territory of supposed optimality or provides multiple disconnected regions of optimality. In either case, if a second test is carried out, whether the second result is consistent with the first in the first case is always judged successful or in the second case is impossible to judge.

For example, if the scheme addresses a spectrum of possibilities from "LV first by 120 ms" to "RV first by 80 ms" and declares that "LV first by 80 ms to RV first by 40 ms" are all optimal, then a second test that declares the optimum is "LV first by 40 ms to RV first by 80 ms" is judged a match—even though in both cases they cover half the range.

In another example, if the first test declares the optimum to be "LV first by 120 ms or RV first by 40 ms" and the second test declares it "LV first by 40 ms or RV first by 80 ms," they may at first be considered almost concordant (due to the near match of RV 40 ms and RV 80 ms) but on further reflection it becomes clear that almost any finding on the second test would be considered a perfect or near match.

So singularity is a vital prerequisite, but how exactly should reproducibility itself be judged?

1. Independent data sets acquired separately

The key to reproducibility is the identification of equivalence or near-equivalence of VV delay optimum by independent observers who acquire separate data blinded to each other's findings. It is grossly inadequate to ask 2 observers to examine the same acquired set of data (it makes no more sense than asking 2 observers to look at the same reading displayed on a blood pressure machine and call it reproducibility).

The enemy of optimization is biologic variability that is continually producing fluctuations in any measured variable. In this environment, there is great opportunity for differences between observations at different VV delays to be the result of these natural biologic fluctuations and not the VV delay itself. For this reason, the 2 operators should acquire separate data. If under these circumstances they obtain the same optimum, then the scheme is sufficiently robust to overcome this noise.

2. Blinding

In clinical practice, most workers have an inherent recognition that the techniques they use are less good than claimed, although they rarely voice this concern. The principal hallmark of the presence of this gestalt knowledge is the behavior of peeking at previous results before making a new measurement. This happens in assessment of LV function and of valvular function[22] and is even condoned in guidelines.

When practitioners conduct peeking, to ensure that values make physiologic sense in the context they are recognizing that the noise in the measurement is so great that they have to select between the various measurements, using some external knowledge in order to achieve an expected pattern. In such an environment, once they conduct one optimization, they tend to tune the results of the second to match the results of the first.

A simple solution to this is to ask 2 independent operators to conduct entirely separate optimizations on the same patient immediately successively without the 2 operators communicating or viewing each other's data. Alternatively, the process could be automated so that the human tendency to manipulate the interpretation of one set of data to match that of the other is avoided.

Again, although this process of testing reproducibility takes a little forethought to understand why it is necessary, its actual execution is easy and quick.

3. Willingness to publish unpleasant results

Individuals testing reproducibility should be willing to publish the findings even if they do not fit their prejudice or a department's liking. It should not be assumed that findings that discord with prejudice are incorrect. Instead, it may be the failure of previous workers to report findings that may have resulted in the present worker having a wrong prejudice. In any case, a biologic observation is a biologic observation and not an assay of the staff member, so no shame should be accrued from realizing that a scheme is not reproducible.

4. Calculate and display the relevant variable, not an irrelevant one

When the data of the 2 optimizations are collected in a handful of patients, the relevant calculation is the SD of difference between the optimal VV delays. This is carried out by listing the VV delay selected by operator 1 in the first column, the VV delay selected by operator 2 in the second column, and the difference in the third column. The difference should be signed (ie, if operator 2 picked a more positive VV delay in a particular patient, it would be marked as a positive difference; meanwhile if that operator picked a more negative VV delay in another patient, it would be marked as a negative difference).

On average (unless an operator is biased toward reporting a higher or lower value consistently), the mean of those differences tends to be distributed at approximately 0. The relevant question is how wide that distribution is, which can be conveniently calculated as the SD of those differences. There are several variables that there is no point in calculating.

Whether operator 1 and operator 2 are significantly different

It is of no use to calculate whether operator 2 reports a significantly higher optimum or not than operator 1. This is only of interest if there was a concern that one operator had a consistent tendency to pick higher or lower values. If they were both selecting purely randomly, without making any biologic measurement, they would have no difference in their mean optima (because they are drawn from identical distribution) even though such an optimization process would be completely useless.

What proportion of patients is within the 95% Bland-Altman CI bands?

There is essentially no point reporting this because the CI bands are designed to capture approximately 95% of the cases on a parametric basis. Deviations from 95% occur by chance due to the shapes of the distribution and give no useful information on the reliability of the technique.

Difference in LVOT VTI or other measurement between settings

The question is how widely the repeat VV optima are distributed, not the measured consequences on the VTI or other physiologic variables. Although it might be intuitively attractive for a clinician to report whether operator 1 and operator 2 generated similar physiologic consequences, selecting settings entirely at random, even with physiology that is strongly dependent on VV delay, results in a near-0 difference between the 2 operators. Again this is because the physiologic responses are drawn from the same distribution, not because the VV delays are equal.

Step 3: Is the Value Identified as Optimal Biologically Plausible?

For any scheme that passes both singularity and reproducibility criteria, it is time to test its physiologic plausibility. For example, a scheme that always defines the optimum VV delay in women as RV first by 60 ms and in men as LV first by 80 ms would meet criteria of singularity and reproducibility, because each patient is always allocated a consistent value, but would not be biologically plausible.

There are several aspects to biologic plausibility. A scheme that for most patients picked RV first by a high degree (eg, 60 ms or 80 ms) would suffer from the apprehension that it is delivering largely RV pacing, which, as is known from trials, such as DAVID, is likely harmful.[16]

Plotting the distribution of optima obtained may give clues to plausibility. It would be expected, from induction from the concept behind BVP, that VV optima most commonly are in the vicinity of VV 0 ms or slightly left first. It would be expected that RV first or very extreme LV first would be identified as optimal in only a minority of patients.

This 3-step process (singularity, reproducibility, and plausibility) can be checked inexpensively and can be conducted for multiple variables in the same study without loss of power. The authors have conducted such a study for markers that are electrical (QRS duration), flow based (LVOT VTI), and pressure based (noninvasive beat-by-beat blood pressure) to show how it could work in this screening process.[23]

Step 4: Does the Optimization Method Result in Improvements in Cardiac Function?

Singular, reproducible, and plausible optimization schemes are still not yet necessarily ready for large-scale trailing.

Optima based on intracardiac measurements need not necessarily agree with each other or produce overall improvements in cardiac function, because there are many potential variables, and maximization of one may be at the expense of another. Outside the heart, however, what generates pressure is what generates flow, so these 2 variables tend to be affected in the same direction by any change in VV delay timing. All other peripherally measured variables are downstream consequences of pressure and/or flow and, therefore, are likely to be affected concordantly. It is implausible for a peripheral variable to have a VV delay optimum that is substantially different from the optimum for pressure and flow.

Optimization should be expected to deliver an increment in cardiac function. The size of the increment can be determined in relation to the status at a reference VV delay, such as 0 ms. For example, if a VV delay of LV first 60 ms is identified as optimal, it can be compared with VV 0 ms in order to determine the magnitude of the increment in blood pressure or flow that is gained by programming the optimized setting. It is important to ensure that if using a measure of cardiac function to both identify the optimal delay and assess the impact of programming the optimal delay, that separate measurements are used to identify the optimal VV delay from those used to determine the hemodynamic impact. Otherwise, there is likely to be a positive bias, which results in an overestimation of the magnitude of improvement in cardiac function.[24] Therefore, one set of measurements should be made to identify the optimal delay and separate measurements made to compare this optimal delay with the reference.

Step 5: Choosing an Optimization Scheme

After these stages, only methods that identify a singular optimum, are reproducible, and are plausible are left. They have good agreement with measures of cardiac function. It is likely that optimization methods demonstrating these properties will show clustering with regard to the VV delay identified as optimal. These schemes will therefore show good agreement with each other with regard to the VV delay determined as optimal. Each scheme would be already validated against all the others in that cluster. With all schemes in the cluster reporting similar optima, any one of the schemes could be chosen for clinical use, perhaps based on cost or local convenience.

No endpoint trials need be carried out before this stage. At this stage, if 2 different measures of cardiac function consistently identify different optima, to assist in choosing between the schemes it may be helpful to conduct a clinical trial. **Box 1** shows the process for identifying a reliable scheme for optimization of VV delay.

HAZARDS OF JUDGING A BOOK BY ITS COVER OR AN ARTICLE BY ITS TITLE

Several different methods have been proposed to guide VV delay optimization. Although little recognized, it is not sufficient to settle on a parameter and measure it at each setting, choosing the setting with the best value, because the measurements may vary spontaneously with time due to natural biologic fluctuation. If thought is not applied, these biologic fluctuations may be mistaken for the effect of VV delay; thereby, a random VV delay setting may unknowingly become selected.

The protocol used to acquire data needs careful planning so that enough steps are taken to minimize the effects of biologic variability. If these steps have not been taken, then the findings may be incorrect. If the planning has not been carried out, then the investigators will not have realized

Box 1
Process for identifying a reliable scheme for optimization of VV delay

Step 1: Does the proposed optimization scheme identify a singular optimal value?

Step 2: Is it reproducible?

Step 3: Is the value identified as optimal biologically plausible?

Step 4: Does the optimization method result in improvements in cardiac function?

Step 5: Choosing an optimization scheme

that they need to take these steps. If signal has been overwhelmed by noise, a study's investigators are unlikely to report it (they may not even know). The only sign of this that a reader can realistically expect to see is the absence of evidence of meticulous quantification of natural biologic variability by the investigators.

It is tempting to classify articles on optimization by their choice of variable measured for optimization (eg, VTI of Doppler, pulse pressure, or LV dP/dt_{max}). But the crucial distinction is not the choice of variable but the choice to measure the variable sufficiently precisely to make the optimization singular, reproducible, and plausible.[25] For each variable there is noise. By measuring (not guessing) the magnitude of the noise, it is possible to calculate how many replicate measurements are required for an optimization of any desired degree of precision.[26,27]

If the steps taken to minimize the effect of noise have not been carefully planned, then even measures that have the potential to be excellent candidates as a means for guiding optimization may fail.

dP/dt_{max}, for example, has strong theoretic grounds for being a good marker of cardiac function. Many different protocols have been used for acquiring invasive dP/dt_{max} to guide AV delay optimization. Some investigators have simply used a single 30-second recording and not compared this to a reference setting[28] whereas others have compared single measurements of calculation of the relative change in dP/dt_{max} with a reference setting[29] and others have used multiple measurements of the relative change.[30–32] Reproducibility is poor if only single measurements are made and is much improved by making multiple measurements.[25]

The foregoing makes it clear that it is insufficient to choose a marker that has strong a priori validity, and insufficient to simply measure it invasively. It is essential that carefully preplanned steps are taken to minimize the effect of noise that occurs due to background spontaneous variations that occur even in dP/dt_{max} measurements.

It is not only the parameter proposed as an optimization marker but also the way in which it is recorded (ie, precisely what noise reduction steps are included and quantitatively how these were decided on) that determines whether it can be a reliable method to guide optimization.

EXAMPLES OF VARIABLES THAT CAN BE MEASURED FOR OPTIMIZATION

A wide variety of variables can be proposed for optimization, including electrical, pressure-based, and flow-based.

LVOT VTI

The intuitively most attractive variable to maximize while optimizing VV delay is cardiac output.[33–35] At a fixed heart rate, this is equivalent to maximizing stroke volume. For a constant outflow tract diameter, this is also equivalent to maximizing stroke distance or VTI. Typically this is recorded noninvasively using Doppler echocardiography, although it can be recorded invasively using a flow wire.[36] At each pacemaker setting, a sample of pulsed wave Doppler traces is acquired from the LVOT, while keeping the probe position constant between settings. It is often recommended to average the VTIs of 3 beats, although articles describing the technique commonly show the process carried out on a single beat per setting. Increments of 20 ms in the VV delay are commonly recommended. The VV delay setting that yields the highest VTI is selected as the optimum.

The authors' group has assessed noninvasive outflow tract VTI as a tool for VV delay optimization in AF.[23] Six consecutive beats of LVOT flow were acquired (**Fig. 1**). The average of the 6 beats was taken as the value for that setting. The authors assessed singularity, reproducibility, and plausibility of the data.

Singularity

The number of optimizations in which there is a single peak of clearly maximum VTI (judged from the raw points, not the curve) is few. Applying curve fitting increases the proportion but there are still many of the 40 optimizations in which the curves are noncurved or inverted. Each inverted curve is noise rather than physiologically meaningful, but what may not be obvious is that it has a counterpart that is correctly oriented but also noise, because it is the nature of random noise to be equal in each direction. Therefore, the number of curves that are biologic meaningful may be as few as 50% or less of those acquired.

Reproducibility

In **Fig. 1**, it can be seen that only 9 of the 20 patients tested have a pair of curves that are both correctly oriented. In the remaining 11, it is not possible to establish reproducibility. In the 9, most have fairly good agreement between the optima indicated by the 2 curves. This is an example of the phenomenon explained earlier: in the absence of strong singularity, there is little point in addressing reproducibility of the optimum. The SD of difference was 34 ms.

Biologic Plausibility

There is no point addressing biologic plausibility because singularity is poor as is reproducibility.

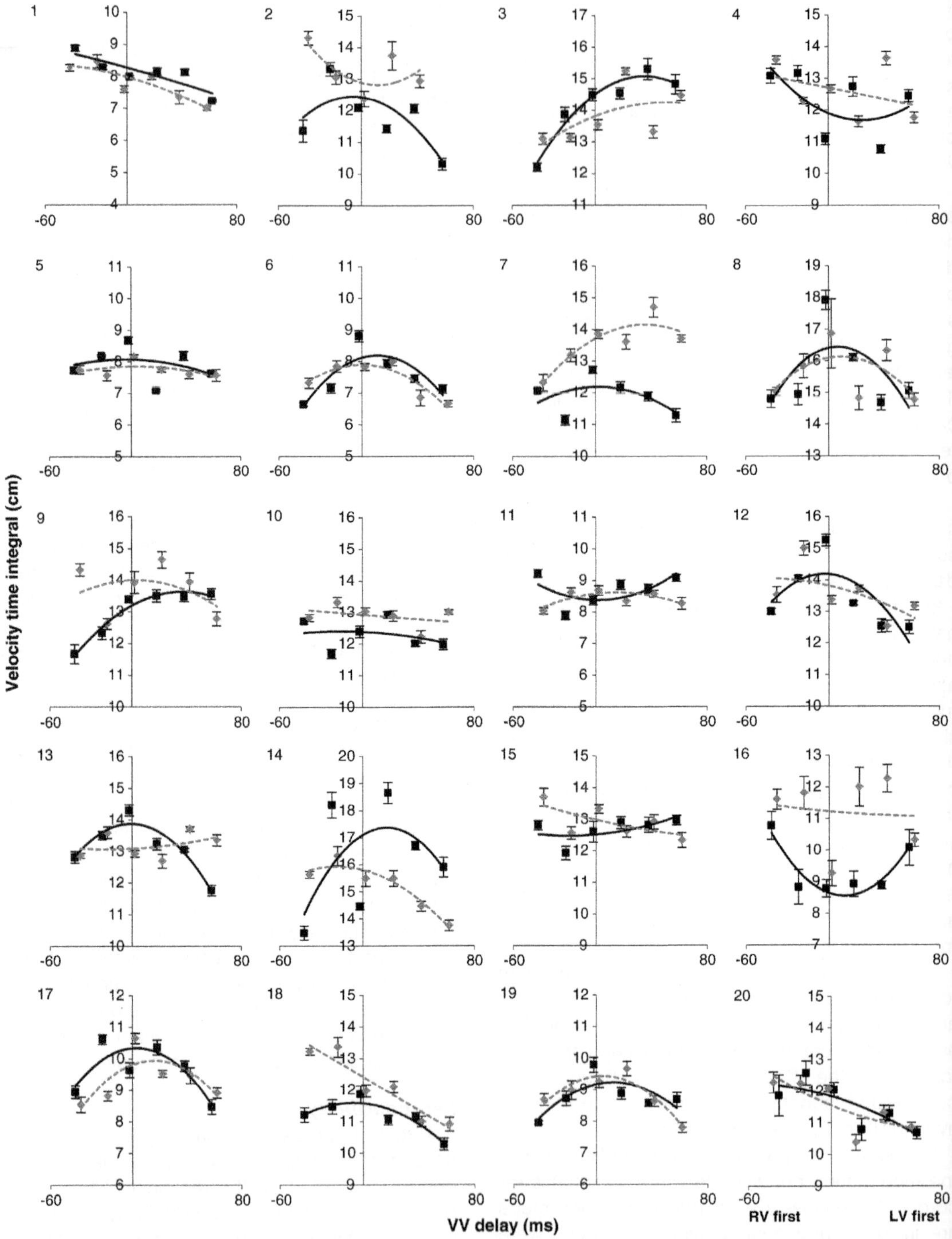

Fig. 1. Data from 20 patients who had VV delay optimization performed twice on the same day, using LVOT VTI Data for the first optimization is displayed in black and the second in gray. A parabola was fitted and the peak o the parabola was considered to represent the optimal VV delay (optimum = largest VTI). (*From* Kyriacou A Li Kam Wa ME, Pabari PA, et al. A systematic approach to designing reliable VV optimization methodology assessment of internal validity of echocardiographic, electrocardiographic and haemodynamic optimization o cardiac resynchronization therapy. Int J Cardiol 2012 Mar 26. [Epub ahead of print]; with permission.)

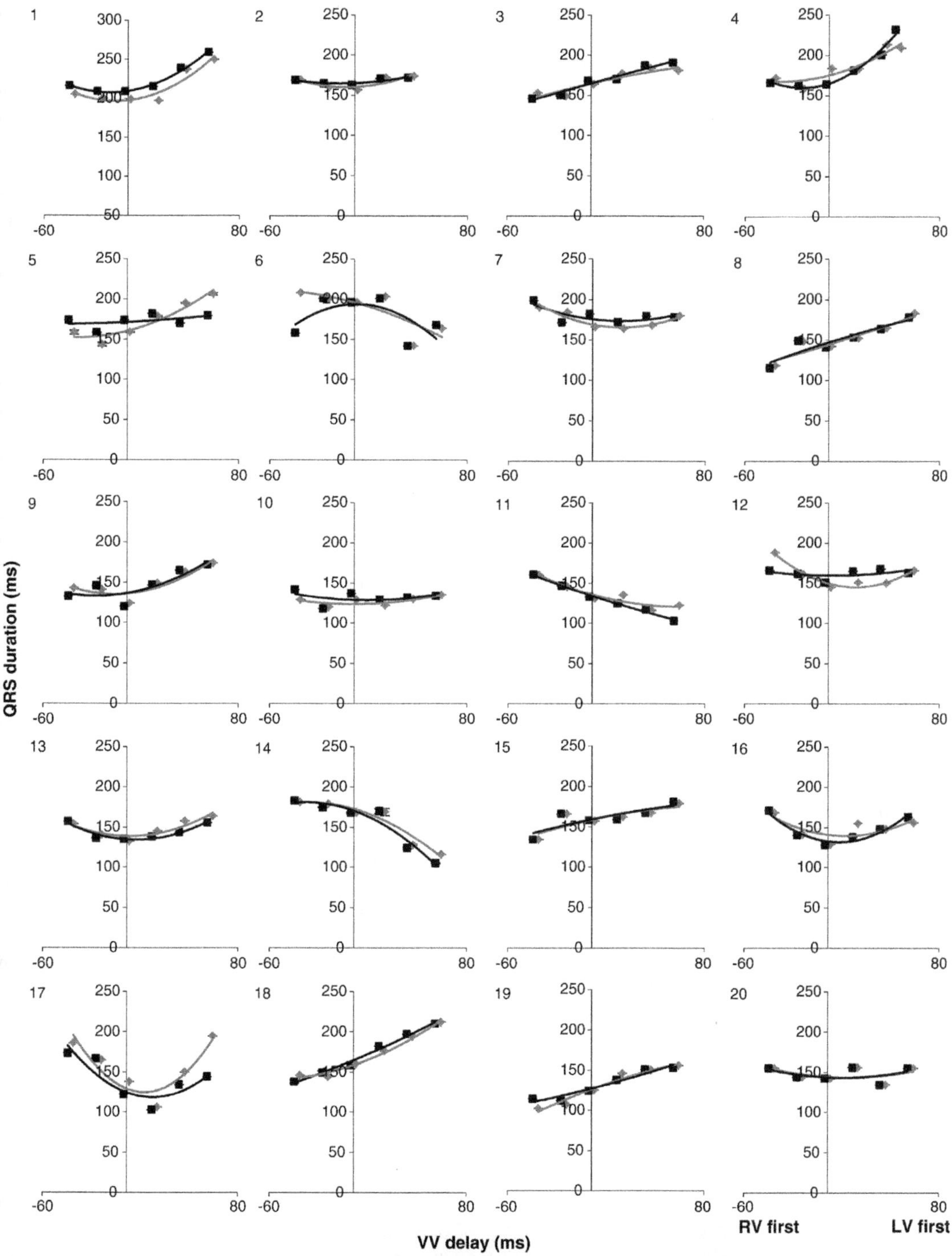

Fig. 2. Data from 20 patients who had VV delay optimization performed twice on the same day, using 12-lead ECG QRS width. Data for the first optimization is displayed in black and the second optimization is displayed in gray. A parabola was fitted for optimization session and the trough of the parabola was considered to represent the optimal VV delay (optimum = narrowest QRS). (*From* Kyriacou A, Li Kam Wa ME, Pabari PA, et al. A systematic approach to designing reliable VV optimization methodology: assessment of internal validity of echocardiographic, electrocardiographic and haemodynamic optimization of cardiac resynchronization therapy. Int J Cardiol 2012 Mar 26. [Epub ahead of print]; with permission.)

This analysis does not show that measurement of flow is doomed to be ineffective for VV optimization. It only shows that the protocol carried out, measuring 6 beats, cannot reliably identify a singular or reproducible optimum. It is entirely possible that an approach that averaged more beats might vanquish the noise sufficiently to make the approach feasible. This does not seem, however, to have yet been tested. Efforts to optimize VV delay by LVOT VTI have often claimed to use 3 beats per setting, and lectures have sometimes shown examples using only 1 beat per setting. It is hard to understand how such attempts could be anything other than futile.

QRS Minimization

With wide QRS a prime criterion for implantation of CRT, it is intellectually attractive to aim to adjust VV delay in a manner to restore QRS width to as close as possible to a normal narrow duration.

Whether competitive narrowing of QRS is a physiologically ideal target is not known, but the authors' experiments may have cast some light.

Singularity

QRS duration can easily be measured precisely, as readily seen from the error bars in **Fig. 2** too narrow to see in many cases (just visible for the gray). In almost every case, there is a clear optimum (ie, VV delay which minimizes QRS duration).

Reproducibility

The replicate data sets are closely concordant, as evidenced by the almost overlapping curves in many cases.

Biologic Plausibility

The concern for QRS duration is that some of the VV delays identified as apparently optimal, in terms of QRS minimization, are not VV delays that spring to mind as physiologically desirable. For example, in patients 3, 5, 8, 15, 18, and 19, the VV delay consistently selected as optimal by both replicate VV optimization processes was RV first by 60 ms. If 30% of cases require such extreme RV preactivation for optimality, then some of the understanding of the mechanism of CRT and cardiac function must be incorrect. **Fig. 3** shows plot of the distribution of VV delays identified as optimal using QRS minimization.

Pressure

The authors' group has conducted a series of experiments over the past 10 years on the potential for using blood pressure, which can be measured beat-to-beat noninvasively, as a marker for optimization of BVPs.[30–32] Pressure has the advantage over flow in that it can be acquired automatically with no human intervention required, which makes it more convenient than echo Doppler.

Singularity

Most of the 40 optimizations shown in **Fig. 4** identified a clear optimum VV delay.

Reproducibility

The test-retest variability of the optimum by this BP protocol was an SD of differences of 10.2 ms.

Plausibility

Eighteen of the 20 patients showed on both optimization sessions an optimum that was in the central region that biologically might appear most plausible. No post hoc data editing took place.

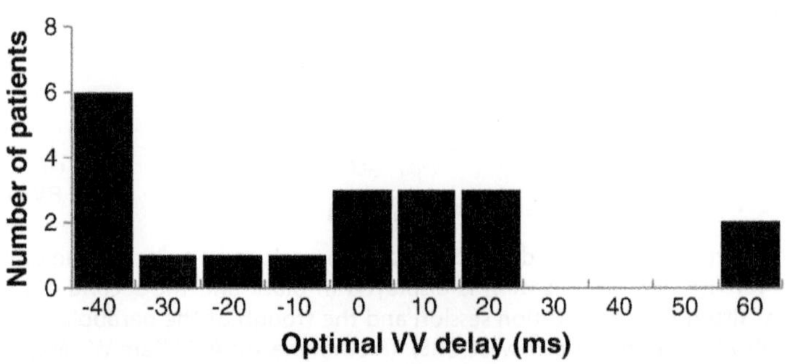

Fig. 3. Plot of the distribution of VV delays identified as optimal using QRS minimization. A high proportion of optima with significant (−40 ms) RV pre-excitation was identified as optimal. (*From* Kyriacou A, Li Kam Wa ME, Pabari PA, et al. A systematic approach to designing reliable VV optimization methodology: assessment of internal validity of echocardiographic, electrocardiographic and haemodynamic optimization of cardiac resynchronization therapy. Int J Cardiol 2012 Mar 26. [Epub ahead of print]; with permission.)

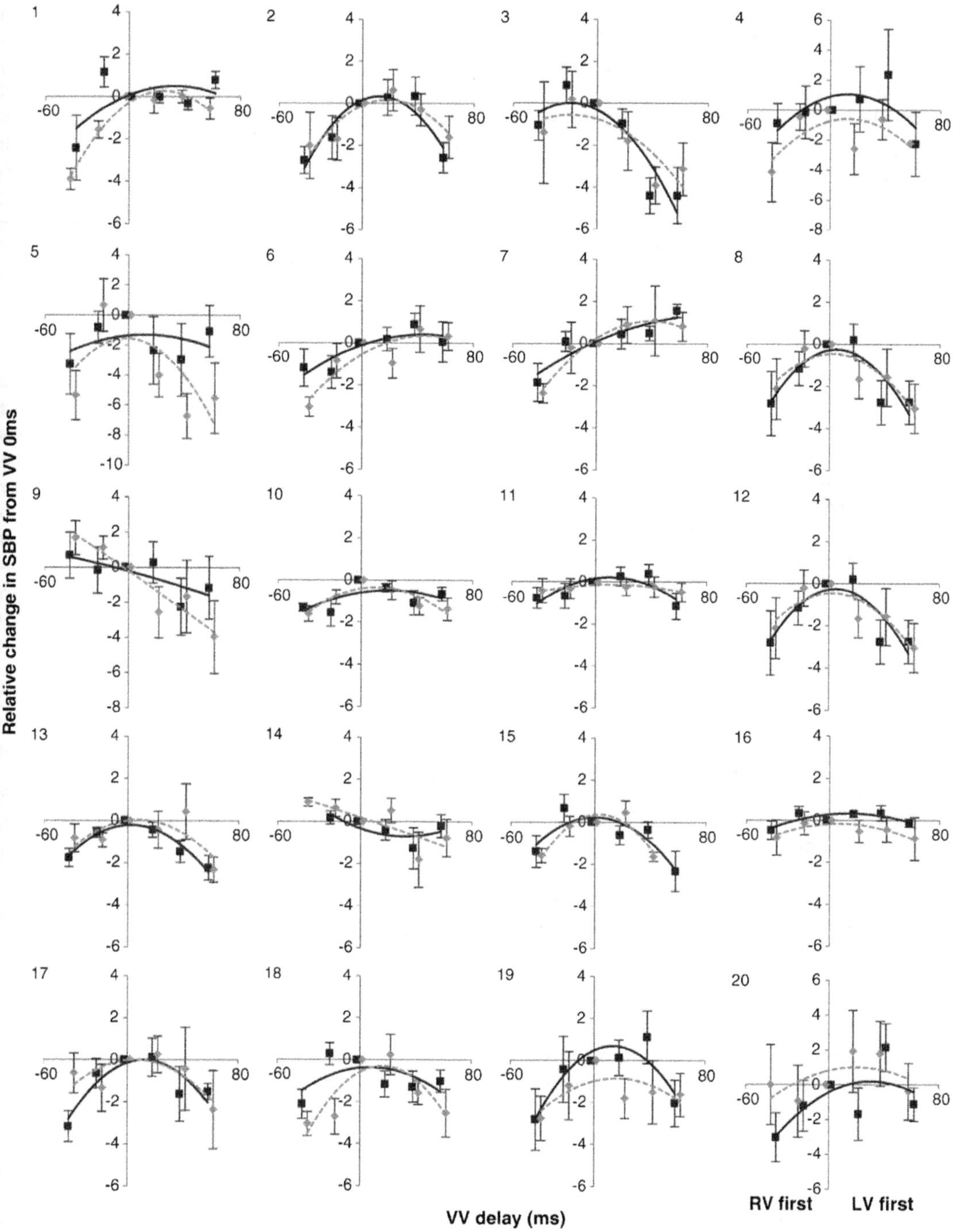

Fig. 4. Data from 20 patients who had VV delay optimization performed twice on the same day, using noninvasive systolic blood pressure (SBP). In order to minimize noise, each tested VV delay was compared with the reference VV delay of 0 ms and the relative change in systolic blood pressure was calculated by subtracting the mean SBP of the 10 beats immediately after the transition from the 10 beats immediately before the transition. A mean of 8 replicate measurements was used. Data for the first optimization is displayed in black and the second optimization is displayed in gray. A parabola was fitted in all optimization sessions and the peak of the parabola was considered to represent the optimal VV delay (optimum = highest relative SBP). (*From* Kyriacou A, Li Kam Wa ME, Pabari PA, et al. A systematic approach to designing reliable VV optimization methodology: assessment of internal validity of echocardiographic, electrocardiographic and haemodynamic optimization of cardiac resynchronization therapy. Int J Cardiol 2012 Mar 26. [Epub ahead of print]; with permission.)

IS TIME SPENT OPTIMIZING VV DELAY RATHER THAN SIMPLY PROGRAMMING SIMULTANEOUS RV AND LV PACING LIKELY TO DELIVER CLINICAL USEFUL IMPROVEMENTS IN CARDIAC FUNCTION?

Although many clinicians consider it not worthwhile to optimize VV delay, the articles that report the results of VV optimization characteristically indicate large increments in physiologic variables measured. How can these be reconciled?

There is a serious trap into which it is easily possible to fall when optimizing VV delay by maximizing a physiologic variable. Consider an extreme case where the biologic variable measured has no relation to VV delay at all and only shows random biologic variability. If N settings are tested, 1 of which is the 0 VV delay that is the reference state, then because of natural variability, there is always 1 VV delay whose measurement is highest. On average, in 1 out of N cases, this is VV 0; in the remaining (N-1)/N cases, it is some other delay. Thus, as more settings are tested, the greater the chance that a non-0 setting will be selected as optimal.

But the problem has even worse ramifications. Clinicians mindful of the need for clinical audit might attempt to calculate the average benefit in the variable achieved by VV optimization. Because, in each case, they would use the increment from VV 0 ms to the optimal VV delay, and in each case that increment would be positive (except in the 1/N cases, in which it is 0 because the VV 0-ms setting happened by chance to give the highest measurement), the increment would be a list of exclusively positive numbers (with a few 0s). Necessarily, such a list would be statistically significantly larger than 0.

Therefore, in any statistical test, the optimization process would seem to have statistically significantly increased the measurement, such as of LVOT VTI, even though in reality the optimization was no more than selecting a VV delay setting at random. In real life, VV delay may be making a contribution, but the size of it is unknown unless special steps are taken to eradicate the noise component.

Therefore, estimating the increment achieved by VV optimization must not be carried out using data that have wide error bars. Using a high degree of replication, such as can be achieved with pressure, and curve fitting to minimize the effect of noise,[27] it is possible to visualize the effect of adjusting VV delay and gauge the likely magnitude of contribution of moving VV delay away from 0 ms.

From the authors' AF study of VV optimization, it seems that in most cases the optimum VV delay gives systolic blood pressure less than 1 mm Hg higher than would be achieved by VV 0-ms pacing. Because blood pressure is approximately 100 mm Hg, the authors interpret this as an increment in cardiac output or stroke volume of less than 1%. To put this into context, simply switching on CRT (in sinus rhythm) to optimal AV delay (in patients in SR) increases blood pressure by approximately 6%. Thus, the amount gained by most patients from VV optimization is less than one-sixth the effect of CRT itself.

SUMMARY

VV delay optimization is a fascinating and potentially hazardous pursuit. The fascination lies in that the process of comparing multiple settings is the acid test of the resynchronization hypothesis, largely unacknowledged by the clinical and scientific community. Lack of a visible prominent effect of VV adjustment on hemodynamics is proof that either the resynchronization concept is plain wrong, or the measurement protocol design is so vulnerable to error that it cannot detect this important effect. The hazard lies in the widespread failure to perceive natural biologic variability, which is often mistaken for failure of the operator to make measurements correctly. Measurement variability causes false optima to appear with VV delay adjustment and makes the size of the optimization benefit become exaggerated.

Using sensitive (narrow-error-bar) methods, VV delay optimization produces small increments in hemodynamic effects over and above programming a nominal setting of VV 0 ms.

REFERENCES

1. Dickstein K, Bogale N, Priori S, et al. The European cardiac resynchronization therapy survey. Eur Heart J 2009;30:2450–60.
2. Molhoek SG, Bax JJ, Bleeker GB, et al. Comparison of response to cardiac resynchronization therapy in patients with sinus rhythm versus chronic atrial fibrillation. Am J Cardiol 2004;94:1506–9.
3. Gasparini M, Auricchio A, Regoli F, et al. Four-year efficacy of cardiac resynchronization therapy on exercise tolerance and disease progression. The importance of performing atrioventricular junction ablation in patients with atrial fibrillation. J Am Coll Cardiol 2006;48:734–43.
4. Kies P, Leclercq C, Bleeker GB, et al. Cardiac resynchronisation therapy in chronic atrial fibrillation: impact on left atrial size and reversal to sinus rhythm. Heart 2006;92:490–4.
5. Delnoy PP, Ottervanger JP, Luttikhuis HO, et al. Comparison of usefulness of cardiac resynchronization therapy in patients with atrial fibrillation and

heart failure versus patients with sinus rhythm and heart failure. Am J Cardiol 2007;99:1252–7.

6. Ferreira AM, Adragao P, Cavaco DM, et al. Benefit of cardiac resynchronization therapy in atrial fibrillation patients vs patients in sinus rhythm: the role of atrio-ventricular junction ablation. Europace 2008;10: 809–15.
7. Gasparini M, Auricchio A, Metra M, et al. Long-term survival in patients undergoing cardiac resynchronization therapy: the importance of performing atrio-ventricular junction ablation in patients with permanent atrial fibrillation. Eur Heart J 2008;29: 1644–52.
8. Tolosana JM, Hernandez Madrid A, Brugada J, et al. Comparison of benefits and mortality in cardiac resynchronization therapy in patients with atrial fibrillation versus patients in sinus rhythm. Am J Cardiol 2008;102:444–9.
9. Dong K, Shen WK, Powell BD, et al. Atrioventricular nodal ablation predicts survival benefit in patients with atrial fibrillation receiving cardiac resynchronization therapy. Heart Rhythm 2010;7:1240–5.
10. Khadjooi K, Foley PW, Chalil S, et al. Long-term effects of cardiac resynchronisation therapy in patients with atrial fibrillation. Heart 2008;94:879–83.
11. Wilton SB, Leung AA, Ghali WA, et al. Outcomes of cardiac resynchronization therapy in patients with versus those without atrial fibrillation: a systematic review and meta-analysis. Heart Rhythm 2011;8: 1088–94. http://dx.doi.org/10.1016/j.hrthm.2011.02. 014.
12. Wilton SB, Kavanagh KM, Aggarwal SG, et al. Association of rate-controlled persistent atrial fibrillation with clinical outcome and ventricular remodelling in recipients of cardiac resynchronization therapy. Can J Cardiol 2011;27(6):787–93. http://dx.doi.org/ 10.1016/j.cjca.2011.06.004.
13. Leclercq C, Walker S, Linde C, et al. Comparative effects of permanent biventricular and right-univentricular pacing in heart failure patients with chronic atrial fibrillation. Eur Heart J 2002;23(22): 1780–7.
14. Linde C, Leclercq C, Rex S, et al. Long-term benefits of biventricular pacing in congestive heart failure: results from the MUltisite STimulation in cardiomyopathy (MUSTIC) study. J Am Coll Cardiol 2002;40: 111–8.
15. Healey JS, Hohnloser SH, Exner DV, et al, RAFT Investigators. Cardiac resynchronization therapy in patients with permanent atrial fibrillation: results from the Resynchronization for Ambulatory Heart Failure Trial (RAFT). Circ Heart Fail 2012; 5:566–70.
16. Wilkoff BL, Cook JR, Epstein AE, et al, Dual Chamber and VVI Implantable Defibrillator Trial Investigators. Dual-chamber pacing or ventricular backup pacing in patients with an implantable defibrillator: the Dual Chamber and VVI Implantable Defibrillator (DAVID) Trial. JAMA 2002;288: 3115–23.
17. Mullens W, Grimm RA, Verga T, et al. Insights from a cardiac resynchronization optimization clinic as part of a heart failure disease management program. J Am Coll Cardiol 2009;53:765–73.
18. Kyriacou A, Pabari P, Francis D. Cardiac resynchronization therapy is certainly cardiac therapy, but how much resynchronization and how much atrio-ventricular delay optimization? Heart Fail Rev 2012; 17:727–36.
19. Kamath GS, Cotiga D, Koneru JN, et al. The utility of 12-lead Holter monitoring in patients with permanent atrial fibrillation for the identification of nonresponders after cardiac resynchronization therapy. J Am Coll Cardiol 2009;53:1050–5.
20. Ganesan AN, Brooks AG, Roberts-Thomson KC, et al. Role of AV nodal ablation in cardiac resynchronization in patients with coexistent atrial fibrillation and heart failure a systematic review. J Am Coll Cardiol 2012;59(8):719–26.
21. Daubert JC, Saxon L, Adamson PB, et al, European Heart Rhythm Association, European Society of Cardiology, Heart Rhythm Society, Heart Failure Society of America, American Society of Echocardiography, American Heart Association, European Association of Echocardiography, Heart Failure Association. 2012 EHRA/HRS expert consensus statement on cardiac resynchronization therapy in heart failure: implant and follow-up recommendations and management. Heart Rhythm 2012;9(9):1524–76.
22. Finegold JA, Manisty CH, Cecaro F, et al. Choosing between velocity-time-integral ratio and peak velocity ratio for calculation of the dimensionless index (or aortic valve area) in serial follow-up of aortic stenosis. Int J Cardiol 2012. [Epub ahead of print].
23. Kyriacou A, Li Kam Wa ME, Pabari PA, et al. A systematic approach to designing reliable VV optimization methodology: assessment of internal validity of echocardiographic, electrocardiographic and haemodynamic optimization of cardiac resynchronization therapy. Int J Cardiol 2012. [Epub ahead of print].
24. Pabari PA, Willson K, Stegemann B, et al. When is an optimization not an optimization? Evaluation of clinical implications of information content (signal-to-noise ratio) in optimization of cardiac resynchronization therapy, and how to measure and maximize it. Heart Fail Rev 2011;16:277–90.
25. Whinnett ZI, Francis DP, Denis A, et al. Comparison of different invasive hemodynamic methods for AV delay optimization in patients with cardiac resynchronization therapy: implications for clinical trial design and clinical practice. Int J Cardiol 2013. http://dx.doi.org/10.1016/j.ijcard.2013.01.216.

26. Francis DP. How to reliably deliver narrow individual-patient error bars for optimization of pacemaker AV or VV delay using a "pick-the-highest" strategy with haemodynamic measurements. Int J Cardiol 2013;163:221–5. http://dx.doi.org/10.1016/j.ijcard.2012.03.128.
27. Francis DP. Precision of a Parabolic Optimum Calculated from Noisy Biological Data, and Implications for Quantitative Optimization of Biventricular Pacemakers (Cardiac Resynchronization Therapy). Applied Mathematics 2011;2:1497–506.
28. Perego GB, Chianca R, Facchini M, et al. Simultaneous vs sequential biventricular pacing in dilated cardiomyopathy: an acute hemodynamic study. Eur J Heart Fail 2003;5:305–13.
29. Bogaard MD, Doevendans PA, Leenders GE, et al. Can optimization of pacing settings compensate for a non-optimal left ventricular pacing site? Europace 2010;12:1262–9.
30. Whinnett ZI, Davies JE, Willson K, et al. Haemodynamic effects of changes in AV and VV delay in cardiac resynchronisation therapy show a consistent pattern: analysis of shape, magnitude and relative importance of AV and VV delay. Heart 2006;92:1628–34.
31. Whinnett ZI, Briscoe C, Davies JE, et al. The atrioventricular delay of cardiac resynchronization can be optimized hemodynamically during exercise and predicted from resting measurements. Heart Rhythm 2008;5:378–86.
32. Whinnett ZI, Nott G, Davies JE, et al. Efficiency, reproducibility and agreement of five different hemodynamic measures for optimization of cardiac resynchronization therapy. Int J Cardiol 2008;129:216–26.
33. Waggoner AD, de las Fuentes L, Davila-Roman VG. Doppler echocardiographic methods for optimization of the atrioventricular delay during cardiac resynchronization therapy. Echocardiography 2008;25(9):1047–55.
34. Boriani G, Muller CP, Seidl KH, et al. Randomized comparison of simultaneous biventricular stimulation versus optimized interventricular delay in cardiac resynchronization therapy. The Resynchronization for the Hemodynamic Treatment for Heart Failure Management II implantable cardioverter defibrillator (RHYTHM II ICD) study. Am Heart J 2006;151:1050–8.
35. Leon AR, Abraham WT, Brozena S, et al. Cardiac resynchronization with sequential biventricular pacing for the treatment of moderate-to-severe heart failure. J Am Coll Cardiol 2005;46:2298–304.
36. Kyriacou A, Whinnett ZI, Sen S, et al. Improvement in coronary blood flow velocity with acute biventricular pacing is predominantly due to an increase in a diastolic backward-travelling decompression (suction) wave. Circulation 2012;126:1334–44.

The Role of Ablation of the Atrioventricular Junction in Patients with Heart Failure and Atrial Fibrillation

Eszter M. Vegh, MD[a], Nitesh Sood, MD[b], Jagmeet P. Singh, MD, PhD, DPhil[a,*]

KEYWORDS

• AV junction ablation • Cardiac resynchronization therapy • Therapy refractory atrial fibrillation

KEY POINTS

- Ablation of the atrioventricular junction (AVJ) is a technically easy procedure that is safe and has a high success rate as an intervention for effective ventricular rate control in patients in symptomatic atrial fibrillation.
- AVJ ablation has been reported to improve quality of life, left ventricular ejection fraction, and exercise duration in patients with symptomatic atrial fibrillation and minimize the incidence of inappropriate shocks.
- Because right ventricular pacing after AVJ ablation may result in a decrease in left ventricular function and worsening of heart failure symptoms, there is increasing evidence to support the effectiveness of cardiac resynchronization therapy in atrial fibrillation populations.
- After receiving resynchronization therapy, AVJ ablation increases the proportion of biventricular pacing and thereby improves the response to cardiac resynchronization therapy in this cohort of patients.

INTRODUCTION

Heart failure (HF) and atrial fibrillation (AF) are at epidemic proportions in the modern world. HF affects more than 5 million Americans and is one of the leading causes of morbidity and mortality.[1] Similarly, more than 2 million people in the United States and a similar number in Europe have AF, with an increasing prevalence in the aging population. Based on Framingham follow-up data, the current lifetime risks for development of AF are 1 in 4 for men and women 40 years of age and older.[2]

AF is a common precipitating factor for HF decompensation in patients with both preserved and depressed left ventricular ejection fraction (LVEF).[3,4] AF also portends an adverse long-term prognosis in such patients.[5] Moreover, the incidence of AF increases with an increasing severity of HF: the incidence being 4% in patients with New York Heart Association (NYHA) functional class I,[3] 10% to 27% in NYHA II to III,[6] and increasing to 50% in patients with NYHA class IV HF.[7] AF has also been associated with an increased incidence of both appropriate and inappropriate implantable cardioverter defibrillator (ICD) shocks, both of which have been associated with HF decompensation and mortality in patients with cardiomyopathy.[8,9]

Rate and rhythm control strategies have both been shown to ameliorate symptoms of AF in

Disclosures: EMV and NS have no disclosures. JPS: Lectures, consulting and research grants from Biotronik, Boston Scientific, Medtronic, Sorin Group, and St. Jude Medical.

[a] Cardiac Arrhythmia Service, Massachusetts General Hospital, Harvard Medical School, 55 Fruit Street, Boston, MA 02114, USA; [b] Division of Cardiology, Lahey Clinic, Tufts University, 41 Burlington Mall Road, Burlington, MA 01805, USA
* Corresponding author.
E-mail address: jsingh@partners.org

Heart Failure Clin 9 (2013) 489–499
http://dx.doi.org/10.1016/j.hfc.2013.07.003

eligible symptoms. Although a strategy of rhythm control has been reported to improve ejection fraction and quality of life in some series,[10] there is no conclusive evidence to suggest that rate control is inferior to rhythm control in patients with HF and irreversible systolic dysfunction.[11–13] This is particularly relevant to some older populations with AF and HF, who may not be suitable for aggressive treatment with antiarrhythmic drugs or catheter ablation.

The strategy of "Ablate and Pace" using atrioventricular junction (AVJ) ablation is an accepted but underused treatment option for patients with symptomatic, drug refractory AF. It is supported by a substantial amount of literature accumulated over a period of greater than 30 years and has recently proved to be an effective strategy to ensure optimal biventricular pacing in patients with AF and cardiomyopathy, undergoing cardiac resynchronization therapy.[14–17]

HISTORY OF AVJ ABLATION

AVJ ablation was first performed in 1981 in a patient suffering from recurrent episodes of drug refractory, symptomatic AF.[18] Scheinman[19] published a report of 5 cases of AVJ ablation in 1982. An electrode catheter was positioned via a transvenous approach at the site of largest His bundle potential. A series of direct current (DC) defibrillation shocks (300–500 J) were delivered until atrioventricular (AV) block was achieved. Four of the 5 patients continued to have AV block, whereas one patient died suddenly at 5.5 weeks after the procedure.[19] Soon after, Gallagher and colleagues[20] reported their results with DC shock-induced AVJ ablation in a series of 9 patients. After being established in canine experiments, radiofrequency ablation gathered ground in the late 1980s, and soon superseded DC shock ablation for the AVJ.[21]

ABLATION OF AVJ: DIFFERENT TECHNIQUES

The goal of AVJ ablation is to achieve conduction block in the compact AV node ideally with a stable junctional escape rhythm after ablation. The actual ablation procedure is technically simple with a low risk of complications as well as a high early and long-term success rate (>98%).[22]

Right-sided Approach

The right-sided method is nearly always attempted first and accounts for most cases. Catheters are typically introduced via a transvenous femoral approach into the right atrium. After mapping a His bundle potential in the right ventricular septal region, the ablation catheter is withdrawn slowly toward the right atrium with a clockwise torque. At the optimal location for ablation, a larger atrial than ventricular electrogram and a His bundle potential should be recorded. Ablation at the proximal part of the conduction apparatus (ie, toward the atrium) is preferred to allow for a junctional rather than a ventricular escape rhythm. Radiofrequency energy is delivered usually for 30 to 60 seconds at temperatures typically of 55 to 70°C at a maximum of 60 W. Early nodal acceleration during ablation suggests an effective ablation lesion (**Fig. 1**).

Left-sided Approach

A highly calcified AV node and/or edema after an unsuccessful right-sided ablation attempt may necessitate a left-sided approach to AVJ ablation. The ablation catheter is introduced through the femoral artery or transseptally to the left side of the ventricular membranous septum. Anatomically this lies immediately inferior to the right fibrous trigone and the junction of the right and the noncoronary cusps of the aortic valve. The penetrating bundle of His enters the left ventricular (LV) outflow tract in this region and is not protected by the central fibrous body. Sousa and colleagues[23] first described this method using 20 to 36 W of energy for 15 to 30 seconds. Later, Marshall and colleagues reported no major complications with high energy, temperature, and duration, similar to a right-sided ablation. Nevertheless, vascular complications, the risks associated with transseptal puncture, and the need for peri-procedural anticoagulation increase the theoretical risk associated with this left-sided approach.

Modification of the Slow Pathway

AF has been associated with AV node remodeling and preferential conduction over the slow AV nodal pathway.[24] Thus, modification of the slow pathway has been explored as an alternative strategy for rate control in patients with drug refractory, symptomatic AF. A few small, single-center studies have reported similar reductions in ventricular rate,[25] but this technique is not routinely used due to a higher resumption of conduction.

Approach from Superior Veins

Some operators have explored ablation of the AV node through access from the cephalic/axillary/subclavian venous system at the time of pacemaker implant.[26] This approach has been reported to reduce both the procedure and the fluoroscopy times, with similar procedural efficacy.[26] This approach may also reduce potential femoral vascular complications and is an alternative for patients with

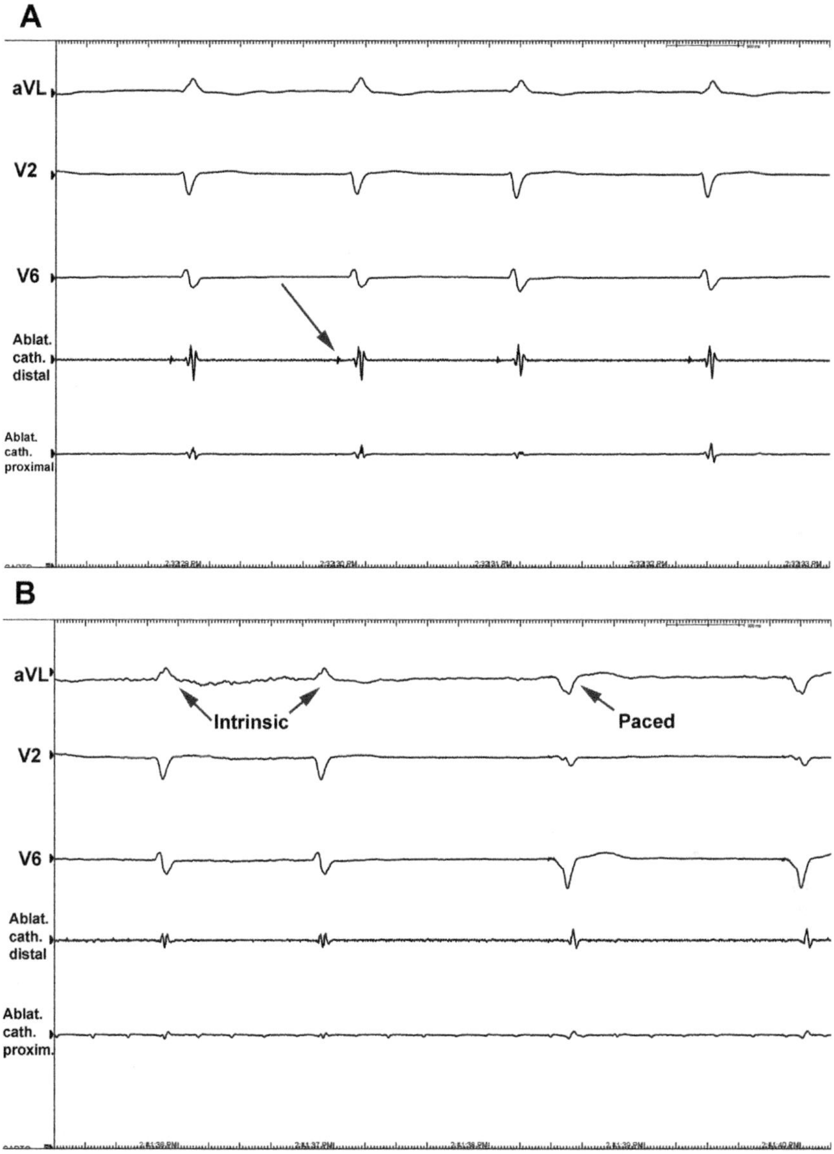

Fig. 1. Electrocardiographic representation of AVN ablation. (*A*) Registered potentials: the arrow points to the His signal. (*B*) The patient attained complete AV block after 3 seconds of ablation. The alteration of QRS morphology indicates the modified activation sequence.

an inferior vena cava filter (which does not provide an absolute contraindication), obstruction, or other issues that limit access from the inferior veins.

BENEFITS OF AVJ ABLATION

Ablation of the AVJ leads to several clinical benefits, although through mechanisms that are not completely understood. Presumably the most important component is prevention of tachycardia-mediated cardiomyopathy. In experimental models, chronic rapid ventricular pacing has been demonstrated to induce biventricular failure. Myocardial energy depletion, ischemia, cellular, and extracellular remodeling and abnormalities of calcium regulation were observed and considered plausible mechanisms. End-stage HF status was reached within 3 to 5 weeks of right ventricular (RV) pacing in dogs; however, the process was reversible in the first 1 to 2 weeks.[27] A second mechanism for the benefit of AVJ ablation is via the regularization of R-R intervals. Clinically, lone AF has been shown to cause LV dysfunction and idiopathic cardiomyopathy, which is reversible after AVJ ablation.[28–30] Clark and colleagues[31] assessed invasive hemodynamics pre- and post-AVJ ablation comparing irregular

R-R intervals during AF to RV paced rhythm with the preablation mean rate. Irregular R-R intervals (representing altering durations between two ventricular beats) demonstrated a significantly decreased cardiac output (4.4 ± 1.6 vs 5.2 ± 2.4 L/min, *P*<.01), increased pulmonary capillary wedge pressure (17 ± 7 vs 14 ± 6 mm Hg, *P*<.002), and increased right atrial pressure (10 ± 6 vs 8 ± 4 mm Hg, *P*<.05) when compared with the paced group at preablation mean heart rate.

Pharmacologic rate control is the first line of treatment of rate control in AF. However, after an unsuccessful trial of medical treatment, AVJ ablation is a reasonable next option.[32] In the Ablate and Pace Trial, 156 highly symptomatic persistent and paroxysmal AF patients were treated with AVJ ablation. At the 12 months follow-up, the authors reported an improved quality of life but no statistically significant change in LVEF and exercise capacity compared with baseline. Notably, the authors reported 23 deaths (5 classified as sudden cardiac death, SCD; 14.7%) in 156 patients included in this study.[28] Subsequently, Ozcan and colleagues[29] reported long-term survival after AVJ ablation. Patients with AF undergoing AVJ ablation were compared with age-matched and sex-matched control subjects free of AF and consecutive AF patients receiving only pharmacologic therapy. A total of 250 patients were followed for a mean period of 3.5 years. The authors observed a similar survival in AVJ-ablated patients as in the general population and AF patients treated with pharmacologic rate control. However, mortality in subjects treated with AVJ ablation was significantly elevated in patients with underlying heart disease. A meta-analysis published by the authors' group examined the safety, efficacy, and effectiveness of AVJ ablation versus pharmacologic treatment of rate control in AF. The authors' analyses showed that, compared with subjects receiving pharmacotherapy, those receiving AVJ ablation obtained a statistically significant improvement in quality-of-life indices and LVEF, and a modest but statistically nonsignificant improvement in functional status and echocardiographic variables. Periprocedural complications were relatively rare, with the incidence of death being 0.27%, malignant arrhythmia 0.57%, that the authors considered too low to draw any safety conclusions. No significant differences were found between all-cause mortality in AVJ ablation versus medical therapy for rate control of AF.[22]

PACING AFTER AVJ ABLATION

Deleterious Effects of RV Pacing

Multiple studies have reported increased numbers of HF hospitalizations and enhanced mortality associated with high percentage of RV pacing (>40%).[33–35] Long-term follow-up of the MADIT-II study reported increased mortality in ICD patients with a high percentage of RV pacing.[36] RV pacing has been shown to result in abnormal activation sequence leading to both electrical and mechanical interventricular dyssynchrony.[37,38] RV pacing has also been associated with worsening diastolic dysfunction and increased levels of inflammatory markers.[39,40]

Evidence for Biventricular Versus RV Pacing in Patients with Preserved Systolic Function (LVEF >45%)

RV pacing after AVJ ablation may result in a decrease in LVEF and worsening of HF symptoms.[15,41] Recent studies have evaluated the potential benefit of a universal biventricular pacing approach after AVJ ablation. The PAVE Study Group randomized patients to either CRT-P (cardiac resynchronization therapy-pacemaker) or RV pacing after AVJ ablation (n = 101 vs 81). Patients treated with CRT-P had a significant improvement in 6-minute walk distance (82.9 ± 94.7 m vs 61.2 ± 90.0 m, *P* = .04), and higher ejection fraction (46 ± 13% vs 41 ± 13%, *P* = .03) 6 months after ablation when compared with the RV paced group. This improvement in 6-minute walk time was higher in patients with more advanced HF (LVEF ≤45% and NYHA II/III symptoms).[41]

Brignole and colleagues[15] recently published the results of a similar study, whereby they hypothesized a superiority of CRT (n = 97) versus RV (n = 89) pacing in reducing HF events in patients with permanent AF undergoing AVJ ablation. During their median follow-up of 20 months, there was a decreased incidence of a composite endpoint of HF hospitalization, worsening symptoms, and mortality in the CRT group. In multivariable analyses, CRT remained the single independent predictor of a lack of HF events. This effect was seen in patients irrespective of ejection fraction. Recent 2-year data from the Pacing to Prevent Cardiac Enlargement trial, that compared biventricular to right ventricular pacing in patients with normal ejection fraction and sinus bradycardia, echoed similar effects on the prevention of deleterious LV remodeling in patients receiving biventricular compared to RV pacing.[42]

Biventricular Versus RV Pacing in Patients with Depressed Systolic Function

Current guidelines recommend biventricular pacing in patients with irreversible cardiomyopathy with LVEF ≤35% undergoing AVJ ablation for AF or who otherwise meet criteria for CRT-D.[32]

Patients with tachycardia-mediated cardiomyopathy with an LVEF ≤35% should be initially implanted with RV pacing lead only.[43]

CLINICAL IMPLICATIONS AND AVJ ABLATION AS A TREATMENT MODALITY: CURRENT GUIDELINES

Current guidelines recommend single-chamber pacemaker implant for patients with normal LV function or reversible LV dysfunction undergoing AVJ ablation for AF.[32] Biventricular defibrillator/pacemaker is indicated in patients with irreversible cardiomyopathy and LVEF of ≤35%. A LV lead upgrade is indicated in patients with LVEF greater than 35% at implant who subsequently develop RV pacing-induced cardiomyopathy and/or HF.

Class II A (Level of Evidence: B)

It is reasonable to use ablation of AV node or accessory pathway to control heart rate when pharmacologic therapy is insufficient or associated with side effects.

Class II B (Level of Evidence: C)

When rate cannot be controlled by pharmacologic therapy or tachycardia-induced cardiomyopathy is suspected, catheter-driven AV node ablation may be considered in patients with AF to control heart rate.

Class III

Catheter ablation of AV node should not be used in AF to control heart rate without a prior trial of medications.

AVJ ABLATION AS A TREATMENT MODALITY

Preserved LVEF Greater than 45%

Symptomatic

AF is a common precipitant of hospitalization in patients with HF with preserved ejection fraction. Loss of atrial systole and irregular R-R intervals are the most likely mechanisms. Patients with AF and HF with preserved ejection fraction tend to be older and mostly not candidates for aggressive rhythm control strategy with anti-arrhythmic drugs or catheter ablation.[31,44] AVJ ablation may be an effective treatment in this patient group after a trial of pharmacologic therapy.

Asymptomatic

Many studies have shown that rate control is equivalent to rhythm control in asymptomatic patients with permanent AF and preserved ejection fraction. Moreover, a recent randomized trial (RACE II) suggested that lenient heart rate control (<110 bpm) may be an optimal strategy for patients with ejection fraction greater than 40%.[45] Thus, patients with asymptomatic permanent AF with preserved ejection fraction may be treated conservatively without aggressive measures. The exercise treadmill test may help with assessing symptoms because, for instance, individuals with rapid ventricular rates during exercise associated with symptoms and/or reduced functional capacity are not truly "asymptomatic." Holter monitors can be used to verify adequate heart rate control over 24 to 48 hours. An "Ablate and Pace" strategy may be appropriate for patients with suboptimal functional capacity, exercise-induced rapid ventricular rates associated with symptoms, inadequate heart rate control (>110 bpm), or those unable to tolerate pharmacologic treatment. In current practice, younger patients with symptomatic AF are often considered better candidates for a trial of anti-arrhythmic therapy or catheter ablation of AF.

Patients with Systolic Dysfunction

Symptomatic

Patients with either tachycardia-mediated cardiomyopathy or symptomatic AF and LV dysfunction should be managed aggressively. In such patients, associated comorbidities such as renal and liver dysfunction frequently limit the use of antiarrhythmic medications. Dofetilide and amiodarone may be safe in patients with LV dysfunction but require close monitoring.[46,47] Class IC drugs are contraindicated in patients with structural heart disease.[48] Sotalol should be used with caution especially in severely depressed LV dysfunction and advanced NYHA class.[49] Notably, dronedarone was recently reported to be associated with increase risk of mortality in patients with LV dysfunction and HF.[50]

A prospective randomized study compared AVJ ablation and biventricular pacing to catheter ablation for patients with AF and LV dysfunction. This study included patients with drug refractory AF, LVEF less than 40% that were at least NYHA class II/III. Patients with normal sinus rhythm after catheter ablation demonstrated a greater improvement in ejection fraction (35% vs 28%), 6-minute walk distance (340 m vs 297 m), and quality-of-life indices. The success rate for pulmonary vein isolation in this study was 88% with anti-arrhythmic drugs and 71% without anti-arrhythmic drugs at 6 months.[51] However, other studies reported variable results with catheter ablation for AF in patients with LV dysfunction.[52–54] Notably, the lack of a standardized ablative approach, frequent need for repeat procedures, and lack of robust data demonstrating benefit makes catheter ablation less attractive as a first-line approach to patients with AF and LV dysfunction. Catheter ablation for AF may be more likely to benefit selected groups of patients, such as those with tachycardia-related cardiomyopathy and paroxysmal or early persistent AF; this is currently being investigated in a prospective trial (CASTLE-HF).[55] Until further data are available, AVJ ablation and biventricular pacing remain a viable and beneficial approach in the treatment of symptomatic drug/ablation refractory AF in patients with LV dysfunction.

Asymptomatic

Even in asymptomatic patients, AF is associated with worse prognosis (CHARM).[56] Pharmacologic rate versus rhythm control was tested in a prospective randomized trial in patients with paroxysmal and persistent AF and HF with an LVEF less than 35% (AF-CHF). The rhythm control strategy with amiodarone and electrical cardioversion showed no benefit, and conversely, reported increased hospitalizations during follow-up.[13] The authors recommend Holter monitor and exercise treadmill test to ascertain symptoms and adequate heart rate control. A trial of sinus rhythm after cardioversion may also be attempted in such patients, to ascertain differences in functional status between sinus rhythm and AF. Truly asymptomatic patients with adequate heart rate control have not been reported to benefit from aggressive rhythm control or by a strategy of AVJ ablation and biventricular pacing. It is essential to evaluate the often subtle symptoms carefully that may arise from AF in patients with irreversible systolic dysfunction and HF. Of note, a lenient rate control strategy has not been extensively evaluated in the HF and cardiomyopathy populations, because patients with ejection fraction less than 40% were excluded from the RACE II trial.[45] Indeed, one study showed an increase in HF hospitalizations in patients with cardiomyopathy and AF whose average ventricular rate was greater than 90 bpm in a 1-month period.[57] Thus, ventricular rate–related symptoms should be carefully assessed in the reduced ejection fraction group.

Prevention of Appropriate ICD Shocks

Many studies have shown that AF is associated with a higher incidence of appropriate shocks in patients with an ICD.[58] This finding has been reported in patients with persistent AF, whereas episodes of paroxysmal AF have also been shown to precede appropriate ICD shocks in 20% of patients.[59] Studies suggest that exacerbations in HF, with electrophysiological abnormalities, mechano-electrical feedback from hemodynamic compromise, rate-related ischemia, ventricular arrhythmias associated with use of anti-arrhythmic drugs, and sympatho-excitation from heart rate irregularity are possible contributing mechanisms for this association.[58–60] These patients frequently have added comorbidities like renal dysfunction, diabetes, and hypertension, hence limiting the choices and dosages of pharmacologic rate control.

Prevention of Inappropriate ICD Shocks

Subanalyses of 2 major primary prevention trials (MADIT-II and SCD-HeFT) have reported an association between inappropriate shocks with increased mortality during follow-up.[8,9] AF remains the most prominent cause of inappropriate ICD shocks.[60–62] A large population-based cohort study of the LATITUDE database demonstrated that this increase in mortality was only seen in patients who received inappropriate shocks for AF.[63] Patients who received inappropriate shocks for other reasons (eg, sensing problems, supraventricular tachyarrhythmias) lacked a similar increase in mortality.[59,63] Hence, it may very well be that the additive effect of AF and shocks is responsible for this association.

Accordingly, patients that receive either appropriate or inappropriate ICD shocks secondary to AF should be aggressively considered for AVJ ablation or rhythm control strategy for management of AF.

Treating Ineffective Biventricular Pacing

Biventricular pacing has been demonstrated to reduce composite endpoint of mortality and HF in patients with cardiomyopathy and AF.[17,64–66] However, this requires a high percentage of biventricular pacing to optimize the response to CRT.[67] AF in patients with native conduction decreases true biventricular capture. The combined effects of AF and decreased percentage of biventricular pacing are additive in increasing mortality.[68,69] The presence of biventricular fusion (hybrid between paced and intrinsic QRS morphologies) and pseudofusion (pacing artifact delivered but intrinsic QRS morphology not altered) can artificially elevate the apparent percentage of biventricular pacing, yet without the benefits of true cardiac resynchronization.[70] Although the cutoff for percentage of biventricular pacing in reducing mortality was recently described in a large cohort of patients (>98.7%),[67] a similar cutoff for patients with AF and biventricular fusion has not been reported.

AVJ ablation has been reported to improve survival and functional status in patients with AF implanted with cardiac resynchronization therapy.[15,17,71] Ganesan and colleagues[14] reported a review and meta-analysis of clinical studies examining the impact of AVJ ablation in CRT-AF patients. This study included 6 trials and compared CRT-AF patients with and without AVJ ablation. Patients without AVJ ablation had higher all-cause (RR 0.42) and cardiovascular (RR 0.44) mortality. Heterogeneity in assessment of functional status precluded definite conclusion for this outcome.[14] Gasparini and colleagues[17] also found a significant increase in the LVEF of patients with CRT and AF with versus without AVJ ablation (37.1 vs 23.7% at 1 year, 39.5 vs 25.0% at 4-year follow-up).

Accordingly, patients with CRT and AF who are deemed to be nonresponders should undergo a careful assessment of true biventricular pacing, which may include a 24- to 48-hour Holter monitor to assess the percentage of paced beats that may truly be fused with intrinsic (dyssynchronous) activation. Patients who fail to respond clinically to resynchronization therapy with a suboptimal percentage of biventricular pacing should be treated aggressively to increase this percentage. Pharmacologic approaches with AV nodal blocking agents is the first-line treatment. Adverse effects of these medications are common in patients with advanced cardiomyopathy and HF. Lack of effective AV node blockade or adverse effects of pharmacologic agents should prompt consideration for AVJ ablation in these patients.

COMPLICATIONS OF AVJ ABLATION

Iatrogenic pacemaker dependency is likely to be a primary hesitation in recommending AVJ ablation more universally for rate control in patients with AF. Indeed, pacemaker dysfunction or loss of capture from lead dislodgment or fracture could be fatal in such patients. However, in a recent meta-analysis of AVJ ablation in AF, the authors' group found the incidence of lead failure as low as 0.23%.[22] Ganesan and colleagues[14] also did not report any major complications secondary to pacemaker dysfunction in their recent meta-analysis.

As an invasive procedure, AVJ carries inherent risks of femoral vascular complications, such as bleeding, hematoma, fistula, and venous thrombosis. Rare complications include intracardiac shunt, cardiac perforation, pericardial tamponade, tricuspid valve regurgitation, infection, and even death. The incidence of complications is approximately 3%, but with major complications is less than 2%.[72] According to the NASPE Prospective Voluntary Registry only 5 significant complications were reported during AVJ ablation of 646 patients, whereby the overall success rate was 97.4%.[73]

Sudden cardiac death after AVJ ablation was described in early studies and also in major trials.[19] The Ablate and Pace Trial reported 11 cases of death, and underlying structural heart disease was found to be a major predisposing factor.[28] Ozcan and colleagues[29] reported 4 likely and 3 possible procedure-related SCD cases in 334 AVJ ablation procedures. They found that risk of death was highest in the first 2 days after ablation. Diabetes, NYHA $\geq$2, ventricular arrhythmias present preprocedure, mitral or aortic stenosis, aortic regurgitation, and chronic obstructive pulmonary disease were independent predictors of mortality.

Ventricular tachyarrhythmias and SCD may contribute to mortality after AVJ ablation and are assumed to be triggered by bradycardia and pause-dependent polymorphic ventricular tachycardia.[74] To prevent this phenomenon, Geelen and colleagues[75] compared a postablation lower rate limit for pacing to 90 bpm (n = 235) for the first 1 to 3 months postablation compared with a group of patients (n = 100) with a lower rate limit $\leq$70 bpm. Notably, they found less SCD (0 vs 6 cases) in the higher base rate group despite no significant differences in baseline characteristics between groups. Postablation ventricular fibrillation was observed only during slow ventricular pacing or escape rhythm. Thus, current practice is to set an elevated pacing rate for some months after AVJ ablation, then reduce the rate over time.

It is important to remember clearly that AVJ-ablated patients demand constant ventricular pacing, leading to early battery depletion demanding more frequent generator replacement with its attendant complications.

AVJ ablation does not address AF per se, and patients still require oral anticoagulation according to their risk for stroke as codified in the CHA_2DS_2-VASc score.

LV–right atrial shunt is an extremely rare complication of AVJ ablation. During ablation, the catheter is positioned toward the apex of the triangle of Koch, directly above the septal leaflet of tricuspid valve. This leaflet is 5 to 10 mm more apically located than the mitral valve and above it the superior AV portion of the membranous septum can be found. This membranous septum can be perforated due to radiofrequency ablation in this area.[76] Can and colleagues[77] reported a patient with such an LV-RA shunt and a 76-mm Hg gradient at 5 months with mild to moderate RV dilatation. Nevertheless, this patient remained stable with NYHA I and II HF during follow-up with conservative management.

Of note, AVERT-AF (Atrio-Ventricular Junction Ablation Followed by Resynchronization Therapy in patients with CHF and AF) is a prospective, randomized, multicenter trial examining AVJ ablation versus pharmacologic rate control in CRT-AF population with respect to functional status, quality of life, and survival. The AVERT-AF is designed to test exercise capacity and functional status, as primary endpoints in patients with chronic AF and depressed ejection fraction, regardless of rate or QRS duration. The results are expected soon.[78]

SUMMARY

AVJ ablation is a technically straightforward and relatively safe procedure, with a high success as an intervention to achieve effective ventricular rate control in patients in symptomatic AF. It has been reported to improve quality of life, LVEF, and exercise duration in these patients. There is increasing evidence that supports its effectiveness in the CRT-AF population to improve response to resynchronization. It is important to remember, however, that patients after AVJ ablation become pacemaker-dependent and still require appropriate antithrombotic therapy to prevent stroke.

REFERENCES

1. Roger VL, Go AS, Lloyd-Jones DM, et al. Executive summary: heart disease and stroke statistics–2012 update: a report from the American Heart Association. Circulation 2012;125:188–97.
2. Lloyd-Jones DM, Wang TJ, Leip EP, et al. Lifetime risk for development of atrial fibrillation: the Framingham Heart Study. Circulation 2004;110: 1042–6.
3. Maisel WH, Stevenson LW. Atrial fibrillation in heart failure: epidemiology, pathophysiology, and rationale for therapy. Am J Cardiol 2003;91:8.
4. Rosenberg MA, Manning WJ. Diastolic dysfunction and risk of atrial fibrillation: a mechanistic appraisal. Circulation 2012;126:2353–62.
5. Dries DL, Exner DV, Gersh BJ, et al. Atrial fibrillation is associated with an increased risk for mortality and heart failure progression in patients with asymptomatic and symptomatic left ventricular systolic dysfunction: a retrospective analysis of the SOLVD trials. Studies of Left Ventricular Dysfunction. J Am Coll Cardiol 1998;32:695–703.
6. Pedersen OD, Bagger H, Keller N, et al. Efficacy of dofetilide in the treatment of atrial fibrillation-flutter in patients with reduced left ventricular function: a Danish investigations of arrhythmia and mortality on dofetilide (diamond) substudy. Circulation 2001;104:292–6.
7. Effects of enalapril on mortality in severe congestive heart failure. Results of the Cooperative North Scandinavian Enalapril Survival Study (CONSENSUS). The CONSENSUS Trial Study Group. N Engl J Med 1987;316:1429–35.
8. Daubert JP, Zareba W, Cannom DS, et al. Inappropriate implantable cardioverter-defibrillator shocks in MADIT II: frequency, mechanisms, predictors, and survival impact. J Am Coll Cardiol 2008;51: 1357–65.
9. Poole JE, Johnson GW, Hellkamp AS, et al. Prognostic importance of defibrillator shocks in patients with heart failure. N Engl J Med 2008;359:1009–17.
10. Hagens VE, Crijns HJ, Van Veldhuisen DJ, et al. Rate control versus rhythm control for patients with persistent atrial fibrillation with mild to moderate heart failure: results from the RAte Control versus Electrical cardioversion (RACE) study. Am Heart J 2005;149:1106–11.
11. Bolliger CT, Guckel C, Engel H, et al. Prediction of functional reserves after lung resection: comparison between quantitative computed tomography, scintigraphy, and anatomy. Respiration 2002;69:482–9.
12. Van Gelder IC, Hagens VE, Bosker HA, et al. A comparison of rate control and rhythm control in patients with recurrent persistent atrial fibrillation. N Engl J Med 2002;347:1834–40.
13. Roy D, Talajic M, Nattel S, et al. Rhythm control versus rate control for atrial fibrillation and heart failure. N Engl J Med 2008;358:2667–77.
14. Ganesan AN, Brooks AG, Roberts-Thomson KC, et al. Role of AV nodal ablation in cardiac resynchronization in patients with coexistent atrial fibrillation and heart failure a systematic review. J Am Coll Cardiol 2012;59:719–26.
15. Brignole M, Botto G, Mont L, et al. Cardiac resynchronization therapy in patients undergoing atrioventricular junction ablation for permanent atrial fibrillation: a randomized trial. Eur Heart J 2011;32:2420–9.
16. Dong K, Shen WK, Powell BD, et al. Atrioventricular nodal ablation predicts survival benefit in patients with atrial fibrillation receiving cardiac resynchronization therapy. Heart Rhythm 2010;7:1240–5.
17. Gasparini M, Auricchio A, Metra M, et al. Long-term survival in patients undergoing cardiac resynchronization therapy: the importance of performing atrio-ventricular junction ablation in patients with permanent atrial fibrillation. Eur Heart J 2008;29: 1644–52.
18. Scheinman MA. Reflections on the first catheter ablation of the atrioventricular junction. Pacing Clin Electrophysiol 2003;26:2315–6.
19. Scheinman MM, Morady F, Hess DS, et al. Catheter-induced ablation of the atrioventricular junction to control refractory supraventricular arrhythmias. JAMA 1982;248:851–5.

20. Gallagher JJ, Svenson RH, Kasell JH, et al. Catheter technique for closed-chest ablation of the atrioventricular conduction system. N Engl J Med 1982;306:194–200.
21. Olgin JE, Scheinman MM. Comparison of high energy direct current and radiofrequency catheter ablation of the atrioventricular junction. J Am Coll Cardiol 1993;21:557–64.
22. Chatterjee NA, Upadhyay GA, Ellenbogen KA, et al. Atrioventricular nodal ablation in atrial fibrillation: a meta-analysis and systematic review. Circ Arrhythm Electrophysiol 2012;5:68–76.
23. Sousa J, el-Atassi R, Rosenheck S, et al. Radiofrequency catheter ablation of the atrioventricular junction from the left ventricle. Circulation 1991; 84:567–71.
24. Zhang Y, Mazgalev TN. Atrioventricular node functional remodeling induced by atrial fibrillation. Heart Rhythm 2012;9:1419–25.
25. Williamson BD, Man KC, Daoud E, et al. Radiofrequency catheter modification of atrioventricular conduction to control the ventricular rate during atrial fibrillation. N Engl J Med 1994;331:910–7.
26. Kalaga R, Kahr R, Migeed M, et al. Comparison of single and double vein approaches for His bundle ablation and pacemaker placement for symptomatic rapid atrial fibrillation. J Interv Card Electrophysiol 2009;24:113–7.
27. Shinbane JS, Wood MA, Jensen DN, et al. Tachycardia-induced cardiomyopathy: a review of animal models and clinical studies. J Am Coll Cardiol 1997;29:709–15.
28. Kay GN, Ellenbogen KA, Giudici M, et al. The Ablate and Pace Trial: a prospective study of catheter ablation of the AV conduction system and permanent pacemaker implantation for treatment of atrial fibrillation. APT Investigators. J Interv Card Electrophysiol 1998;2:121–35.
29. Ozcan C, Jahangir A, Friedman PA, et al. Long-term survival after ablation of the atrioventricular node and implantation of a permanent pacemaker in patients with atrial fibrillation. N Engl J Med 2001; 344:1043–51.
30. Wood MA, Brown-Mahoney C, Kay GN, et al. Clinical outcomes after ablation and pacing therapy for atrial fibrillation: a meta-analysis. Circulation 2000; 101:1138–44.
31. Clark DM, Plumb VJ, Epstein AE, et al. Hemodynamic effects of an irregular sequence of ventricular cycle lengths during atrial fibrillation. J Am Coll Cardiol 1997;30:1039–45.
32. Fuster V, Ryden LE, Cannom DS, et al. 2011 ACCF/AHA/HRS focused updates incorporated into the ACC/AHA/ESC 2006 Guidelines for the management of patients with atrial fibrillation: a report of the American College of Cardiology Foundation/American Heart Association Task Force on Practice Guidelines developed in partnership with the European Society of Cardiology and in collaboration with the European Heart Rhythm Association and the Heart Rhythm Society. J Am Coll Cardiol 2011;57:101–98.
33. Wilkoff BL, Cook JR, Epstein AE, et al. Dual-chamber pacing or ventricular backup pacing in patients with an implantable defibrillator: the Dual Chamber and VVI Implantable Defibrillator (DAVID) Trial. JAMA 2002;288:3115–23.
34. Brignole M, Gammage M, Puggioni E, et al. Comparative assessment of right, left, and biventricular pacing in patients with permanent atrial fibrillation. Eur Heart J 2005;26:712–22.
35. Sweeney MO, Ellenbogen KA, Tang AS, et al. Atrial pacing or ventricular backup-only pacing in implantable cardioverter-defibrillator patients. Heart Rhythm 2010;7:1552–60.
36. Barsheshet A, Wang PJ, Moss AJ, et al. Reverse remodeling and the risk of ventricular tachyarrhythmias in the MADIT-CRT (Multicenter Automatic Defibrillator Implantation Trial-Cardiac Resynchronization Therapy). J Am Coll Cardiol 2011;57:2416–23.
37. Bank AJ, Kaufman CL, Burns KV, et al. Intramural dyssynchrony and response to cardiac resynchronization therapy in patients with and without previous right ventricular pacing. Eur J Heart Fail 2010; 12:1317–24.
38. Bank AJ, Schwartzman DS, Burns KV, et al. Intramural dyssynchrony from acute right ventricular apical pacing in human subjects with normal left ventricular function. J Cardiovasc Transl Res 2010;3:321–9.
39. Rubaj A, Rucinski P, Oleszczak K, et al. Inflammatory activation following interruption of long-term cardiac resynchronization therapy. Heart Vessels 2012. http://dx.doi.org/10.1007/s00380-012-0285-y.
40. Fang F, Zhang Q, Chan JY, et al. Deleterious effect of right ventricular apical pacing on left ventricular diastolic function and the impact of pre-existing diastolic disease. Eur Heart J 2011;32:1891–9.
41. Doshi RN, Daoud EG, Fellows C, et al. Left ventricular-based cardiac stimulation post AV nodal ablation evaluation (the PAVE study). J Cardiovasc Electrophysiol 2005;16:1160–5.
42. Chan JY, Fang F, Zhang Q, et al. Biventricular pacing is superior to right ventricular pacing in bradycardia patients with preserved systolic function: 2-year results of the PACE trial. Eur Heart J 2011; 32:2533–40.
43. Tracy CM, Epstein AE, Darbar D, et al. 2012 ACCF/AHA/HRS Focused Update of the 2008 Guidelines for Device-Based Therapy of Cardiac Rhythm Abnormalities: a Report of the American College of Cardiology Foundation/American Heart Association Task Force on Practice Guidelines. J Am Coll Cardiol 2012;60:1297–313.

44. Linderer T, Chatterjee K, Parmley WW, et al. Influence of atrial systole on the Frank-Starling relation and the end-diastolic pressure-diameter relation of the left ventricle. Circulation 1983;67:1045–53.
45. Van Gelder IC, Groenveld HF, Crijns HJ, et al. Lenient versus strict rate control in patients with atrial fibrillation. N Engl J Med 2010;362:1363–73.
46. Torp-Pedersen C, Moller M, Bloch-Thomsen PE, et al. Dofetilide in patients with congestive heart failure and left ventricular dysfunction. Danish Investigations of Arrhythmia and Mortality on Dofetilide Study Group. N Engl J Med 1999;341:857–65.
47. Effect of prophylactic amiodarone on mortality after acute myocardial infarction and in congestive heart failure: meta-analysis of individual data from 6500 patients in randomised trials. Amiodarone Trials Meta-Analysis Investigators. Lancet 1997;350:1417–24.
48. Echt DS, Liebson PR, Mitchell LB, et al. Mortality and morbidity in patients receiving encainide, flecainide, or placebo. The Cardiac Arrhythmia Suppression Trial. N Engl J Med 1991;324:781–8.
49. Waldo AL, Camm AJ, deRuyter H, et al. Effect of d-sotalol on mortality in patients with left ventricular dysfunction after recent and remote myocardial infarction. The SWORD Investigators. Survival With Oral d-Sotalol. Lancet 1996;348:7–12.
50. Kober L, Torp-Pedersen C, McMurray JJ, et al. Increased mortality after dronedarone therapy for severe heart failure. N Engl J Med 2008;358:2678–87.
51. Khan MN, Jais P, Cummings J, et al. Pulmonary-vein isolation for atrial fibrillation in patients with heart failure. N Engl J Med 2008;359:1778–85.
52. Efremidis M, Sideris A, Xydonas S, et al. Ablation of atrial fibrillation in patients with heart failure: reversal of atrial and ventricular remodelling. Hellenic J Cardiol 2008;49:19–25.
53. MacDonald MR, Connelly DT, Hawkins NM, et al. Radiofrequency ablation for persistent atrial fibrillation in patients with advanced heart failure and severe left ventricular systolic dysfunction: a randomised controlled trial. Heart 2011;97:740–7.
54. Dagres N, Varounis C, Gaspar T, et al. Catheter ablation for atrial fibrillation in patients with left ventricular systolic dysfunction. A systematic review and meta-analysis. J Card Fail 2011;17:964–70.
55. Marrouche NF, Brachmann J, CASTLE-AF Steering Committee. Catheter ablation versus standard conventional treatment in patients with left ventricular dysfunction and atrial fibrillation (CASTLE-AF) - study design. Pacing Clin Electrophysiol 2009;32:987–94.
56. Olsson LG, Swedberg K, Ducharme A, et al. Atrial fibrillation and risk of clinical events in chronic heart failure with and without left ventricular systolic dysfunction: results from the Candesartan in Heart failure-Assessment of Reduction in Mortality and morbidity (CHARM) program. J Am Coll Cardio 2006;47:1997–2004.
57. Sarkar S, Koehler J, Crossley GH, et al. Burden o atrial fibrillation and poor rate control detected by continuous monitoring and the risk for heart failure hospitalization. Am Heart J 2012;164:616–24.
58. Fischer A, Ousdigian KT, Johnson JW, et al. The impact of atrial fibrillation with rapid ventricula rates and device programming on shocks ir 106,513 ICD and CRT-D patients. Heart Rhythm 2012;9:24–31.
59. Kleemann T, Hochadel M, Strauss M, et al. Comparison between atrial fibrillation-triggered implantable cardioverter-defibrillator (ICD) shocks and inappropriate shocks caused by lead failure different impact on prognosis in clinical practice J Cardiovasc Electrophysiol 2012;23:735–40.
60. van Rees JB, Borleffs CJ, de Bie MK, et al. Inappropriate implantable cardioverter-defibrillator shocks incidence, predictors, and impact on mortality J Am Coll Cardiol 2011;57:556–62.
61. Saxon LA, Hayes DL, Gilliam FR, et al. Long-term outcome after ICD and CRT implantation and influence of remote device follow-up: the ALTITUDE survival study. Circulation 2010;122:2359–67.
62. Stempniewicz P, Cheng A, Connolly A, et al. Appropriate and inappropriate electrical therapies delivered by an implantable cardioverter-defibrillator effect on intracardiac electrogram. J Cardiovasc Electrophysiol 2011;22:554–60.
63. Powell BD, Asirvatham SJ, Perschbacher DL, et al Noise, Artifact, and Oversensing Related Inappropriate ICD Shock Evaluation: ALTITUDE NOISE Study. Pacing Clin Electrophysiol 2012;35(7) 863–9.
64. Khadjooi K, Foley PW, Chalil S, et al. Long-term effects of cardiac resynchronisation therapy in patients with atrial fibrillation. Heart 2008;94:879–83.
65. Gasparini M, Auricchio A, Regoli F, et al. Four-yea efficacy of cardiac resynchronization therapy on exercise tolerance and disease progression: the importance of performing atrioventricular junction ablation in patients with atrial fibrillation. J Am Coll Cardiol 2006;48:734–43.
66. Hoppe UC, Casares JM, Eiskjaer H, et al. Effect o cardiac resynchronization on the incidence of atria fibrillation in patients with severe heart failure. Circulation 2006;114:18–25.
67. Hayes DL, Boehmer JP, Day JD, et al. Cardiac resynchronization therapy and the relationship o percent biventricular pacing to symptoms and survival. Heart Rhythm 2011;8:1469–75.
68. Gasparini M, Cappelleri A. Atrial arrhythmias afte cardiac resynchronization therapy: an inverse correlation with achieving 100% biventricular pacing and cardiac resynchronization therapy effectiveness. Europace 2010;12:9–10.

69. Gasparini M, Steinberg JS, Arshad A, et al. Resumption of sinus rhythm in patients with heart failure and permanent atrial fibrillation undergoing cardiac resynchronization therapy: a longitudinal observational study. Eur Heart J 2010;31: 976–83.
70. Kamath GS, Cotiga D, Koneru JN, et al. The utility of 12-lead Holter monitoring in patients with permanent atrial fibrillation for the identification of nonresponders after cardiac resynchronization therapy. J Am Coll Cardiol 2009;53:1050–5.
71. Upadhyay GA, Choudhry NK, Auricchio A, et al. Cardiac resynchronization in patients with atrial fibrillation: a meta-analysis of prospective cohort studies. J Am Coll Cardiol 2008;52:1239–46.
72. Hoffmayer KS, Scheinman M. Current role of atrioventricular junction (AVJ) ablation. Pacing Clin Electrophysiol 2013;36:257–65.
73. Scheinman MM, Huang S. The 1998 NASPE prospective catheter ablation registry. Pacing Clin Electrophysiol 2000;23:1020–8.
74. Brandt RR, Shen WK. Bradycardia-induced polymorphic ventricular tachycardia after atrioventricular junction ablation for sinus tachycardia-induced cardiomyopathy. J Cardiovasc Electrophysiol 1995; 6:630–3.
75. Geelen P, Brugada J, Andries E, et al. Ventricular fibrillation and sudden death after radiofrequency catheter ablation of the atrioventricular junction. Pacing Clin Electrophysiol 1997;20:343–8.
76. Sharma AK, Chander R, Singh JP. AV nodal ablation-induced Gerbode defect (LV-RA Shunt). J Cardiovasc Electrophysiol 2011;22:1288–9.
77. Can I, Krueger K, Chandrashekar Y, et al. Images in cardiovascular medicine. Gerbode-type defect induced by catheter ablation of the atrioventricular node. Circulation 2009;119:553–6.
78. Hamdan MH, Freedman RA, Gilbert EM, et al. Atrioventricular junction ablation followed by resynchronization therapy in patients with congestive heart failure and atrial fibrillation (AVERT-AF) study design. Pacing Clin Electrophysiol 2006;29:1081–8.

Ablation of Atrial Tachycardia and Atrial Flutter in Heart Failure

Ayotunde Bamimore, MB, ChB,
Paul Mounsey, BSc, BM BCh, PhD, MRCP*

KEYWORDS

• Tachyarrhythmia • Heart failure • Atrial flutter • Atrial tachycardia • Ablation

KEY POINTS

- Atrial tachycardia (AT) and atrial flutter (AFL) are common tachyarrhythmias in the heart failure population.
- They commonly lead to, exacerbate, and increase the morbidity and mortality associated with heart failure and, thereby, warrant urgent and early definitive therapy in the form of catheter ablation.
- Catheter ablation requires careful patient stabilization and extensive preprocedural planning, particularly with regards to anesthesia, strategy, catheter choice, mapping system, and fluid balance, to increase efficacy and limit adverse effects.
- Heart failure may limit the success of catheter ablation with higher reported recurrence rates and, in selected patients, a hybrid epicardial-endocardial ablation can be considered.

Atrial tachyarrhythmias are common in patients with heart failure and vice versa.[1] Several publications highlight the development of heart failure in patients with poorly controlled atrial tachyarrhythmias as well as the development of atrial arrhythmias in heart failure patients previously known to be in sinus rhythm. The structural, electrophysiologic, and neuroendocrine changes that occur in one facilitate the development of the other, thereby setting up a vicious cycle, such that atrial tachyarrhythmias beget heart failure and heart failure begets atrial tachyarrhythmias. This statement, however true, is an oversimplification of a complex relationship.

Atrial tachyarrhythmias are those tachycardias that are initiated or sustained by the atria and do not require the atrioventricular (AV) node or ventricles for perpetuation. They may be regular or irregular. The irregular atrial arrhythmias are atrial fibrillation (AF) and multifocal AT whereas regular atrial tachyarrhythmias were previously classified as AT and AFL. This outdated classification of regular atrial tachyarrhythmias was based on heart rate and ECG morphology, such that tachycardias with atrial rates equal to or greater than 240 beats per minute (bpm), with an undulating baseline lacking an isoelectric baseline in at least one lead (saw tooth), were classified as AFL and the others lacking these 2 characteristics as AT. Contemporary electrophysiology studies (EPSs) and improvement in mapping techniques have led to a more precise classification based on pathophysiologic mechanisms.[2]

Regular atrial arrhythmias are now classified as

1. Focal ATs (formerly ATs), which have the following characteristics
   - Origin outside the sinus node and from a discrete portion of the atrium (<2 cm^2)

Disclosures: The authors have nothing to disclose.

Division of Cardiology, University of North Carolina, Chapel Hill, 160 Dental Circle, Burnett-Womack Building, CB #7075, Chapel Hill, NC 27599, USA
* Corresponding author.
E-mail address: Paul_mounsey@med.unc.edu

Heart Failure Clin 9 (2013) 501–514
http://dx.doi.org/10.1016/j.hfc.2013.07.002

heartfailure.theclinics.com

- Centrifugal spread of activation from the discrete portion
- Mechanism automatic, triggered activity, or microreentry
- Propagation occurring over a short duration of the cycle length (**Fig. 1**)
- Rate above 100 bpm but less than 240 bpm
- Warming up and cooling down properties

2. Macroreentrant AT (formerly AFL), with the following characteristics
   - Mechanism is macroreentry involving a large portion of the atrium
   - Propagation occurring around an area of fixed or functional barrier
   - Propagation occurring over most of the duration of the cycle length (**Fig. 2**)

For the remainder of this review, AT refers to focal AT and AFL refers to macroreentrant AT, based on the newer classification. This distinction is not often made in publications. Sometimes the new classifications are implied and knowledge of this by readers is assumed, whereas in other instances, writers use the old classification. Some studies group AT and AFL together as ATs, distinguishing them from AF. Further complicating the scenario is that a patient may exhibit each of these various tachyarrhythmias at different times. This confusion in terminologies makes the exact prevalence of AT and AFL in the general population, let alone in heart failure patients, uncertain. Although there is a robust amount of literature on AF (often including AFL) in the general population and in heart failure patients, studies on AT and AFL are sparse. Few studies have made efforts to separate these various atrial arrhythmias and, from this limited information, the following is known. The prevalence of AT has been reported to be 0.34% in an asymptomatic population, rising to 0.46% in a population with symptoms,[3] whereas the prevalence of AFL is largely speculative. The incidence of AFL is, however, reported to be approximately 0.07% in the United States, amounting to 200,000 new cases per year, among which 80,000 patients are diagnosed with AFL only (without AF).[4] These numbers are overshadowed by those of AF, which has a prevalence of 2.2 million in the United States (0.7%–1% of the population) and an incidence that stands at 0.1%.[5] Generally, in cardiac disease states, the

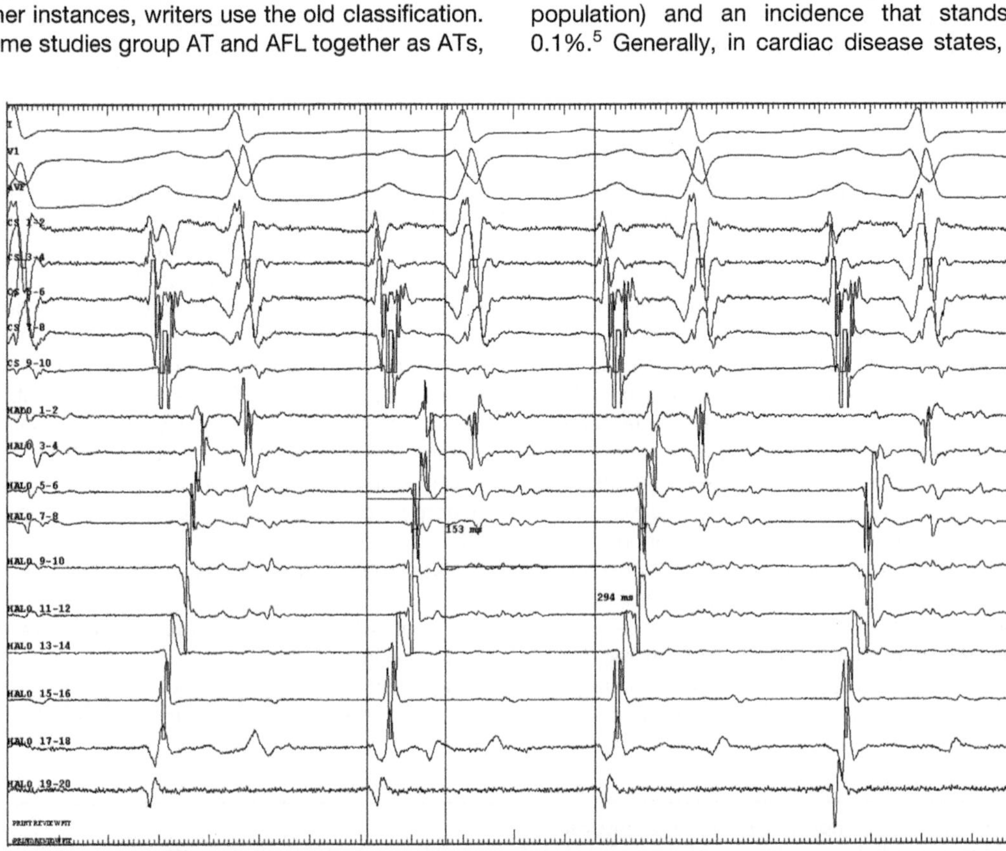

Fig. 1. Surface and intracardiac electrograms at 200 mm/s paper speed, showing a focal AT with a cycle length of 447 ms (153 + 294), which is 134 bpm. Surface leads I, VI, and aVF are shown as well as coronary sinus (CS) leads and Halo catheter leads spanning the crista terminalis in the right atrium. The duration of endocardial activation across large regions of the right atrium (Halo electrodes) and representing the left atrium (CS) is 153 ms, which is only 34% of the entire tachycardia cycle length and is depicted by the first caliper.

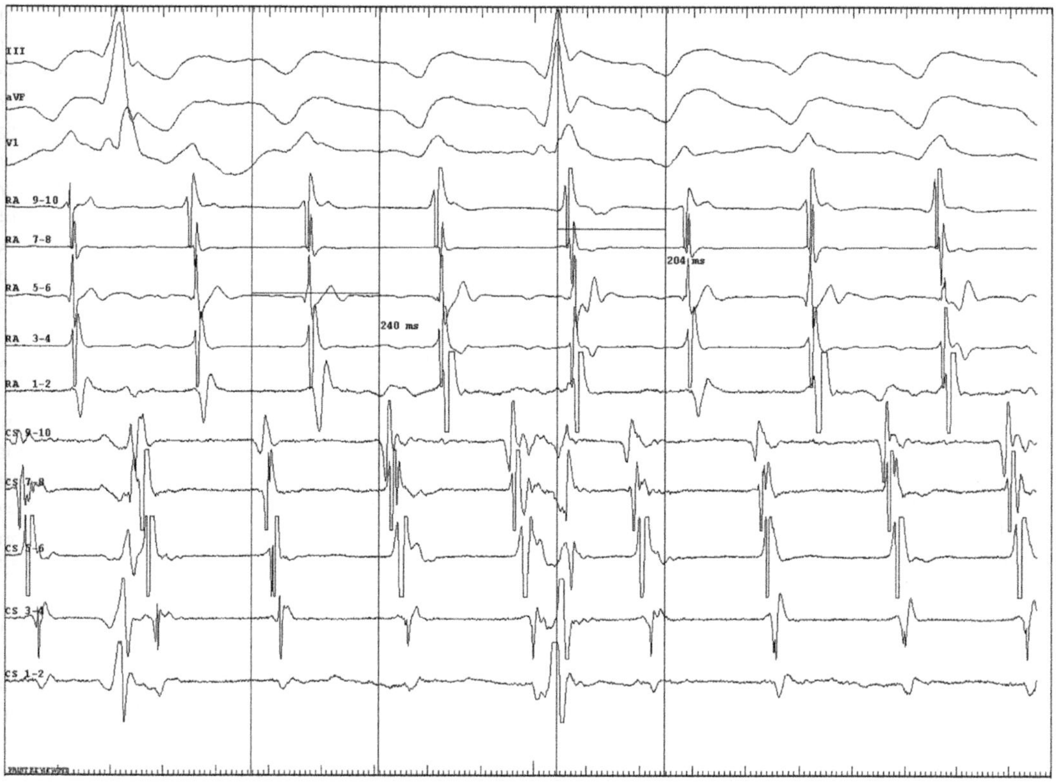

Fig. 2. Surface and intracardiac electrograms at 200 mm/s paper speed, showing macroreentry in the right atrium (typical AFL), with a cycle length of 240 ms (first set of calipers), which is 250 bpm with a 3:1 AV block. Intracardiac leads consist of a 20-pole catheter that has its proximal 10 electrodes (RA 1–2 to RA 9–10) along the right atrium lateral wall and the distal 10 (CS 1–2 to 9–10) in the coronary sinus. Endocardial activation spans a large portion of the entire tachycardia cycle, and its duration depicted by the second caliper is 204 ms, which is 85% of the entire tachycardia cycle length.

prevalence of these arrhythmias increases as corroborated by a study of 917 patients post–acute myocardial infarction, of whom 7% had AF, 3% had AFL, and 3.6% had AT.[6] In heart failure, which may represent a final common pathway for many cardiac conditions, the prevalence of AF is reported to be between 20% and 50% (depending on New York Heart Association class)[7,8] and, although the exact prevalence of AFL and AT are not as well known, their numbers most likely increase as the prevalence of AF increases.

WHY ARE AT AND AFL MORE PREVALENT IN HEART FAILURE PATIENTS?

First, the risk factors for atrial arrhythmias are the same as those for heart failure, so these conditions afflict the same patients. These risk factors include advanced age, hypertension, diabetes, obesity, and cigarette smoking.[4,8,9] In addition, some of the structural changes in the atria of heart failure patients are shared by those with atrial arrhythmias. Wyndham and colleagues[10] excised tissue samples from the culprit AT focus in a patient, and histology revealed markedly increased levels of mononuclear infiltrates and connective tissue. Josephson and colleagues[11] also demonstrated an increase in wall thickness, endocardial thickness, and inflammatory cells as well as increased mesenchymal cells. In addition, they noted multicomponent atrial electrograms around the foci of atrial tachyarrhythmias depicting slow and asynchronous conduction similar to that seen in diseased ventricles in ventricular tachycardia studies. Similar findings are seen in the atria of patients with heart failure and are attributable to myocardial stretch from pressure and volume changes. In essence, the structural and neuroendocrine alterations in heart failure probably facilitate the development of atrial tachyarrhythmias by complex and interrelated mechanisms (discussed in articles elsewhere in this issue).

WHAT ARE THE EFFECTS OF AT AND AFL ON HEART FAILURE?

Tachyarrhythmias with uncontrolled ventricular response can be the sole cause of heart failure in patients with no other risk factors. The first reported case of suspected tachycardia-mediated cardiomyopathy (TCM) was by Gossage and Hicks in 1913[12] and, since then, animal models of chronic atrial pacing mimicking AT have confirmed the predictable development of reversible heart failure.[13]

Given the aforementioned observations, AT and AFL may, therefore, be either the cause or consequence of heart failure, thereby evoking uncertainty and confusion in the management of new patients with both disorders. This scenario may require aggressive treatment of the arrhythmia and subsequent observation for a few months before it can be determined whether a patient has TCM or heart failure due to another cause with concurrent tachyarrhythmia. Sometimes the left ventricle end diastolic dimension may help distinguish between the two, with left ventricular dimension less than or equal to 6.1 cm being 100% sensitive for TCM and 71.4% specific in a patient presenting with heart failure and an apparently new tachyarrhythmia.[14]

Uncertainty and confusion may also be found in scenarios in which heart failure coexists with AT originating from sites close to the sinoatrial node having a positive P-wave axis on ECG leads II, III, and aVF, giving the initial impression of sinus tachycardia secondary to heart failure.[15] It may take several days to weeks of Holter monitoring of the pattern of tachycardia to make the distinction. Patterns of sudden dips in the heart rate to a new lower baseline alternating with sudden jumps to the higher baseline heart rate may be the first clue that the diagnosis is AT rather than sinus tachycardia, which shows more gradual diurnal fluctuations. EPS may be required in difficult cases.

AT and AFL are common causes of heart failure exacerbation and hospitalization. In patients with preexisting heart failure, they may result in further deterioration in ejection fraction, pushing patients with mild systolic dysfunction to severe dysfunction. This worsening in ejection fraction affects the prognosis and could, for example, be of importance in determining whether a patient requires prophylactic implantable cardioverter defibrillator (ICD) therapy.[8]

Uncontrolled ventricular rates in patients with atrial tachyarrhythmias may increase the likelihood of other morbidities, like myocardial infarction, in patients with ischemic cardiomyopathy or unnecessary ICD firing, with its attendant increased mortality.[16] These arrhythmias have often influenced the choice of ICD type in heart failure patients (single ventricular chamber vs dual, atrial, and ventricular chambers) to facilitate supraventricular tachycardia discrimination.[17,18] In patients with cardiac resynchronization therapy, conducted ventricular beats due to AT and AFL reduce biventricular pacing that may reduce its benefit or cause deterioration in patients with prior response.[19] If the percentage of biventricular pacing suddenly drops in-between evaluations, atrial tachyarrhythmias should be sought and it may be prudent to set up a lower detection or monitor-only zone to pick these up. In addition to these comorbidities, the presence of AT and AF in heart failure patients admitted for myocardial infarction portends an almost 2-fold increase in 30-day mortality, more so if the ejection fraction is between 25% and 35%.[20] Lastly, the onset of AT and AFL may be the first indicator of development of hyperthyroidism, pulmonary embolism, or even progression of the underlying myocardial disease.

In addition to the direct effects of AT and AFL on heart failure, there are several indirect effects. AT and AFL complicate the treatment of heart failure patients by typically making them require higher doses of nodal blocking agents, possibly with associated hypotension, by increasing the need for digoxin, anticoagulation, and antiarrhythmic agents along with their attendant risks.

WHAT IMPACT DOES HEART FAILURE HAVE ON THE MANAGEMENT OF AT AND AFL?

The structural and neurohormonal changes in heart failure facilitate the development of AT and AFL, which in turn leads to further adverse remodeling, which in turn predisposes patients to more atrial tachyarrhythmias, thereby setting up a vicious cycle. By so doing, heart failure encourages the development of new atrial tachyarrhythmias while increasing the burden of preexisting AT and AFL and encouraging recurrence.

The presence of heart failure also influences the treatment strategy of atrial tachyarrhythmias. Restoration of sinus rhythm is highly likely to be attempted given that AT and AFL can precipitate and perpetuate acute decompensation and hospitalizations. In heart failure exacerbations, the authors are inclined to promptly cardiovert patients rather than use nodal blocking agents. Cardioversion is useful in AFL but has limited success in AT. If deciding on a conservative strategy of using AV nodal blocking agents, choices are limited to β-blockers and digoxin. Nondihydropyridine calcium channel blockers, commonly used in the general population, are negatively inotropic and, therefore, contraindicated in most patients with systolic dysfunction. Given the high cathecholaminergic state of heart failure decompensation, digoxin is less desirable given its potential morbidity and mortality[21] and reduced efficacy.[22]

Also, because of the high catecholaminergic state of heart failure, higher than usual doses of β- blockers may be needed—a challenge in a population that may already have low blood pressure from multiple drugs and may not be able to tolerate higher doses of β-blockers or may only be able to tolerate them at the cost of reducing or discontinuing other medications, like angiotensin-converting enzyme inhibitors. Not all acutely decompensated patients, however, may immediately be given β-blockers because of pulmonary edema and the risk of initial worsening.[8] Having considered all these factors, a combination of digoxin and β-blockers is often needed.[23]

Lastly, a conservative approach in treating AT and AFL in heart failure patients is more likely to require antiarrhythmic medication, and there are essentially 2 choices with good safety profile in heart failure: amiodarone[24] and dofetilide.[25] This limitation is because commonly prescribed antiarrhythmic class IC agents[26] and sotalol[27] are absolutely and relatively contraindicated in heart failure, respectively. Dronedarone, another widely used drug in the general population, caused new heart failure and death in patients with chronic atrial arrhythmias or decompensated heart failure, so its use is limited in patients with preexisting heart failure.[28]

Multiple challenges, therefore, exist to a pharmacologic therapy of AT and AFL in heart failure.

CONSIDERATIONS FOR THE ABLATION OF AT AND AFL IN HEART FAILURE PATIENTS

There is a need for definitive therapy for AT and AFL in heart failure patients, particularly given the high efficacy of catheter ablation in the general population, with 85% to 90% success in AT and 90% to 93% in AFL.[29–31] Moreover, approximately 10% of patients with atrial tachyarrhythmias in heart failure, after elimination of the arrhythmia, may be essentially cured of heart failure, leading to a retrospective diagnosis of tachycardia-related cardiomyopathy.[15] In essence, heart failure adds an urgency to the treatment of AT and AFL as well as the need for early consideration of definitive therapy.

A caveat to ablation is that its potential complications may be higher in this population, with more comorbidities, impacts of polypharmacy, propensity for renal insufficiency, drug-drug interactions, and other factors. These factors require meticulous preprocedural planning in patients with heart failure, who may initially be too sick for the procedure. Under these circumstances, cardioversion may be a useful temporizing measure. Besides influencing the timing of procedure, the presence of heart failure has an impact on periablation management. Ablation of complex left-sided AT and AFL may last for several hours, a serious challenge in those with preexisting orthopnea and paroxysmal nocturnal dyspnea. This may require preprocedural aggressive diuresis sometimes at the cost of an acceptable temporary worsening of renal function. When this is inadequate, an early evaluation by anesthesia staff may be helpful in planning the procedure.

Other considerations include the presence of ICD and cardiac resynchronization therapy devices in an increasing proportion of heart failure patients, introducing the risk of lead dislodgement. This may inform the choice of diagnostic catheters and the choice of electroanatomic mapping systems. For example, a bulky catheter, like a Halo catheter, which encircles the tricuspid annulus, may not be elected to be used a patients with multiple leads, or a decision may be made to avoid inserting a diagnostic catheter into the coronary sinus of patients with left ventricular leads. Because coronary sinus activation is often used as an intracardiac timing reference, its unavailability requires an alternative reference site or even technology.

The presence of heart failure may also influence the choice of ablation catheters, especially with regards to open irrigation catheters, which add to the periprocedural fluid input. This additional fluid load should carefully assessed so that intraprocedure or postprocedure additional diuretics may be given as needed.

Once these scenarios and the peculiarities of AT and AFL in heart failure patients have been addressed, there should be few differences between ablation of these arrhythmias in patients with heart failure compared with those without.

ABLATION OF AT

Success in the ablation of AT depends on an understanding of the arrhythmia mechanism. ATs have been localized to several predictable areas of the atria and surrounding structures with the following frequencies (**Table 1**).[32]

Rarely, ATs have also been localized to the noncoronary aortic cusp,[33] superior vena cava (SVC),[34] or the ligament of Marshall.[35] These AT foci are typically 2 cm^2 or less in area, and the aim of catheter ablation is to identify the site of

Table 1
Distribution of the anatomic locations of foci of atrial tachycardias in both atria

Right Atrium	Distribution
Crista terminalis	31%
Tricuspid annulus	22%
Perinodal tissue	11%
Coronary sinus os	8%
Interatrial septum	<1%
Right atrial appendage	<1%
Total	73%
Left Atrium	**Distribution**
Pulmonary veins	19%
Superior mitral annulus	4%
Coronary sinus body	2%
Interatrial septum	<1%
Left atrial appendage	<1%
Roof	<1%
Total	27%

earliest atrial activation, apply radiofrequency energy, and eliminate them.

Localizing Atrial Tachycardias

The surface P-wave morphology of the AT may be helpful in predicting the site of origin and hence help in planning the procedure using algorithms that have been developed. **Fig. 3** shows an adapted and simplified algorithm that partially summarizes the elegant work of Kalman and colleagues.[32]

There are exceptions to the rule and that most algorithms are developed in patients with clear isoelectric baselines, resulting in undistorted P waves and mostly normal hearts, so extrapolation to patients with structural abnormalities with distortion from chamber enlargement may render ECG prediction less reliable.

Induction and Mapping of ATs

Mapping of a focal AT entails recording electrograms from various parts of the atrial endocardium, with the aim of localizing the earliest point of activation, which is consistent with the point of origin. This point usually precedes the surface P wave by 38 $\pm$ 7 ms in duration.[36]

At the time of EPS, if tachycardia is not present, then it may have to be induced by pacing rapidly in the atrium (burst pacing) or programmed extra stimuli. Isoproterenol or other sympathomimetic agents may need to be given in addition to these protocols to induce tachycardia. Antiarrhythmic agents should be discontinued at least 5 half-lives before EPS when possible and limiting sedation as much as possible may also facilitate tachycardia initiation.

Multielectrode diagnostic catheters are placed in the heart, which can simultaneously record signals from different regions of the heart to give a general idea of the activation sequence. For example, a 20-electrode catheter (Halo) can be wrapped along the lateral wall of the right atrium partly overlapping the crista terminalis. Propagation along this Halo catheter enables determining if the lateral wall is activated before the septum or determining if the activation sequence proceeds from a superior to inferior direction or vice versa. A catheter with between 4 and 10 electrodes is usually placed in the coronary sinus, which interrogates the proximal portion of the os all the way to the area around the mitral annulus on the left side. Coronary sinus propagation enables determining if AT activation is from left atrium to right atrium or vice versa. Once the chamber of origin of the tachycardia is known, a roving catheter can then be used to interrogate the area of interest in detail until the earliest point of activation is found. This area of earliest activation may also demonstrate low and multicomponent voltage indicative of an abnormal focus. Radiofrequency ablation (RFA) is applied at a power of 30 W to 50 W for approximately 30 to 60 seconds. Termination of tachycardia and an inability to reinitiate it approximately 30 minutes after the last RFA application is a good indicator of success.

Other forms of mapping include 3-D electroanatomic mapping (**Fig. 4**), which involves reconstruction of the shell of the atria on which the activation sequence of the tachycardia is superimposed to identify and target the area of earliest activation for RFA.[37]

Finally, if the tachycardia cannot be reproduced in an electrophysiology laboratory in a patient with previously documented AT, the ECG can be used to initially predict the area of origin and then a roving catheter can be moved around the large initial area of interest with intermittent atrial pacing until P-wave morphologies similar to that of the clinical tachycardia (pace mapping) are reproduced. This area is then targeted for ablation.[38]

ABLATION OF ATRIAL FLUTTER

Ablation of macroreentrant atrial tachyarrhythmia differs from AT in that there is no discrete focus to be identified and targeted for RFA but rather a critical isthmus that permits sustenance of the tachycardia, which can be interrupted with a line of RFA lesions. Ablation of AFL is thus targeted to the precise circuit along which the wave front o

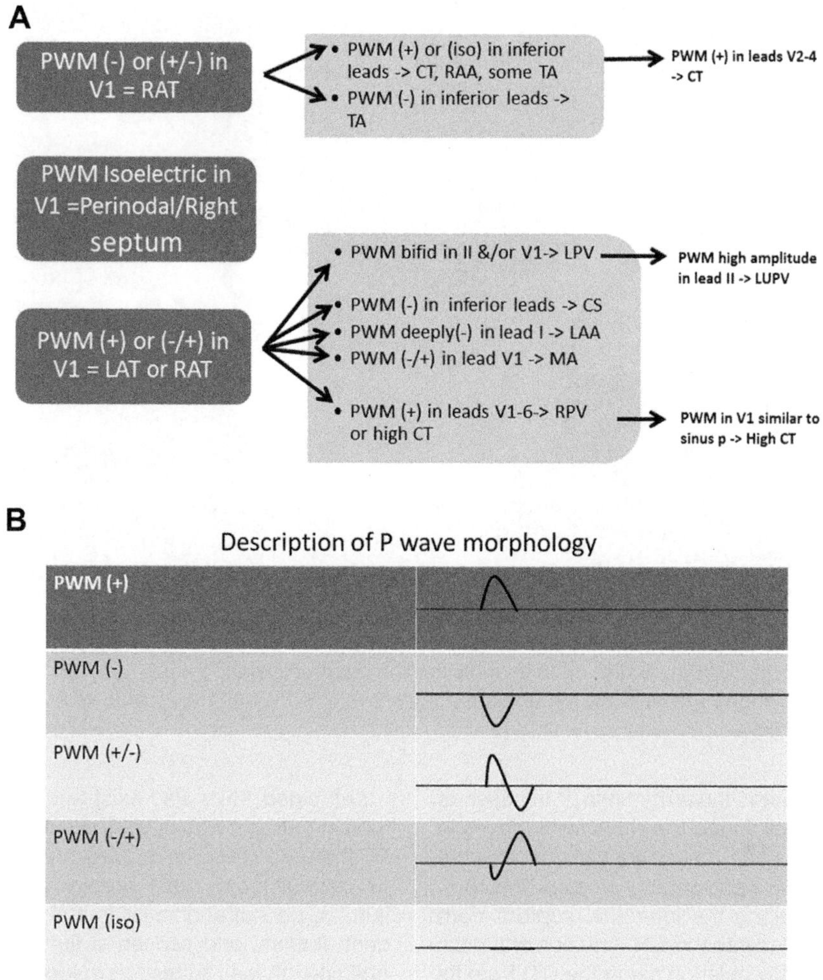

Fig. 3. (*A*) A modified and simplified algorithm showing how ECG P-wave morphology (PWM) can be used to predict the anatomic site of origin of ATs. This partially summarizes the work of Kistler and colleagues.[32] (*B*) A table with visual representation of different P-wave morphologies. CT, Crista terminalis; LAT, left atrial tachycardia; LUPV, left upper pulmonary vein; MA, Mitral annulus; RAA, right atrial appendage; RAT, right atrial tachycardia; RPV, right pulmonary vein.

the tachycardia conducts (**Figs. 5–7**). The boundaries of such circuits are typically formed by regions of functional or anatomic conduction block. Multiple circuits have been described in the right and left atria, with the most common in the right atrium and responsible for the initiation of typical AFL. AFLs are classified into the following[2]:

1. Counterclockwise cavotricuspid isthmus (CTI)–dependent right AFL (typical flutter)
2. Clockwise CTI–dependent right AFL (reverse typical flutter)
3. Lesion macroreentrant AT (scar-related AFL)
4. Left atrial macroreentrant tachycardia (left AFL)

The circuit along which typical flutter travels involves the crista terminalis as it runs along the lateral wall of the right atrium, extending from the SVC superiorly to the inferior vena cava (IVC) inferiorly. Its continuation inferiorly blends with the anterior lip of the IVC and the eustachian ridge, which extends medially from the IVC toward the interatrial septum, all forming a single continuous unit that in turn forms the posterior limit of what is known as the CTI. The anterior limit of the CTI is the annulus of the tricuspid valve. The wave front of typical flutter ascends in a counterclockwise fashion caudocranially along the interatrial septum to the roof of the right atrium and courses anterior to the crista terminalis to descend along the right atrial lateral wall. Its path is then funneled into the CTI, which is the narrowest portion of the circuit and is also the area of slow conduction that permits the wavelength of the arrhythmia to fit into the fixed circuit and still have an excitable

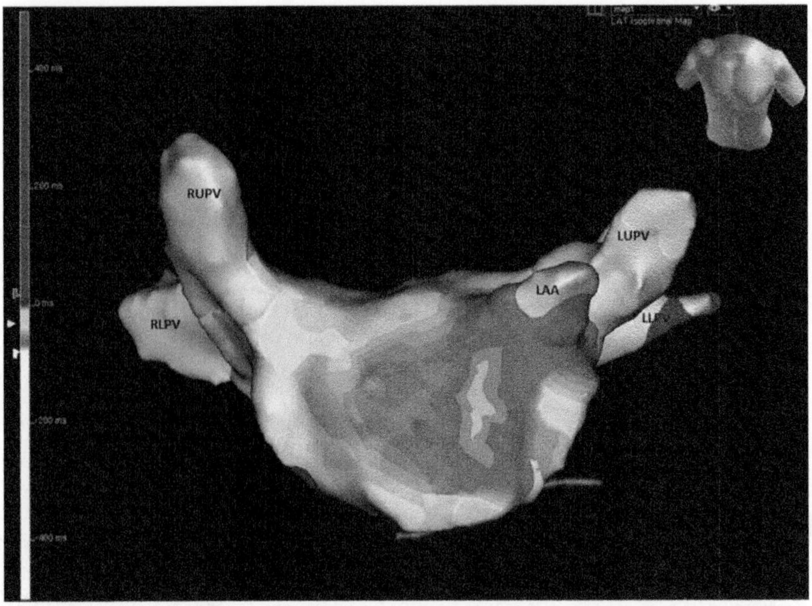

Fig. 4. Electroanatomic map of the left atrium showing the activation pattern of a left AT with a radial spread from the anterior wall of the atrium. Point of earliest activation is the white spot followed by the region in red, then orange, then yellow, and so on. Blue indicates the latest activated regions. LAA, left atrial appendage; LLPV, left lower pulmonary vein; LUPV, left upper pulmonary vein; RLPV, right lower pulmonary vein; RUPV, right upper pulmonary vein.

gap that perpetuates the arrhythmia.[39] In cases of the reverse typical flutter, the wave front moves in a clockwise fashion caudocranially along the lateral wall of the right atrium, crosses the roof, and descends along the interatrial septum from where it is funneled into the CTI. Ablation of typical flutter is essentially ablation along the CTI from its anterior to its posterior limit[40] with the aim of creation of a line of bidirectional block.[41]

Lesion macroreentrant atrial tachyarrhythmias are those with circuits around anatomic scars in the atrium. Commonly these scars are from atriotomies, septal patches for ASD repairs, suture lines, and scar formed by previous ablation. In these scenarios, the goal of EPS is to identify the circuit, delineate the narrowest portion, and then attempt to create a line of RFA lesions along this narrow isthmus in such a way that one connects at both ends to nonconducting structures. For example, a line of RFA lesions may be created from the anatomic line of scar to the SVC, the IVC, or the tricuspid annulus.

Several other described flutters include a lower loop reentry flutter, which rotates around the IVC, traversing the CTI anteriorly and the low posterior right atrium posteriorly. This is a variant of typical flutter and can be ablated along the CTI. An upper loop reentry flutter rotates around the SVC. Mixed variants (double loop or figure of 8) are essentially a combination.[2]

Left-sided AFLs also exist and these are common in patients who have had catheter or surgical AF therapy. These have been arbitrarily classified as peripulmonary vein reentry (roof-dependent) flutters, perimitral annular (mitral isthmus–dependent) flutters, and periseptal flutters (see **Fig. 7**). Ablating these flutters requires mapping and applying RFA lesions along narrowest and/or most accessible portion of the circuit.[42]

ALTERNATIVES TO ABLATION OF AT/AFL: ABLATION OF THE AV NODE

"Ablate and pace" is an old strategy that involved AV nodal ablation with implantation of a dual-chamber permanent pacemaker and was reserved for patients refractory to all medications. It produced excellent relief of symptoms[43] but has been largely overtaken by the advent of catheter ablation. In the current state of electrophysiology, few patients who are intolerant of or allergic to multiple medications and also not amenable to catheter ablation may qualify for it. With increasing knowledge of the deleterious effects of chronic right ventricular pacing, however, particularly in patients with cardiomyopathies,[44] biventricular pacemaker implantation has become the preferred mode because it prevents worsening of heart failure and reduces hospitalization.[45]

A

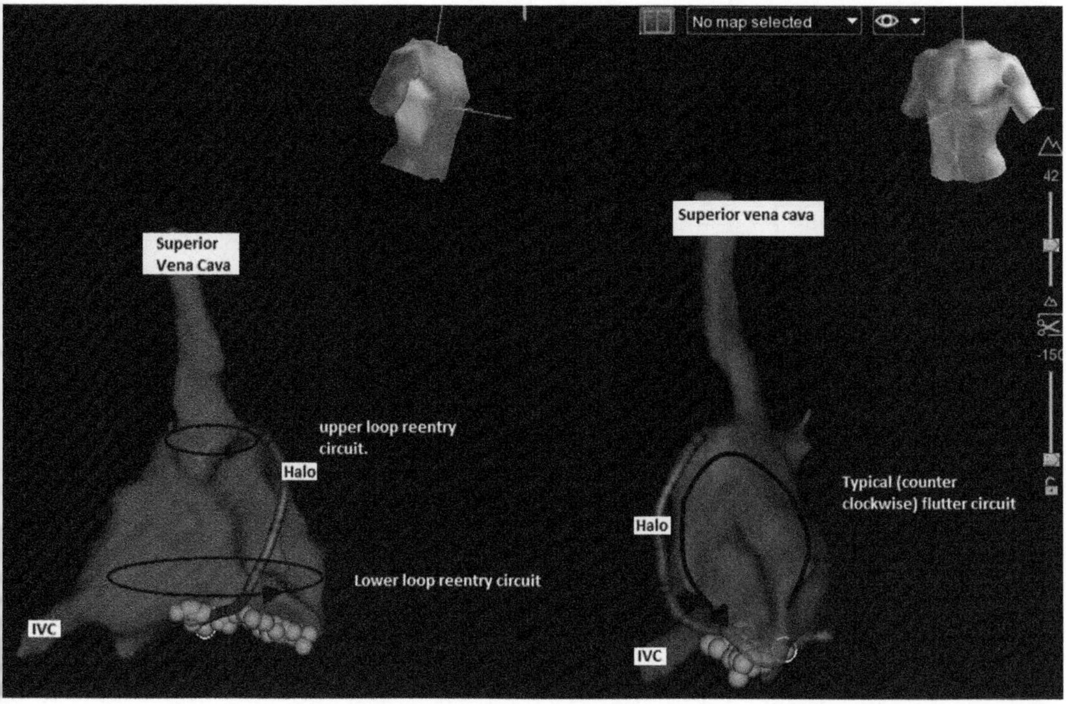

B

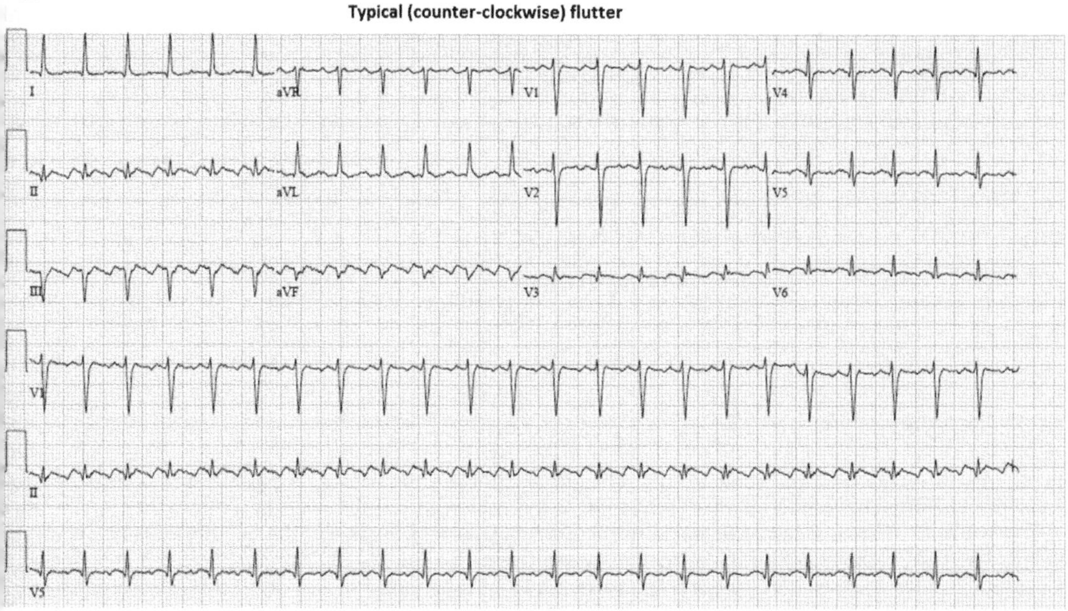

'ig. 5. (*A*) Electroanatomic map of the right atrium showing the activation pattern of a typical counterclockwise lutter circuit, an upper loop reentry, and a lower loop reentry flutter circuit. The reverse typical flutter runs clock-vise instead of counterclockwise along the same circuit. The blue spheres represent RFA lesions created along the CTI. Halo, Halo catheter hugging crista terminalis. (*B*) Surface ECG of a patient showing typical counterclockwise CTI-dependent) flutter.

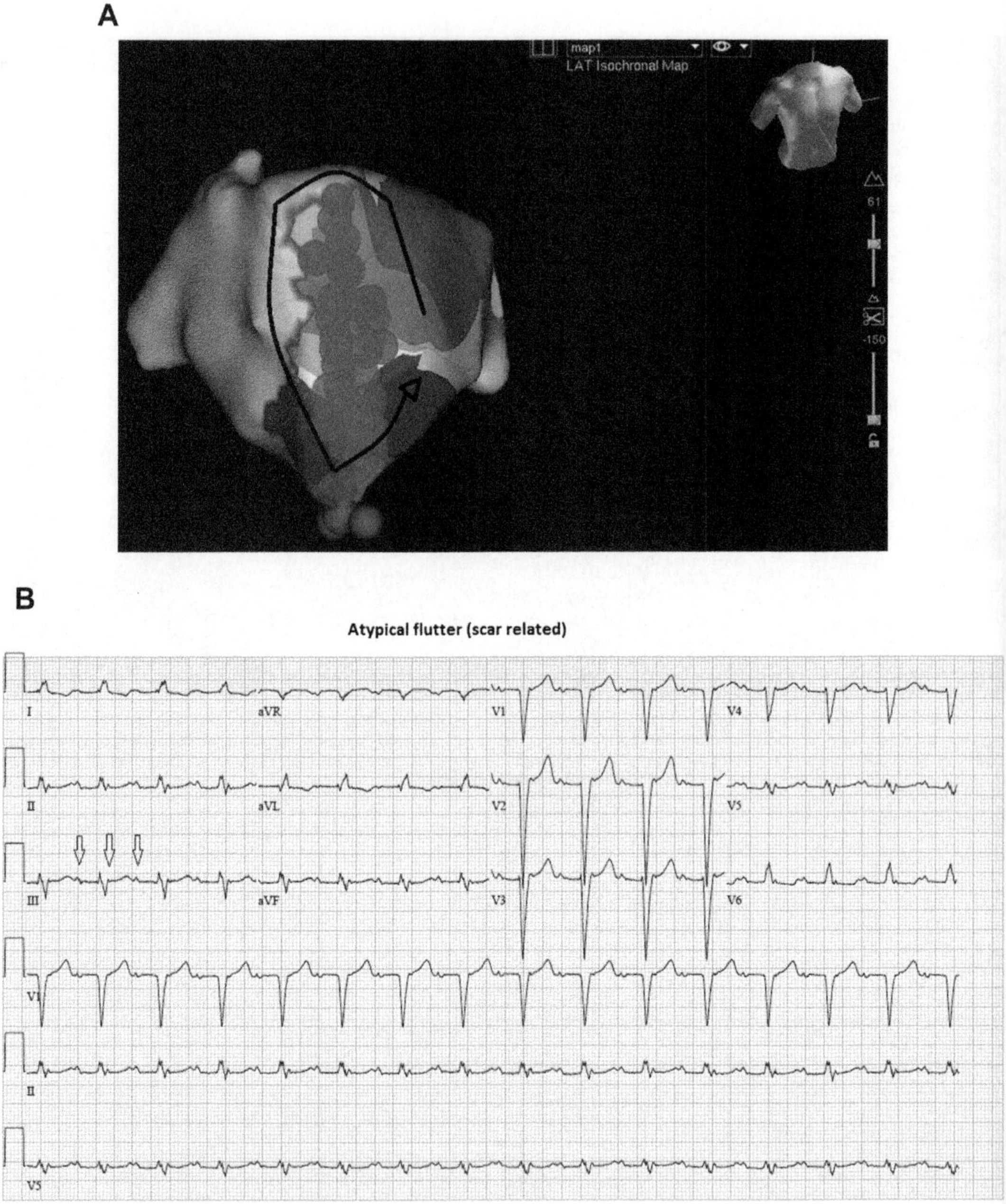

Fig. 6. (*A*) Electroanatomic mapping of the right atrium showing the activation pattern of a scar-related AFL along the lateral wall. Point of earliest activation is the region in red followed by yellow, then green, then blue, and purple. There is a gap of excitable tissue (*gray*) between the head and the tail of the arrow, indicating the head and tail, respectively, of the arrhythmia wave front. The line of red dots represents the area of scar in this instance made by prior RFA lesions. (*B*) A surface ECG of a patient showing atypical flutter secondary to a right atriotomy scar. The arrows point to positive flutter waves in lead III.

WHEN AFL IS REALLY AF

In patients with atypical AFL, in particular arising from the left atrium after a prior AF ablation, mapping not uncommonly reveals a much disorganized rhythm, which is actually AF rather than AFL. Redo AF ablation may be scheduled in such patients with the understanding that the success of catheter ablation in heart failure patients with recurrent persistent AF is at best modest. More extensive ablation is usually

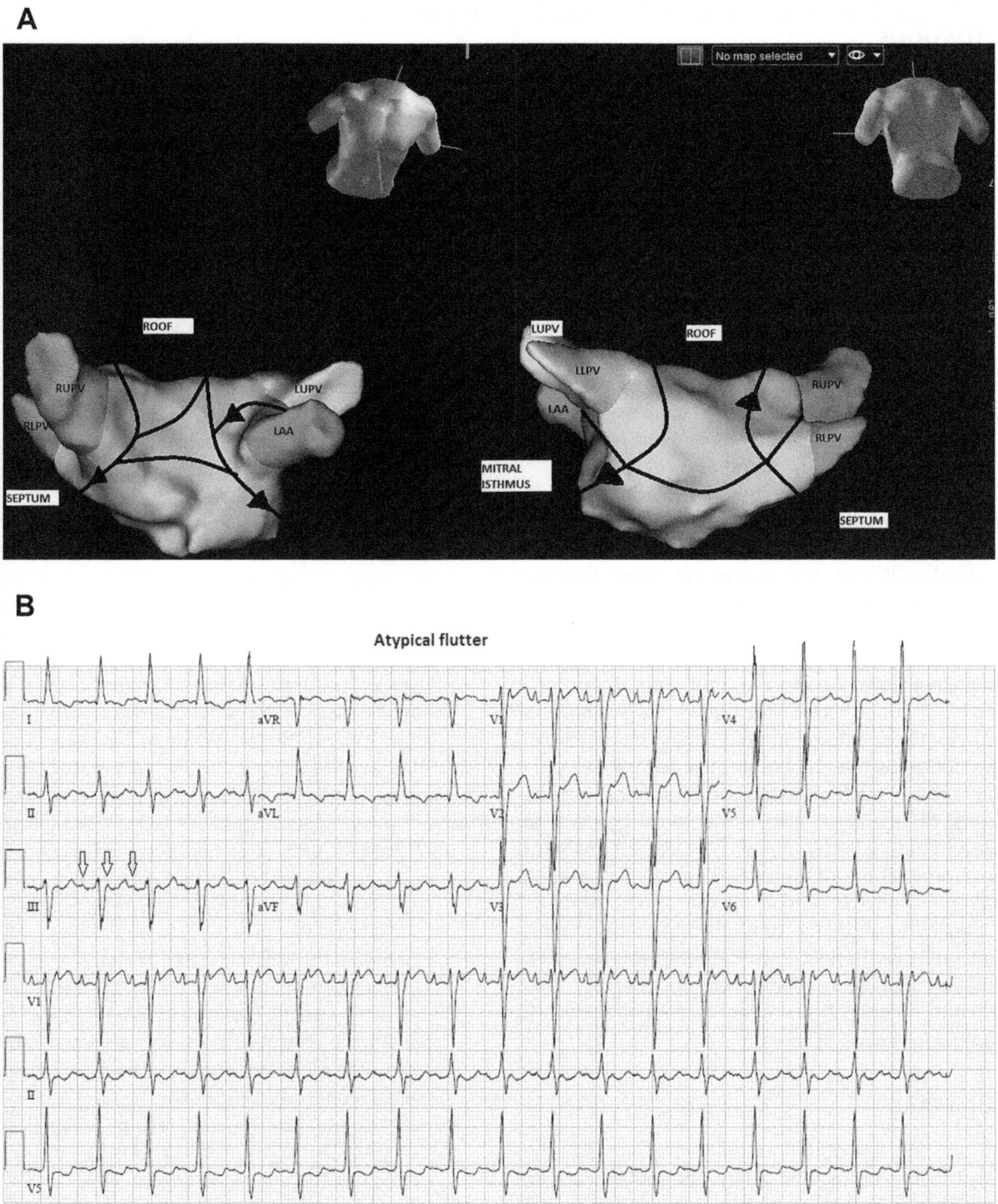

Fig. 7. (*A*) Electroanatomic anatomic map of the anterior and posterior surfaces of the left atrium showing some of the possible multiple paths/circuits of a left AFL. LAA, left atrial appendage; LLPV, left lower pulmonary vein; LUPV, left upper pulmonary vein; RLPV, right lower pulmonary vein; RUPV, right upper pulmonary vein. (*B*) A surface ECG of a patient showing atypical flutter, which in this case was a left AFL. The arrows point to positive flutter waves in lead III.

required in such patients and a hybrid epicardial-endocardial catheter ablation may offer an increased efficacy, particularly when performed simultaneously rather than in a staged fashion. The largest cohort that underwent this strategy to date was reported by Gehi and colleagues.[46] They reported a 66% rate of freedom from arrhythmia 12 months post–single hybrid procedure in spite of an average left atrial size of 5.1 cm. This is a promising result.

ABLATION OF AT AND AFL IN CHALLENGING SITUATIONS

AT and typical AFL have been reported as the most common supraventricular arrhythmias occurring late after cardiac transplantation. Typical AFLs tend to occur in the donor heart whereas the ATs commonly originate from the recipient atria or perisuture areas. Ablations have been successfully performed by delivering RFA to CTI in cases of AFL and by ablation of atrioatrial electrical connections across anastomotic suture lines or ablation of the foci of origin in either the donor or recipient atria without prohibitive complications.[47] Similarly, AT originating from the anastomotic pulmonary veins of donors propagating across suture lines into the atria of lung transplant recipients have been reported and ablated by pulmonary vein isolation.[48]

Patients with congenital heart diseases and heart failure commonly develop atrial tachyarrhythmias. The challenges in these cases include understanding of the congenital heart disease and its hemodynamic consequences and of the altered anatomy that may render certain areas inaccessible. Ablation in this cohort requires extensive planning and a multidisciplinary approach. Concomitant corrective surgeries and arrhythmia substrate ablation may be useful in this cohort as may be preemptive techniques during surgery, such as extension of surgical cuts to areas of anatomic and physiologic barriers to prevent future arrhythmias. Success of catheter ablation is in the range of 80% to 90%[49] in such patients, with a 10% to 25% risk for recurrence.[50]

Finally, to show the breadth of patient population that may benefit from catheter ablation, AFL ablation has been performed successfully and without complications even in patients on left ventricular assist devices.[51]

SUMMARY

AT and AFL are common tachyarrhythmias in the heart failure population. They commonly lead to, exacerbate, and increase the morbidity and mortality associated with heart failure and, thereby, warrant urgent and early definitive therapy in the form of catheter ablation. Catheter ablation requires careful patient stabilization and extensive preprocedural planning, particularly with regards to anesthesia, strategy, catheter choice, mapping system, and fluid balance, to increase efficacy and limit adverse effects. Heart failure may limit the success of catheter ablation with higher reported recurrence rates[52] and, in selected patients, a hybrid epicardial-endocardial ablation can be considered.

REFERENCES

1. Markides V, Peters NS. Mechanisms underlying the development of atrial arrhythmias in heart failure. Heart Fail Rev 2002;7:243–53.
2. Saoudi N, Cosio F, Waldo A, et al. Classification of atrial flutter and regular atrial tachycardia according to electrophysiologic mechanism and anatomic bases: a statement from a joint expert group from the Working Group of Arrhythmias of the European Society of Cardiology and the North American Society of Pacing and Electrophysiology. J Cardiovasc Electrophysiol 2001;12:852–66.
3. Poutiainen AM, Koistinen MJ, Airaksinen KE, et al. Prevalence and natural course of ectopic atrial tachycardia. Eur Heart J 1999;20:694–700.
4. Granada J, Uribe W, Chyou PH, et al. Incidence and predictors of atrial flutter in the general population. J Am Coll Cardiol 2000;36:2242–6.
5. Fuster V, Rydén LE, Cannom DS, et al, American College of Cardiology, American Heart Association Task Force, European Society of Cardiology Committee for Practice Guidelines, European Heart Rhythm Association, Heart Rhythm Society. ACC/AHA/ESC 2006 guidelines for the management of patients with atrial fibrillation: full text: a report of the American College of Cardiology/American Heart Association Task Force on practice guidelines and the European Society of Cardiology Committee for Practice Guidelines (Writing Committee to Revise the 2001 guidelines for the management of patients with atrial fibrillation) developed in collaboration with the European Heart Rhythm Association and the Heart Rhythm Society. Europace 2006;8:651–745.
6. Liberthson RR, Salisbury KW, Hutter AM, et al. Atrial tachyarrhythmias in acute myocardial infarction. Am J Med 1976;60:956–60.
7. Savelieva I, Camm AJ. Atrial fibrillation and heart failure: natural history and pharmacological treatment. Europace 2003;5:S5–19.
8. Hunt SA, Abraham WT, Chin MH, et al, American College of Cardiology, American Heart Association Task Force on Practice Guidelines, American College of Chest Physicians, International Society for Heart and Lung Transplantation, Heart Rhythm Society. ACC/AHA 2005 Guideline Update for the Diagnosis and Management of Chronic Heart Failure in the Adult: a report of the American College of Cardiology/American Heart Association Task Force on Practice Guidelines (Writing Committee to Update the 2001 Guidelines for the Evaluation and Management of Heart Failure): developed in collaboration with the American College of Chest Physicians and the International Society for Heart and Lung Transplantation: endorsed by the Heart Rhythm Society. Circulation 2005;112:154–235.

9. Kannel WB, Wolf PA, Benjamin EJ, et al. Prevalence, incidence, prognosis, and predisposing conditions for atrial fibrillation: population-based estimates. Am J Cardiol 1998;82:2N–9N.
10. Wyndham CR, Arnsdorf MF, Levitsky S. Successful surgical excision of focal paroxysmal atrial tachycardia. Observations in vivo and in vitro. Circulation 1980;62:1365–72.
11. Josephson ME, Spear JF, Harken AH, et al. Surgical excision of automatic atrial tachycardia: anatomic and electrophysiologic correlates. Am Heart J 1982;104:1076–85.
12. Gossage AM, Braxton Hicks JA. On auricular fibrillation. QJM 1913;6:435–40.
13. Whipple GH, Sheffield LT, Woodman EG, et al. Reversible congestive heart failure due to rapid stimulation of the normal heart. Proc New Engl Cardiovasc Soc 1961–1962;20:39–40.
14. Jeong YH, Choi KJ, Song JM, et al. Diagnostic approach and treatment strategy in tachycardia-induced cardiomyopathy. Clin Cardiol 2008;31:72–8.
15. Medi C, Kalman JM, Haqqani H, et al. Tachycardia-mediated cardiomyopathy secondary to focal atrial tachycardia: long-term outcome after catheter ablation. J Am Coll Cardiol 2009;53:1791–7.
16. Poole JE, Johnson GW, Hellkamp AS, et al. Prognostic importance of defibrillator shocks in patients with heart failure. N Engl J Med 2008;359:1009–17.
17. Dorian P, Philippon F, Thibault B, et al. Randomized controlled study of detection enhancements versus rate-only detection to prevent inappropriate therapy in a dual-chamber implantable cardioverter-defibrillator. Heart Rhythm 2004;1:540–7.
18. Friedman PA, McClelland RL, Bamlet WR, et al. Dual-chamber versus single-chamber detection enhancements for implantable defibrillator rhythm diagnosis: the detect supraventricular tachycardia study. Circulation 2006;113:2871–9.
19. Gasparini M, Galimberti P, Ceriotti C. The importance of increased percentage of biventricular pacing to improve clinical outcomes in patients receiving cardiac resynchronization therapy. Curr Opin Cardiol 2013;28:50–4.
20. Pedersen OD, Bagger H, Køber L, et al, TRACE Study Group. Impact of congestive heart failure and left ventricular systolic function on the prognostic significance of atrial fibrillation and atrial flutter following acute myocardial infarction. Int J Cardiol 2005;100:65–71.
21. The effect of digoxin on mortality and morbidity in patients with heart failure. The Digitalis Investigation Group. N Engl J Med 1997;336:525–33.
22. Sarter BH, Marchlinski FE. Redefining the role of digoxin in the treatment of atrial fibrillation. Am J Cardiol 1992;69:71G–81G.
23. Khand AU, Rankin AC, Martin W, et al. Carvedilol alone or in combination with digoxin for the management of atrial fibrillation in patients with heart failure? J Am Coll Cardiol 2003;42:1944–51.
24. Singh S, Fletcher RD, Fisher S, et al. Congestive heart failure: survival trial of antiarrhythmic therapy (CHF STAT). The CHF STAT Investigators. Control Clin Trials 1992;13:339–50.
25. Møller M, Torp-Pedersen CT, Køber L. Dofetilide in patients with congestive heart failure and left ventricular dysfunction: safety aspects and effect on atrial fibrillation. The Danish Investigators of Arrhythmia and Mortality on Dofetilide (DIAMOND) Study Group. Congest Heart Fail 2001;7:146–50.
26. Preliminary report: effect of encainide and flecainide on mortality in a randomized trial of arrhythmia suppression after myocardial infarction. The Cardiac Arrhythmia Suppression Trial (CAST) Investigators. N Engl J Med 1989;10:406–12.
27. Pratt CM, Camm AJ, Cooper W, et al. Mortality in the survival with ORal D-sotalol (SWORD) trial: why did patients die? Am J Cardiol 1998;81:869–76.
28. Connolly SJ, Camm AJ, Halperin JL, et al. Dronedarone in high-risk permanent atrial fibrillation. N Engl J Med 2011;365:268–76.
29. Xia Y, Ju WZ, Chen ML, et al. Catheter ablation of focal atrial tachycardia: the topographic distribution and long-term outcome. Zhonghua Xin Xue Guan Bing Za Zhi 2012;40:231–6 [in Chinese].
30. Pérez FJ, Schubert CM, Parvez B, et al. Long-term outcomes after catheter ablation of cavo-tricuspid isthmus dependent atrial flutter: a meta-analysis. Circ Arrhythm Electrophysiol 2009;2:393–401.
31. Lee G, Sanders P, Kalman JM. Catheter ablation of atrial arrhythmias: state of the art. Lancet 2012;380:1509–19.
32. Kistler PM, Roberts-Thomson KC, Haqqani HM, et al. P-wave morphology in focal atrial tachycardia: development of an algorithm to predict the anatomic site of origin. J Am Coll Cardiol 2006;48:1010–7.
33. Ouyang F, Ma J, Ho SY, et al. Focal atrial tachycardia originating from the non-coronary aortic sinus: electrophysiological characteristics and catheter ablation. J Am Coll Cardiol 2006;48:122–31.
34. Dong J, Schreieck J, Ndrepepa G, et al. Ectopic tachycardia originating from the superior vena cava. J Cardiovasc Electrophysiol 2002;13:620–4.
35. Polymeropoulos KP, Rodriguez LM, Timmermans C, et al. Images in cardiovascular medicine. Radiofrequency ablation of a focal atrial tachycardia originating from the Marshall ligament as a trigger for atrial fibrillation. Circulation 2002;105:2112–3.

36. Chen SA, Chiang CE, Yang CJ, et al. Radiofrequency catheter ablation of sustained intra-atrial reentrant tachycardia in adult patients. Identification of electrophysiological characteristics and endocardial mapping techniques. Circulation 1993;88:578–87.
37. Natale A, Breeding L, Tomassoni G, et al. Ablation of right and left ectopic atrial tachycardias using a three-dimensional non fluoroscopic mapping system. Am J Cardiol 1998;82:989–92.
38. Singh B, Sapra R, Gupta RK, et al. Pace mapping for the localization of focal atrial tachycardia arising near the mitral annulus. Indian Heart J 2004;56:58–60.
39. Feld GK, Fleck RP, Chen PS, et al. Radiofrequency catheter ablation for the treatment of human type 1 atrial flutter. Identification of a critical zone in the reentrant circuit by endocardial mapping techniques. Circulation 1992;86:1233–40.
40. Fischer B, Haissaguerre M, Garrigues S, et al. Radiofrequency catheter ablation of common atrial flutter in 80 patients. J Am Coll Cardiol 1995;25:1365–72.
41. Moreira JM, Alessi SR, Rezende AG, et al. Catheter ablation of atrial flutter. Electrophysiological characterization of posterior and septal isthmus block. Arq Bras Cardiol 1998;71:37–47 [in Portuguese].
42. Jaïs P, Shah DC, Haïssaguerre M, et al. Mapping and ablation of left atrial flutters. Circulation 2000;101:2928–34.
43. Kay GN, Ellenbogen KA, Giudici M, et al. Ablate and Pace Trial: a prospective study of catheter ablation of the AV conduction system and permanent pacemaker implantation for treatment of atrial fibrillation. APT Investigators. J Interv Card Electrophysiol 1998;2:121–35.
44. Wilkoff BL, Dual Chamber and VVI Implantable Defibrillator Trial Investigators. The Dual Chamber and VVI Implantable Defibrillator (DAVID) Trial rationale, design, results, clinical implications and lessons for future trials. Card Electrophysiol Rev 2003;7:468–72.
45. Brignole M, Botto G, Mont L, et al. Cardiac resynchronization therapy in patients undergoing atrioventricular junction ablation for permanent atrial fibrillation: a randomized trial. Eur Heart J 2011;32:2420–9.
46. Gehi AK, Mounsey JP, Pursell I, et al. Hybrid epicardial-endocardial ablation using a pericardioscopic technique for the treatment of atrial fibrillation. Heart Rhythm 2013;10:22–8.
47. Li YG, Grönefeld G, Israel C, et al. Radiofrequency catheter ablation in patients with symptomatic atrial flutter/tachycardia after orthotopic heart transplantation. Chin Med J (Engl) 2006;119:2036–41.
48. Nazmul M, Munger TM, Powell BD. Atrial tachycardia originating from a donor pulmonary vein in a lung transplant recipient. Circulation 2011;124:1288–9.
49. Lam W, Friedman RA. Electrophysiology issues in adult congenital heart disease. Methodist Debakey Cardiovasc J 2011;7:13–7.
50. Akar JG, Kok LC, Haines DE, et al. Coexistance of type I atrial flutter and intra-atrial re-entrant tachycardia in patients with surgically corrected congenital heart disease. J Am Coll Cardiol 2001;38:377–84.
51. Maury P, Delmas C, Trouillet C, et al. First experience of percutaneous radio-frequency ablation for atrial flutter and atrial fibrillation in a patient with HeartMate II left ventricular assist device. J Interv Card Electrophysiol 2010;29:63–7.
52. Landolina M, Cantù F, De Ferrari GM, et al. The role of invasive electrophysiology in the management of patients with chronic heart failure. Heart Fail Monit 2002;3:49–59.

Catheter Ablation of Atrial Fibrillation in Heart Failure

Senthil Kirubakaran, MRCP, MD[a,*],
Mark D. O'Neill, DPhil, FRCP, FHRS[b]

KEYWORDS

• Atrial fibrillation • Catheter ablation • Heart failure • Impaired ventricular function

KEY POINTS

- Modest efficacy rates (50%–88%) have been reported for rhythm control of AF with catheter ablation over the short term in patients with heart failure.
- Maintenance of sinus rhythm after ablation is associated with improvements in ventricular systolic function (reverse ventricular remodeling); NHYA functional class; and quality of life.
- Equivalent improvements in ventricular function are seen in patients with paroxysmal and persistent AF.
- Greater improvements in ventricular function are seen in patients with idiopathic cardiomyopathy.
- Reverse ventricular remodeling occurs even in patients with controlled ventricular rates during AF before catheter ablation.
- Efficacy of catheter ablation for AF is less than in patients with normal ventricular function with the requirement for more procedures.
- Some evidence shows catheter ablation of AF to be superior to optimal rate control with greater improvements in exercise tolerance, NYHA functional class, and reverse ventricular remodeling.
- Patient selection for catheter ablation of AF is reasonable in selected patients with heart failure and should be made after considering such factors as the degree and cause of ventricular dysfunction, the underlying atrial substrate, atrial size, and coexisting comorbidities.

INTRODUCTION

Atrial fibrillation (AF) and heart failure (HF) are two epidemics of cardiovascular disease. They often coexist, with their interaction creating a vicious pathophysiologic circle where HF promotes AF and vice versa. This is a considerable therapeutic challenge, with an integrated approach to the management of each condition required to achieve the most favorable outcome for the patient. Although well-established pharmacologic and nonpharmacologic treatments are used for the treatment of HF, the availability of efficacious and safe antiarrhythmic drugs for the treatment of AF in patients with HF is limited. Catheter ablation is an effective treatment for patients with AF in the absence of significant structural heart disease. This article discusses the role of catheter ablation for the treatment of AF in patients with HF.

TREATMENT OF AF IN HF

The adverse hemodynamic, electrophysiologic, and structural effects of AF in patients with HF and the associated morbidity and increased mortality emphasize the importance of identifying and treating AF in these patients. Analysis of the Cardiac Resynchronisation in Heart Failure trial showed the prevalence of AF in the HF population in those with no prior documented history of AF to

No conflicts of interest.

[a] Cardiothoracic Department, Guy's and St Thomas' NHS Trust, Westminster Bridge Road, London SE1 7EH, UK;
[b] Divisions of Imaging Sciences and Biomedical Engineering and Cardiovascular Medicine, Medical Engineering Centre, 3rd Floor, Lambeth Wing, St. Thomas' Hospital, London SE1 7EH, UK
* Corresponding author.
E-mail address: senthilk1uk@yahoo.co.uk

Heart Failure Clin 9 (2013) 515–532
http://dx.doi.org/10.1016/j.hfc.2013.07.006
1551-7136/13/$ – see front matter

heartfailure.theclinics.com

be 39% (159 of 404 patients), with 22% detected only using device-based diagnostic telemetry.[1] Furthermore, an estimated 5% to 10% of HF hospitalization is caused by the development of new AF or associated rapid ventricular rates.[2–4] This together with the detrimental effects on left ventricular ejection fraction (LVEF) highlights the importance of intensive screening for AF in this population group to initiate strategies to improve treatment with pharmacologic agents or catheter ablation. However, despite these adverse effects, controversy exists as to whether patients with HF respond better to rhythm restoration or ventricular rate control.

The Atrial Fibrillation Investigation of Rhythm Management (AFFIRM) and Rate Control versus Electrical Cardioversion of Persistent Atrial Fibrillation studies showed no difference in the development of HF or hospitalization for HF[5,6] between a rate or rhythm control strategy. Similarly, three other prospective randomized trials (How to Treat Chronic Atrial Fibrillation,[7] Strategies of Treatment of Atrial Fibrillation,[8] and Pharmacologic Intervention in Atrial Fibrillation[9]) showed equivalent outcomes in both arms. However, extrapolation of these results specifically to patients with HF should be done with caution, because the number of patients with HF in these studies was small. The Atrial Fibrillation and Congestive Heart Failure (AF-CHF) was the first randomized prospective trial to assess rhythm and rate control for AF in patients with HF. After a mean follow-up of 3 years, the investigators found no difference in mortality, hospitalization for HF, and stroke between the two groups.

Although these studies have shown equivalent outcomes for rhythm and rate control strategies, the potential benefits of sinus rhythm (SR) might have been offset by the limited efficacy and potentially deleterious effects of antiarrhythmic drugs. Currently, the available pharmacologic agents for rhythm control in patients with HF are amiodarone, sotalol, and dofetilide. The DIAMOND-CHF study showed dofetilide to be an effective class III antiarrhythmic agent in patients with HF.[10] However, despite this finding there was no associated mortality benefit with dofetilide treatment in patients with HF. Amiodarone seems to be the most effective agent; however, its use has been associated with the increased risk of symptomatic bradycardia requiring implantation of a permanent pacemaker[11] and has not been found to reduce mortality in this population group.[12] Upstream therapies with angiotensin receptor blockers and 3-hydroxy-3-methylglutaryl coenzyme A reductase inhibitors seem to have a modest success at reducing AF in patients with HF, because of their possible effects on structural remodeling.[13–17]

Despite the use of these antiarrhythmic drugs, the recurrence rate of AF after successful cardioversion is as high as 44% to 67% after 1 year.[18] Further support for the development of either more efficacious pharmacologic agents or the use of nonpharmacologic treatments came from further analysis of the AFFIRM and AF-CHF trials. The AFFIRM study showed that maintenance of SR was associated with a 47% reduction in the risk of death, whereas the use of antiarrhythmic drugs and the presence of congestive cardiac failure increased the risk of death by 49%, thus reversing the benefit of SR.[19] Post hoc analysis of the AFFIRM and AF-CHF trials demonstrated better survival rates in patients who remained in SR.[19] Further evidence for the maintenance of SR in patients with HF comes from the CAFE II Study comparing rate versus rhythm control with amiodarone and cardioversion in which a greater proportion of rhythm control patients had improved LVEF, quality of life, and natriuretic peptide levels.[20] Restoration and maintenance of SR with pharmacologic agents and electrical cardioversion has also been shown to improve ventricular function in patients with idiopathic cardiomyopathy.[21,22] These findings together with the adverse prognostic effects of AF in patients with HF have been one of the major drivers in developing more efficacious rhythm control approaches to AF in patients with HF to interrupt the vicious circle of AF and HF progression.[23–25]

Stulak and colleagues[26] evaluated whether improved rhythm control for AF in patients undergoing the Cox-Maze procedure improves ventricular function and functional status in a cohort of patients with HF. They reported 97% success rates in treating AF in the 37 patients with ventricular dysfunction. Improved rhythm control was associated with a significant improvement in LVEF (43%–55%; $P<.01$), which correlated with an improvement in functional status. However, the Cox-Maze procedure is an invasive procedure associated with significant complications. This study did, however, strengthen the argument for improved rhythm control strategies in the HF population.

One promising approach is catheter ablation. Over a decade ago, Haissaguerre and colleagues[27] made the pivotal discovery that focal discharges from the pulmonary veins (PVs) initiate AF and ablation of these triggers prevented AF in up to 70% of patients.[28] However, the frequent existence of multiple foci, inconsistencies in PV firing during the procedure, and the high incidence of PV stenosis led to an empiric approach to electrically isolate all the PVs from the left atrium using either a segmental ostial approach[29] or wide anatomic circumferential antral ablation.[30] Numerous studies have since demonstrated the efficacy and safety of PV isolation (PVI) in patients with paroxysmal AF in those who failed antiarrhythmic therapy.[31–36] However, patients with persistent and long-standing persistent AF frequently have significant atrial electrophysiologic and structural changes responsible for arrhythmia maintenance for which PVI alone has been shown to be an ineffective ablation strategy.[37–40] Since then, further approaches with modest success rates have been reported by different groups, including ablation of complex fractionated atrial electrograms (CFAE), which are thought to represent critical sites of slow and discontinuous conduction[38,41]; a stepwise approach including PVI, linear ablation, and CFAE[39,42,43]; ganglionated plexi ablation[44,45]; and ablation of focal rotors[46,47] thought to be responsible for sustaining persistent AF. Although durable PVI remains the building block of an effective catheter ablation procedure for AF, there is consensus that this alone is inadequate for the treatment of patients with nonparoxysmal AF.

CATHETER ABLATION OF AF IN HF SECONDARY TO LV DYSFUNCTION

The efficacy and safety of catheter ablation for AF was then extended to patients with impaired LV function and HF where the prevalence of AF is higher (**Table 1**). In 2004, Chen and colleagues[48] retrospectively reviewed 377 patients who had undergone catheter ablation for AF. A total of 94 of these patients had impaired LV function, defined as an LVEF of less than 40%, of which 56% of patients had persistent AF. Despite the high proportion of patients with persistent AF, only PVI was performed. After a single procedure, the AF recurrence rate was 27%, which was higher compared with those with normal LV function (13%; *P*<.05). A total of 85% of these patients underwent a second procedure to reisolate the PVs. After a mean follow-up of 14 months, 74% of patients had no AF recurrences off antiarrhythmic drugs. More importantly, the improvement in rhythm control was associated with a trend to an increased LVEF of 4.6% along with an improved quality of life. Complication rates did not differ between patients with reduced and normal ventricular function.

A prospective study by Hsu and colleagues[49] published in the same year also evaluated the efficacy and effects of restoration and maintenance of SR by catheter ablation of AF in 58 patients with LV dysfunction. A total of 91% of patients had persistent AF with a mean duration of 80 ± 45 months and mean New York Heart Association (NYHA) class of 2.3 ± 0.5 and LVEF 35 ± 7%.[49] Contrary to the previous study, left atrial (LA) linear ablation was performed between the two superior PVs (roof line) and from the mitral valve annulus to the left PV (mitral isthmus line) in addition to PVI. A total of 50% of patients required a second procedure because of AF recurrence. After a mean follow-up of 12 ± 7 months, 78% of patients with HF remained in SR compared with 84% in the control group with normal ventricular function (*P* = .34). This was associated with a significant decrease in mean NYHA class by 0.9, improved quality of life as assessed using the Short Form-36 questionnaire, and improved exercise capacity. Maintenance of SR was associated with reverse ventricular remodeling with overall improvements in LVEF of 21% and reductions in LV size, with the greatest improvements seen in the first 3 months after the ablation. Reverse ventricular remodeling occurred irrespective of the cause of LV dysfunction; however, a greater improvement was seen in those with isolated dilated cardiomyopathy compared with those with concurrent structural heart disease (LVEF increase of 24 ± 10% and 16 ± 14%, respectively; *P*<.001). Consistent improvements in ventricular function were also seen in patients with persistent AF with poor and adequate rate control, with greater improvements in LVEF seen in those with poor rate control (LVEF increase 23 ± 10% and 17 ± 15%, respectively; *P*<.001). As to be expected, the only variable associated with no improvement of LVEF was AF recurrence; however, among the 12 patients with AF recurrence, four patients still had an improvement in LVEF because of a reduction in AF burden with ablation converting persistent to paroxysmal AF.

This study highlighted an important finding: regardless of the cause of HF or prior rate control, improvements of ventricular function were seen in all groups, with the greatest improvement in those patients with poor ventricular rate control and the absence of coexisting structural heart disease. Of these patients, 92% had significant improvements in LVEF suggesting that most patients with AF and idiopathic cardiomyopathy have some degree of tachycardia-induced cardiomyopathy, further strengthening the argument for recognition of this patient group and consideration for rhythm control with catheter ablation.

Two years later, a similar smaller prospective study by Tondo and colleagues[50] with a different ablation strategy of PVI, mitral, and cavotricuspid isthmus lines confirmed these findings in 40 patients with LV dysfunction and AF. After a mean follow-up of 14 ± 2 months, 87% of patients with impaired LV function were in SR with significant improvements in LVEF of 14 ± 2%, exercise

Table 1
Summary of clinical trials examining the efficacy and safety of catheter ablation for AF in patients with impaired left ventricular function

	Chen et al,[48] 2004		Hsu et al,[49] 2004		Tondo et al,[50] 2006		Gentlesk et al,[51] 2007		Nademanee et al,[57] 2008	Lutomsky et al,[52] 2008	
Groups	Low LVEF	Normal LVEF	Low LVEF	Normal LVEF	Low LVEF	Normal LVEF	Low LVEF	Normal LVEF	Low LVEF	Low LVEF	Normal LVEF
Sample size	94	283	58	58	40	65	67	299	129	18	52
Mean age (y)	57 ± 8	55 ± 11	56 ± 10	56 ± 10	57 ± 10	56 ± 8	54	54	67	56.4 ± 10.6	58.5 ± 8.9
Paroxysmal AF	41%	55%	9%	9%	25%	23%	70%	82%	40%	100%	100%
Ischemic HD	—	—	21%	9%	25%	29%	18%	9%	—	17%	15%
Valvular HD	16%	13%	16%	5%	25%	18%	9%	5%	17%	—	—
Mean AF duration (mo)	72 ± 48	60 ± 24	80 ± 45	79 ± 53	36 ± 12	48 ± 12	67	71	40	—	—
Mean NYHA class	2.72	1.06	2.3 ± 0.5	1.3 ± 0.5	2.8 ± 0.1	—	—	—	—	—	—
Mean LVEF (%)	36 ± 8	54 ± 3	35 ± 7	66 ± 7	33 ± 2	64 ± 6	42 ± 9	61 ± 6	31 ± 7	41 ± 6.5	60 ± 6
Mean LA diameter (mm)	47 ± 8	45 ± 5	50 ± 7	46 ± 6	48 ± 4	44 ± 3	44 ± 7	48 ± 6	—	—	—
Ablation type	PVI ± CTI	PVI ± CTI	PVI ± LINES	PVI ± LINES	PVI ± Mitral ± CTI	PVI ± Mitral + CTI	PVI	PVI	CFAE	PVI	PVI
Complications (%)											
Procedure deaths	0	0	0	0	0	0	—	—	0	0	0
Stroke	2	1	2	2	0	0	—	—	5	0	0
Tamponade	0	0	2	0	0	2	—	—	9	0	0
Periprocedure pulmonary edema	1	0	—	—	—	—	—	—	—	0	0
Procedure duration (min)	—	—	218 ± 65	232 ± 90	225 ± 48	234 ± 50	—	—	—	—	—
Mean follow-up (mo)	14 ± 6	15 ± 8	12 ± 7	12 ± 6	14 ± 2	14 ± 2	20	20	27	6	6
AF recorded after first procedure	27%	13%	—	—	45%	29%	—	—	—	50%	27%
Mean number procedures	1.2	1.1	1.5	1.5	1.3	1.2	1.6 ± 0.8	1.3 ± 0.5	1.7	1	1

Arrhythmia free off AAD	74%	87%	78%	84%	—	—	—	—	79%	—	—
Arrhythmia free on AAD	—	—	69%	71%	87%	92%	86%	87%	89%	50%	73%
Mean NYHA change	—	—	−0.9	—	—	—	—	—	—	—	—
Mean LVEF change	4.6% (ns)	—	+21 ± 13%	—	+14 ± 2%	—	+14%	—	+10%	+9.8%	−1.8%
Mean change in LV size (LVIDs)	—	—	+8 ± 7 mm	—	—	—	+3 mm	—	—	+2.7 mm (ns)	−0.6 mm
Mean LA change (mm)	—	—	—	—	—	—	—	—	—	—	—
Improvement in exercise capacity	—	—	Yes	Yes	Yes	Yes	—	—	—	—	—
Improvement in QOL	Yes	Yes	Yes	Yes	Yes	Yes	—	—	—	—	—

	Khan et al,[63] 2008		Choi et al,[64] 2010		De Potter et al,[53] 2010		MacDonald et al,[65] 2011		Jones et al,[67] 2013	
Groups	PVI	AVN/BiV	PVI	Drugs for Rhythm Control	Low LVEF	Normal LVEF	PVI	Rate	PVI	Rate
Sample size	41	40	14	13	36	36	22	19	26	26
Mean age (y)	60	61	56 ± 11	63 ± 14	52	51	62	64	64 ± 10	62 ± 9
Paroxysmal AF	49%	55%	67%	73%	39%	—	0	0	0	0
Ischemic HD	—	—	33%	40%	25%	—	50%	47%	38%	27%
Valvular HD	—	—	—	—	11%	—	—	—	—	—
Mean AF duration (mo)	48	47	44 ± 34	56 ± 46	44	78	44	64	23 ± 22	24 ± 29
Mean NHYA class	—	—	1.7 ± 0.8	2 ± 0.8	—	—	2.9 ± 0.4	2.9 ± 0.4	2.46 ± 0.5	2.5 ± 0.5
Mean LVEF (%)	27 ± 8	29 ± 7	37 ± 6	34 ± 11	41 ± 8	63 ± 5	16 ± 7	20 ± 6	22 ± 8	25 ± 7
Mean LA diameter (mm)	49 ± 5	47 ± 6	45 ± 7	48 ± 9	42 ± 6	42 ± 5	—	—	50 ± 6	46 ± 7
Ablation type	PVI ± LINES ± CFAE	NA	PVI	NA	PVI + LINES	PVI + LINES	PVI ± CFAE ± LINES	NA	PVI + LINES + CFAE	NA
Complications (%)										
Procedure deaths	0	0	0	0	0	0	0	0	0	0

(*continued on next page*)

Table 1
(continued)

Groups	Khan et al,[63] 2008		Choi et al,[64] 2010		De Potter et al,[53] 2010		MacDonald et al,[65] 2011		Jones et al,[67] 2013	
	PVI	AVN/BiV	PVI	Drugs for Rhythm Control	Low LVEF	Normal LVEF	PVI	Rate	PVI	Rate
CVA	0	0	0	0	0	1 (TIA)	1	0	0	0
Tamponade	1	0	1	NA	0	0	2	0	1	0
Intraprocedure pulmonary edema	1	0	0	NA	0	0	1	0	1	NA
Procedure duration (min)	—	—	—	NA	—	—	205	NA	333 ± 61	NA
Mean follow-up (mo)	6	6	16 ± 13	16 ± 13	14	17	6	6	12	12
AF recurrence after first procedure	—	100%	27%	60%	50%	55.6%	50%	100%	31%	—
Mean number procedures	1.2	NA	—	NA	1.4	1.4	—	NA	—	NA
Arrhythmia free off AAD	71%	0%	73%	—	—	—	—	—	92%	NA
Arrhythmia free on AAD	88%	0%	—	40%	69.4%	69.4%	50%	0%	—	NA
Mean NYHA change	—	—	−0.4 (P<.01)	−0.2 (P = ns)	—	—	—	—	—	—
Mean LVEF change	+8 ± 8%	−1 ± 4%	+13%	+2% (P = ns)	+8%	—	+4.5 ± 11%	+2.8 ± 6.7%	+10.9 ± 11%	+5.4 ± 8.5%
Mean change in LV sizes	—	—	—	—	—	—	20 ± 50 ml	10 ± 32 ml	—	—
Improvement in exercise capacity	Yes (P<.001 cf AVN and BiVp)	Yes	—	—	—	—	No	No	Yes ($V_{O_{2max}}$)	No
Improvement in QOL	Yes (P<.01 cf AVN and BiVp)	Yes	—	—	—	—	No	No	Yes	No

Abbreviations: AAD, antiarrhythmic drugs; AVN, atrioventricular node; BiVp, biventricular pacing; CTI, cavo-tricuspid isthmus; CVA, (cerebrovascular accident); LA, left atrial; LVID, left ventricular internal dimension; NYHA, New York Heart Association; QOL, quality of life; TIA, transient ischemic attack.

capacity, and quality of life. There were no significant differences in outcomes between the HF and control groups, apart from a higher proportion of patients with HF on antiarrhythmic drugs, 38% compared with 23%, respectively.

Gentlesk and colleagues[51] prospectively evaluated the effect of PVI on LVEF in 67 patients with AF (70% paroxysmal) and decreased LVEF ≤50%). Isolation of the PVs was performed followed by ablation of non-PV triggers, which were identified after administration of isoproterenol and atrial burst pacing. After 20 months of follow-up, AF control defined as freedom from AF or greater than 90% reduction in AF burden determined using transtelephonic monitoring was 86%. This compared favorably with those patients with normal LV function, although more repeat procedures were required (1.6 ± 0.8 vs 1.3 ± 0.6; P<.05). This was associated with a significant improvement in LVEF (from 42 ± 9% to 56 ± 8%; P<.001), with more than 70% of patients returning to normal ventricular function (EF>55%) at 20 months follow-up (**Fig. 1**). Furthermore, assessments were made of LA function, with a significant increase in LA ejection fraction observed 6 months after catheter ablation and SR maintenance (from 0.32 ± 0.11 to 0.54 ± 0.18; P<.01), which supports the hypothesis that improvement in LVEF might in part be a result of improved atrial transport function.

Similar to Hsu and colleagues,[49] the improvement in ventricular function was not confined to those with poor ventricular rate control, with 88% of the patients having adequate rate control during AF before the ablation, which was defined as heart rates of less than 100 bpm for less than 50% of the

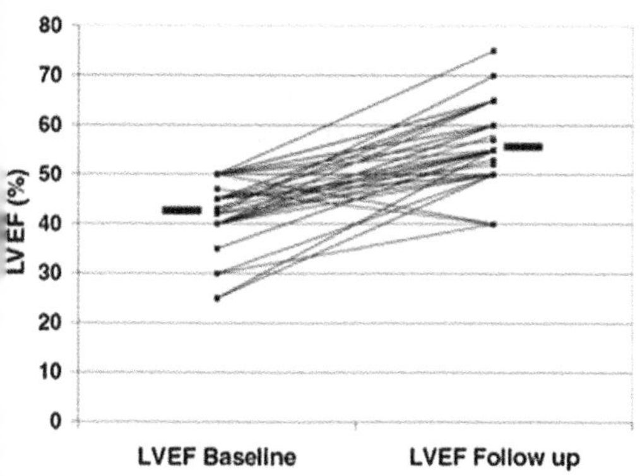

Fig. 1. Effect of PVI on left ventricular function in 67 patients with idiopathic cardiomyopathy. Mean increase in LVEF from 42 ± 9% to 57 ± 7%; P<.001. (*From* Gentlesk PJ, Sauer WH, Gerstenfeld EP, et al. Reversal of left ventricular dysfunction following ablation of atrial fibrillation. J Cardiovasc Electrophysiol 2007;18:12; with permission.)

time using transtelephonic monitoring for 2 to 3 weeks. These authors concluded that even when AF is not persistent, with well-controlled ventricular rates, reverse ventricular remodeling still occurs and highlighted the presence of an underrecognized group of patients with cardiomyopathy that would benefit by improved rhythm control with catheter ablation.

Similar findings were reported by Lutomsky and colleagues[52] who examined the impact of PVI on cardiac function using cardiac magnetic resonance imaging (CMRI) in patients with paroxysmal AF and impaired LV systolic function. Seventy patients with short periods of AF, defined as less than 24 hours, underwent CMRI before and 6 months after PVI. After a mean follow-up of 152 days, patients with impaired LVEF had lower success rates compared with those with preserved ventricular function (50% vs 73%; P<.05); however, a significant improvement in LVEF was seen (41 ± 6% to 51 ± 12%; P = .004). Interestingly, some patients with previously normal ventricular function who developed AF recurrence after catheter ablation had impaired LV function in follow-up, further supporting the important deleterious impact of AF on ventricular function. The authors concluded that even short periods of paroxysmal AF in patients with HF might have a detrimental effect on LVEF.

The reported success rates for catheter ablation for AF in patients with HF are inferior to patients without structural heart disease, with higher recurrence rates and more redo procedures required. To identify whether this is a consequence of LV dysfunction itself or confounding factors, such as LA size, AF duration, and AF type, a case control matching design study was performed by De Potter and colleagues.[53] In this study 36 patients with depressed LV function (LVEF<50%) and 36 patients with normal LVEF were matched for age, LA size, AF duration, and AF type. Circumferential PV ablation together with a roof, inferior LA, and mitral isthmus lines were performed. A successful outcome was defined as freedom from AF or any episode of AF or atrial flutter episodes of less than 30 seconds. After a mean follow-up of 16 months and a mean of 1.4 procedures, 69.4% had successful outcomes in both groups. There were no differences in outcomes or complication rates between the two groups suggesting that impaired LV systolic function itself is not a predictor of poor success rates or outcomes after catheter ablation. LA size was found to be the only predictor of AF recurrence after ablation: mean LA size was 40.9 ± 5.5 mm in the successful group and 44.7 ± 5.3 mm in the unsuccessful group (P<.01) and reflects more advanced atrial remodeling in the HF population. This has recently been confirmed in a study assessing the degree of atrial remodeling using CMRI,[54] where patients with LV systolic dysfunction displayed a comparatively greater degree of structural remodeling quantified using late gadolinium MRI than patients with normal LVEF. LA size has been identified as an independent predictor of AF recurrence after catheter ablation in patients with preserved ventricular function with a traditional upper limit of 55 mm being used for exclusion from catheter-based therapies for AF and enrollment for clinical trials.[55,56] As with previous studies in the HF population, reverse ventricular remodeling was evident in those patients who maintained SR after catheter ablation, with an increase in mean LVEF from 42.1% to 56.5% (*P*<.001) after 6 months. Those patients with idiopathic cardiomyopathy had the largest increase in LVEF.

Following Nadamanee and colleagues initial study describing an alternative approach to AF ablation, in which CFAE were targeted with high procedural success rates, this approach was used in high-risk patients with AF, similar to the cohort studied in the AFFIRM trial.[41,57] The cohort of 771 patients was at least 65 years old or had at least one or more risk factors for a stroke (hypertension, diabetes, structural heart disease, prior stroke or transient ischemic attack, or HF and LVEF ≤40%). A total of 129 patients had impaired LV systolic function with a mean LVEF of 30% in a more elderly population group compared with the previous studies described. A total of 60% of patients had persistent AF and the ablation strategy consisted of electrogram guided (CFAE) ablation alone. After a mean follow-up of 27 months, the AF recurrence rate after multiple procedures was 11%. Similar to previous studies, a significant improvement in LVEF was seen in those who maintained SR from 31 ± 7% to 41 ± 13% (*P*<.001) compared with those who remained in AF (24 ± 8% to 23.5 ± 9%; *P* = ns). Multivariate analysis and Cox regression analysis showed SR to be an independent predictor of a favorable prognosis. This was demonstrated in patients with both preserved and impaired LV systolic function (**Fig. 2**). The authors concluded the improvement in LV function in the HF cohort after maintenance of SR resulted in improved survival.

Rhythm Control with Catheter Ablation Versus Rate Control in Patients with Depressed Ventricular Systolic Function

Although the studies described have clearly shown improvements in ventricular function with catheter ablation of AF, more modest improvements were observed in studies using the "ablate and pace" strategy.[58–61] Greater improvements have been seen in patients who received a biventricular (BiV) pacemaker and AV node (AVN) ablation.[62] Although this approach provides effective rate control with evidence of reverse ventricular remodeling, it does not restore atrioventricular synchrony, and atrial systole has a significant contribution to cardiac output. The Pulmonary Vein Antrum Isolation versus AV Node Ablation with Biventricular Pacing for the Treatment of Atrial Fibrillation in Patients with Congestive Heart Failure (PABA-CHF) randomized multicenter trial was therefore undertaken to compare PVI and AVN ablation with BiV pacing in patients with depressed ventricular function, with an LVEF of less than 40% with NYHA Class II or III symptoms.[63] A total of 81 patients underwent randomization with 41 undergoing PVI with or without linear lines and fractionated electrogram ablation and 40 BiV

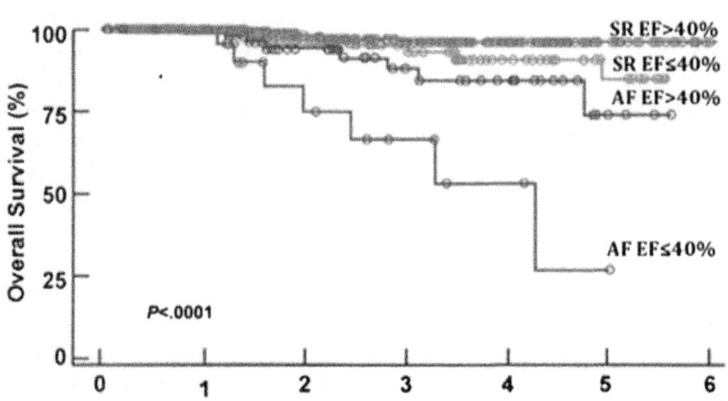

Fig. 2. Kaplan-Meier survival curves for four patient groups after catheter ablation for AF: (1) SR and EF >40%, (2) SR and EF ≤40%, (3) AF and EF >40%, and (4) AF and EF ≤40%. (*From* Nademanee K, Schwab MC, Kosar EM, et al. Clinical outcomes of catheter substrate ablation for high-risk patients with atrial fibrillation. J Am Coll Cardiol 2008;51:847; with permission.)

pacing and AVN ablation. Both groups were matched in terms of LVEF, LA size, type of AF, and age. At 6 months follow-up, all the patients in the AVN ablation and pacing group were in AF, whereas 88% of patients in the PVI group had no AF recurrence with antiarrhythmic drugs. Furthermore, progression of AF (from paroxysmal to persistent to long-standing persistent) did not occur in any of the patients undergoing PVI but occurred in 30% of those who underwent AVN ablation and pacing. Conversely, all the patients in persistent AF before ablation who had AF recurrence were only having paroxysms of AF, compared with 5% in the AVN ablation and BiV pacing group. The change in ventricular function and atrial size during follow up was significantly different between the two groups. At 6 months, the mean LVEF increased by 8 ± 8% compared with a decrease of 1 ± 4% in the AVN ablation and pacing group ($P<.001$). Similarly, the LA internal diameter decreased in the PVI group by 0.4 ± 0.3 cm and increased in the AVN ablation and pacing group by 0.1 ± 0.2 cm ($P<.001$). The improved maintenance of SR with PVI, and therefore reverse ventricular remodeling effects, were associated with greater improvements in function capacity measured during a 6-minute walk test and quality of life compared with AVN ablation and pacing and adds further support for the important contribution of atrial systole to cardiac output in patients with depressed ventricular function. Further analysis showed that greater improvements in LVEF, functional capacity, and quality of life were seen in patients with persistent AF undergoing PVI compared with the paroxysmal patients with AF. Complication rates were similar in both groups. In the PVI group, one patient had pericardial tamponade and two had PV stenosis and pulmonary edema. In the BiV pacing group, one patient had lead dislodgement and one had a pneumothorax. The authors concluded that rhythm control with catheter ablation and PVI provided superior morphologic and functional improvements compared with the best rate control strategy with AVN ablation and BiV pacing. The finding of greater benefit in patients with persistent AF compared with paroxysmal AF contradicts current beliefs that patients with persistent AF have advanced disease, particularly impaired ventricular function, which precludes them from catheter ablation. In light of these trials, one might argue that patients with persistent AF and HF have more to gain from catheter ablation because of the greater improvements in ventricular function, functional class, and quality of life.

Following these studies demonstrating the benefits of catheter ablation for AF in patients with HF, three studies were reported comparing conventional rate or rhythm control with pharmacologic agents and catheter ablation. Choi and colleagues[64] performed a retrospective case control trial to evaluate cardiac function and outcomes in patients with LV dysfunction treated with either catheter ablation or conventional medication with rate and rhythm control strategies. Two groups consisting of 14 patients in the catheter ablation group and 13 in the medication group were evenly matched in terms of age, NYHA class, LVEF, AF duration, AF type, and LA size. After a mean follow-up of 16 ± 13 months, 73% of patients treated with catheter ablation remained in SR, which was associated with a significant improvement in LVEF from 37% to 51% and improvements in NYHA functional class. Conversely, only 40% of control subjects remained in SR, and showed no change in LVEF or NHYA functional class on follow-up echocardiography.

After this, another study was conducted to compare a rhythm control strategy by catheter ablation against rate control using pharmacologic agents in patients with more severe impairment of LV function and persistent AF.[65] Twenty patients were randomized to catheter ablation and 18 to medical rate control. At the end of the 6-month follow-up period, SR was maintained in 50% of patients in the ablation group and 0% in the rate control group. Comparison between the two strategies revealed no significant difference in change in LVEF or LV dimensions, 6-minute walk test, or quality of life when measured using the Kansas City Cardiomyopathy Questionnaire and Minnesota Living with Heart Failure Questionnaire. These results are contrary to the previous beneficial results reported in patients undergoing catheter ablation. The authors commented that maintenance of SR in their study was lower than previous studies (50% compared with 78%–96%), which was because the study group recruited, which was older, had more severe systolic dysfunction and longer AF durations. These clinical characteristics are associated with atrial dilatation and fibrosis and decreased procedural success.[66] In view of these findings they performed a post hoc analysis to identify whether patients in SR demonstrated any improvements in cardiac structure or function. They identified significant improvements in LVEF, which occurred within 1 week of SR; however, this was not associated with any improvement in exercise capacity or quality of life. They speculated that the improvement in LV function observed might have been as a consequence of measuring LVEF in SR rather than AF, because there were no other observed improvements in functional exercise capacity or N-terminal prohormone of brain natriuretic peptide (NT-proBNP) and the improvement in LVEF was observed 1 week after catheter ablation when significant reverse ventricular remodeling is unlikely to occur.

More recently, Jones and colleagues[67] conducted a single-center prospective randomized control trial comparing catheter ablation with rate control for persistent AF. Fifty-two patients met the inclusion criteria of LVEF less than or equal to 35% assessed using radionucleotide ventriculography, NYHA Class II to IV, and on optimal HF medical therapy. Appropriate rate control, defined as a mean resting heart rate less than or equal to 80 bpm and after a 6-minute walk test of less than or equal to 110 bpm was achieved in 96% of patients in the rate control group at 3 months. A stepwise catheter ablation strategy was used that included PVI; linear lesions (roof, mitral, and cavotricuspid isthmus); and CFAE ablation. The 1-year arrhythmia-free survival was 72% after a single ablation procedure and after multiple procedures it was 92%. There was one serious procedural complication requiring emergency pericardiocentesis and sternotomy to repair a perforation at the atrioventricular groove. Other complications included one groin hematoma, one chest infection 2 weeks postablation, and one patient with postprocedural pulmonary edema. In keeping with previous studies, catheter ablation and maintenance of SR was associated with reverse structural and functional remodeling with a significant decrease in LA and RA area and an increase in LVEF at 12 months. When compared with stringent rate control, the primary end point of peak VO_2 had increased significantly in the ablation group and decreased in the rate control group (difference + 3.07 ml/kg/min; 95% confidence interval, 0.56–5.59; $P = .018$). For the secondary end points, ablation also improved quality-of-life scores assessed using the Minnesota questionnaire ($P = .019$) and decreased brain natriuretic peptide (BNP) ($P = .045$), and showed nonsignificant trends toward improved 6-minute walk test ($P = .095$) and EF ($P = .055$). This study reported high success rates after catheter ablation that may reflect the younger cohort of patients enrolled with a high proportion of nonischemic cardiomyopathy. Although these are promising results, ablation procedures were extensive with mean procedure times of 333 $\pm$ 61 minutes and ablation times of 80 $\pm$ 19 minutes. Nevertheless, this study demonstrates that maintenance of SR after catheter ablation in patients with HF in the short term is associated with greater improvements in symptoms, neurohormonal status, and objective physiologic exercise capacity compared with rate control for persistent AF.

Meta-analysis

The results of these clinical trials represent a heterogenous group of patients with different ages, AF types and durations, ablation strategy, and follow-up, and therefore outcomes of AF ablation in patients with HF are difficult to analyze. Two meta-analyses were performed to assess the role of catheter ablation for AF in patients with HF. The first performed by Wilton and colleagues[68] compared the safety and efficacy of AF ablation in patients with and without LV dysfunction. They reported that those with ventricular dysfunction were 1.5 times more likely to have AF recurrences after a single ablation procedure compared with those with preserved ventricular function. However, after repeat procedures, similar success rates were reported in both groups without increased risk or complication rates. It is not surprising that repeat procedures are required in those with ventricular dysfunction because of the more complex atrial substrate and larger atrial size. Reassuringly, this does not seem to be associated with increased risk; however, the previously mentioned studies are small with incomplete reporting in some of the studies. The consistent finding of improved LVEF after catheter ablation and maintenance of SR in the studies was highlighted by this meta-analysis and is an important finding. After catheter ablation, patients with LV dysfunction experienced an absolute improvement in LVEF of 11% (95% confidence interval, 7%–14%) (**Fig. 3**).

A second meta-analysis reviewed nine studies (of which six were common to both meta-analyses) with 354 patients, of which four were cohort studies, three case controlled, and two randomized controlled studies.[69] Study patients were mainly male with a mean age of 49 to 62 years with moderately impaired LV systolic function with LVEF range from 35% to 43%. Similar to the previous meta-analysis, LVEF improved after ablation by a mean difference of 11.1% (**Fig. 4**) with the presence of coronary artery disease being inversely related to LVEF improvement ($P<.0001$). This meta-analysis found no association between the degree of LVEF improvement and the proportion of patients with persistent or paroxysmal AF.

Complication rates were reported in seven out of the nine studies and out of the 268 patients who underwent AF ablation, 18 developed complications (6.7%), which included four strokes (1.5%), five pericardial effusions/tamponade (1.9%), two episodes of periprocedural pulmonary edema (0.8%), two cases of pulmonary stenosis (0.8%), three with minor groin bleeding (1.2%), and one patient required readmission 1 week after

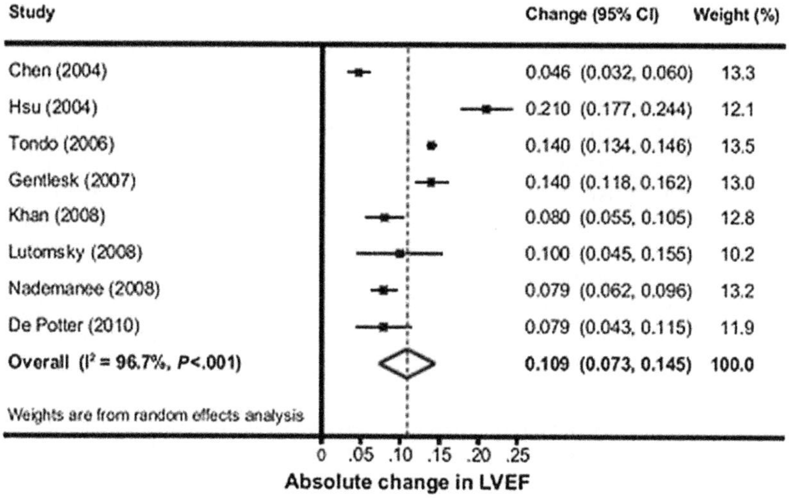

ig. 3. Meta-analysis of absolute change in LVEF after catheter ablation for AF in patients with impaired ventricular systolic function. (*From* Wilton SB, Fundytus A, Ghali WA, et al. Meta-analysis of the effectiveness and safety of catheter ablation of atrial fibrillation in patients with versus without left ventricular systolic dysfunction. Am J Cardiol 2010;106:1289; with permission.)

ischarge with HF. Quality of life was not assessed n this meta-analysis because of the heterogeneity n the measures used in the studies.

The evidence suggests that improved rhythm ontrol with catheter ablation in patients with HF s feasible and moderately efficacious in the short erm (between 60% and 88%) and is associated vith reverse atrial and ventricular remodeling[70] nd improved ventricular systolic function, which mproves exercise capacity and quality of life. he improvement in ventricular function might n part be related to improved ventricular rate ontrol and rhythm regularization. There is some vidence that regularization of ventricular rhythm independent of rate can improve hemodynamics. In two studies, after AVN ablation, regular right ventricular pacing at equivalent ventricular rates to that observed during AF was associated with improved cardiac outputs, decreased filling pressures, and improved LVEF.[71,72] The mechanism for reversal of arrhythmia-induced cardiomyopathy may be similar to that observed after suppression[73] and ablation[74] of frequent ventricular ectopy. However, rate or rhythm regularization alone cannot explain all the observed results. For example, the PABA-CHF trial comparing AVN ablation and BiV pacing with PVI demonstrated no improvements in LVEF in those treated with BiV pacing. In addition,

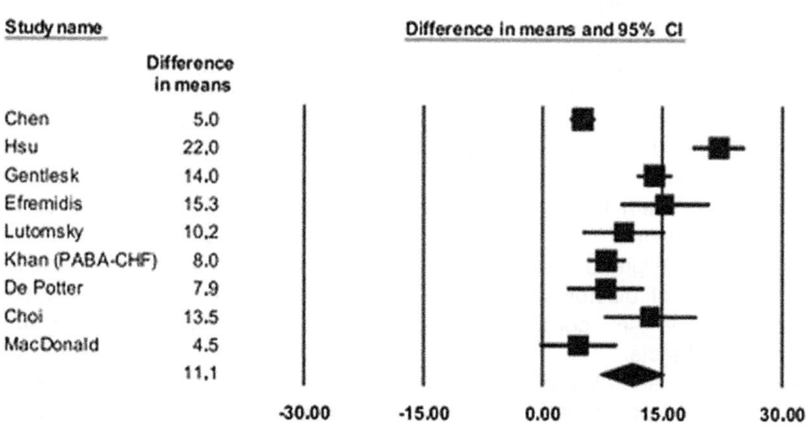

ig. 4. Change in left ventricular systolic function after catheter ablation for AF. The *diamond* represents the nean difference in LVEF, and width is 95% confidence interval. (*From* Dagres N, Varounis C, Gaspar T, et al. Catheter ablation for atrial fibrillation in patients with left ventricular systolic dysfunction. A systematic review and neta-analysis. J Card Fail 2011;17:967; with permission.)

consistent improvements in LV function were seen in patients with adequate ventricular rate control or short (<24 hours) episodes of AF.[49,51,52,67] Another possible explanation for the improvement in LV function might be related to technical issues with quantification of LVEF in SR and AF and the use of nonmasked operators. Calculation of LVEF during AF is associated with an underestimation of LVEF because of beat-beat variability.[75] For example, the PABA-CHF study comparing catheter ablation and CRT with AVN ablation was comparing LVEF postintervention in SR and AF, with 12% of patients in AF after catheter ablation compared with 100% after Cardiac Resynchronisation Therapy (CRT) and AVN ablation, which might have influenced the improvements in LVEF observed. However, two studies did perform baseline and follow-up LVEF measurements during SR and found equivalent increases in LVEF after catheter ablation comparable with the other studies.[51,52] Another explanation for an improvement in LVEF could be improved atrial transport function associated with SR, which was suggested by the improvement in LA function after catheter ablation in two studies.[51,76]

Another important consideration when interpreting changes in LVEF is the imaging modality used. Most of the studies used transthoracic echocardiography, which measures LVEF during one cardiac cycle. However, nuclear imaging is a more reliable modality for LVEF assessment in AF because its value is calculated by measuring a composite beat created during 20 minutes of recorded heartbeats.

Catheter Ablation for AF and Effects on Diastolic Function

Isolated diastolic HF or HF with preserved LV dysfunction accounts for 30% to 50% of patients with HF and is associated with AF particularly in the elderly.[77–83] A substudy of the CHARISMA trial also identified the association of diastolic dysfunction with new-onset AF and vascular events after myocardial infarction.[78] The severity and degree of diastolic dysfunction seem to be associated with risk for the development of AF.[82] A study by Jais and colleagues[81] highlighted the significant differences in measures of diastolic function in patients labeled as "lone AF" compared with age-matched control subjects.

Frequently the onset of AF in these patients is associated with significant hemodynamic effects caused by the presence of impaired LV relaxation and reduced LV filling further exposed by the loss of atrial contractility. The mechanism for the increase in incidence of AF in patients with diastolic HF is incompletely understood, but in part is related to the common etiologies, the presence of raised ventricular filling pressures and associated atrial stretch, dilatation, and contractile dysfunction. An increasing LA pressure and volume is positively correlated with the degree and severity of diastolic dysfunction.[84,85] This increase in LA pressure and size creates a favorable substrate for the maintenance of AF by increasing dispersion of refractoriness and alterations in anisotropic and conduction properties.

There is now favorable evidence on the efficacy of catheter ablation for AF in patients with LV systolic dysfunction; however, studies with isolated diastolic dysfunction are limited. The first prospective trial was in 2005 by Reant and colleagues[86] who evaluated 48 patients with paroxysmal and persistent AF and diastolic dysfunction. Compared with healthy control subjects in SR, LA dimensions were greater and measures of diastolic function using echocardiography and tissue Doppler were reduced. After catheter ablation that involved PVI and linear lesions and a mean follow-up of 11 months, reverse morphologic LA remodeling and improvements in LV diastolic function were observed. This study suggested that in part impaired diastolic function caused by AF and maintenance of SR with catheter ablation could potentially reverse this process. In 2011 Cha and colleagues[87] evaluated and compared the long-term efficacy of catheter ablation for AF in patients with normal LV function and abnormal diastolic and systolic function. One year after ablation, elimination rates for AF off antiarrhythmic drugs were 84% in those with normal LV function and 62% and 75% with abnormal LV systolic function and diastolic function, respectively. However after a 5-year follow-up period the success rates in patients were poor, with only 33% of patients free from AF in the systolic dysfunction group and 40% in the diastolic dysfunction group (**Fig. 5**).

Similar to previous studies, those patients with LV systolic dysfunction had a significant increase in LVEF from 35% to 56% with AF recurrence being a predictor of reverse LV remodeling. However fewer patients had improvements in diastolic function, with only 30% demonstrating an improvement compared with 49% in those with systolic dysfunction. The authors concluded that AF ablation in patients with diastolic dysfunction is relatively efficacious after 1 year; however, in the long term arrhythmia recurrence was high. They acknowledged in this study that patients with diastolic dysfunction were older with a high proportion of comorbidities, such as hypertension, and suggested that during longer follow-up, progression of diastolic dysfunction and redevelopment

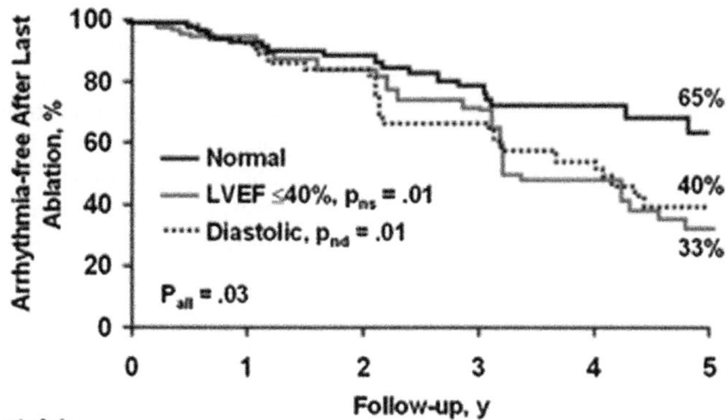

No. at risk						
Normal	100	73	53	39	26	15
EF≤40%	111	86	66	43	19	10
Diastolic	156	116	83	43	27	12

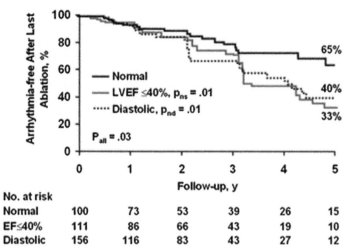

Fig. 5. Long-term freedom from AF recurrence after ablation in patients with left ventricular systolic and diastolic dysfunction. (*From* Cha YM, Wokhlu A, Asirvatham SJ, et al. Success of ablation for atrial fibrillation in isolated left ventricular diastolic dysfunction: a comparison to systolic dysfunction and normal ventricular function. Circ Arrhythm Electrophysiol 2011;4:728; with permission.)

of the vulnerable substrate may predispose to AF recurrence. One year later, Hu and colleagues[88] assessed the relationship between diastolic dysfunction, LA substrate quantified by measuring atrial voltages, and efficacy of catheter ablation in patients with paroxysmal AF. As in the previous study, patients with diastolic dysfunction were older. Patients with diastolic dysfunction had significantly lower atrial voltages compared with those with normal ventricular function after adjusting for age and hypertension. After catheter ablation, AF recurrence in those with diastolic dysfunction was higher at 30% compared with 10% in the normal LV function group. Further analysis also showed that low atrial voltages were predictors of AF recurrence after ablation.

Thus, the presence of atrial structural remodeling, in particular atrial fibrosis, is associated with poorer outcomes after catheter ablation because of a favorable substrate for the maintenance of reentry circuits and sites for non-PV ectopy and could explain the higher recurrence rates of AF in patients with diastolic dysfunction.[89,90]

PATIENT SELECTION FOR CATHETER ABLATION FOR AF IN PATIENTS WITH HF

Although the current studies suggest modest efficacy rates with catheter ablation of AF in patients with HF, these are largely based on cohort studies in experienced high-volume centers with significant heterogeneity in patient selection and outcome measures. The studied population in most studies was selected and not representative of the average patient with HF with concomitant AF (eg, patients were frequently younger and with a relatively high LVEF). Therefore, generalized recommendations on catheter ablation for all patients with AF in the HF population cannot be made; however, based on the current available evidence, highly selective patients should be considered on an individual basis. The studies do, however, highlight several important factors, which are relevant when selecting patients for catheter ablation.

As with patients with normal ventricular function, LA dilatation is an important predictor of AF recurrence in the HF population secondary to more advanced structural remodeling and atrial fibrosis. In the general population LA diameters of greater than 55 mm have more recently been excluded from catheter ablation and in the HF population LA diameters greater than 45 mm in two studies have been associated with AF recurrence and poorer outcomes.

Baseline LVEF is also an important factor and as alluded to previously many studies demonstrating reasonable outcomes at 1 year recruited patients with an average LVEF between 35% and 45%. MacDonald and colleagues[65] who recruited patients with a lower LVEF reported poorer outcomes with catheter ablation compared with previous studies and therefore highlighted the importance of LVEF for patient selection.

Although shorter AF durations have been reported as a predictor of success after catheter ablation for persistent AF in patients with preserved LVEF, the AF durations in the current studies have been variable, between 36 and 80 months, with similar efficacy rates. Contrary to studies on catheter ablation in patients with preserved LV systolic function, patients with persistent AF seemed to derive significant benefit from catheter ablation and one might argue have more to gain, because these patients are more likely to have an associated tachycardia-induced cardiomyopathy, which potentially could be reversed by catheter ablation and maintenance of SR.

Finally, the cause of ventricular dysfunction has been shown to be a predictor of success, with patients diagnosed with idiopathic cardiomyopathy having greater success rates and reverse remodeling after catheter ablation, which is likely related to a higher proportion of patients with a tachycardia-induced cardiomyopathy in this group.

Patients with HF and AF are a challenging group. It is important to recognize that AF is one aspect of the management of the patient with HF. Patients should be treated with optimal HF medical therapy before considering catheter ablation analogous to patient selection for CRT. When deciding on a nonpharmacologic strategy for the treatment of AF in these patients one must formulate an estimate for the likelihood of maintaining SR incorporating the previously mentioned factors and coexisting comorbidities. Additional information on the underlying atrial substrate from advanced imaging modalities may be useful to further assess the likelihood of success after catheter ablation. For example, Akkaya and colleagues[54] recently showed a greater improvement in LVEF after catheter ablation in patients with HF in those with less atrial remodeling assessed using late gadolinium CMRI.

Catheter ablation in the HF population is associated with longer procedure and higher fluoroscopy times, more repeat procedures, and complication rates reported by some studies as high as 13%. Although the studies have reported modest success rates, the follow-up of these patients is limited and between 6 and 20 months. In keeping with previous studies on catheter ablation of AF[91] the success rates are likely to diminish during longer follow-up. Therefore, thorough discussions with the patient at the outset about short-term success rates, requirement for multiple procedures, complication rates, and unproved long-term success rates are important before deciding on catheter ablation for AF in patients with HF.

SUMMARY

Current evidence is supportive for a beneficial role in maintenance of SR in patients with HF with AF by catheter ablation. Catheter ablation for AF seems to be superior to rate control and pharmacologic rhythm control. The benefit is not restricted to type of AF (paroxysmal or persistent); however, greater benefit is seen in patients with idiopathic dilated cardiomyopathy where AF is a significant contributor to depressed ventricular function and symptoms. The studies have demonstrated improved rhythm control with better quality of life and reverse ventricular and atrial remodeling. Given the increased morbidity and mortality associated with AF in the presence of HF, one would expect improved ventricular function after catheter ablation to be associated with improvements in these parameters. However, no large-scale trials have been reported demonstrating a mortality benefit with catheter ablation in this patient cohort, because none of the studies were robust or powered sufficiently to assess mortality differences. Larger trials are required, such as the ongoing CASTLE-AF and RAFT-AF trials, to evaluate whether catheter ablation of AF in patients with HF is associated with improved mortality compared with conventional treatment. This has been recognized in the 2012 Consensus Statement on catheter ablation of AF, which states that "catheter ablation of AF is reasonable in highly selected patients with HF."[92]

REFERENCES

1. Hoppe UC, Casares JM, Eiskjaer H, et al. Effect of cardiac resynchronization on the incidence of atrial fibrillation in patients with severe heart failure. Circulation 2006;114:18–25.
2. Michalsen A, Konig G, Thimme W. Preventable causative factors leading to hospital admission with decompensated heart failure. Heart 1998;80:437–41.
3. Tsuyuki RT, McKelvie RS, Arnold JM, et al. Acute precipitants of congestive heart failure exacerbations. Arch Intern Med 2001;161:2337–42.
4. Chin MH, Goldman L. Factors contributing to the hospitalization of patients with congestive heart failure. Am J Public Health 1997;87:643–8.
5. Wyse DG, Waldo AL, DiMarco JP, et al, The Atrial Fibrillation Follow-up Investigation of Rhythm Management (AFFIRM) Investigators. A comparison of rate control and rhythm control in patients with atrial fibrillation. N Engl J Med 2002;347:1825–33.
6. Blackshear JL, Safford RE. AFFIRM and RACE trials: implications for the management of atrial fibrillation. Card Electrophysiol Rev 2003;7:366–9.
7. Opolski G, Torbicki A, Kosior DA, et al. Rate control vs rhythm control in patients with nonvalvular persistent atrial fibrillation: the results of the Polish How to Treat Chronic Atrial Fibrillation (HOT CAFE) Study. Chest 2004;126:476–86.

8. Carlsson J, Miketic S, Windeler J, et al. Randomized trial of rate-control versus rhythm-control in persistent atrial fibrillation: the Strategies of Treatment of Atrial Fibrillation (STAF) study. J Am Coll Cardiol 2003;41:1690–6.
9. Hohnloser SH, Kuck KH, Lilienthal J. Rhythm or rate control in atrial fibrillation–Pharmacological Intervention in Atrial Fibrillation (PIAF): a randomised trial. Lancet 2000;356:1789–94.
10. Moller M, Torp-Pedersen CT, Kober L. Dofetilide in patients with congestive heart failure and left ventricular dysfunction: safety aspects and effect on atrial fibrillation. The Danish Investigators of Arrhythmia and Mortality on Dofetilide (DIAMOND) Study Group. Congest Heart Fail 2001;7:146–50.
11. Weinfeld MS, Drazner MH, Stevenson WG, et al. Early outcome of initiating amiodarone for atrial fibrillation in advanced heart failure. J Heart Lung Transplant 2000;19:638–43.
12. Roy D, Talajic M, Nattel S, et al. Rhythm control versus rate control for atrial fibrillation and heart failure. N Engl J Med 2008;358:2667–77.
13. Pedersen OD, Bagger H, Kober L, et al. Trandolapril reduces the incidence of atrial fibrillation after acute myocardial infarction in patients with left ventricular dysfunction. Circulation 1999;100:376–80.
14. Swedberg KP, Coen-Solal A. Prevention of atrial fibrillation in symptomatic chronic heart failure by candesartan: results of the CHARM study. J Am Coll Cardiol 2004;43(Suppl A):222A.
15. Wachtell K, Lehto M, Gerdts E, et al. Angiotensin II receptor blockade reduces new-onset atrial fibrillation and subsequent stroke compared to atenolol: the Losartan Intervention For End Point Reduction in Hypertension (LIFE) study. J Am Coll Cardiol 2005;45:712–9.
16. Young-Xu Y, Jabbour S, Goldberg R, et al. Usefulness of statin drugs in protecting against atrial fibrillation in patients with coronary artery disease. Am J Cardiol 2003;92:1379–83.
17. Shiroshita-Takeshita A, Brundel BJ, Burstein B, et al. Effects of simvastatin on the development of the atrial fibrillation substrate in dogs with congestive heart failure. Cardiovasc Res 2007;74:75–84.
18. Lafuente-Lafuente C, Mouly S, Longas-Tejero MA, et al. Antiarrhythmic drugs for maintaining sinus rhythm after cardioversion of atrial fibrillation: a systematic review of randomized controlled trials. Arch Intern Med 2006;166:719–28.
19. Corley SD, Epstein AE, DiMarco JP, et al. Relationships between sinus rhythm, treatment, and survival in the Atrial Fibrillation Follow-Up Investigation of Rhythm Management (AFFIRM) Study. Circulation 2004;109:1509–13.
20. Shelton RJ, Clark AL, Goode K, et al. A randomised, controlled study of rate versus rhythm control in patients with chronic atrial fibrillation and heart failure: (CAFE-II Study). Heart 2009;95:924–30.
21. Peters KG, Kienzle MG. Severe cardiomyopathy due to chronic rapidly conducted atrial fibrillation: complete recovery after restoration of sinus rhythm. Am J Med 1988;85:242–4.
22. Van Gelder IC, Crijns HJ, Blanksma PK, et al. Time course of hemodynamic changes and improvement of exercise tolerance after cardioversion of chronic atrial fibrillation unassociated with cardiac valve disease. Am J Cardiol 1993;72:560–6.
23. Benjamin EJ, Levy D, Vaziri SM, et al. Independent risk factors for atrial fibrillation in a population-based cohort: the Framingham Heart Study. JAMA 1994;271:840–4.
24. Poole-Wilson PA, Swedberg K, Cleland JG, et al. Comparison of carvedilol and metoprolol on clinical outcomes in patients with chronic heart failure in the Carvedilol Or Metoprolol European Trial (COMET): randomised controlled trial. Lancet 2003;36:7–13.
25. Middlekauff HR, Stevenson WG, Stevenson LW. Prognostic significance of atrial fibrillation in advanced heart failure. A study of 390 patients. Circulation 1991;84:40–8.
26. Stulak JM, Dearani JA, Daly RC, et al. Left ventricular dysfunction in atrial fibrillation: restoration of sinus rhythm by the Cox-maze procedure significantly improves systolic function and functional status. Ann Thorac Surg 2006;82:494–500 [discussion: 500–1].
27. Haissaguerre M, Jaise P, Sha D, et al. Spontaneous initiation of atrial fibrillation by ectopic beats originating in the pulmonary veins. N Engl J Med 1998;339:659–66.
28. Haissaguerre M, Jais P, Shah DC, et al. Electrophysiological end point for catheter ablation of atrial fibrillation initiated from multiple pulmonary venous foci. Circulation 2000;101:1409–17.
29. Oral H, Scharf C, Chugh A, et al. Catheter ablation for paroxysmal atrial fibrillation: segmental pulmonary vein ostial ablation versus left atrial ablation. Circulation 2003;108:2355–60.
30. Pappone C, Oreto G, Rosanio S, et al. Atrial electroanatomic remodeling after circumferential radiofrequency pulmonary vein ablation: efficacy of an anatomic approach in a large cohort of patients with atrial fibrillation. Circulation 2001;104:2539–44.
31. Wilber DJ, Pappone C, Neuzil P, et al. Comparison of antiarrhythmic drug therapy and radiofrequency catheter ablation in patients with paroxysmal atrial fibrillation: a randomized controlled trial. JAMA 2010;303:333–40.
32. Wazni OM, Marrouche NF, Martin DO, et al. Radiofrequency ablation vs antiarrhythmic drugs as first-line treatment of symptomatic atrial fibrillation: a randomized trial. JAMA 2005;293:2634–40.

33. Pappone C, Rosanio S, Augello G, et al. Mortality, morbidity, and quality of life after circumferential pulmonary vein ablation for atrial fibrillation: outcomes from a controlled nonrandomized long-term study. J Am Coll Cardiol 2003;42:185–97.
34. Ouyang F, Bansch D, Ernst S, et al. Complete isolation of left atrium surrounding the pulmonary veins: new insights from the double-Lasso technique in paroxysmal atrial fibrillation. Circulation 2004;110: 2090–6.
35. Haissaguerre M, Shah DC, Jais P, et al. Mapping-guided ablation of pulmonary veins to cure atrial fibrillation. Am J Cardiol 2000;86:9K–19K.
36. Nair GM, Nery PB, Diwakaramenon S, et al. A systematic review of randomized trials comparing radiofrequency ablation with antiarrhythmic medications in patients with atrial fibrillation. J Cardiovasc Electrophysiol 2009;20:138–44.
37. Elayi CS, Di Biase L, Barrett C, et al. Atrial fibrillation termination as a procedural endpoint during ablation in long-standing persistent atrial fibrillation. Heart Rhythm 2010;7:1216–23.
38. Elayi CS, Verma A, Di Biase L, et al. Ablation for longstanding permanent atrial fibrillation: results from a randomized study comparing three different strategies. Heart Rhythm 2008;5:1658–64.
39. Haissaguerre M, Hocini M, Sanders P, et al. Catheter ablation of long-lasting persistent atrial fibrillation: clinical outcome and mechanisms of subsequent arrhythmias. J Cardiovasc Electrophysiol 2005;16:1138–47.
40. Oral H, Knight BP, Tada H, et al. Pulmonary vein isolation for paroxysmal and persistent atrial fibrillation. Circulation 2002;105:1077–81.
41. Nademanee K, McKenzie J, Kosar E, et al. A new approach for catheter ablation of atrial fibrillation: mapping of the electrophysiologic substrate. J Am Coll Cardiol 2004;43:2044–53.
42. Haissaguerre M, Sanders P, Hocini M, et al. Catheter ablation of long-lasting persistent atrial fibrillation: critical structures for termination. J Cardiovasc Electrophysiol 2005;16:1125–37.
43. O'Neill MD, Wright M, Knecht S, et al. Long-term follow-up of persistent atrial fibrillation ablation using termination as a procedural endpoint. Eur Heart J 2009;30:1105–12.
44. Nakagawa H, Scherlag BJ, Patterson E, et al. Pathophysiologic basis of autonomic ganglionated plexus ablation in patients with atrial fibrillation. Heart Rhythm 2009;6:S26–34.
45. Lu Z, Scherlag BJ, Lin J, et al. Autonomic mechanism for initiation of rapid firing from atria and pulmonary veins: evidence by ablation of ganglionated plexi. Cardiovasc Res 2009;84:245–52.
46. Narayan SM, Krummen DE, Shivkumar K, et al. Treatment of atrial fibrillation by the ablation of localized sources: CONFIRM (Conventional Ablation for Atrial Fibrillation With or Without Focal Impulse and Rotor Modulation) trial. J Am Col Cardiol 2012;60:628–36.
47. Narayan SM, Patel J, Mulpuru S, et al. Focal impulse and rotor modulation ablation of sustaining rotors abruptly terminates persistent atrial fibrillation to sinus rhythm with elimination on follow-up a video case study. Heart Rhythm 2012;9:1436–9
48. Chen MS, Marrouche NF, Khaykin Y, et al. Pulmonary vein isolation for the treatment of atrial fibrillation in patients with impaired systolic function J Am Coll Cardiol 2004;43:1004–9.
49. Hsu LF, Jais P, Sanders P, et al. Catheter ablation for atrial fibrillation in congestive heart failure N Engl J Med 2004;351:2373–83.
50. Tondo C, Mantica M, Russo G, et al. Pulmonary vein vestibule ablation for the control of atrial fibrillation in patients with impaired left ventricular function. Pacing Clin Electrophysiol 2006;29:962–70.
51. Gentlesk PJ, Sauer WH, Gerstenfeld EP, et al. Reversal of left ventricular dysfunction following ablation of atrial fibrillation. J Cardiovasc Electrophysiol 2007;18:9–14.
52. Lutomsky BA, Rostock T, Koops A, et al. Catheter ablation of paroxysmal atrial fibrillation improves cardiac function: a prospective study on the impact of atrial fibrillation ablation on left ventricular function assessed by magnetic resonance imaging Europace 2008;10:593–9.
53. De Potter T, Berruezo A, Mont L, et al. Left ventricular systolic dysfunction by itself does not influence outcome of atrial fibrillation ablation. Europace 2010;12:24–9.
54. Akkaya M, Higuchi K, Koopmann M, et al. Higher degree of left atrial structural remodeling in patients with atrial fibrillation and left ventricular systolic dysfunction. J Cardiovasc Electrophysio 2013;24(5):485–91.
55. Berruezo A, Tamborero D, Mont L, et al. Pre-procedural predictors of atrial fibrillation recurrence after circumferential pulmonary vein ablation. Eur Heart J 2007;28:836–41.
56. McCready JW, Smedley T, Lambiase PD, et al. Predictors of recurrence following radiofrequency ablation for persistent atrial fibrillation. Europace 2011;13:355–61.
57. Nademanee K, Schwab MC, Kosar EM, et al. Clinical outcomes of catheter substrate ablation for high-risk patients with atrial fibrillation. J Am Col Cardiol 2008;51:843–9.
58. Wood MA, Brown-Mahoney C, Kay GN, et al. Clinical outcomes after ablation and pacing therapy for atrial fibrillation: a meta-analysis. Circulation 2000 101:1138–44.
59. Kay GN, Ellenbogen KA, Giudici M, et al. The Ablate and Pace trial: a prospective study of catheter ablation of the AV conduction system and

permanent pacemaker implantation for treatment of atrial fibrillation. APT Investigators. J Interv Card Electrophysiol 1998;2:121–35.
60. Ozcan C, Jahangir A, Friedman PA, et al. Long-term survival after ablation of the atrioventricular node and implantation of a permanent pacemaker in patients with atrial fibrillation. N Engl J Med 2001; 344:1043–51.
61. Brignole M, Menozzi C, Gianfranchi L, et al. Assessment of atrioventricular junction ablation and VVIR pacemaker versus pharmacological treatment in patients with heart failure and chronic atrial fibrillation: a randomized, controlled study. Circulation 1998;98:953–60.
62. Doshi RN, Daoud EG, Fellows C, et al. Left ventricular-based cardiac stimulation post AV nodal ablation evaluation (the PAVE study). J Cardiovasc Electrophysiol 2005;16:1160–5.
63. Khan MN, Jais P, Cummings J, et al. Pulmonary-vein isolation for atrial fibrillation in patients with heart failure. N Engl J Med 2008;359:1778–85.
64. Choi AD, Hematpour K, Kukin M, et al. Ablation vs medical therapy in the setting of symptomatic atrial fibrillation and left ventricular dysfunction. Congest Heart Fail 2010;16:10–4.
65. MacDonald MR, Connelly DT, Hawkins NM, et al. Radiofrequency ablation for persistent atrial fibrillation in patients with advanced heart failure and severe left ventricular systolic dysfunction: a randomised controlled trial. Heart 2011;97:740–7.
66. Oakes RS, Badger TJ, Kholmovski EG, et al. Detection and quantification of left atrial structural remodeling with delayed-enhancement magnetic resonance imaging in patients with atrial fibrillation. Circulation 2009;119:1758–67.
67. Jones DG, Haldar SK, Hussain W, et al. A randomized trial to assess catheter ablation versus rate control in the management of persistent atrial fibrillation in heart failure (ARC-HF). J Am Coll Cardiol 2013;61:1894–903.
68. Wilton SB, Fundytus A, Ghali WA, et al. Meta-analysis of the effectiveness and safety of catheter ablation of atrial fibrillation in patients with versus without left ventricular systolic dysfunction. Am J Cardiol 2010;106:1284–91.
69. Dagres N, Varounis C, Gaspar T, et al. Catheter ablation for atrial fibrillation in patients with left ventricular systolic dysfunction. A systematic review and meta-analysis. J Card Fail 2011;17:964–70.
70. Efremidis M, Sideris A, Xydonas S, et al. Ablation of atrial fibrillation in patients with heart failure: reversal of atrial and ventricular remodelling. Hellenic J Cardiol 2008;49:19–25.
71. Clark DM, Plumb VJ, Epstein AE, et al. Hemodynamic effects of an irregular sequence of ventricular cycle lengths during atrial fibrillation. J Am Coll Cardiol 1997;30:1039–45.
72. Verma A, Newman D, Geist M, et al. Effects of rhythm regularization and rate control in improving left ventricular function in atrial fibrillation patients undergoing atrioventricular nodal ablation. Can J Cardiol 2001;17:437–45.
73. Duffee DF, Shen WK, Smith HC. Suppression of frequent premature ventricular contractions and improvement of left ventricular function in patients with presumed idiopathic dilated cardiomyopathy. Mayo Clin Proc 1998;73:430–3.
74. Yarlagadda RK, Iwai S, Stein KM, et al. Reversal of cardiomyopathy in patients with repetitive monomorphic ventricular ectopy originating from the right ventricular outflow tract. Circulation 2005; 112:1092–7.
75. Schneider J, Berger HJ, Sands MJ, et al. Beat-to-beat left ventricular performance in atrial fibrillation: radionuclide assessment with the computerized nuclear probe. Am J Cardiol 1983;51:1189–95.
76. Lemola K, Desjardins B, Sneider M, et al. Effect of left atrial circumferential ablation for atrial fibrillation on left atrial transport function. Heart Rhythm 2005; 2:923–8.
77. Kosiuk J, Van Belle Y, Bode K, et al. Left ventricular diastolic dysfunction in atrial fibrillation: predictors and relation with symptom severity. J Cardiovasc Electrophysiol 2012;23:1073–7.
78. Jons C, Joergensen RM, Hassager C, et al. Diastolic dysfunction predicts new-onset atrial fibrillation and cardiovascular events in patients with acute myocardial infarction and depressed left ventricular systolic function: a CARISMA substudy. Eur J Echocardiogr 2010;11:602–7.
79. Elesber AA, Redfield MM. Approach to patients with heart failure and normal ejection fraction. Mayo Clin Proc 2001;76:1047–52.
80. Moon J, Rim SJ, Cho IJ, et al. Left ventricular hypertrophy determines the severity of diastolic dysfunction in patients with nonvalvular atrial fibrillation and preserved left ventricular systolic function. Clin Exp Hypertens 2010;32:540–6.
81. Jais P, Peng JT, Shah DC, et al. Left ventricular diastolic dysfunction in patients with so-called lone atrial fibrillation. J Cardiovasc Electrophysiol 2000;11:623–5.
82. Tsang TS, Barnes ME, Gersh BJ, et al. Risks for atrial fibrillation and congestive heart failure in patients >/=65 years of age with abnormal left ventricular diastolic relaxation. Am J Cardiol 2004;93: 54–8.
83. Tsang TS, Gersh BJ, Appleton CP, et al. Left ventricular diastolic dysfunction as a predictor of the first diagnosed nonvalvular atrial fibrillation in 840 elderly men and women. J Am Coll Cardiol 2002; 40:1636–44.
84. Tsang TS, Barnes ME, Gersh BJ, et al. Left atrial volume as a morphophysiologic expression of left

ventricular diastolic dysfunction and relation to cardiovascular risk burden. Am J Cardiol 2002;90: 1284–9.
85. Pritchett AM, Mahoney DW, Jacobsen SJ, et al. Diastolic dysfunction and left atrial volume: a population-based study. J Am Coll Cardiol 2005; 45:87–92.
86. Reant P, Lafitte S, Jais P, et al. Reverse remodeling of the left cardiac chambers after catheter ablation after 1 year in a series of patients with isolated atrial fibrillation. Circulation 2005;112: 2896–903.
87. Cha YM, Wokhlu A, Asirvatham SJ, et al. Success of ablation for atrial fibrillation in isolated left ventricular diastolic dysfunction: a comparison to systolic dysfunction and normal ventricular function. Circ Arrhythm Electrophysiol 2011;4:724–32.
88. Hu YF, Hsu TL, Yu WC, et al. The impact of diastolic dysfunction on the atrial substrate properties and outcome of catheter ablation in patients with paroxysmal atrial fibrillation. Circ J 2010;74(10):2074–8.
89. Akoum N, Daccarett M, McGann C, et al. Atrial fibrosis helps select the appropriate patient and strategy in catheter ablation of atrial fibrillation: a DE-MRI guided approach. J Cardiovasc Electrophysiol 2011;22:16–22.
90. Verma A, Wazni OM, Marrouche NF, et al. Pre-existent left atrial scarring in patients undergoing pulmonary vein antrum isolation: an independent predictor of procedural failure. J Am Coll Cardiol 2005;45:285–92.
91. Tilz RR, Rillig A, Thum AM, et al. Catheter ablation of long-standing persistent atrial fibrillation: 5-year outcomes of the Hamburg Sequential Ablation Strategy. J Am Coll Cardiol 2012;60:1921–9.
92. Calkins H, Kuck KH, Cappato R, et al. 2012 HRS/EHRA/ECAS Expert Consensus Statement on Catheter and Surgical Ablation of Atrial Fibrillation: recommendations for patient selection, procedural techniques, patient management and follow-up, definitions, endpoints, and research trial design. Europace 2012;14:528–606.

Surgical Treatment of Atrial Fibrillation in the Heart Failure Population

Stephen R. Large, MA, MS, FRCS, FRCP, MBA*,
Samer A.M. Nashef, MB ChB, FRCS, PhD

KEYWORDS

• Atrial fibrillation • Heart failure • Maze procedure • Surgery • Treatment

KEY POINTS

- Surgery to correct a structural heart valve problem can restore sinus rhythm in approximately one-fifth of patients with atrial fibrillation (AF), and the addition of a maze procedure will increase this proportion.
- Evidence shows that the maze procedure may restore atrial function in some patients and may have beneficial effects on functional symptoms and prognosis.
- The addition of a maze procedure for patients with AF undergoing valve or coronary surgery adds little risk and may be beneficial.
- The role of the maze procedure as an isolated treatment for lone AF in the context of heart failure with no structurally correctable cause is unknown.
- Future progress will determine the appropriate indications for treatment and the risks and benefits of any intervention.

INTRODUCTION

Atrial fibrillation (AF) is common, affecting approximately 2% of the population, with this proportion increasing with age.[1] It brings with it an irregular pulse, a loss of coordinated atrial contraction, a 5-fold increase in the risk of stroke, a doubling of mortality, worsening quality of life, and a progression from occasional (paroxysmal) to continuous (persistent) AF. Structural changes are seen in atria with AF (myocyte hypertrophy, fibrosis, inflammation, and apoptosis)[2] and, with a poorly controlled ventricular rate, changes typical of dilated cardiomyopathy are seen. AF is a strong and independent risk factor for the development of heart failure, and both conditions frequently coexist, partly because of overlapping risk factors.[3] In addition to this association, AF reduces cardiac function by reducing ventricular filling through both loss of atrial contraction and reduced diastolic interval time. This impairment of cardiac pumping action adds fatigue, dizziness, and breathlessness to palpitations in the panoply of symptoms attributable to AF.

Heart failure is also common, and its prevalence also increases with age. It affects at least 10% of the population older than 70 years and has been defined by the European Society of Cardiology as "an abnormality of cardiac structure or function leading to failure of the heart to deliver oxygen at a rate commensurate with the requirements of the metabolizing tissues, despite normal filling pressures (or only at the expense of increased filling pressures)".[3] Its natural history is progressive and the outcome is not good, with survival worsening with increasing severity of heart failure, so much so that patients with drug-resistant advanced heart failure (New York Heart

---

Disclosures: The authors have nothing to disclose.
Papworth Hospital, Cambridge CB23 3RE, UK
* Corresponding author.
E-mail address: srl24@cam.ac.uk

Heart Failure Clin 9 (2013) 533–539
http://dx.doi.org/10.1016/j.hfc.2013.07.012
1551-7136/13/$ – see front matter

heartfailure.theclinics.com

Association class IV) can expect a survival rate of only 8% at 2 years.[4] Two mechanisms are thought to account for this: further events leading to myocyte death, such as recurrent myocardial infarction, and myocardial injury, resulting in activation of the renin-angiotensin-aldosterone and sympathetic nervous systems. These systemic responses themselves lead to further myocardial injury, producing a pathophysiologic vicious cycle, resulting in many of the clinical features of the heart failure syndrome, including myocardial electrical instability.[5]

The symptoms and signs of heart failure have some similarity to those of AF. The 2 conditions coexist at a prevalence between 10% and 50% (**Fig. 1**).[6,7] The probability exists that when combined with AF, the prognosis of heart failure worsens. Certainly the likelihood of stroke increases by a further 3.5-fold when AF and heart failure combine.

MANAGEMENT OF AF IN HEART FAILURE

The management of patients with AF with and without coexisting heart failure follows a series of steps:

1. Identification of correctable predisposing causes
2. Identification of features that favor a rhythm control or a rate control strategy
3. Assessment of thromboembolism risk and implementation of prophylaxis

The treatment of AF per se requires the iden tification of treatable causes (hyperthyroidism electrolyte disorders, uncontrolled hypertension mitral valve disease, ischemic heart disease) and precipitating factors (recent surgery, chest infec tion, exacerbation of chronic pulmonary disease acute myocardial ischemia, acute alcohol excess) Treatment directed at the predisposing cause has a variable likelihood of success in correcting AF Surgery has a role to play in this regard, especially with cardiac structural and ischemic presenta tions, and is addressed in the following section.

If AF cannot be corrected through treating an underlying cause, pharmacologic managemen of rate, rhythm, and thromboembolic risk is re quired. Counterintuitively, the pharmacologic pur suit of sinus rhythm in patients with AF does no seem to improve long-term survival, perhaps even being associated with slightly worse prog nosis than merely controlling heart rate. Six trials have failed to show any improvement in prognosis with rhythm control.[8–13] The unadjusted hazard ratio for the rhythm-control group, compared with the rate-control group, was 1.06 (95% confi dence interval [CI], 0.86–1.30). Most of those in the rhythm-management group were on amiodar one. Perhaps the complexities of drug therapy and the circumstances that led to AF and hear failure are too much to expect stable sinus rhythm to be consistently and safely achieved. If AF is permanent, the risk of stroke can be quantified using a scoring system that guides appropriate anticoagulation.[14] The main hazard of long-term

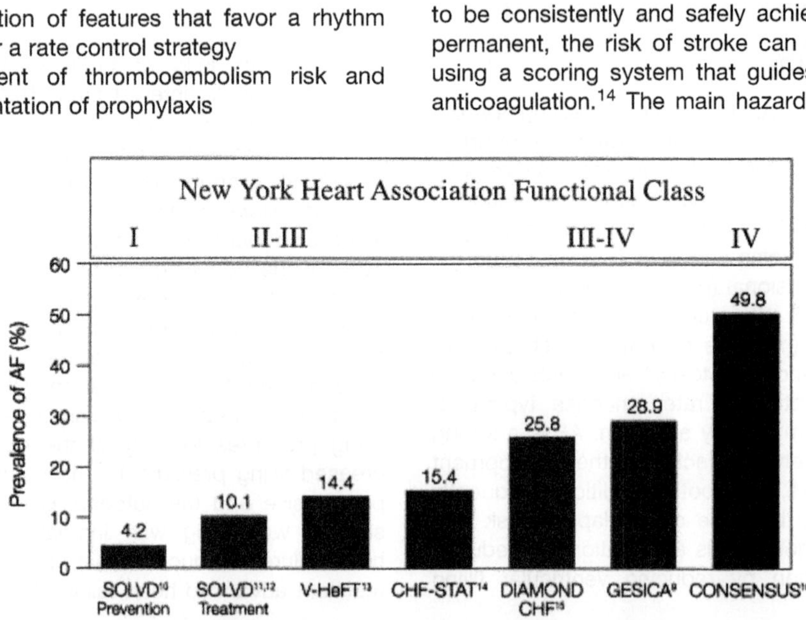

Fig. 1. Prevalence of atrial fibrillation (AF) in several major heart failure trials. CHF-STAT, Congestive Heart Failure Survival Trial of Antiarrhythmic Therapy; CONSENSUS, Cooperative North Scandinavian Enalapril Survival Study DIAMOND CHF, Danish Investigations of Arrhythmia and Mortality on Dofetilide Congestive Heart Failure study GESICA, Grupo de Estudio de la Sobrevida en la Insuficiencia Cardiaca en Argentina; SOLVD, Studies of Left Ventricular Dysfunction; V-HeFT, Vasodilator in Heart Failure Trial. (*From* Maisel WH, Stevenson LW. Atrial fibrillation in heart failure: epidemiology, pathophysiology, and rationale for therapy. Am J Cardiol 2003;91(6):2; with permission.)

anticoagulant therapy is bleeding. The risk of anticoagulant-related bleeding can also be quantified using a similar clinical tool, HAS-BLED (H, hypertension; A, abnormal liver or renal function; S, stroke history; B, bleeding predisposition; L, labile INR [international normalised ratio]; E, elderly [age 65 years and older]; D, drugs or alcohol usage),[15] which identifies patients at higher risk. It is possible, of course, that the "holy grail" of sinus rhythm in patients presenting with AF and heart failure can be achieved with a surgical approach.

SURGICAL TREATMENT IN HEART FAILURE AND AF

Heart failure from a variety of causes can be treated well with surgery. Correction of structural abnormalities of the heart, such as replacing a stenotic or regurgitant aortic valve or correcting mitral regurgitation through valve repair or replacement, often abolishes all of the symptoms and signs of heart failure, and can be associated with a markedly improved prognosis. Even coronary artery bypass grafting may improve some of the symptoms of heart failure in selected patients with hibernating, viable myocardium. The effects of correction of a structural valve defect on coexisting AF are less certain. In mitral regurgitation complicated by AF, correcting the valve lesion will restore sinus rhythm in 21% of patients.[16] The rate of sinus rhythm restoration correlated inversely with left ventricular end-systolic diameter. This effect is not commonly seen in patients with AF who have revascularization for myocardial ischemia.

A direct surgical approach to AF is a recent development. Because of an incomplete understanding of its pathophysiology, AF was not regarded as a surgical condition until recently.

Several major breakthroughs have occurred in understanding of the mechanisms of AF. The first is the observation by Haïssaguerre and colleagues[17] that AF often originates in the vicinity of the pulmonary veins. Surgery that is specifically directed at AF began in the 1980s when Williams and colleagues[18] described left atrial isolation. This procedure electrically isolated the fibrillating left atrium from the rest of the heart. Guiraudon and colleagues[19] developed a "corridor" procedure, effectively isolating both atria but leaving intact the connection between the sinoatrial and atrioventricular nodes. Of course, a feature of both the left atrial isolation and the corridor procedure is that the left atrium continues to fibrillate.

In 1987, James Cox[20] proposed the construction of an electrical "maze" throughout the left and right atria. The principle behind this operation is that through electrically isolating the pulmonary veins from the atrial body, and partitioning atrial tissues into a maze in which the "paths" are narrow enough to block the large (≈5 cm: **Fig. 2**) macroreentry circuits, AF can be surgically abolished and sinus rhythm restored.

CURRENT SURGICAL APPROACHES IN AF

The lines of electrical isolation in the maze procedure have been extensively studied since the technique was introduced in 1987. Several modifications to the maze lesion set have been proposed and accepted. One set of lesions in common use

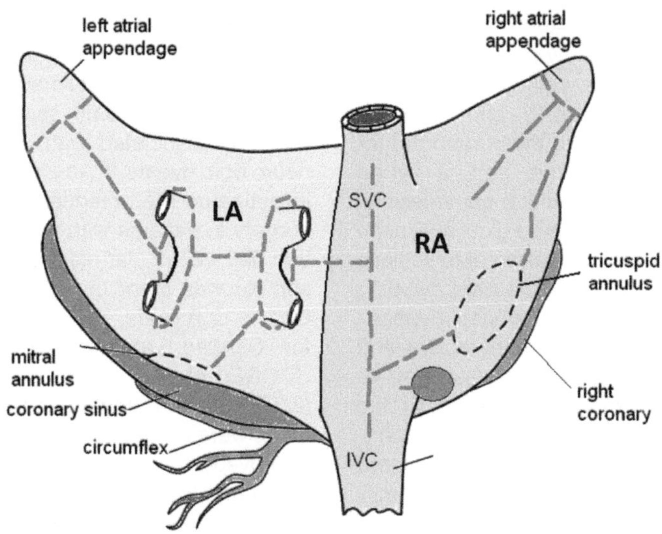

Fig. 2. A maze procedure lesion set: the posterior aspect of the atria is shown. The bold broken lines show the lesion set. IVC, inferior vena cava; LA, left atrium; RA, right atrium; SVC, superior vena cava.

nowadays is illustrated in **Fig. 2**. The maze procedure was originally performed by cutting and resuturing atrial tissue along prescribed lines (the "cut-and-sew" maze). Despite reports of a high rate of restoration of electrical sinus rhythm, the cut-and-sew maze procedure never achieved widespread use, possibly because it is a major cardiac operation that requires full median sternotomy and cardiopulmonary bypass, and the extensive suture lines are time-consuming with a predictably substantial bleeding risk. Attention was therefore focused on replacing surgical cuts with electrical isolation achieved through other means, such as radiofrequency, cryotherapy, and even electrocautery. A multitude of devices were developed and marketed to this end, and the number of modified maze procedures performed worldwide increased sharply.

The complete maze procedure, whether achieved using the cut-and-sew method or with the aid of an energy device, still requires median sternotomy and cardiopulmonary bypass to allow access to the mitral and tricuspid annuli, which mark the end point of some of the maze isolation lines. In an attempt to reduce the magnitude of the operation, alternative and less-invasive approaches have been described.

Pulmonary vein isolation instead of the full maze procedure has been proposed based on Haïssaguerre's finding that the pulmonary vein region is responsible for most AF triggers. This procedure is less complex than a full maze, and can be achieved using a port-access approach, which avoids median sternotomy and cardiopulmonary bypass. Some have combined this approach with left atrial appendage exclusion with a view to reducing further the risk of thromboembolism, and with vagal denervation, in an attempt to increase effectiveness. These less-invasive techniques have been reported to achieve sinus rhythm restoration rates of between 52% and 80% at 1 year,[21,22] markedly inferior to those reported for the full maze. To address this gap, a hybrid approach[23] was proposed in which some lesions are created using a port-access surgical approach and others percutaneously in an attempt to achieve as complete a lesion set as possible while avoiding median sternotomy and cardiopulmonary bypass.

The maze procedure, with its many guises and methods of delivery, can now be considered to be firmly established as part of the modern cardiac surgeon's armamentarium. However, no consensus exists on the optimal surgical approach to AF. A full surgical maze procedure undoubtedly has the highest level of effectiveness, but in the context of heart failure, such an invasive procedure should be approached with caution in view of the limited cardiac functional reserve. If surgical treatment is being contemplated for AF in heart failure, the decision must take account of both the effectiveness of the proposed approach and its attendant risk.

Before addressing the role of the maze procedure as a treatment for AF in the setting of heart failure, the state of the evidence must be appreciated for its effectiveness in AF generally. In isolated symptomatic longstanding AF, wherein the predominant symptoms are fatigue and troublesome palpitations, no doubt exists that the maze procedure is effective in reducing symptoms and, probably, thromboembolic risk.[24] The restoration of sinus rhythm varies between 50% and more than 95%, and the success rate depends on several factors. The highest success rates are achieved in AF of relatively recent onset in otherwise normal atria without excessive enlargement, in the absence of other cardiac lesions, in paroxysmal rather than persistent AF, and are enhanced by the completeness of the lesion set created by the maze procedure. However, even in chronic longstanding AF, the maze procedure has a higher success rate of restoring sinus rhythm than percutaneous, open, or port-access pulmonary vein isolation.[25]

A recent review of Cox's own experience[20] with this procedure in lone AF reported an attendant mortality of 1.4% and a freedom from AF of 93% at 1 year and 84% at 10 years. The incidence of stroke was 0.5% at 10 years, with all patients in stable sinus rhythm free of oral anticoagulants.

The incidence of stroke was similarly low after a successful surgical maze procedure in 433 patients. This finding was independent of the $CHADS_2$ (C, congestive heart failure; H, hypertension; A, age 75 years and older; D, diabetes mellitus; S_2, prior stroke [or transient ischemic attack or thromboembolism]) score and warfarin use, but was associated with diabetes and previous neurologic events.[26] Ad and colleagues[27] recently investigated the potential benefit from Cox maze surgery in patients with impaired ventricular function (left ventricular ejection fraction $\leq$40%). The sample was small (n = 42) with a mean age of 61.1 $\pm$ 12.9 years, and additive European System for Cardiac Operative Risk Evaluation (EuroSCORE) of 7.5 $\pm$ 3.1. One operative death (2.3%) and no strokes or transient ischemic attacks were reported at follow-up. Ejection fraction improved from 30% $\pm$ 5.0% to 45% $\pm$ 13.0% at a mean of 1.5 $\pm$ 11.3 months after surgery. The return to sinus rhythm at the time of follow-up echocardiography was 86% (35 of 40 patients). The physical functioning and health-related quality of life scores improved (37.0 ± 12.3 to 46.8 ± 9.1; P = .02) at 12 months with a significant reduction n symptom severity. The Kaplan-Meier major event-free survival rate at 24 months was 87% CI, 80.4–91.6; the events considered were redo valve replacement, ventricular assist device implantation, or death).

Therefore, reasonable evidence exists that a maze procedure is effective in restoring sinus rhythm and may allow the withdrawal of anticoagulation in patients in whom this restoration is achieved, and that this can be performed without an attendant increase in the rate of thromboembolic events, but none of this evidence is from randomized controlled trials. Reasons exist to be circumspect in considering this evidence. Patients who are offered major cardiac surgery for AF are almost certainly fitter than the general population with AF. The clinical outcomes achieved in this selected group may not be replicated in typical patients with AF and heart failure, who tend to be older, with structural or myocardial abnormalities. These patients would be symptomatic for a multitude of reasons,[12] perhaps with the heart failure playing a greater role in symptomatology than the AF itself.

Two questions must be answered. The first is whether surgical correction of AF can be justified as a concomitant procedure in patients with AF undergoing major cardiac surgery, such as valve and coronary operations. This question will be answered by the results of further prospective studies, such as the adjunct maze study (the Amaze Trial) to determine whether a maze procedure has added value beyond the production of a regular R-R interval. The second is whether surgical correction of AF as a lone procedure is associated with survival and event-free benefits in patients with heart failure. The answer to this question is unknown, even in patients without heart failure. Much of the anticipated benefits will derive from the restoration of atrial function, which should intuitively be associated with a reduced risk of stroke. Several studies have indicated that some restoration of atrial function can occur[24,28] after surgical maze procedures, but more information is needed to determine whether these benefits justify the risk of a major cardiac intervention in elderly patients in heart failure.

Finally, heart failure and AF may represent a "chicken-and-egg" scenario. Many conditions associated with heart failure are also associated with AF, with documented mechanisms for the effect of mitral lesions and myocardial ischemia on atrial function. However, AF may also cause heart failure, such as through tachycardia-induced cardiomyopathy and, in some patients, atrioventricular valve annular dilatation as a result of the AF and its attendant volume loading and increased atrial and ventricular diastolic pressure. If such a pathophysiologic mechanism is responsible for heart failure, then an argument can be made to manage the AF surgically as a method of heart failure treatment, but much more evidence is needed.

Surgical correction of AF in a well-defined group of patients seems to produce a robust, drug-free cardioversion to sinus rhythm. Evidence shows that this is reasonably safe and effective surgery. Data on maze surgery in the setting of heart failure are limited, but those that are available seem to indicate favorable outcomes, which would mean that the failure of pharmacologic rhythm control in AF may simply reflect the shortcomings and adverse effects of the currently available drugs for rhythm control.

SUMMARY

Surgery to correct a structural heart valve problem can restore sinus rhythm in approximately one-fifth of patients with AF. The addition of a maze procedure will substantially increase this proportion. In patients with troublesome palpitations, the maze procedure can be performed safely and is symptomatically effective. From the viewpoint of effective cardiac function, evidence indicates that the maze procedure may restore some atrial function in some patients, and may be proven in the future to have beneficial effects on functional symptoms and perhaps even prognosis, but the risk/benefit equation remains to be determined. In patients with AF who are undergoing valve or coronary surgery, the addition of a maze procedure adds little risk and may be of benefit, and it is reasonable to assume that this will also apply to the heart failure subset. The role of the maze procedure as an isolated treatment for lone AF in the context of heart failure with no structurally correctable cause is unknown. Future progress in this field will determine the appropriate indications for treatment and the risks and benefits of any intervention, and is likely to require a multidisciplinary approach involving both electrophysiologists and cardiac surgeons.

REFERENCES

1. Kirchhof P, Auricchio A, Bax J, et al. Outcome parameters for trials in atrial fibrillation: executive summary. Recommendations from a consensus conference organized by the German Atrial Fibrillation Competence NETwork (AFNET) and the European Heart Rhythm Association (EHRA). Eur Heart J 2007;28: 2803–17.

2. Frustaci A, Chimenti C, Bellocci F, et al. Histological substrate of atrial biopsies in patients with lone atrial fibrillation. Circulation 1997;96:1180–4.
3. Dickstein K, Cohen-Solal A, Filippatos G, et al, ESC Committee for Practice Guidelines (CPG). ESC Guidelines for the diagnosis and treatment of acute and chronic heart failure 2008: the Task Force for the diagnosis and treatment of acute and chronic heart failure 2008 of the European Society of Cardiology. Developed in collaboration with the Heart Failure Association of the ESC (HFA) and endorsed by the European Society of Intensive Care Medicine (ESICM). Eur Heart J 2008;29:2388–442.
4. Rose E, Gelijns A, Moskowitz A, et al, Randomized Evaluation of Mechanical Assistance for the Treatment of Congestive Heart Failure (REMATCH) Study Group. Long-term use of a left ventricular assist device for end-stage heart failure. N Engl J Med 2001; 345:1435–43.
5. Hohnloser SH, Kuck KH, Lilienthal J. Rhythm or rate control in atrial fibrillation—Pharmacological Intervention in Atrial Fibrillation (PIAF): a randomised trial. Lancet 2000;356:1789–94.
6. McMurray J, Adamopoulos S, Anker S, et al. ESC guidelines for the diagnosis and treatment of acute and chronic heart failure 2012. The Task Force for the Diagnosis and Treatment of Acute and Chronic Heart Failure 2012 of the European Society of Cardiology. Developed in collaboration with the Heart Failure Association (HFA) of the ESC. Eur Heart J 2012; 33:1787–847.
7. Maisel WH, Stevenson LW. Atrial fibrillation in heart failure: epidemiology, pathophysiology, and rationale for therapy. Am J Cardiol 2003;91(6):2–8.
8. Wyse DG, Waldo AL, DiMarco JP, AFFIRM Investigators. A comparison of rate control and rhythm control in patients with atrial fibrillation. N Engl J Med 2002; 347:1825–33.
9. Van Gelder IC, Hagens VE, Bosker HA, et al. A comparison of rate control and rhythm control in patients with recurrent persistent atrial fibrillation. N Engl J Med 2002;347:1834–40.
10. Carlsson J, Miketic S, Windeler J, et al, STAF Investigators. Randomized trial of rate-control versus rhythm control in persistent atrial fibrillation. J Am Coll Cardiol 2003;41:1690–6.
11. Opolski G, Torbicki A, Kosior DA, et al. Rate control vs rhythm control in patients with nonvalvular persistent atrial fibrillation: the results of the Polish How to Treat Chronic Atrial Fibrillation (HOT CAFE) study. Chest 2004;126:476–86.
12. Roy D, Talajic M, Nattel S, et al, Atrial Fibrillation and Congestive Heart Failure Investigators. Rhythm control versus rate control for atrial fibrillation and heart failure. N Engl J Med 2008;358:2667–77.
13. Ogawa S, Yamashita T, Yamazaki T, et al. Optimal treatment strategy for patients with paroxysmal atrial fibrillation: J-RHYTHM study. Circ J 2009;73 242–8.
14. Lip G, Nieuwlaat R, Pisters R, et al. Refining clinica risk stratification for predicting stroke and thrombo embolism in atrial fibrillation using a novel risk factor-based approach the euro heart survey on atrial fibrillation. Chest 2010;137(2):263–72.
15. Pisters R, Lane DA, Nieuwlaat R, et al. A nove user-friendly score (HAS-BLED) to assess 1-yea risk of major bleeding in patients with atrial fibrilla tion: the Euro Heart Survey. Chest 2010;138(5) 1093–100.
16. Large SR, Hosseinpour AR, Wisbey C, et al. Spontaneous cardioversion and mitral valve repair: a role for surgical cardioversion (Cox-maze)? Eur J Cardiothorac Surg 1997;11(1):76–80.
17. Haïssaguerre M, Jaïs P, Shah DC, et al. Spontaneous initiation of atrial fibrillation by ectopic beats originating in the pulmonary veins. N Engl J Med 1998;339(10):659–66.
18. Williams J, Ungerleider R, Lofland G, et al. Left atria isolation: new treatment for supra-ventricular ar rhythmias. J Thorac Cardiovasc Surg 1980;80(3) 373–80.
19. Leitch J, Klein G, Yee R, et al. Sinus node—atrio ventricular node isolation: long term results of the Corridor operation for atrial fibrillation. J Am Coll Cardiol 1991;17(4):970–5.
20. Weimar T, Schena S, Bailey M, et al. The Cox-maze procedure for lone atrial fibrillation a single-cente experience over 2 decades. Circ Arrhythm Electrophysiol 2012;5:8–14.
21. Bagge L, Blomstrom P, Nilsson L, et al. Epicardia off-pump pulmonary vein isolation and vagal dener vation improve long-term outcome and quality of life in patients with atrial fibrillation. J Thorac Cardiovasc Surg 2009;137:1265–71.
22. Wang JG, Li Y, Shi JH, et al. Treatment of long lasting persistent atrial fibrillation using minimally invasive surgery combined with irbesartan. Ann Thorac Surg 2011;91:1183–9.
23. Muneretto C, Bisleri G, Bontempi L, et al. Successfu treatment of lone persistent atrial fibrillation by means of a hybrid thoracoscopic-transcathete approach. Innovations (Phila) 2012;7:254–8.
24. Cox J, Ad N, Palazo T, et al. Impact of the maze procedure on stroke rate in patients with atria fibrillation. J Thorac Cardiovasc Surg 1999;118(5) 833–40.
25. Edgerton J, Edgerton Z, Weaver T, et al. Minimally invasive pulmonary vein isolation and partial auto nomic denervation for surgical treatment of atria fibrillation. Ann Thorac Surg 2008;86(1):35–8.
26. Pet M, Robertson JO, Bailey M, et al. The impact o CHADS(2) score on late stroke after the Cox maze procedure. J Thorac Cardiovasc Surg 2013;146(1) 85–9.

27. Ad N, Henry L, Hunt S. The impact of surgical ablation in patients with low ejection fraction, heart failure, and atrial fibrillation. Eur J Cardiothorac Surg 2011;40(1):70–6.

28. Aikawa M, Watanabe H, Shimokawa T, et al. Preoperative left atrial emptying fraction is a powerful predictor of successful maze procedure. Circ J 2009; 73(2):269–73.

Index

Note: Page numbers of article titles are in **boldface** type.

Heart Failure Clin 9 (2013) 541–544
http://dx.doi.org/10.1016/S1551-7136(13)00074-3
1551-7136/13/$ – see front matter

H

I

L

M

N

O

P

R

S

United States Postal Service

Statement of Ownership, Management, and Circulation
(All Periodicals Publications Except Requestor Publications)

1. Publication Title: Heart Failure Clinics
2. Publication Number: 0 2 5 - 0 5 5
3. Filing Date: 9/14/13
4. Issue Frequency: Jan, Apr, July, Oct
5. Number of Issues Published Annually: 4
6. Annual Subscription Price: $224.00
7. Complete Mailing Address of Known Office of Publication (*Not printer*) (*Street, city, county, state, and ZIP+4®*)
   Elsevier Inc.
   360 Park Avenue South
   New York, NY 10010-1710

   Contact Person: Stephen R. Bushing
   Telephone (Include area code): 215-239-3688
8. Complete Mailing Address of Headquarters or General Business Office of Publisher (*Not printer*)
   Elsevier Inc., 360 Park Avenue South, New York, NY 10010-1710
9. Full Names and Complete Mailing Addresses of Publisher, Editor, and Managing Editor (*Do not leave blank*)

Publisher (*Name and complete mailing address*)
Linda Belfus, Elsevier, Inc., 1600 John F. Kennedy Blvd. Suite 1800, Philadelphia, PA 19103-2899

Editor (*Name and complete mailing address*)
Barbara Cohen-Kligerman, Elsevier, Inc., 1600 John F. Kennedy Blvd. Suite 1800, Philadelphia, PA 19103-2899

Managing Editor (*Name and complete mailing address*)
Adrianne Brigido, Elsevier, Inc., 1600 John F. Kennedy Blvd. Suite 1800, Philadelphia, PA 19103-2899

10. Owner (*Do not leave blank. If the publication is owned by a corporation, give the name and address of the corporation immediately followed by the names and addresses of all stockholders owning or holding 1 percent or more of the total amount of stock. If not owned by a corporation, give the names and addresses of the individual owners. If owned by a partnership or other unincorporated firm, give its name and address as well as those of each individual owner. If the publication is published by a nonprofit organization, give its name and address.*)

Full Name	Complete Mailing Address
Wholly owned subsidiary of	1600 John F. Kennedy Blvd., Ste. 1800
Reed/Elsevier, US holdings	Philadelphia, PA 19103-2899

11. Known Bondholders, Mortgagees, and Other Security Holders Owning or Holding 1 Percent or More of Total Amount of Bonds, Mortgages, or Other Securities. If none, check box → ☐ None

Full Name	Complete Mailing Address
N/A	

12. Tax Status (*For completion by nonprofit organizations authorized to mail at nonprofit rates*) (*Check one*)
    The purpose, function, and nonprofit status of this organization and the exempt status for federal income tax purposes:
    ☐ Has Not Changed During Preceding 12 Months
    ☐ Has Changed During Preceding 12 Months (*Publisher must submit explanation of change with this statement*)

PS Form **3526**, September 2007 (Page 1 of 3 (Instructions Page 3)) PSN 7530-01-000-9931 **PRIVACY NOTICE**: See our Privacy policy in www.usps.com

13. Publication Title: Heart Failure Clinics
14. Issue Date for Circulation Data Below: July 2013

15. Extent and Nature of Circulation		Average No. Copies Each Issue During Preceding 12 Months	No. Copies of Single Issue Published Nearest to Filing Date
a. Total Number of Copies (*Net press run*)		203	176
b. Paid Circulation (By Mail and Outside the Mail)	(1) Mailed Outside-County Paid Subscriptions Stated on PS Form 3541. (*Include paid distribution above nominal rate, advertiser's proof copies, and exchange copies*)	60	56
	(2) Mailed In-County Paid Subscriptions Stated on PS Form 3541 (*Include paid distribution above nominal rate, advertiser's proof copies, and exchange copies*)		
	(3) Paid Distribution Outside the Mails Including Sales Through Dealers and Carriers, Street Vendors, Counter Sales, and Other Paid Distribution Outside USPS®	12	10
	(4) Paid Distribution by Other Classes Mailed Through the USPS (e.g. First-Class Mail®)		
c. Total Paid Distribution (*Sum of 15b (1), (2), (3), and (4)*) ►		72	66
d. Free or Nominal Rate Distribution (By Mail and Outside the Mail)	(1) Free or Nominal Rate Outside-County Copies Included on PS Form 3541	61	60
	(2) Free or Nominal Rate In-County Copies Included on PS Form 3541		
	(3) Free or Nominal Rate Copies Mailed at Other Classes Through the USPS (e.g. First-Class Mail)		
	(4) Free or Nominal Rate Distribution Outside the Mail (Carriers or other means)		
e. Total Free or Nominal Rate Distribution (Sum of 15d (1), (2), (3) and (4))		61	60
f. Total Distribution (Sum of 15c and 15e) ►		133	126
g. Copies not Distributed (See instructions to publishers #4 (page #3)) ►		70	50
h. Total (Sum of 15f and g)		203	176
i. Percent Paid (15c divided by 15f times 100) ►		54.14%	52.38%

16. Publication of Statement of Ownership
    ☐ If the publication is a general publication, publication of this statement is required. Will be printed in the **October 2013** issue of this publication. ☐ Publication not required

17. Signature and Title of Editor, Publisher, Business Manager, or Owner
    Stephen R. Bushing – Inventory /Distribution Coordinator
    Date: September 14, 2013

I certify that all information furnished on this form is true and complete. I understand that anyone who furnishes false or misleading information on this form or who omits material or information requested on the form may be subject to criminal sanctions (including fines and imprisonment) and/or civil sanctions (including civil penalties).

PS Form **3526**, September 2007 (Page 2 of 3)

Printed and bound by CPI Group (UK) Ltd, Croydon, CR0 4YY
03/10/2024
01040301-0015